THE HOUSEFLY

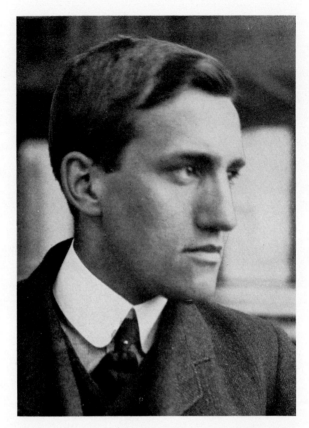

C. Gordon Hewitt, D.Sc., F.R.S.C., Dr. Hewitt was perhaps the greatest single contributor to a scientific understanding of the biology and sanitary importance of *Musca domestica*. His researches culminated in 1914 in the publication of *The House-fly . . . Its Structure, Habits, Development, Relation to Disease and Control*. Photograph supplied by Division of Illustration, Science Service, Department of Agriculture, Canada.

The Housefly

ITS NATURAL HISTORY,

MEDICAL IMPORTANCE,

AND CONTROL

Luther S. West

Professor and Head of Department of Biology,
Northern Michigan College of Education;
Major, Medical Service Corps, U.S.A.R.

Comstock Publishing Company

INC.

ASSOCIATED WITH CORNELL UNIVERSITY PRESS

Ithaca, New York, 1951

PRINTED IN THE UNITED STATES OF AMERICA BY THE
VAIL-BALLOU PRESS, INC., BINGHAMTON, NEW YORK

DEDICATED TO my father, Norman Luther West, onetime rural school teacher, whose practical knowledge of woodcraft, agriculture, and health science has served as an inspiration for the professional careers of his two sons.

Foreword

PLINY in his *Natural History* wrote, "It is an arduous task to give novelty to what is ancient, authority to what is new, interest to what is obsolete, light to what is obscure, charm to what is loathesome, and credit to what is dubious." To such a task Professor West has devoted five years of intensive observation, study, drawing, and writing, and he has produced an outstanding treatise on a subject of much importance. The unusual difficulties inherent in the preparation of the text are suggested by the fact that this is the first comprehensive work on the housefly to appear in English in thirty-six years. Yet pertinacious filth-feeding and filth-breeding *Musca domestica* is probably the most widely distributed as well as the most dangerous insect closely associated with man. Paradoxically, not many scientists or laymen can with certainty recognize this species at sight, common though it is. So this is a much-needed text and reference book of great value to civil and military physicians and sanitarians, to public health officers, to biologists, to students, and to all who are interested in natural history.

Luther West has won distinction in both civil and military life. During World War II, I became acquainted with him when he was Chief of Medical Entomology at the Army Medical School in Washington, where his clear, practical, and precise lectures were unexcelled. He is a talented teacher, as is apparent throughout the pages which follow.

While, as Professor West states in his first chapter, the period of friendly tolerance of flies has never really been terminated, yet most of us now, like Sir John Lubbock in the nineteenth century, think of houseflies as "winged sponges spreading hither and thither to carry out the foul behests of contagion." But throughout much of the world the fly rules man to an unbelievable extent. As an example, I can cite a village that I visited in the Near East in 1949, where 50 per cent of the people are blind in one or both eyes because of fly-borne trachoma. I have also been in overseas communities where regularly a third of the babies die before they are a year old, chiefly, it seemed to me, because of fly-borne bowel infections. Millions still accept houseflies as an inevitable part of fate; yet, of course, quoting Woods Hutchinson, "We must not blame God for the fly. . . . The fly is the resurrection, the reincarnation of our own dirt and carelessness."

DDT and the newer economic toxicants have shown much usefulness against flies but, as Professor West makes clear, they do not replace, but supplement, sanitary measures. The housefly is a resourceful antagonist. It carries in its genes an incredible bag of tricks. Apparently destroyed in a community by DDT, it blossoms forth with a 10,000-fold resistance; then, seemingly defeated by benzene hexachloride, it reappears with a powerful immunity; finally, sent down dramatically by chlordane, it rises once more, invincible in the face of all three toxicants. The problem of housefly and pest-mosquito resistance to organic poisons is growing more formidable each year.

Let no one expect an easy victory over houseflies. Probably the best way to deal with the housefly is to expunge its breeding places and to prevent their formation. However, such environmental sanitation is costly and difficult, and it comes very slowly in underdeveloped areas. Much more research and sanitary endeavor are required before we can hope for decisive results in the prevention of fly-borne illness throughout the world. Hence the great significance at home and abroad of Professor West's book.

Here is a timely monograph, scholarly, practical, and well-balanced, dealing with each phase of the subject—morphology, physiology, behavior, life history, taxonomy, distribution, ecology, relation to disease, usefulness in the laboratory and in nature, techniques in the field, museum, and laboratory, control measures, prevention, and bibliography—and having a fine historical flavor throughout. This treatise will not only fulfill the need for readily accessible and authoritative information about houseflies, but it will stimulate further study and, all in all, will be a notable contribution toward the welfare of mankind.

PAUL F. RUSSELL, M.D.

The Rockefeller Foundation,
International Health Division

Preface

An actually existing fly is more important than a possibly existing angel.—Emerson, Letter to Moncure D. Conway

NO comprehensive treatment of the housefly and its importance to man has appeared in the English language since Hewitt's excellent volume, published by the Cambridge University Press in 1914. This came three years after *The House Fly, Disease Carrier* . . . , prepared by the noted American entomologist L. O. Howard, a volume which, though not intended as a scientific monograph, has served American biologists and sanitarians as an authoritative work of reference for nearly forty years. Mention should likewise be made of Graham-Smith's *Flies in Relation to Disease: Non-blood-sucking Flies,* 1914, which, although it treats of many species in addition to *Musca domestica,* contains particularly valuable information concerning muscoid structure and biology. All three of the foregoing volumes are, however, long since out of print. This fact, combined with the newer knowledge of control procedure, renders it imperative that a modern account of this long-time enemy of human welfare be prepared for the information of all concerned.

During World War II it was particularly apparent that medical men and health workers generally were eager to master and utilize a much greater knowledge of medical entomology than library facilities in this or other countries ordinarily made possible. This observation convinced the writer that the bringing together of the hitherto scattered information concerning a species which has probably been responsible for more human misery than any other insect would be not only a desirable but a very practical undertaking. The present volume is the result of such an effort, and is presented, with all its faults, in the hope that it may serve a useful purpose in improving the health and happiness of man.

The standards of civilization cannot be maintained without constant vigilance, and basic to this is a state of mind capable of envisioning even higher ideals than have yet been realized. It is probably true that more people are influenced by habit and custom than by logic, practical instruction, or even personal experience. If it is possible to surround the rising generation with an environment relatively free from flies and fly-borne filth, communities of the future will perhaps insist upon surroundings which are both pleasing and sanitary, and which they will not willingly relinquish, even under stress. Constant re-education of youth cannot, therefore, be neglected, and constitutes one of the principal reasons for the publication of this volume. The present undertaking, however imperfect, is above all else an attempt to serve an obvious international need in the field of sanitary education.

While the book is intended primarily for the use of public health officers, Army and Navy medical personnel, experiment station workers, college and university staff members, and students of animal biology, a deliberate attempt has been made to reduce technical language to a minimum in the hope that it may also find a place in school and public libraries and thus be of firsthand value to all intelligent citizens who may be interested in natural history, sanitation, or public health. The somewhat elementary introduction to taxonomy and nomenclature, for example, contained in Chapter V, was written with this end in view.

Work on the manuscript began during the final year of World War II, but the greater portion of the actual writing has been accomplished since the author's return to civil life.

Thanks are due to General George R. Callender, formerly Assistant Commandant of the Army Medical School, and to Doctor Paul F. Russell, then Chief of Parasitology, Army Medical School, for the use of facilities at the Army Medical Center, including permission to maintain a large colony of *Musca domestica* and to utilize the services of U.S. Army technicians.

Without the use of library facilities at Cornell University, the completion of the book would have been virtually impossible. In this connection, the author especially wishes to express his appreciation for the personal assistance of Doctor Marjorie Ruth Ross, librarian in the Entomological Department.

For many years Doctor Robert Matheson, now Emeritus Professor of Entomology at Cornell University, has assisted his former students with helpful criticism and sound advice. The author is especially grateful for the use of Doctor Matheson's laboratory during the summers of 1946 and 1947 and for permission to consult his private collection of entomological books and papers.

For unrestricted access to the Cornell University collections, for office space, and for the use of optical and other equipment during two summers, thanks are due to Doctor Charles E. Palm, Head of the Department of Entomology at Cornell University, and to Doctor Henry Dietrich, curator of the collection.

The author is particularly grateful to Doctor Walter H. Schaefer, of the Department of Biology at Northern Michigan College, for the critical reading of several chapters and for numerous helpful suggestions. Acknowledgments are also due Mr. Walter Forsberg, for painstaking work in connection with the preparation of the illustrations, in which Mrs. Donald MacVean and Miss Betsey West also assisted. The author likewise wishes to thank Miss Alice West for her very welcome assistance in preparing the bibliography for the publisher.

Special thanks should be accorded the author's wife, Beatrice Ryan West, for her wise counseling as to arrangement and style, and for the unselfish devotion of her time to the reading and correction of the proof.

LUTHER S. WEST

Marquette, Michigan
November, 1950

Contents

THE HOUSEFLY

CHAPTER I

Flies and Men:
Introductory and Historical

And there came a grievous swarm of flies into the house of Pharaoh, and into his servants' houses, and into all the land of Egypt, and the land was corrupted by this kind of flies.—Exodus 8:24 (Douay version)

HOUSEFLIES and related species appear to have forced themselves upon the attention of man in all periods of recorded history. That flies were a nuisance and a menace to health among ancient peoples is borne out not only by the above quotation but by numerous other sources.

Herms (1944) points out that as early as 1577 Mercurialis took note of the habits of flies as they passed back and forth between individuals ill of plague and the food of healthy persons, and suggested that the "virus" of the disease was possibly transmitted in this way. Herms also calls attention to the opinion advanced by Soares de Souza in 1587, and again by Bancroft in 1769, that flies might have to do with the transmission of yaws, the experimental demonstration of which was not forthcoming until the work of Castellani, in 1907.

Sydenham in 1666 made the observation that if insects, and especially houseflies, were abundant in summer, the fall months were usually unhealthy.

It appears that Montfils in 1776 considered flies as possible distributors of anthrax, though it was not until nearly a hundred years later that Raimbert (1869) caused the disease in guinea pigs by inoculating them with a suspension of pulverized wings, proboscides, and other parts of the bodies of nonblood-sucking flies.[1]

---

[1] While experimental procedures of this type have little, if any, direct bearing on the possibility of transmission in nature, they have their place in demonstrating that the pathogen is actually on or in the body of the insect host, and lead the way to a more precise understanding of how transmission may, in fact, take place. Thus, while it is generally conceded that some lesion or abrasion must exist for the anthrax bacillus to

In 1824 a case of gastric myiasis was reported in an English lady, and though the descriptions of the maggot are exaggerated and even fantastic, there seems no reason to doubt the authenticity of the observation itself (Lelean, 1904).

In 1871 Sir John Lubbock (later Lord Avebury) warned that flies which alight on decomposing matter carry such material with them through the air, and in the same year Leidy published, in the *Proceedings of the Academy of Natural Sciences of Philadelphia,* his convictions that flies were important in the spread of gangrene in hospitals during the American Civil War.

In 1873 Nicholas published a short note entitled "The Fly in Its Sanitary Aspect," and from this time on there appears to have been increasing attention paid to the possible association of flies with disease, though scientific interest in the subject did not come sharply to a focus for another twenty-five years.

Thorough study of the life history of the housefly began around 1896, with the work of L. O. Howard, who continued his observations for many years and repeatedly called attention to the fly's potential vectorship of filth- and food-borne disease. It was Howard who strongly advocated the designation "typhoid fly" as most appropriate for a species of such feeding habits.

Particular attention was directed to *Musca domestica* as a disease carrier during the period of the Spanish-American War. American troops suffered greatly from malaria, yellow fever, and typhoid, and though various species of mosquitoes came to be identified as the only vectors of yellow fever and malaria, enteric infections such as cholera, typhoid, amoebiasis, bacillary dysentery, and the milder diarrheas were clearly recognized as filth-borne infections. The prevalence of typhoid fever particularly forced the medical department of the army to give careful attention to all possible factors that might be concerned with the spread of enteric diseases, and the housefly was found to be of great importance in this connection. Doctor V. C. Vaughan (1899) made the telling observation that flies, crawling over the food of soldiers, frequently carried on their legs and bodies particles of lime which they could have picked up only while feeding on feces in latrines.

British medical authorities encountered similar health problems and made similar observations in connection with the South African wars.

By this time interest in the medical importance of the housefly was becoming widespread, and in 1907 Newstead published his preliminary report on the habits, life cycle, and breeding places of the common housefly, *Musca domestica,* as observed in the city of Liverpool. Newstead made various sug-

---

gain access to the human host, it is just such lesions or abrasions to which nonbloodsucking flies are naturally attracted and into which by proboscis, feet, or fecal droplet they may easily introduce the organism concerned.

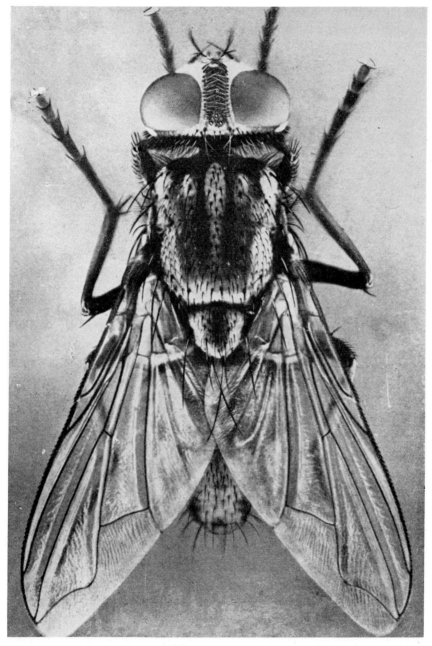

Figure 1. Dorsal view of *Musca domestica,* male specimen. (Photograph by N. A. Cobb; copyright, National Geographic Society.)

gestions as to the best means of checking its increase, and followed with other reports containing additional data in 1908 and 1909.

Also in 1909 Nuttall and Jepson published a summary of existing knowledge concerning the transmission of infective diseases by nonbiting flies, with particular emphasis on typhoid and cholera. Their paper includes the following significant statement: "In potential possibilities the droppings of one fly may, in certain circumstances, weigh in the balance as against buckets of water or of milk."

Thus, during the early years of the present century, the occurrence of enteric infections came to be associated more and more, in the minds of thoughtful people, with the presence of filth-feeding flies. This association was and is particularly evident in temperate regions during the late summer and early fall when flies, more than any other factor, appear to be responsible for the rise in frequency of such infections.

But a convinced attitude is by no means general even today, and that many human beings actually harbor a friendly feeling for the fly, at least under certain circumstances, cannot be denied. When not excessively numerous their presence has usually been not only tolerated but even "enjoyed"! Witness references to "tickling little baby's nose" in the lighter poetry of grandma's day! Again, the esthetic pleasure one derives from the hum of flies on a hot summer afternoon is known to all who have a love of rural things and who recall with nostalgic clearness the sounds as well as the sights and smells of a childhood that did its daydreaming in the setting of a sunlit barnyard or vine-covered veranda where insect life seemed as inevitable a part of nature's background as were sunshine, clouds, and rain.

This very association of flies with agricultural and domestic environments, however, serves to remind us that broadly speaking man himself has made the housefly (Cobb, 1910b). For, if it were not for the food, protection, and breeding places found about human habitations, *Musca domestica* might be a rare and unusual species today. It is, in fact, becoming so in communities where the stabling of animals is forbidden and garbage is promptly removed; were it not for the unbelievable fecundity of the few who manage to be about during the spring and early summer, the hordes that characterize late summer and early fall in so many regions of the world might well become insignificant, at least in the more urban communities of temperate zones.

The world as a whole, however, is far from realizing this degree of progress, and just as millions of the inhabitants of Egypt, Palestine, Arabia, and other Near Eastern lands live, dress, and carry on generally much as did their ancestors some two or three thousand years ago, so do flies furnish a buzzing accompaniment to it all, while babies die of dysentery almost as monotonously as in the days of Joshua, Herod, or Mohammed!

CHANGING ATTITUDES

We have seen how ancient and medieval peoples suffered from fly-borne scourges in their day and how not a few comprehended the relationship between the presence of many flies and the prevalence of human disease. This was true before the etiology of specific enteric diseases was even remotely understood. With the work of Louis Pasteur and the growth of the germ theory of disease, more exact concepts of the role of flies in disease transmission were made possible, and attention came to be focused sharply upon the nonbloodsucking filth-feeding Diptera, of which *Musca domestica* is the best known and most important.

To give a more understandable picture of the evolution of human attitude toward sanitary science in general and fly-borne infection in particular, I shall review briefly the changes in public opinion in the United States from the colonial period to the present time.

The Period of Friendly Tolerance (Early Times to ?)

This period lasted a long time and has never really been terminated. As Doane (1910) puts it, "A few of them [flies] were nice things to have around, to make things seem homelike. . . . Those that were knocked into the coffee or the cream could be fished out; those that went into the soup or the hash were never missed." He goes on to point out that flies were considered splendid things with which to amuse the baby! The fact that they fed frequently on refuse of all kinds gave them a favorable reputation as scavengers, and when they had finished these "duties" they gave an impression of great cleanliness by assiduously brushing their heads and bodies with their legs.

Not until the rise of the science of bacteriology could it be otherwise. Most people had no concept of the existence of microorganisms, to say nothing of their exceedingly small size and the possibility that a million or more might be carried at the same time by a single insect. And wherever man is ignorant today, the same attitude prevails. Neither is such ignorance confined to the tribesmen of Africa or Arabia, or the inhabitants of the Pacific isles. Within the shadow of the great universities of highly civilized peoples, the masses know little of these things. Protected as most of us are by the existence of well-drawn ordinances and the watchful eye of organized health departments, we subscribe to the generally accepted practices of the community, with scarcely a thought as to the rationale of our procedures or the costly historical

experiences that lie back of the relative security we now enjoy. We coast on
the momentum imparted by our predecessors. Realizing this, we have little
right to be critical of the complacence of our great-grandfathers. They made
the most of their environment and got some enjoyment from it, even if they
did pay a great price in a high infant mortality and unnecessary infections
throughout their lives.

The Period of Incrimination (1875–1900)

This period has its roots much farther back. As usual with the growth of
new convictions, scattered investigators were far ahead of the general public.
Interesting facts regarding the existence and distribution of microorganisms
were recorded in laboratories and published in technical journals, but there
was little or no publicity in the popular press; physicians continued to be much
more interested in treating the sick than in preventing sickness, and not a
few were frankly skeptical of the whole germ theory of disease.

It is difficult to say how long this state of affairs might have continued had
not stern necessity served to arouse popular opinion and focus attention upon
what should have been obvious. The experiences of American soldiers during
the Spanish-American War and of British military units in South Africa
provided the stimulus. The findings of military commissions were not only
made the basis of real changes of policy in military administration but were
echoed and re-echoed in daily press and other popular literature until even the
man on the street became at least dimly aware of the cause of typhoid fever
and other intestinal disorders, of the necessity for prompt and proper disposal
of human excrement, and of the great capacity of filth-feeding flies to convey
contamination to human food.

The Period of Popular Education (1900–1915)

Real education of the public was achieved during the period between 1900
and 1915. Government bulletins and circulars, reports of state entomologists,
and other publications more or less reliable found their way into the public
schools and were made the basis of indirect education in the home through
the medium of the children. Farmers and others took to screening windows,
to improving the condition of privies, and to providing the latter where none
had existed before. Real progress was made, especially in the field of keeping
flies away from foodstuffs. Keeping them from feeding on filth was of course
more difficult, and any general attempt to prevent their production by special
handling of the manure produced on farms was rather far in the future, but
the educational idea was sound, public understanding was improving, and it
was a period of increasing regard for public health.

The year 1910 witnessed perhaps the greatest concentration of published titles dealing with the housefly of any year before or since. Popular magazines and daily newspapers carried stories and articles calculated to arouse public interest, while more technical journals in the field of medical and biological science contained serious discussions and reports of scientific observations. Emphasis was strongest on public health education, and it was certainly needed.

There seems, however, to have been an overselling of the idea. Once an intelligent citizen has been convinced of something, he does not particularly care to hear or read an endless repetition of the argument. He would much prefer to be treated to additional and more helpful facts. This period reminds us of the thirty years following the publication of Darwin's *Origin of Species* (1859). There was then much excitement and controversy over the evolution idea, but real research was crowded into the background and the relatively few high-grade investigations that got into print were largely ignored by pro-Darwinians and anti-Darwinians alike. The neglect of Mendel's discovery of dominance, segregation, and independent assortment is a case in point. Not until a new generation arose was emphasis on laboratory and field experiment properly restored, resulting as everyone knows in the birth of the science of genetics and a scientific approach to evolutionary problems.

And so with sanitary science in the early years of the present century. This was not the fault of the leaders in scientific research, who endeavored earnestly to maintain a proper balance between the popular and the technical, and took care not to neglect the latter. L. O. Howard, as chief of the Bureau of Entomology, U.S. Department of Agriculture, planned and encouraged researches on the life history and ecological relations of flies, especially as related to possible methods of control. At the same time he wrote many popular articles, and finally combined the educational and technical most successfully in his volume *The Housefly, Disease Carrier* . . . (1911a), which has been referred to elsewhere. C. G. Hewitt published many items, both in British and Canadian journals. Hewitt's efforts culminated in 1914 in a dual release, consisting of his four-hundred-page monograph, *The Housefly* Musca domestica *Linn.,* and a smaller, nontechnical volume, *House-flies and How They Spread Disease*. E. E. Austen, who published several technical papers on the relation of flies to disease, was content to prepare, for the general information of the public, a single pamphlet [2] that included instruction in current methods of control. During this period Graham-Smith conducted several investigations

---

[2] This document (1913) was made the basis for later releases under similar titles in 1920, 1926, 1928, and 1939, the last revised by Professor Smart.

on the bacterial flora of fecal-feeding flies and brought together his extensive knowledge of the morphology, life history, and medical importance of non-bloodsucking Diptera in the well-known volume published in 1914.

W. S. Patton seems to have made no attempt to popularize the subject at any time in his career. As a matter of fact, most of Patton's excellent contributions were published at least a decade later.

But once popular interest had been aroused, imagination tended to outstrip the facts. The housefly seems to have become regarded by journalists as the criminal of the ages, and its elimination or suppression was heralded as the panacea for most human ills.

Conservative educators, physicians, and others naturally resented this extreme attitude and endeavored to substitute a moderate viewpoint. Some even opposed the whole idea of fly-borne disease on the grounds that there was a scarcity of exact scientific proof. Controversy raged. Research was neglected, or the results of investigations were twisted to support previously established prejudice. Finally the reading public grew tired of sensational publicity in which repetition was the most outstanding feature. When war came to Europe in 1914 it provided new interests for both editors and readers, and the period of excessive publicity for the fly and her misdemeanors was at an end.

The Period of False Security (1915–1940)

It might almost be said that public interest collapsed like a pricked balloon. Scientific research also did a little resting on its oars. The monographs had been written, and an era had come to an end. Protection from typhoid and paratyphoid was available in the form of vaccines and this assured the safety of the troops in the field; at least it was supposed to do so. Civilian populations particularly tended to be neglectful of conditions that a decade earlier they would not have been allowed to forget. Sporadic attempts were made by state health and education departments to maintain sanitary instruction in the schools, but in America, at least, there was a peculiar and not easily understandable trend away from health education generally, so pronounced that a generation may be said to have grown to maturity without even the most elementary knowledge of the physiological activities of their own bodies. It was a generation of specialists, and only the specialist in applied biology was expected to acquire such knowledge or to have use for it.

The twenty-five-year period of which we are speaking may be divided into three successive parts: (a) the period of World War I, (b) the period of post-war prosperity, and (c) the period of depression and social legislation.

Considerable interest in medical entomology was stimulated of course by

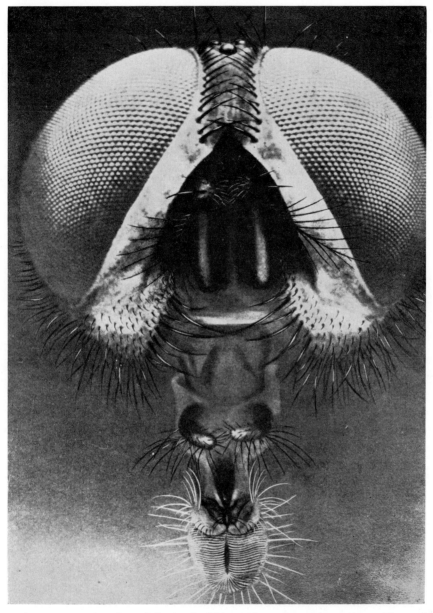

Figure 2. Anterior view of the head of *Musca domestica;* male specimen. The oral disc is thrust forward and slightly upward, thereby disclosing the prestomal cavity, between the two labella. (Photograph by N. A. Cobb; copyright, National Geographic Society.)

World War I, the bloodsucking species of insects being chiefly responsible. The prostration by malaria of both Allied and German armies in the region of the Dardanelles, and more particularly in Greek Macedonia, for approximately a two-year period called renewed attention to the role of the anopheline mosquito in the dissemination of the world's most important parasitic disease, while the relation of the body louse to both typhus and trench fever commanded the attention of a number of the world's leading medical officers and entomologists. Diseases capable of transmission by filth-feeding insects were of secondary importance, largely because the bulk of the fighting took place in geographical areas where such infections have rarely been of paramount interest.

Of course military authorities were faced with the usual problems created by the milder diarrheas, and in certain regions the more serious dysenteries gave concern. Dudgeon (1919) pointed out that in Macedonia these diseases were most prevalent when flies were most abundant, with the incidence of disease showing an appropriate lag behind the peak of fly production. Thus the marked increase in flies during April and May was associated with much dysentery in May and June. Similarly a second seasonal increase in flies, from September through November, was followed by dysentery of equal severity. Again, Buxton (1920) found in lower Mesopotamia that the housefly was a major factor in the distribution of intestinal disorders, as shown by the fact that over 60 per cent of the flies captured carried human feces. Four per cent carried human intestinal parasites; 0.5 per cent, *Endamoeba histolytica*. He stated that this was considered a "well-sanitated" area, but that bowel disorders were regrettably numerous.

J. N. Ross (1916), in giving his impressions of the Gallipoli campaign, stated that infections were undoubtedly transmitted by flies to the food consumed by the troops, since it was impossible to keep the food fly-free. Likewise Taylor (1919), in his study of bacillary dysentery in the Salonica Command, noted that the incidence of the disease corresponded with the prevalence of flies, being greatest from spring to early summer and again from late summer to early fall. Taylor experimented with both Flexner and Shiga bacilli and determined that houseflies could carry both types. He also found a certain percentage of wild-caught flies harboring dysentery bacilli.

A somewhat belated publication by Simmons (1923) called attention to severe epidemics of dysentery, influenza, and pneumonia among the personnel of the American Expeditionary Forces in the Department of Landes, in southwestern France, in 1918. There had been considerable neglect in regard to sanitary matters, and flies abounded. Simmons considered the severity of the influenza and pneumonia outbreaks to be due in part to the weakening of the men by fly-borne dysentery. It is interesting to note that Simmons advocated the utilization of professional entomologists in the capacity of commissioned officers, a policy that was to be employed very successfully in World War II.

Nevertheless, as mentioned previously, a sense of security had been established by the discovery of vaccines for typhoid, paratyphoid, and cholera, and interest in common flies as disease distributors was at a rather low ebb. This disinterest was perhaps but a natural reaction after the very great publicity given the "typhoid" fly during the decade between 1905 and 1915. People had become a bit surfeited with what one writer called the "repetitious babble of sentiment in dealing with flies," and were doubtless a little relieved to have the clamor subside. Then too, the increasing substitution of automobiles for horse-drawn vehicles had resulted in a decreased amount of available manure, the medium most preferred by the housefly in nature for its breeding activities. As city dwellers began to appreciate the desirability of an environment without flies, ordinances were put into effect forbidding or discouraging the keeping of animals within corporate limits, the enforcement of which fell naturally into the hands of the responsible few, while the majority of the citizenry ceased to feel any serious concern for improving the environment.

Flies actually emerged from World War I in the guise of friends and benefactors! The old observation that wounds which had become *flyblown* frequently healed more quickly than wounds not so infested bloomed again in connection with hot summer days, trench warfare, and the necessity of leaving the wounded in no man's land until darkness made the work of stretcher-bearers relatively safe. It was but a step from the observations of the battlefield to the deliberate use of sterile maggots for the treatment of stubborn infections, particularly lesions associated with osteomyelitis. Later discovery of the specific secretions (allantoin and urea) by which the larvae accomplished this seeming miracle eventually made use of the living maggots quite unnecessary, but for upwards of twenty years maggot therapy received enthusiastic support from a goodly portion of the medical profession.

The period immediately following World War I saw no very great advances in the *techniques* of sanitary science; but in civilized countries and especially in urban centers there was achieved a considerable improvement in sanitary *standards*. It was a period of unprecedented prosperity, and many families built new homes or moved to better ones. Residences were screened that had not before been so protected. Privies were replaced by septic tanks in suburban areas, and many communities launched plans for sewage and garbage disposal plants, for removal of pollution from rivers, and for other sanitary improvements.

In strictly rural areas of the United States the only real progress was accomplished in connection with dairy husbandry, where legal standards concerning the bacterial content of milk soon demonstrated the economic advantage of a dairy barn being as free as possible from contaminating flies. In most of the warmer countries of the world relatively little attention was given to fly sanitation, though the Health Organization of the League of Nations sponsored the publication of a number of researches, and some excellent studies were carried on by experimental workers in various European countries.

The economic depression that began in 1929 and continued for nearly ten years demonstrated how intimately sanitary practices relate to the standard of living. Unemployed families drifted from urban centers to abandoned farms and attempted subsistence farming, often unsuccessfully. Families that had been accustomed to screens and sanitary plumbing found themselves living in tar-paper shacks in backwoods areas under truly primitive conditions. Those who did not migrate found property maintenance increasingly difficult, and gradual demolition of habitations and other buildings was the inevitable result. Fortunately, before too long, social legislation was passed which, though costly in the extreme, saved large fractions of the population from destitution and malnutrition and probably from epidemic disease as well. Employment was created for millions, and in many cases municipalities were assisted to complete hospitals, sewage disposal plants, and other health-conserving enterprises.

Sanitary standards were clearly on the upgrade when hostilities broke out in 1939. Even so, the military leaders of the various belligerent nations were far from being adequately prepared to cope with the sanitary problems of World War II. As in all previous wars, casualties from disease greatly exceeded in number the casualties from battle. Victory for either side depended, more than civilians realized, on the solution of health problems among the troops, and no expense was spared in the race to control malaria, filariasis, typhus, and the dysenteries. It was a period in which medical entomology became once more a field of vital interest.

The Period of Stern Necessity (1940–1945)

With the advent of World War II, attention became focused very abruptly upon the tropics in which, for a time at least, it appeared that the bulk of the fighting must take place. Malaria, filariasis, scrub typhus, and schistosomiasis each occupied the center of the stage in definitive areas, but dysentery, espe-

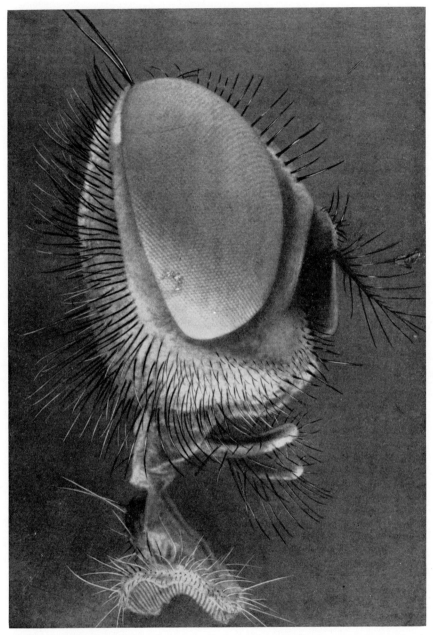

Figure 3. Right lateral view of the head of *Musca domestica*. Antennae and proboscis are particularly well shown. Both structures are important in sensory perception. (Photograph by N. A. Cobb; copyright, National Geographic Society.)

cially of the bacillary type, was recognized in almost all theaters as a serious military problem. Contaminated food or water was always involved. In the moist tropics flies were not as great a factor in this contamination as in the countries usually described as "hot and dry" (Egypt, Arabia, Iraq, and Iran).

The sanitary habits of native populations proved to be the principal stumbling block in achieving satisfactory fly control. Good discipline could and did insure proper disposal of human waste where military personnel were concerned, but education of the natives was often difficult, sometimes impossible. In this, the troops of the U.S.S.R. which guarded the northern end of the supply route into their country from the Persian Gulf were perhaps most successful, though the methods there employed were sometimes severe to the point of ruthlessness.

In areas of active hostilities, where sanitary practices inevitably break down at least to some extent, the direct use of insecticidal sprays constituted the sanitarians' principal tool—pyrethrum, lethane, or thanite about mess halls and barracks, and sodium arsenite for treating unburied cadavers and the bodies of animals.

The advent of DDT proved a veritable godsend to medical department officers and changed the picture materially during the latter period of the war. The unusual residual effect that characterizes this insecticide causes most surfaces to remain toxic to flies and other insects for many days, sometimes months, after a single application. The properties and shortcomings of DDT will be discussed at length in another chapter. It is sufficient to say that, both during the war and since the cessation of hostilities, many large-scale investigations have been carried out at experiment stations, by government agencies, by commercial interests, and by private individuals in various parts of the world, and that economic entomology has most assuredly entered a new period of endeavor by reason of the development of DDT and compounds related to it.

Aftermath and Outlook (1945 on)

There is no doubt but that our scientific knowledge of medical entomology is now far greater than it has ever been. Our weakness lies in the fact that this knowledge is locked in the minds and filing cases of comparatively few people. It should be a challenging fact that during the past quarter of a century, while scientific data concerning the biology of medically important species has grown apace, popular education concerning insect-borne diseases, which as we have said reached almost artificial heights before 1915, has been permitted to languish. The average citizen in the United States today, though far better educated generally than his predecessors of a generation previous, is often quite lacking in the most elementary knowledge of medical entomology and its significance in human welfare. Flies, to be sure, are regarded as undesirable for *esthetic* reasons, and this is excellent as it leads to their general suppression, especially in more cultured homes. The proper rationale, however, is lacking in most instances, and people tend therefore to be satisfied merely with a reduction in numbers, not realizing that a single specimen at the picnic table may be the carrier of typhoid bacilli just obtained from human feces or of tubercle bacilli from sputum deposited nearby.

What is needed is a reawakening of individual responsibility in this, as in so many other fields of human interest. It is the author's hope that in a very modest way the present volume will contribute to that end.

PURPOSE AND SCOPE OF THE PRESENT WORK

The chapters that follow will treat of the biology of *Musca domestica* and other filth-feeding flies from a number of important aspects. External morphology will be discussed in sufficient detail to make clear all structures used in species recognition. Internal morphology will be given equal consideration, as basic to an understanding of food habits, reproduction, and adaptation to environment. The taxonomic relation of *Musca domestica* to others of the genus and to muscoid species generally will be discussed in some detail, in accordance with accepted principles of zoological classification, especially as employed by students of the Order Diptera.

The economic, medical, and public-health aspects will of course be given major emphasis. External and internal morphology will be interpreted in terms of structures favoring dissemination of infectious organisms. The life history of the fly will be scrutinized in terms of ecological factors that make possible both the multiplication of the species and the distribution of disease.

Methods used in research procedures will be described, and the value of *Musca domestica* as an experimental organism will be given due consideration. All known methods of fly control will be listed and the more valuable procedures will be discussed at length. Natural or biological control measures will be contrasted with artificial methods both on an emergency and on a long-range basis.

It is sincerely hoped that the reader, by reason of this many-sided approach, may not only acquire a deeper insight into some of the "defects" of our modern civilization but may also gain a better appreciation of the need, not only for unlimited research, but also for constant educational effort in the field of public health. Should the nations of the world again take up arms against

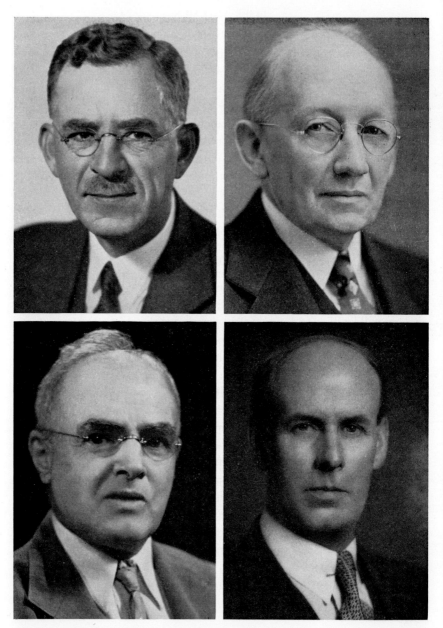

Figure 4. American public health educators. *Upper left:* W. B. Herms. *Lower left:* W. A. Riley. *Upper right:* O. A. Johannsen. *Lower right:* Robert Matheson. These scholars, each a distinguished investigator in his own right, found time in the midst of strenuous careers to compile the immense and widely scattered literature in the field of medical entomology and so render important information available to American students and clinicians. Sufficient recognition is rarely given to this type of service.

one another we may well look for the widespread destruction of most of those sanitary conveniences that now render our lives reasonably safe from communicable disease. Without sewers or water mains we would soon be surrounded by filth-borne organisms of many kinds, some of them of the most dangerous kind. And should the enemy resort to biological warfare, the list of dangerous protozoa, bacteria, viruses, and rickettsias against which we would be obliged to protect ourselves might be unexpectedly long. It is quite conceivable that insects, including flies, might be intentionally employed on an extensive scale by belligerent nations to introduce disease among stricken populations. In such a setting, medical entomology would hold at least as important a place as it has ever held in the history of the race.

The present compilation is probably justified for no other reason than that well over two thousand references to *Musca domestica* have appeared in the literature since the publication of any comprehensive monograph in the English language.[3] Should a more practical justification be demanded, however, such can undoubtedly be found in the enormous amount of human suffering that has existed and will exist as a result of the natural activities of common flies.

BLOODSUCKING AND NONBLOODSUCKING FLIES

Since there is always confusion in the minds of many as to whether common flies can "bite," it may be well to point out that medical interest is about equally divided between the bloodsucking and nonbloodsucking forms. In the first category are the mosquitoes with their known relationship to malaria, yellow fever, dengue, and filariasis. Somewhat related to the mosquitoes are the sand flies (*Phlebotomus*) and the punkies (*Culicoides*). The first genus carries pappataci fever, verruga, and several types of leishmaniasis. The latter is the vector of two rather benign tropical roundworms, *Acanthocheilonema perstans* and *Mansonella ozzardi*. Flies of the genus *Simulium* convey the tropical roundworm *Onchocerca volvulus*, while the tabanid genus *Chrysops* is intermediate host for *Loa loa*. Both *Chrysops* and *Tabanus* are known to be mechanical transmitters of tularemia. Among the muscoid flies, *Glossina* is the well-known vector of African trypanosomiasis (several kinds), the same parasites being also capable of mechanical transmission by the stable fly, *Stomoxys*.

[3] Dr. Mathias Thomsen's comprehensive report of researches on houseflies and stable flies, published in Danish in 1938, is a valuable and beautifully illustrated work. In Spanish, the modest but very practical volume by Dr. Luis Nájera Angulo, published in 1947, is highly informative, especially in regard to inexpensive methods of control.

Over and against these bloodsucking species are the various genera of filth-feeding and filth-breeding flies. The genus *Musca*, concerning which this volume has most to do, is unquestionably the most important. But there are other genera of more or less similar habit. Species of *Calliphora, Lucilia, Phormia, Muscina, Anthomyia, Fannia,* and *Sarcophaga* are attracted both by foul substances and by odors of the human table, and thus have frequent opportunity to transmit pathogenic organisms by mouth parts, feet, fecal discharges, and body hairs.

The particular diseases capable of transmission by nonbloodsucking flies, while not as many as those conveyed by biting species, probably involve at least as large a portion of the earth's surface, and before the development of typhoid and cholera vaccines ran a strong race in the matter of mortality. Even today there is no more frequent cause of infant death in the entire world than the intestinal infections. This is particularly true in the drier countries of western Asia.

In addition to the role played by adult flies in the dissemination of filth-borne infection, we have the spectacle of some twenty or thirty species manifesting the ability to spend the larval period as parasites upon or within the human body, where they cause more or less anxiety, discomfort, and distress. With almost no exception, these are the larvae of forms that are nonbloodsucking in the adult state, a fact that considerably increases the medical importance of the nonbloodsucking groups. If we add to this list the botflies of domestic animals and of the game animals in which man is interested, the medical and veterinary importance of the nonbiting Diptera becomes significant indeed.

CHAPTER II

External Morphology

INCLUDING THE ORGANS OF COPULATION AND OVIPOSITION

Something in the insect seems to be alien to the habits, morals and psychology of this world, as if it had come from some other planet, more monstrous, more energetic, more insensate, more atrocious, more infernal than our own.—Maurice Maeterlinck, J. H. Fabre et son oeuvre

IF IT were possible to enlarge a fly to the size of a mastodon, the full implication of the above quotation would be apparent to all concerned. According to his temperament, the observer might well be astonished, delighted, or even terrified as the functional significance of the creature's locomotor, sensory, and ingestive structures dawned upon his consciousness. Even one who has observed this and related species through the microscope hundreds and perhaps thousands of times never quite gets used to viewing the monster with her all-seeing eyes, her sensitive, aristate antennae, and the host of bristles and spines which adorn almost every part of her exterior. The following account of the fly's superficial structures is not written, however, to stimulate the imagination. It aims merely to acquaint the reader with those anatomical terms that will best serve him in his subsequent understanding of the fly's taxonomic position, behavior, and relation to disease.

A word as to the fly's place in the animal kingdom will be in order. The housefly is first an insect, and as such manifests all the important morphological features of the Class Hexapoda. Second, it is an arthropod, lacking none of the structures characteristic of that phylum. Beyond this, the fly is an animal, whose sensory, locomotor, food-taking, and reproductive structures adapt it, after the manner of all species, for successful continuance within a limited variety of environmental conditions.

It should be remembered that a knowledge and understanding of external body characters is basic to an appreciation of all other aspects of an animal's biology. Determination to genus and species depends, primarily, on externally visible structures. Size, shape, and structure of the mouth parts determine the feeding habits of the species and indicate at once whether it is a consumer of solid or liquid materials, a parasite, or a scavenger. The presence or absence of wings and their number and character, when present, not only assist in classifying to group but permit a fairly accurate conjecture as to the nature of locomotion and the probable migratory range. Hairs, tubercles, and the glandular apertures sometimes associated with them have a very real connection with the mechanical transmission of disease organisms, while the same structures, if borne on the feet, serve to determine the type of surface (rough, smooth, vertical, inverted) over which the insect can successfully make its way.

GENERAL DESCRIPTION

Musca domestica is a medium-sized, mouse-gray insect, usually 6 to 7 mm. in length, with a wing span approximately twice this distance. When at rest, however, the wings are directed somewhat posteriorly, so as to give to the fly a triangular appearance when viewed from above. The wings, otherwise clear and transparent, are somewhat yellowish at the base.

As with some 750,000 other species of insects, the fly's body is composed of three easily recognized parts: (1) the head, a subspherical unit of which the most conspicuous feature is a pair of relatively enormous compound eyes; (2) the thorax, or central portion, which bears both legs and wings; and (3) the abdomen, which consists of five readily visible segments and which terminates in structures peculiar to the sex of the individual. Head, thorax, and abdomen are of approximately equal width (1.9 to 2.2 mm.), but both neck and waistline are remarkably reduced, the former especially, an arrangement that provides for extreme flexibility and permits almost complete rotation of the head.

THE HEAD

In anterior view (Fig. 2) the following head structures may be seen: The large compound eyes, purplish brown in color, occupy either side of the head and appear very slightly bean-shaped, due to the faintly sinuous outline of their inner margins. The surface of each compound eye is divided into approximately 4,000 facets, each irregularly hexagonal in outline. Each facet functions as a lens, permitting light to stimulate the visual unit (ommatidium) immediately beneath. In the housefly the surface of the compound eye is free from hair. Certain related species show marked pilosity. At the very top of the head (vertex), situated in a small triangle with the point directed forward, may be seen the three ocelli, or simple eyes, the surface of which is not divided into facets. Extending from the vertex forward to the base of the antennae is a dull-black stripe, the frontal vitta. In male specimens the vitta practically fills the space between the eyes. In females the front is much wider, and though the vitta is much wider also, particularly above, there remains on either side

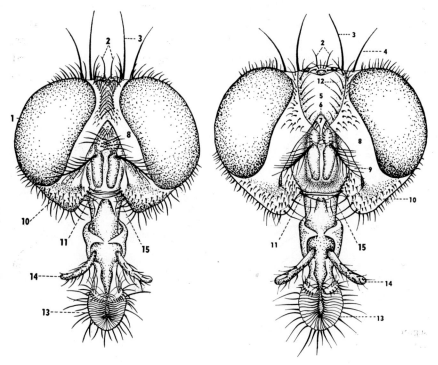

Figure 5. *Musca domestica.* Cephalic views of head. *Left:* Male. *Right:* Female. *1,* compound eye; *2,* postvertical bristles; *3,* inner vertical bristle; *4,* outer vertical bristle; *5,* front; *6,* frontal suture; *7,* frontal lunule; *8,* sides of face; *9,* facial ridge; *10,* cheek (gena); *11,* antenna; *12,* inner vertical row of frontal bristles; *13,* labella; *14,* palpus; *15,* oral vibrissae.

a definite area of a light golden color, separating the vitta from the eyes. These sides of the front are continuous with the "sides of the face," which in males extend but a short distance upward from the facial depression. The lower portion of the face, on either side, consists of a rather swollen area, the gena, which is easily recognized by the large number of downwardly directed, bristly hairs. The genae are sometimes referred to as cheeks and are approximately one-third of the eye height.

The two antennae lie in the facial depression, already mentioned. The basal segment, close to the frontal vitta, is ringlike and quite obscure. The second, twice as long as broad, is blackish brown in color and bears a number of irregular, short, black hairs, one stouter and longer than the rest. The second antennal segment is distinctly cleft on the outer side. The third segment, fully four times as long as broad, is shaped somewhat like a fat knife blade. It is dark in color and is covered with a fine silvery-golden pile. Near its base and slightly external to the anterior edge arises the bristlelike arista, as long as the antenna itself and bearing, both above and below, fairly long hairs (*spinulae*) that make the arista more conspicuous than the segment to which it is attached. The usual arrangement for these spinules is seven above and five below. The

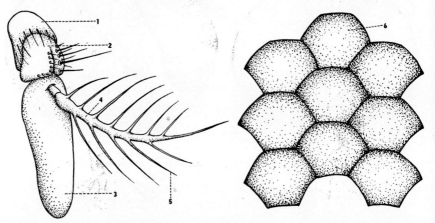

Figure 6. Important sensory structures. *Left:* Antenna (right side), showing three segments and plumose arista. *Right:* Several facets from the surface of a compound eye. *1,* scape; *2,* pedicel; *3,* first flagellar segment; *4,* arista; *5,* hairs of arista; *6,* individual facet.

distal third of the arista is bare, as is the under surface near the base. The arista itself is actually three-segmented, but the two basal units are so tiny that one or both may be easily overlooked. The whole structure is usually interpreted as homologous with the fourth, fifth, and sixth segments of more primitive antennal types. The antennae of houseflies are the same in both sexes. The three basal segments (Fig. 6) are sometimes called the scape, the pedicel, and the first flagellar segment (Patton, 1930). Due to the great terminal development of the last, the arista of houseflies and of a very large number of related species comes to be dorsal rather than terminal to this segment.

Each antenna lies more or less in a cradle of its own, the triangular facial depression being divided by a low but distinct carina, more evident when the antennae are removed.

The facial ridges mark the boundaries of the facial depression on either side and on its lower portion each bears a number of bristlelike, black hairs, the strongest of which are designated as oral vibrissae. Slightly external to the facial ridge may be seen on either side a definite groove, the ptilinal suture, which, curving upward, becomes continuous with its counterpart of the op-

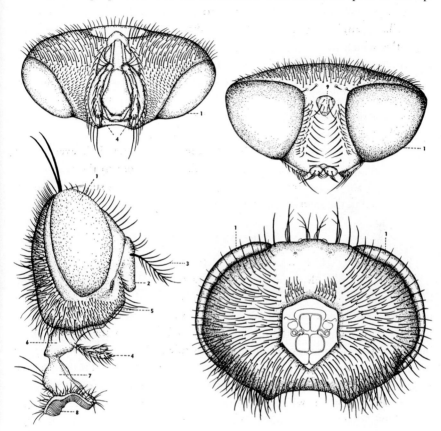

Figure 7. Special views of the head. *Upper left:* Ventral aspect. *Upper right:* Dorsal aspect. *Lower left:* Lateral aspect. *Lower right:* Caudal aspect. *1,* compound eye; *2,* third antennal segment; *3,* arista; *4,* palpi; *5,* oral margin; *6,* rostrum; *7,* haustellum; *8,* labella; *9,* ocellar triangle.

posite side. At the apex of the curve may be seen a diamond- or lunule-shaped area where closure is not quite complete. This suture marks the line of disappearance of the ptilinum, a saclike protuberance that assisted the fly in extricating itself from the puparium, after which it was withdrawn into the head.

A distinct "lip" (oral margin) separates the facial depression from the base of the proboscis.

Besides the oral vibrissae, certain other conspicuous bristles have been given names. Just behind the ocellar triangle are the two posterior verticals. To the right and left of these are the very large inner vertical bristles. Still more lateral in position are the robust outer verticals. The ocellar bristles arise from the ocellar triangle. The principal pair is directed forward. The heavy rows of bristles which mark the lateral margins of the vitta are known as frontals (above) and transfrontals (below). Taken together, the frontals and transfrontals are said to constitute the inner vertical row. Between these and the compound eyes are the relatively weak frontoorbitals, present only in the female. The upper portions of the sides of the face bear a few fine hairs, scarcely discernible in the male.

The posterior surface of the head is termed the occiput. It is everywhere more or less hairy. The hairs and bristles that arise close to the base of the proboscis are sometimes referred to as the "beard." The term succiput is sometimes applied to the inferior portion of the posterior surface.

THE PROBOSCIS

The proboscis, which when extended for feeding may be as long as the head height, can be almost completely retracted, so that sometimes only the bulblike oral lobes (labella) are exposed. The extended proboscis may be seen to consist of three successive parts: (1) the rostrum, a more or less triangular portion (lateral view) with the base attached broadly to the head; (2) an intermediate portion somewhat more expanded distally than basally, the haustellum; and (3) the terminal labella, already mentioned. The two labella together form a heart-shaped structure that the fly presses against any substance or surface on which it desires to feed. Parallel transverse ridges (pseudotracheae) characterize the free surface of the labella and it is through pores in these structures that the food material is drawn into the channel that leads to the alimentary tract. A more detailed account of labial structure will be given in Chapter III, where a complete discussion of the feeding process will be found.

From the anterior surface of the rostrum arise the two club-shaped maxillary palpi. In the housefly these range from dark brown to black and bear a number of irregular, dark hairs.

THE THORAX

The middle portion of the fly's body is composed of three segments, the prothorax, mesothorax, and metathorax, each of which bears a pair of legs. Only the mesothorax, however, is adorned with wings, a fact that explains the extraordinary development of this segment, especially on the dorsal side. In fact, when viewed from above, the thorax of all muscoidean flies appears to consist almost entirely of mesonotum. In houseflies this is subdivided as follows.

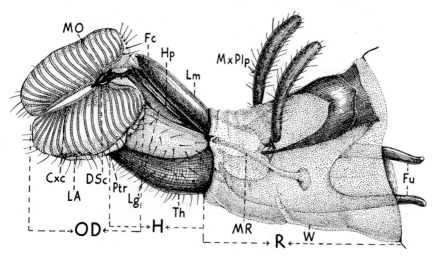

Figure 8. The proboscis of *Musca domestica,* frontolateral view. *Lg,* labial gutter. Other labeling as in Figure 25. (Matheson, *Medical Entomology;* Comstock Publishing Co.)

A transverse suture (Fig. 9) separates the prescutum from the scutum (Curran, 1934), while a second suture, more posterior, marks the boundary line between the mesonotum (proper) and its posterior extension, the scutellum. The three areas thus delineated are progressively narrower from front to rear, the scutellum having almost the outline of an equilateral triangle. Just behind the head, on either side, are the humeral callosities. More posterior, opposite the transverse suture are the lens-shaped notopleural areas. Just in front of the scutellum on either side is the postalar callus, filling in the posterolateral angle of the mesonotum. All surfaces are rather heavily beset with hairs, the larger and coarser of which have been given names. Thus the humeral callosity bears the humeral bristles, while just behind those are the post-humerals. In line with these, but farther back, are the presuturals, while be-

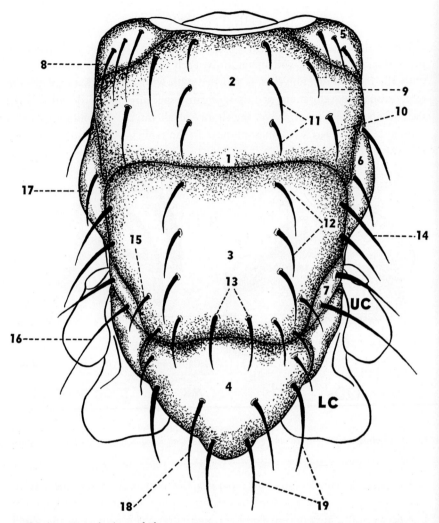

Figure 9. Dorsal view of thorax. *1,* transverse suture; *2,* prescutum; *3,* scutum; *4,* scutellum; *5,* humeral callosity; *6,* notopleura; *7,* postalar callus; *8,* humeral bristles; *9,* posthumeral bristle; *10,* presutural bristle; *11,* anterior dorsocentral bristles; *12,* posterior dorsocentral bristles; *13,* acrostical bristles; *14,* supra-alar bristles; *15,* intra-alar bristles; *16,* postalar bristles; *17,* notopleural bristles; *18,* discal scutellar bristle; *19,* marginal scutellar bristles; *UC,* upper calypter; *LC,* lower calypter.

hind the suture, in the same sequence, lie the intra-alars. Postalar bristles occupy the postalar callosities. Interior to the posthumerals are the dorsocentrals, while in the medial dorsal position most muscoids have two rows of acrostical bristles. These are represented in the housefly, however, by only a single pair, just in front of the scutellum. Dorsocentral and acrostical bristles are referred to as anterior and posterior according to whether they lie before or behind the transverse suture. Scutellar bristles are designated as discal or marginal, according to position.

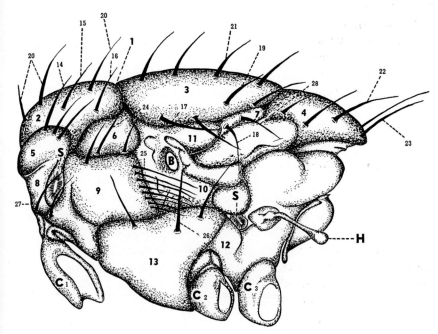

Figure 10. Lateral view of thorax. *1*, transverse suture; *2*, prescutum; *3*, scutum; *4*, scutellum; *5*, humeral callosity; *6*, notopleura; *7*, postalar callus; *8*, propleura; *9*, mesopleura; *10*, pteropleura; *11*, supra-alar groove; *12*, hypopleura; *13*, sternopleura; *14*, humeral bristles; *15*, posthumeral bristles; *16*, presutural bristles; *17*, supra-alar bristles; *18*, postalar bristles; *19*, intra-alar bristles; *20*, anterior dorsocentral bristles; *21*, posterior dorsocentral bristles; *22*, discal scutellar bristles; *23*, marginal scutellar bristles; *24*, notopleural bristles; *25*, mesopleural bristles; *26*, sternopleural bristles; *27*, propleural bristle; *28*, postalar bristles. *B*, base of wing; *C 1, 2, 3,* Coxae of prothoracic, mesothoracic, and metathoracic legs; *H*, halter; *S*, spiracles.

In general it may be said that the chaetotaxy of *Musca domestica* is much less definite than that of certain other muscoid flies, specifically *Calliphora, Sarcophaga,* and various genera of the family Tachinidae.

In lateral view the thoracic structure appears somewhat more complicated; nevertheless, the various sclerites are not difficult to recognize. Pronotum, notopleura, humeral callus, mesonotum, and scutellum are easily differentiated. The propleura extends ventrad from the humeral callus. The mesopleura lies just below the notopleura, while the posterior portion of the lateral

surface is made up largely of the pteropleural sclerite. The hypopleura lies behind the middle coxa, the sternopleura just in front. Bristles borne on any of
these areas take their names from the sclerite concerned. Thus the housefly has
one large and several lesser propleural bristles, with a similar aggregation of
mesopleurals closely adjacent, a fairly regular row of mesopleurals along the
posterior margin of that sclerite, a weak tuft of pteropleurals, and three strong
sternopleurals, one in front and two behind. In this species (and family)
hypopleurals are absent.

Connecting the scutellum with the dorsal portion of the first abdominal
segment is the dark, shiny, convex, hairless metanotum. If we follow Hewitt
and consider this the postscutellum of the mesothorax, then the true metanotum is represented by a slender, pointed process on either side, extending
upward from the epimeron of the metathorax and lying upon a membranous
area, the mesophragma. Just anterior to this, on either side is a peculiar
knobbed hair, the halter. The halteres of flies are considered homologous with
the second pair of wings borne by the metathorax of most insects. They are
vestigial structures, no longer used for locomotion. They do, however, function
as sensory organs and are useful in maintaining equilibrium. (See Chapter
III.) The base of each halter is somewhat conical in shape, and on this portion
are borne a number of chordotonal sense organs. These constitute the basal
sensorium of Patton and others. Their structure may be properly understood
only by microscopic examination of a histological preparation. The shank or
medial portion of the halter is slender and rodlike; the terminal portion is
expanded into a spherical knob of which the basal portion has a wall distinctly
thicker than that of the extremity.

Two breathing pores, or spiracles, are also present on the lateral surface of
the thorax, one in the suture between the propleura and mesopleura, the other
just below the halter. They have thickened lips and to a limited extent may
be opened or closed by the action of special muscles.

The dorsal surface of the thorax is of a changeable silvery-gold pollinose
coloration, but this is interrupted to produce the effect of four longitudinal
black stripes, practically parallel. These are most conspicuous just behind the
head, fading to evanescence before reaching the scutellum. They are best seen
when viewed from above, with the head of the specimen away from the observer. These four lines distinguish common houseflies from a number of
other muscoids, the closest approximation being found in certain species of
Sarcophaga, which, however, may be recognized by the presence of hypopleural bristles and by certain peculiarities of abdominal coloration and body
shape.

Laterally, the thoracic sclerites may be described as dark, with most of the surface thinly covered by a gray pollinose sheen, not very evenly spread.

APPENDAGES OF THE THORAX

The Wings

The "root" of the wing attaches just in front of the scutellar bridge and directly above the pteropleural bristles.

Overlapping the base of the wing is a small, hairy, scalelike plate or cap, the tegula. Some authors prefer to consider the term tegula synonymous with squama or calypter. In the present volume, however, it will be applied only to the structure just described.

The wing membrane itself averages 6.2 mm. long by 2.48 mm. wide, and except for the supporting veins is transparent throughout. Viewed beneath the binocular dissecting scope under reflected light, the wing surface shows

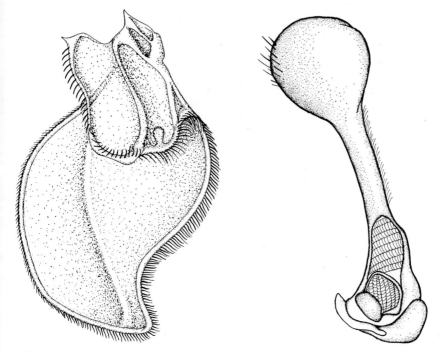

Figure 11. Accessory wing structures. *Left:* Right squama (alula, calypter), lateral view. Note that smaller, basal portion is folded over so that its morphologically ventral surface is uppermost. *Right:* Halter, or balancing organ, believed to be homologous with the metathoracic wing of other orders. Note chordotonal sense organs (basal sensoria) in proximal region.

many iridescent areas, with delicate shades of green and pink predominating. This is due to the refraction of light by many wrinkles and corrugations, microscopic in size.

The growth and development of the wing buds in the pupal stage will be discussed more fully in Chapter IV. It is sufficient to say here that the so-called veins, which are so conspicuous in the adult state and which function primarily for support, represent for the most part the paths of tracheal trunks that served the respiratory needs of the wing bud during the developmental period. In adult life a limited amount of blood circulates between the wing membranes, following the course of major veins (E. Thomsen, 1938), but the distal portion especially tends to become dry, brittle, and relatively lifeless. If worn or broken, the wing cannot be regenerated or replaced.

Of the eight original tracheal trunks, six are represented by persistent longitudinal veins, the first and third anal veins being no longer indicated in the higher Diptera.

Margins and angles of the wing. That margin of the wing which is the more robust and which is directed forward during flight is called the costal margin, or simply costa. Since the outline of the wing is slightly suggestive of a triangle, the posterior margin may be divided into an outer margin that extends from the apex to a point opposite the greatest width of the wing, and an inner margin that curves forward to the axillary lobe. Both posterior margins are adorned by numerous marginal hairs or "fringe scales," regularly arranged. With three margins it is also possible to conceive of three angles, the humeral angle at the base of costa, the apical angle at the extreme tip of the wing, and a poorly defined anal angle where the inner and outer margins meet.

The membrane of the wing base is termed the axillary membrane (Comstock, 1940). The posterior margin of this area is somewhat thickened, being supported by a chitinous extension from the posterior lateral angle of the notum, called the axillary cord. In the housefly and related forms this region of the wing is much complicated by an expansion of the axillary membrane, which results in the creation of a yellowish opaque lobe or scale which overlies the halter and is a conspicuous feature of thoracic morphology. This is called the squama, alula, or calypter. The fact that the wing base is so much narrower than the wing itself requires the basal third of the squama to be folded upon the distal portion in such a manner that the dorsal surfaces of the two are brought together. Thus there are really two squamae on either side, a smaller, "upper" squama, with its morphologically ventral surface uppermost, and a larger, "lower" unit, normal in position. Both are bounded by the axillary cord.

Adjacent to the squamae but more nearly in the plane of the wing itself is

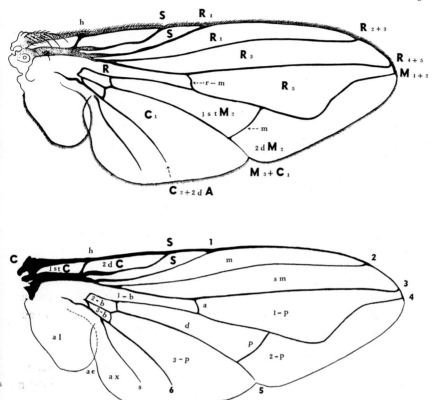

Figure 12. Upper: Wing of *Musca domestica*. Labeling of veins and cells is in accordance with Comstock-Needham system. The costal vein and the two costal cells are not lettered. *A*, anal veins; *C*, cubitus and cubital cells; *M*, media and medial cells; *R*, radius and radial cells; *S*, subcosta, vein and cell; *h*, humeral cross vein; *m*, medial cross vein; *r–m*, radiomedial cross vein. *Lower:* Wing of *Musca domestica*. Labeling is in accordance with accepted usage among dipterologists. *C*, costal vein and cells (*1st, 2d*); *S*, subcostal (auxiliary) vein and cell; *1, 2, 3, 4, 5, 6*, first to sixth longitudinal veins; *m, sm*, marginal and submarginal cells; *1-p, 2-p, 3-p*, first, second, and third posterior cells; *1-b, 2-b, 3-b*, first, second, and third basal cells; *a*, anterior cross vein; *al*, axillary lobe; *ae*, axillary excision; *ax*, axillary cell; *d*, discal cell; *h*, humeral cross vein; *p*, posterior cross vein; *s*, spurious (third anal) vein.

the axillary lobe. This is merely a portion of the anal region, set off by a notch on the inner posterior margin. This notch is termed the axillary excision.

Venation. Along the costal margin runs the costal vein. It continues almost to the apex, where it terminates abruptly. Throughout its course the costal vein is covered by short, black spines, coarser near the base. Just beyond the humeral cross vein and again at the termination of the subcostal vein, the costa is reduced in diameter and somewhat lighter in color. Such points are sometimes referred to as "fractures," especially if the interruption is at all conspicuous. The remaining longitudinal veins are as follows:

The subcostal vein is rather pale and runs in the trough of a definite furrow in the wing membrane. It extends for about two-fifths of the length of the wing before joining the costal margin. At less than half the distance from the base, subcosta is connected with costa by the somewhat oblique humeral cross vein, already mentioned.

It is customary among students of the Diptera to refer to the remaining longitudinal veins by number, rather than by name. The first longitudinal vein, which runs confluent with subcosta for a short distance at the base, has a total length of approximately half of the wing. Halfway along the thickened basal portion, one or two small black bristles may be seen. The vein itself runs along the crest of a definite ridge, in contrast with the "valley" position of subcosta. There is a definite tendency for the veins to alternate in this regard; hence some entomologists refer to alternate convex (ridge-following) and concave (furrow-following) veins in describing specimens. The second and third longitudinal veins are both branches of the radial vein of general entomologists. This system (in which vein one is also included) shares a common origin with subcosta, as indicated above. The second and third units, which are sometimes referred to collectively as the radial sector, run a short distance as a single vein, then separate, taking somewhat divergent courses to the anterior margin, slightly in advance of the apical angle.

The central vein of the wing (longitudinal vein 4) has an inconspicuous connection with the anterior veins at the base, then runs a straight course for nearly four-fifths of its length. On approaching the margin, however, it swings forward and unites with the tip end of costa, a little behind the termination of vein 3 and just before the apex. In certain muscoid genera (*Gasterophilus*) this final bend does not occur, and in other groups (*Anthomyia, Stomoxys, Muscina*) various intermediate conditions prevail. In *Glossina* the course of vein 4 is much distorted due to the more distal position of the small anterior (radiomedial) cross vein. Vein 4 is believed to be homologous with the first two branches of the medial vein of primitive groups.

Vein 5 has no fundamental origin with the anterior veins but is, nevertheless, anchored to vein 4 by two connections close to the base and a third near the outer margin. The first of these connections, usually quite obscure, probably represents the posterior arculus of authors. The second marks the path of the third and fourth branches of media as they proceed caudally to fuse with parts of cubitus. The third is a true cross vein, uniting the two principal branches of media. In the housefly it is slightly sinuous and bounds the outer margin of the discal cell. Vein 5 continues to the margin, where the point of termination is marked by a definite notch.

The sixth longitudinal vein has a common origin with the fifth, but diverges rather sharply, coming to an end in the anal region without attaining the margin. The cross vein that unites it to vein 5 near the base is believed homologous with the second branch of cubitus, which has a tendency to fuse with one or more anal veins in a number of highly evolved groups. There is evidence (Fig. 12) that the first anal vein of primitive species has been reduced practically to oblivion and that it is the second anal vein in reality which has persisted as longitudinal vein 6 and with which cubitus is now fused.

A shadow, or fold, posterior to vein 6 may usually be seen. It is referred to as the spurious vein, and may possibly be homologous with the third anal vein of other groups.

The spaces between the wing veins are termed cells. Cells are referred to as "open" if they are bounded at any point by the wing margin, and "closed" if surrounded entirely by veins. According to the Comstock-Needham system (1898) of naming the veins, all cells are designated according to the vein just preceding. Thus the humeral cross vein divides the first from the second costal cell. Similarly, the open cell bounded anteriorly by subcosta becomes the subcostal cell. All the others, however, have been given special names according to position, as the application of the Comstock-Needham system to dipterous wings has not proved very satisfactory for taxonomic purposes. The marginal cell is that which lies between longitudinal veins 1 and 2, while the submarginal lies similarly between veins 2 and 3. Following around the margin we have then a series of posterior cells, the first (which is also called the apical cell) lying between veins 3 and 4, the second posterior between veins 4 and 5, and the third posterior between veins 5 and 6. Posterior to vein 6 is the axillary cell, sometimes more or less divided by the so-called spurious vein. In the interior of the wing are four closed cells, the largest of which, bounded by veins 4 and 5 and the large posterior cross vein, has already been referred to as the discal cell. The largest of the remaining three lies between the basal portions of veins 3 and 4, and is terminated by the small or anterior cross vein. It is called the first basal cell. The second and third basal cells lie between veins 4 and 5 and between veins 5 and 6, respectively. Figure 12 (upper) shows the veins and cells labeled according to the Comstock-Needham system, and Figure 12 (lower) according to prevailing usage among dipterologists.

The Legs

The six legs of a fly are all essentially similar. Each consists of a basal coxa, a small, triangular trochanter, an elongated and comparatively robust femur, a tibia of about the same length as the femur but more slender throughout, the

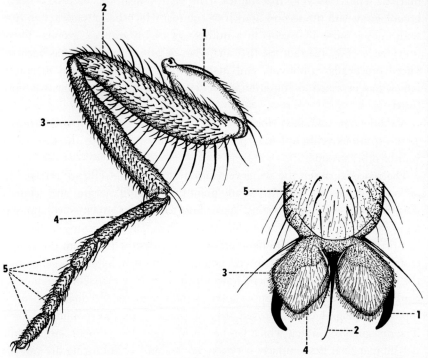

Figure 13. Leg of the housefly. *Left:* Caudal aspect of left anterior leg. *1,* coxa; *2,* femur; *3,* tibia; *4,* basitarsus; *5,* remaining segments of tarsus. *Right:* Terminal portion of last tarsal segment. *1,* claw; *2,* empodium; *3,* pulvillus; *4,* tenent hairs; *5,* fifth tarsal segment.

distal extremity being of greater diameter than the proximal, and a five-segmented tarsus. The first tarsal segment (basitarsus) is much longer than the others. This condition is best developed on the third pair of legs.

The anterior coxae are the largest and are rather typically fusiform, or boat-shaped. The second and third pairs of coxae are smaller and the sclerites composing them are more distinct from one another. The femora of the prothoracic legs are shorter and stouter than those of the mesothoracic and metathoracic pairs. An interesting adaptation is found on the anterior tibiae, which are a little shorter than those of the intermediate and posterior legs.

On the mesial surface of each fore tibia is a row of closely set setae, rather orange in color, which the fly uses in combing particles of dirt from the hairs and setae of the general body surface. A similar arrangement is found on the first tarsal segments of the third pair of legs. This provides for the grooming of the posterior portions of the body.

The foot of the fly is especially interesting. Its structure has been the subject of study and speculation for many years (Hepworth, 1854; Merlin, 1897, 1905). The fifth tarsal segment bears a pair of curved claws (ungues), which are used in clinging to rough surfaces. At the base of each claw and ventral thereto is a bladderlike structure called a pulvillus, which in turn bears a large number of tiny, glandular hairs. These hairs, by reason of the secretion which exudes at or near their tips, are continually wet and sticky, a condition that enables the fly to cling to vertical or even inverted surfaces. For this reason they are called tenent hairs.

Between the bases of the two pulvilli is a tapering, bristlelike structure, the empodium. It remains to be shown whether the empodium exercises any special sensory function. In addition, ventral to the pulvilli are the single median and two lateral foot plates, small, scalelike structures rather easily overlooked.

All segments of the legs bear a considerable number of hairs, bristles, or spines. Especially conspicuous are certain spines found on the shank and distal extremity of the tibia. In many groups of Diptera these are of taxonomic importance.

THE ABDOMEN

The first abdominal segment is considerably reduced, being visible only on the ventral side, but the second, third, fourth, and fifth are well developed. The dorsal sclerites (tergites) not only constitute the entire dorsal surface but the lateral as well, and, turning under, extend a considerable distance toward the mid-ventral line. True pleural sclerites are absent, but there is considerable expanse of pleural membrane between the tergites and the narrow sternites, which all lie in the median ventral line. The first of the sternites is somewhat fork-shaped; the second, roughly quadrangular, with its greatest width anterior. The third and fourth are narrower, while the fifth broadens distally to support the genitalia.

In the female, the visible abdominal spiracles are ten in number, five on either side. They are best seen in ventral view and are located close to the ventral margin of the five conspicuous tergites. Due to the fusion of the tergites of segments 1 and 2, the first two spiracles of either side appear to be located on a single segment. In the male there are two additional pairs, on the rudimentary sixth and seventh segments.

The ventral position of the union of tergites with sternites is more characteristic of museum specimens or of flies that have not fed. In a fresh, well-fed specimen, in gravid females, and in flies distended by *Empusa* fungus, the appearance is more often as in Figure 14. In this illustration the conjunctival fold, which connects the sternites with the tergites, has been distended by internal pressure and the sclerites are no longer in contact.

The basal half of the abdomen, especially on the lateral surface, is fre-

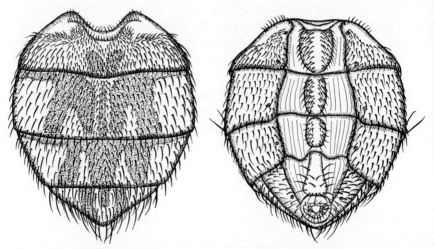

Figure 14. Abdomen of *Musca domestica;* female specimen. *Left:* Dorsal aspect. *Right:* Ventral aspect. Note extensive conjunctival areas. The ovipositor is withdrawn.

quently yellowish or transparent buff in color. This feature is usually more pronounced in males than in females. The median dorsal region of the anterior segments is marked by a brown or blackish longitudinal band. The rest of the abdominal surface is brownish gray with a yellowish pollinose sheen.

THE OVIPOSITOR

The small number of visible abdominal segments is obviously a specialized condition, as the primitive number of abdominal segments in insects is believed to be eleven. In the housefly and a great many other similar forms, a number of terminal segments have been telescoped posteriorly to form the genital structures. This is very apparent when a female fly extrudes her ovipositor (Fig. 15), an organ nearly as long as the preceding portion of the

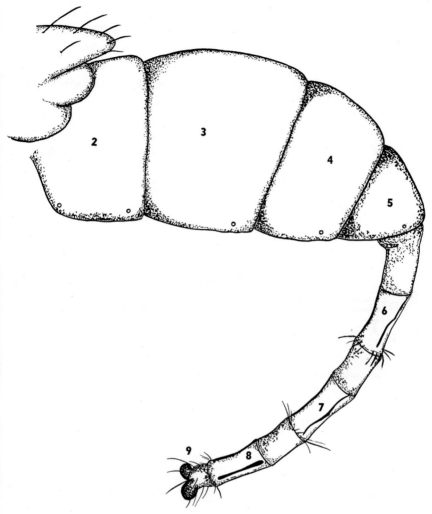

Figure 15. Female abdomen with ovipositor extended. Abdominal segments are numbered. Intermediate sections consist of conjunctival membrane that folds upon itself when the ovipositor is telescoped within the body.

abdomen. It is not difficult to demonstrate that four distinct segments have been utilized in this connection, giving a total of nine persisting segments in the female abdomen. In males Awati (1916a) has shown that ten are represented, at least vestigially, though only eight may be readily accounted for.

One can easily cause the ovipositor to extend by pressing gently on the abdomen of the freshly killed fly. Six joints or sections may be recognized. The first, third, fifth, and sixth represent true segments of the body; the second and fourth are composed wholly of intersegmental membrane. Only the ninth segment has tergite and sternite of a normal type. These are usually referred to as the supra-anal and subanal plates. The former bears caudally a pair of button-shaped cerci, which, as Patton (1930) points out, are really the persistent appendages of segment 11, no longer present. The subanal plate is heart-shaped or arrow-shaped. It bears no appendages.

In each of segments 6, 7, and 8 the tergite is represented by a pair of longitudinal chitinous rods, those of segment 6 joining anteriorly to form an Inverted Y. The sternite in each of these segments consists of a single chitinous rod, usually more slender than those representing the tergites. These vestigial sclerites of segments 6 to 8 show great variation within the species.

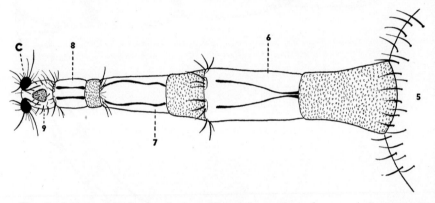

Figure 16. Ovipositor in dorsal view. Note how tergites of segment six approach one another to form a Y-shaped pattern. Ninth segment bears arrow-shaped subanal plate and two button-shaped cerci (*C*). Segments are numbered as in Figure 15.

The female genital aperture is located at the anterior margin of the ninth sternite, between segments 8 and 9.

THE MALE GENITALIA

The external genitalia of male houseflies consist of the variously modified sclerites of abdominal segments 6, 7, 8, 9, and 10. These are normally withdrawn into the fifth segment to the extent that very little can be seen from a lateral approach. Viewed caudally, however, certain parts are not difficult to distinguish.

The nomenclature of the various structures has been much confused, due to the fact that modern morphologists recognize a rotation of the segments of which earlier workers were not aware. We thus have a double system of terminology, the earlier of which might well be discarded were it not for the fact that in using the classical literature (e.g. Hewitt, 1914a) the student finds it necessary to understand the older concepts. We shall therefore here

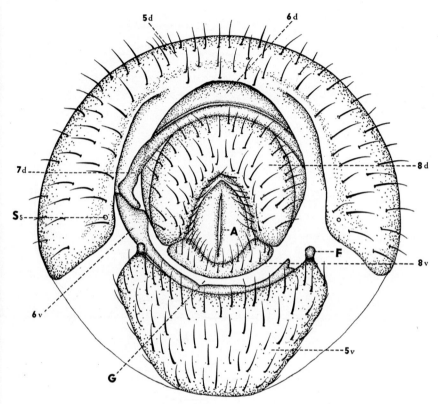

Figure 17. Caudal view of male abdomen. *A*, anal aperture; *F*, primary forceps; *G*, aperture to genital atrium; *S5*, spiracle of segment five; *5d, 6d, 7d, 8d*, dorsal arches of respective segments; *5v, 6v, 8v*, ventral arches of respective segments. Labeling is in accordance with interpretation of Hewitt and other early workers. Consult text for discussion of more recent concepts. (Adapted from Hewitt, *The House-Fly* [Cambridge University Press, 1914], and from dissection.)

describe the male genital structures in two ways: first, as understood by Hewitt and contemporaries; second, as interpreted by Hardy (1944).

Older Concepts of Genital Morphology

If one imagines himself looking directly at the anal aperture (shown in Fig. 17 as a vertical slit), the dorsal arch of the eighth (?) abdominal segment will be seen to surround the anus on all but the ventral side. This sclerite may

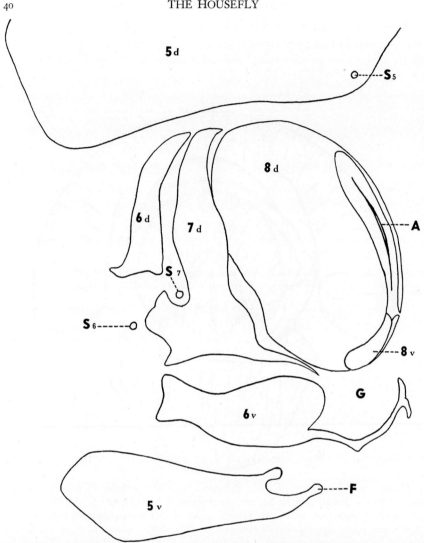

Figure 18. Near-lateral view of terminal segments of male. Tergite and sternite of segment five have been moved apart to disclose other structures. *S5, S6, S7,* spiracles of respective segments. Other lettering as in Figure 17. (Adapted from Hewitt, *The House-Fly* [Cambridge University Press, 1914], and from dissection.)

be said to form the apex of the abdomen. Joining with the dorsal arch on either side, and forming the ventral border of the anal membrane, is the ventral arch of the same segment, so deeply notched in the center as to appear like two convex sclerites joined by a narrow bridge. Such in fact was Hewitt's own interpretation of its origin. This unit serves to separate the anal area from the entrance to the genital atrium, which lies immediately below. The sclerites of this (eighth?) segment, like those of the first five, bear setae.

The seventh dorsal arch lies above the eighth and appears as a narrow, curving sclerite much more heavily developed on the left side than on the right. The ventral arch of the seventh segment consists of a pair of curved sclerites not visible from this approach. (These constitute the inner claspers or secondary forceps.)

The dorsal arch of the sixth segment lies above that of the seventh and is similar to it, save that there is no asymmetrical prolongation to the left. The ventral arch of the sixth segment is a nonsymmetrical sclerite, enlarged on the left side into a spatulate plate that extends forward as shown in Figure 18. The remainder of the sclerite consists of a narrow bar that borders the genital atrium on the ventral side and terminates in a bifurcation at the right. This barlike portion lies more or less in the arms of the fifth sternite, which is deeply excavated on its posterior border.

The lateral angles of the fifth sternite are each prolonged into a definite process somewhat knoblike at the tip. The two taken together are sometimes called the *primary forceps.*

Let us now suppose that the above-described structures have been relaxed and drawn out by appropriate technique (see Chapter XVI) from their telescoped position within the confines of segment 8. All parts will thereby become visible in lateral view. Figure 18, already referred to, makes the relationships reasonably clear. Especially striking is the manner in which the left side of the seventh dorsal arch extends forward in a beaklike process. This separation of the parts also demonstrates the presence of two more abdominal spiracles, which are believed to pertain to segments 6 and 7.

The penis, or intromittent organ (aedeagus, phallosome, mesosome), is a complicated structure lying just dorsal to the ventral arch of segment 7, which in turn, due to its migration forward, rests normally upon the corresponding sclerite of segment 5. The body of the penis is composed of the so-called median sclerite, which is roughly semicircular in outline, the convex border being directed downward. From either corner there extends upward an alar process. Against the base of each alar process, on the outer side, rests the lateral extremity of the dorsal arch of segment 8. The tips of the alar processes articulate with the lateral portion of the anterior border of the two sclerites making up the ventral arch of segment 7. These two sclerites constitute the secondary forceps. They are not connected ventrally. Each articulates laterally with the margin of the eighth dorsal arch.

The functional portion of the penis, sometimes called the theca, articulates with the median sclerite by means of two small chitinous nodules. These are the cornetti of Berlese (1902). The theca, which is hollow, is continuous at its base with the ejaculatory duct. Just dorsal to the point where the ejacula-

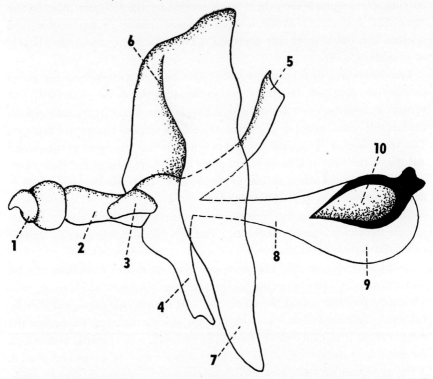

Figure 19. Left lateral view of penis and adjacent structures. *1,* glans; *2,* theca; *3,* left chitinous nodule; *4,* superior apophysis; *5,* inferior apophysis; *6,* body of the penis; *7,* left alar process; *8,* ejaculatory duct; *9,* ejaculatory sac; *10,* ejaculatory apodeme. (Adapted from Hewitt, *The House-Fly* [Cambridge University Press, 1914], and from dissection.)

tory duct enters the theca is a cylindrical sclerite, the superior apophysis. A similar structure, the inferior apophysis, extends downward and forward from the ventral side. The theca terminates in a rather delicate, hyaline enlargement, the glans, shaped somewhat like an inflated cockscomb and bearing at its curved extremity the opening of the ejaculatory duct.

No attempt will be made here to homologize the above description with the terminology employed by Aldrich (1916) concerning the genitalia of the Sarcophagidae. Aldrich's system is very useful, however, in determining species in that family and should be studied by anyone interested in the genital structures of muscoid flies.

Awati (1916a), who studied the genitalia with reference to specific differences in the genus *Musca,* took exception to several points in Hewitt's interpretation, especially the recognition of segment 8, which Awati considered to have disappeared in calyptrate Muscidae. The segment that bears the anus he considered to be the tenth; that on which the genital aperture is found, the ninth. The eighth segment, when present (which Awati admits to be true in all lower Diptera), he termed the "pre-genital" segment. Awati used the supposed absence of this segment to explain the forward position of the genital aperture, which he considered to lie just behind the fifth (or sixth) abdominal somite in the males of *Musca* and related forms. Because the female sex aperture lies between segments 8 and 9, Awati thought it improbable that the position of the genital outlet could be used in determining homologies, as Lowne (1870) attempted to do. Awati was convinced, on the other hand, that the anus, which according to his (and later) interpretations occurs on segment 10 in both sexes, is of great importance in this respect. He also relied heavily on the seven pairs of spiracles in homologizing segmental structures.

The chitinous bodies, which Hewitt regarded as representing the sternite of the genital segment, Awati considered to be the cerci of the segment following, as he believed the sternite of the genital segment to have disappeared in modern forms.

Again, the inner claspers of Hewitt, which that author believed to be modified portions of the seventh sternite, Awati regarded as appendages of the genital segment and homologous with the valvulae externae of blowflies as described by Lowne.

The anal segment, as Awati would have it, is represented only by the anal cerci (superior claspers), which serve to hide the other genital structures from external view.

Awati noted the tendency to asymmetry, especially in segment 7 (Hewitt's segment 6), but, like Hewitt, did not perceive that a rotation of the structures might be involved. In spite of the many differences of opinion of these two authors, their interpretations are therefore similar in that both attempted to assign names to the various elements in their natural (definitive) position. Let us now consider a more modern concept.

Theory of Rotation

It is customary to refer to the eighth and ninth segments of the male, together with their appendages, as the hypopygium. Feuerborn (1922), in studying the genitalia of muscoid flies, came to the conclusion that the entire hypopygium in this group had undergone an evolutionary rotation of 360 degrees. His evidence was derived largely from the fact that the distal portion of the ejaculatory duct makes a complete loop around the rectum before attaining the exterior. (See Chapter III.) Richards (1927) accepted this inter-

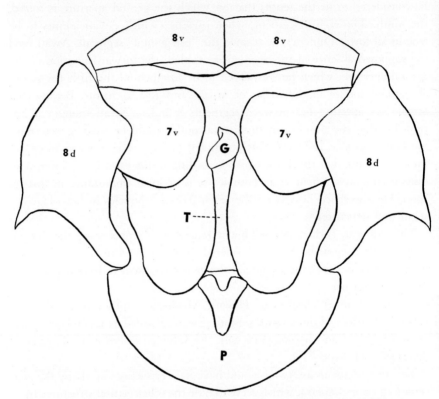

Figure 20. Ventral view of terminal segments of male. Ventral arch of fifth segment has been removed. *P*, body of penis; *G*, glans; *T*, theca; *7v*, ventral arch of seventh segment. Right and left portions (secondary forceps), which are normally ventral to the penis, have been spread apart, to show that organ. *8d, 8v*, dorsal and ventral arches of eighth segment.

pretation for lack of a better one, but was frankly puzzled as to how it might have taken place. Finally Hardy (1944), who had previously studied the copulatory positions of various groups of Diptera (1935), made a special examination of the terminal sclerites of *Calliphora,* from which he derived an interpretation which is probably correct in most respects and which will be discussed further in this place.

The gist of Hardy's concept is that in the Muscoidea the fourth and fifth segments have remained normal, the sixth has rotated 60 degrees, the seventh 120 degrees, the eighth 180 degrees, and the ninth 360 degrees. The tenth, of course, is vestigial. He points out that the tergites do not all correspond with

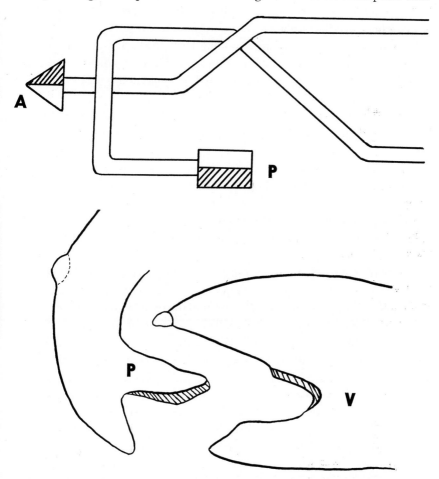

Figure 21. Rotation of male genitalia; diagrammatic. Morphologically dorsal surfaces are shaded. *Upper:* Relation of digestive and genital tracts. Penis (*P*) is represented by quadrangle, anus (*A*) by triangular element. *Lower:* Relation of penis (*P*) to vagina (*V*) at time of copulation. (Adapted from Hardy, 1944.)

the underlying sternites, as might be expected from so extensive a disturbance. The terminology that he uses may be best understood by a study of Figure 22. As there depicted, the "forceps" are seen to belong to the ninth segment, the "accessory plate" to segment 8, the "aedeagus" to segment 7, and the "ventral plate" to segment 5. The so-called "phallic pouch" pertains to segment 6. The anus is interpreted as lying between segments 8 and 9 and is dorsal in position. Unlike some morphologists, Hardy does not consider the "claspers" homologous with similar structures in the Orthorrhapha (see Chapter V), since they are completely lost in the Syrphidae and related forms, which stand between.

To understand adequately the reasoning back of Hardy's interpretation, it is necessary to review briefly the modifications through which the terminal segments of the male appear to have passed in connection with the evolution of the Order Diptera.

The more primitive species are said to have the terminalia erect. In such forms the anal papilla lies above the aedeagus, which is directed toward the rear.

From such ancestors as these, certain groups arose in which the terminalia may be said to be diverted. The terminal segments are loosely and rather flexibly united with one another, so that the male copulatory structures may lie in any position between the erect one and a rotation of 180 degrees to the right. They always assume the last position, however, when copulation takes place.

Closely related to the above are other species in which the inverted position has become more or less fixed, the aedeagus lying permanently above the anal papilla. Feuerborn gave to this condition the term hypopygium inversum.

The next step was the development of a curvilinear relation of the segments, the terminalia being strongly bent to one side (the right) as in present-day Dolichopodidae and Syrphidae. The several segments may be said to lie in a series along a curved median line. Both tergites and sternites undergo a spiral twisting, so that the sternites come to lie on the posterior or outer curve. The tergites, since they lie along the inner curve, are correspondingly reduced. It is interesting that the tracheae within (see Chapter III) show a corresponding spiral twist from left to right. The aedeagus, which in more primitive times was directed posteriorly, is by this manipulation made to extend anteriorly. In the Syrphidae and related families a pouch develops in the pleurae to receive the aedeagus. This persists in the Muscoidea as a gap between the sternite and tergite of the sixth segment, the two sclerites forming the periphery of the "phallic pouch." (See Fig. 22.)

A subsequent migration of the anus from below the aedeagus to a plane lying above it completed the encirclement of the alimentary canal, and accounts for the present relation of the rectum and the ejaculatory duct. Hardy (1944) considers that while this last modification was in progress the terminal segments realigned themselves so that a curvilinear relation no longer exists in Muscoidean groups. All segments are now once more in linear series. This rectilinear condition differs from the primitive rectilinear, however, in that the aedeagus is directed anteriorly, the result of its original inversion by rotation. Houseflies may therefore be said to possess rectilinear circumverted terminalia.

The effect is as if the entire hypopygium had rotated a full 360 degrees, but this has been accomplished by segments 6, 7, and 8 each revolving approximately 60 degrees.

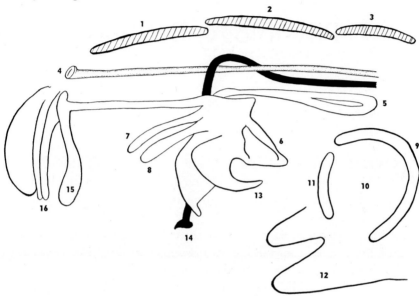

Figure 22. Diagrammatic analysis of the terminal sclerites of a male muscoid fly (*Calliphora*). *1*, sternite of segment eight; *2*, sternite of segment seven; *3*, tergite of segment five; *4*, anus; *5*, apodeme of segment nine; *6*, apodeme of segment eight; *7*, spine; *8*, posterior clasper; *9*, tergite of segment six; *10*, phallic pouch; *11*, sternite of segment six; *12*, sternite of segment five; *13*, anterior clasper; *14*, aedeagus; *15*, accessory plate; *16*, forceps, formed of ninth tergite. (Interpretation according to Hardy, 1944; after Lowne, 1870, and Feuerborn, 1922.)

The writer is of course aware that much difference of opinion still exists among leading morphologists concerning body segmentation in the Diptera. The present work makes no pretense of stating the latest attitude or of arbitrating between authorities. The terminology here employed is merely that which, in the opinion of the writer, will be most easily comprehended by the practical sanitarian and which will enable him to make the best possible use of the great amount of background literature that exists. For a thorough understanding of the complex problems involved and of the reasons for radically divergent interpretations, the reader is referred to the excellent works of Snodgrass (1935) and of Crampton (1941, 1942).

CHAPTER III

Internal Morphology, Physiology, Behavior

Make not thy sport abuses; for the fly that feeds on dung is coloured thereby.—
George Herbert, "The Church Porch"

AS WITH all Arthropoda, the body plan of the housefly is that of a "tube within a tube," the external cylinder being formed by the body wall and its associated musculature, and the internal, by the tissues of the alimentary tract. Between the two is the body cavity, or coelom, which, as in other insects, contains blood and may therefore properly be termed a haemocoel. More or less suspended in the haemocoel are the various appendages of the alimentary canal including the Malpighian tubules, crop, and salivary glands. The body cavity contains likewise the central nervous system, the heart, and the organs of reproduction, while branches of the tracheal system traverse the spaces between the various organs and the body wall. We shall describe the several systems separately, beginning with the alimentary tract.

THE PROBOSCIS

The feeding apparatus of the fly has long been of interest to investigators (e.g. Macloskie, 1880). It is now quite generally accepted that the greater part of the proboscis has been developed from the labium, and not from the maxillae, as Lowne (1870, 1895) considered to be the case. The terminology here used, therefore, is chiefly that of Hewitt (1914a) and Graham-Smith (1914, 1930a), rather than that of Lowne, who proposed special names for various structures to suit his particular interpretation of the morphology. These names would merely be confusing at the present time.

Graham-Smith's paper (1930a), though it deals exclusively with *Calliphora erythrocephala* (*vicina*), is a particularly helpful contribution as it standardizes, so far as may be possible, the nomenclature of Lowne (1890–1895), Patton and Cragg (1913c), and his own previously published works.

As mentioned in Chapter II, the proboscis consists of a conical basal unit, the rostrum, a median section, the haustellum, and a terminal broadened portion, the oral disc or oral sucker, consisting of two distinct lobes termed labella. Between the two labella is the central or prestomal cavity leading to the alimentary canal. This is more or less surrounded by the so-called discal sclerite, which is roughly horseshoe-shaped, with the open side anterior.

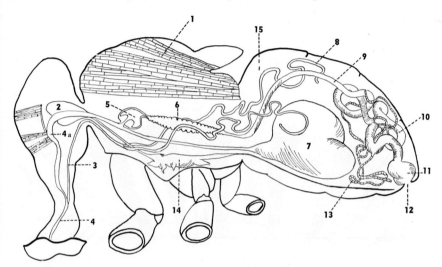

Figure 23. Internal organization of *Musca domestica*. *1,* longitudinal muscles of thorax; *2,* supraoesophageal ganglion; *3,* salivary duct; *4,* pharynx; *4a,* oesophagus; *5,* proventriculus; *6,* stomach; *7,* crop; *8,* salivary gland; *9,* proximal intestine; *10,* distal intestine; *11,* rectum; *12,* anus; *13,* Malpighian tubes; *14,* compound thoracic ganglion; *15,* haemocoel. (Adapted from Patton, 1930.)

Each labellum bears on its ventral surface a number of more or less parallel transverse ridges, the pseudotracheae. These are actually tubes, the inside diameter of which ranges from 0.008 mm. to 0.016 mm. The more anterior six or seven pseudotracheae communicate with a collecting channel that follows the interior border of the labellum to the prestomal cavity mentioned above. The more posterior twelve or thirteen pseudotracheae are served by a similar collecting channel, but the three or four which lie opposite the prestomal aperture communicate directly.

The prestomal cavity itself is bounded on either side by five prestomal teeth. These are borne by the discal sclerite and alternate in position with the pseudotracheae of that region. These teeth form the walls of gutters along which fluids from the above-mentioned collecting tubes pass into the mouth cavity proper. In certain other genera (*Calliphora, Lucilia, Sarcophaga*) three or even four rows of teeth are present, the branches of the intermediate and other sets serving as a floor for the gutters, already mentioned, a function which in the housefly is taken over by a number of chitinized plates.

The external mouth aperture leads to a passageway that traverses the haustellum. Some authors call this the cavity of the prelabrum. The true mouth lies at the juncture of the haustellum and the rostrum. Beyond this lie the prepharyngeal and pharyngeal portions of the rostral cavity. The latter is continuous with the oesophagus.

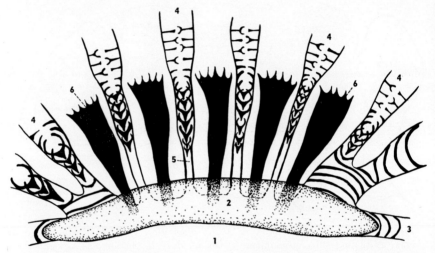

Figure 24. Prestomal teeth and adjacent structures. *1*, Region of the prestomal aperture; *2*, prestomal (discal) sclerite, interior view; *3*, collecting channel; *4*, pseudotracheae; *5*, floor of gutter, formed of chitinous plates; *6*, prestomal teeth. Tips function for rasping. Sides form walls for gutters. (Adapted from several authors and from dissection.)

The proboscis is retractible and when withdrawn is seen to bend sharply at two points—that is, where the haustellum joins the rostrum and where the rostrum joins the head. The food canal is particularly flexible at these points, the lower of which is partially encased by a protective structure, the hyoid sclerite or prepharynx. Its function is to keep the food canal open, regardless of the degree of flexure. Retraction of the proboscis is accomplished by direct muscular action. All parts except the oral sucker are usually made to disappear within the head capsule, and sometimes this part also.

Extension is a somewhat more complicated process. The rostrum is extruded by the distention of certain large air sacs that lie within it. The extension of the more distal parts is accomplished partly by direct muscular action, partly by increased blood pressure. Each labellum contains a sizable haemocoel, the filling of which causes the oral lobe to expand.

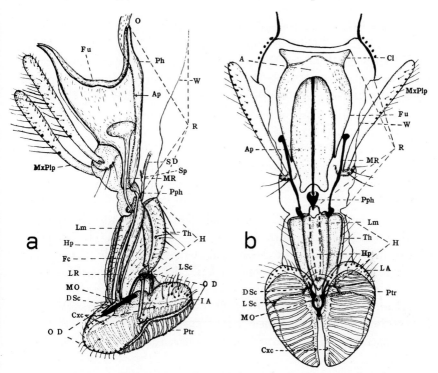

Figure 25. Detailed structure of housefly proboscis. *a:* Lateral interpretation. *b:* Cephalic approach. *A,* anterior arch of fulcrum; *Ap,* anterior wall of pharynx; *Cl,* clypeus; *Cxc,* main collecting channels; *DSc,* discal sclerite; *Fc,* food channel; *Fu,* fulcrum; *H,* haustellum; *Hp,* hypopharynx; *LA,* labellum; *Lm,* labrum; *LR,* labellar rods; *LSc,* labellar sclerite; *MO,* opening to food channel; *MR,* maxillary rods; *MxPlp,* maxillary palpus; *O,* oesophagus; *OD,* oral disc; *Ph,* pharynx; *Pph,* prepharyngeal sclerite; *Ptr,* pseudotracheae; *R,* rostrum; *SD,* salivary duct; *Sp,* salivary pump; *Th,* theca (= mentum); *W,* membranous wall. (Matheson, *Medical Entomology;* Comstock Publishing Co.)

Rostrum, haustellum, and oral sucker will now be described in somewhat greater detail.

The rostrum is covered with a tough, chitinous membrane, continuous with the similar covering of the haustellum. Its internal support consists chiefly of a large stirrup-shaped sclerite, the fulcrum, composed in reality of a number of separate sclerites intimately fused. The pumping pharynx and its dilator muscles lie within this structure. Downward, and forward from the fulcrum, on either side extends a rodlike unit, sinuously curved, the distal extremity of which unites with the base of the labrum, a sclerite that forms the forward wall of the haustellum. These units, the maxillary rods, are believed to be homologous with the stipes of more generalized maxillae. Anterior to each is a small sclerite supporting the maxillary palpus of that side.

The haustellum, which is more or less cylindrical, includes the labium, hypopharynx, and labrum-epipharynx. The first constitutes the posterior wall and is somewhat complicated. The most conspicuous feature is the posteriorly convex theca or *mentum,* which extends from the base of the haustellum to the rodlike labial sclerites of the oral disc. Extending forward from the mentum on either side is a tough membrane that connects with the chitinized anterior surface of the labium. This surface is deeply grooved for the reception of the hypopharynx. It is bounded laterally by the two sturdy labellar rods (paraphyses) that extend from the base of the haustellum to the principal sclerite of the oral disc.

The hypopharynx is blade-shaped and lies in what may be called the labial gutter. Its anterior surface is longitudinally grooved. The lateral margins of the hypopharynx fit closely against those of the labrum-epipharynx, which lies immediately in front and has a longitudinal concavity on the posterior side. The hypopharynx and labrum-epipharynx thus form the walls of a channel for the passage of food. Their tips extend to the mouth opening in the discal sclerite, while their bases, which are fused, surround the true mouth opening that lies above. The hypopharynx also contains the salivary duct.

The oral disc has already been described as consisting of two large labella united medially by the discal sclerite. The latter is firmly united with the distal extremities of the labellar rods. The prestomal cavity continues caudally between the labellar lobes as a fairly deep, median fissure. This becomes much shallower when the lobes are spread apart, and may disappear altogether when they are everted.

Each pseudotrachea is kept dilated by a large number of circular chitinous rings, which are incomplete on the exposed (ventral) surface. Each pseudotracheal ring is expanded at one end but forked at the other. (See Fig. 26.) Adjacent rings alternate in direction, so that the spatulate extremity of any one lies between the bifid extremities of its two neighbors. The two arms of the bifid extremity are curved so as to bound a circular aperture leading to the lumen of the pseudotrachea. These interbifid spaces determine the size of any particles that may be ingested during the ordinary sampling of liquid food. They range from 0.003 to 0.004 mm. in diameter. A funnel-shaped depression leads from the surface of the pseudotrachea to each interbifid space. These are termed interbified grooves. The surface membrane of the labellum is stretched tightly over all parts except the interbifid spaces and along a zigzag fissure that runs the length of the pseudotracheae, uniting the open segments of consecutive interbifid areas. Through this channel, as well as through the circular apertures, the insect may imbibe liquid food.

The terminal portions of the pseudotracheae which open directly into the

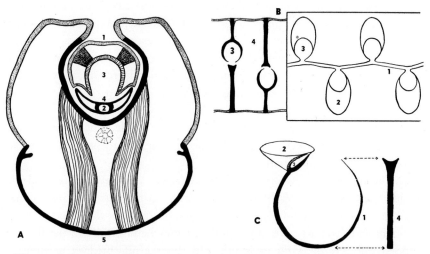

Figure 26. Special details of mouth parts. *A:* Diagrammatic section through haustellum. *1,* labrum; *2,* salivary canal; *3,* food canal; *4,* hypopharynx; *5,* mentum. *B:* Pseudotracheal channel. Right portion shows surface view. At left, integument of labellum is stripped away to expose chitinous rings. *1,* zigzag fissure; *2,* interbifid groove; *3,* interbifid space; *4,* membrane of pseudotracheal channel. *C:* Attachment of interbifid groove to forks of chitinous ring. *1,* chitinous ring, side view; *2,* interbifid groove; *3,* interbifid space; *4,* distal portion of chitinous ring, end view. (Adapted from various authors.)

prestomal cavity lack the feeding apertures of the more exposed areas and therefore function merely as so many collecting tubes.

Graham-Smith (1930a) summarizes his study of the blowfly proboscis by stating that the fly can ingest food material in at least three ways. (1) It can merely suck up liquid food, filtering out the particles of larger size. (2) It can utilize its prestomal teeth to scrape selected surfaces, moistening them, in the meantime, with saliva or with vomitus to produce an emulsion that is subsequently ingested. Or, (3) using neither prestomal teeth nor filtration apparatus, the fly may suck up directly such material as thick sputum or feces, together with helminth ova or any similar particles that these substances may contain.

There is no reason to believe that the housefly is any less versatile. It is, of course, a somewhat smaller insect, which may limit the size of the larger particles ingested. The behavior of the labella in these three different procedures may be described as follows:

1. In feeding by suction and filtration, the commonest method of taking food, suction created by muscular action in the pharynx is employed to draw fluid through the interbifid grooves into the pseudotracheae.

To suck up a thin layer of fluid, the fly causes the labella to separate until they come to lie at right angles to the long axis of the proboscis, one labellum extending to the right, the other to the left. The exposed surfaces, which are the only parts furnished with pseudotracheae, are thus applied lightly to the fluid, which is then sucked in through the interbifid grooves. Any particles too large to pass these apertures are thus filtered out and rejected. Graham-Smith calls this the filtering position. Sometimes the marginal strips of the labella are turned distally to create a rim, and the whole structure is made to resemble a cupping device. When this occurs, the mouth parts may be said to be in the cupping position.

2. The use of the prestomal teeth for scraping and pulverizing food materials involves a considerably wider separation of the labella. If just enough change of position occurs to permit slight use of the teeth, the pseudotracheae will still be in contact with any liquid that may be present, and the filtering process still goes on. Graham-Smith calls this the intermediate position. If, however, the fly finds it necessary to make full use of the teeth for scraping, the labella are folded back still more, so that the pseudotracheal surfaces are completely out of action. This is the true scraping position.

3. A final modification involves the turning back not only of the labellar surfaces but of the teeth themselves, so that the latter point upward, or at least laterally, and are no longer in a position to scarify the food substance. This results, however, in opening the oral aperture, located on the discal sclerite. This aperture is then applied directly to the food, and large amounts of material in suspension may be sucked up directly. Relatively large objects such as the ova of parasitic worms may be ingested in this way. Graham-Smith calls this the direct-feeding position. There is evidence that individual flies differ in their ability to open the mouth aperture sufficiently wide to permit the ingestion of eggs of large diameter.

Salivary Glands

The salivary duct opens into the prestomal cavity. Its terminal portion lies embedded in the substance of the hypopharynx (ligula of older writers), and thus closely parallels the prelabral cavity as far as the level of the prepharyngeal sclerite. From here it extends somewhat more caudally, diverging from the pharynx at a rather acute angle. In this portion of the duct, we find a special mechanism, the salivary syringe, which serves as a pumping organ to force the saliva onward to the hypopharynx. The outline of this organ is controlled by the action of special muscles (Fig. 27). At the distal extremity of the salivary syringe is a one-way valve so arranged that saliva which passes beyond this point may not return toward the salivary glands.

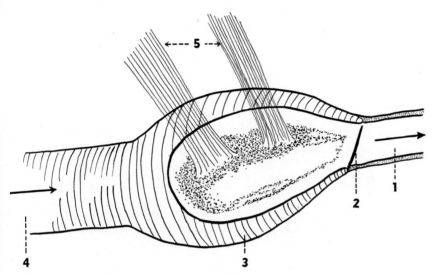

Figure 27. Salivary syringe. *1*, duct to hypopharynx; *2*, one-way valve; *3*, wall of the syringe; *4*, common salivary duct; *5*, muscles controlling pumping action. (Adapted from Matheson, 1944.)

In the cervical region, the duct turns directly caudad and passing ventrally to both oesophagus and nerve ring enters the thoracic cavity. In the prothoracic region the duct divides, one branch continuing caudad on the left side, the other on the right. In so doing, each passes upward around the nerve cord and then proceeds backward, more or less on the level of the mesenteron. At this point, the structure is definitely glandular, and there is considerable looping, which becomes even more pronounced in the abdominal region. The glands may thus be described as coiled tubes, as long or longer than the body of the fly, with a goodly portion of each gland lying in the abdominal cavity. Their diameter is practically uniform throughout. Each is lined by a single layer of epithelial cells of the cuboidal type.

In addition to the principal salivary glands described above (lingual salivary glands), Graham-Smith (1914) recognizes labial salivary glands, lying at the base of the labella and opening into the oral pits.

THE OESOPHAGUS

The muscular pharynx extends vertically to a point just within the head capsule, where it gives rise to the oesophagus. The latter proceeds dorsally to a point on a level with the center of the face, where it turns nearly at right angles and, passing through the nerve ring, enters the thoracic cavity. The oesophagus terminates in the prothorax. At this point it gives rise, on the ventral side, to a straight, slender duct that extends the length of the thorax into the abdomen and there expands into a great sac or bladderlike vesicle, the crop. Crop and channel are sometimes referred to as the oesophageal diverticulum. The crop is definitely bilobed. By contraction of the plain muscles in its walls, the content of the crop may be regurgitated through the mouth. This performance is a very common preliminary to the taking of the food and gives excellent opportunity for the distribution of infectious organisms.

The oesophagus is followed by the proventriculus, a circular, somewhat chitinized, buttonlike structure, rather horizontally disposed, which the oesophagus enters from below. Mouth, pharynx, oesophagus, and proventriculus are all part of the stomodaeum, or fore-gut, which arises by invagination at the anterior extremity during embryonic development, uniting subsequently with the stomach, which is of endodermal origin.

STOMACH AND PROXIMAL INTESTINE

The stomach proper (chyle stomach) extends the length of the thorax without change of direction. Both anterior and posterior extremities are somewhat constricted in diameter. The greatest width is found in the posterior half. The stomach is lined in the anterior and posterior portions with a digestive epithelium of the columnar type. For the greater portion of its length, however, the digestive epithelium is folded in such a way as to form a large number of sacculi or crypts which Hewitt considered homologous with the gastric caeca of Orthoptera and other forms.

Following the stomach is the proximal intestine, which more or less fills the abdominal cavity. It varies considerably in length, but always consists of a number of loops and turns. It is lined by columnar epithelium. The stomach and proximal intestine, taken together, constitute the mid-gut or mesenteron, derived essentially from embryonic entoderm. The term ventriculus is appropriate for the entire mesenteron, though many workers prefer to use it for the chyle stomach only.

At the point where the mid-gut joins the hind-gut are located the Malpighian tubes. There are two principal Malpighian ducts, each of which branches into a pair of tubules. These organs are excretory and drain into the alimentary tract.

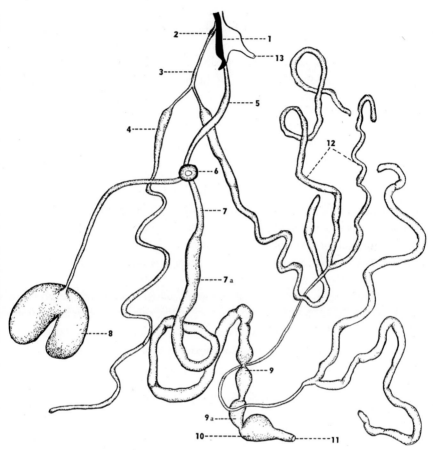

Figure 28. Alimentary canal of adult fly. *1*, pharynx (of head); *2*, salivary syringe; *3*, salivary duct; *4*, salivary gland; *5*, oesophagus; *6*, proventriculus; *7*, stomach; *7a*, proximal intestine; *8*, crop; *9*, distal intestine; *9a*, rectal valve; *10*, rectum; *11*, anus; *12*, Malpighian tubes; *13*, fulcrum (of head). (From dissection and from Matheson, 1944.)

HIND-GUT

All that follows is proctodaeum, derived by invagination from the posterior extremity. Both stomodaeum and proctodaeum are reflexions of the body wall, and as such have a delicate chitinous lining, the intima, which is continuous with the chitin of the exoskeleton. The proctodaeum is divided into an anterior portion, the distal intestine, and a posterior, dilated portion, the rectum. A cone-shaped expansion of the distal intestine just anterior to the rectum has been designated the rectal valve. The anterior portion of the rectum is lined by cubical cells that impart to the intima a tuberculate appearance. The middle portion, which is dilated, contains the four fingerlike, rectal glands, two on either side. The short, terminal portion has thickened muscular walls. The rectum opens to the exterior by way of the anus, which in the male sex appears as a vertical slit, surrounded by the sclerites of the hypopygium. In the female fly, due to the manner in which the segments of the ovipositor are telescoped within the abdomen, the anus is not easily demonstrated from without.

PERISTALSIS

Abbott (1945), who studied especially the crop and adjacent structures in Calliphoridae, states that in the living fly the digestive organs are normally in constant motion. The lobes of the crop contract rhythmically, in alternate fashion, waves of contraction passing anteriorly to the proventriculus. Except when regurgitation takes places, the proventricular sphincter is synchronized to relax at the proper moments and thus permit passage of food into the midgut. From this point waves of contraction pass posteriorly.

The same author found that at a certain narrow point in the hind-gut, which may be considered to function as a valve, waves of reverse peristalsis operate to effect dilation. Strong, irregular contractions of the rectal sac were also observed. These result in cyclical movements of the rectal papillae. They are not of a synchronous character.

SPECIAL SECRETIONS OF THE ALIMENTARY TRACT

Cornwall and Patton (1914), who studied especially the bloodsucking members of this group, found that *Philaematomyia crassirostris* (*insignis*) possesses a powerful anticoagulin in its salivary secretions and another in the mesenteron. The latter is most active 20 to 44 hours after the fly's first blood meal. *Musca nebulo,* however, though closely related, produces neither of these substances. *Musca convexifrons* has no anticoagulin in the salivary glands, but does have a fairly powerful one in the mid-intestine. *Musca pattoni* has both a powerful anticoagulant in the mid-gut and a much weaker one in the saliva. These authors consider this an example of an evolutionary series, the bloodsucking forms having descended, apparently, from nonbloodsucking *Musca*like ancestors. It is perhaps important to note that salivary secretions of bloodsucking muscoids are rarely, if ever, considered irritating to the human skin. Evidence to the contrary, however, has been brought forward by Pavlovskii, Stein, and Buichkov (1932), who found that saliva, as well as certain extracts from the crop of *M. domestica,* contains thermolabile substances which, if introduced into the skin of man, may have an inflammatory effect. The skin must be injured in some way for penetration to take place, hence no irritation is ordinarily noticed in connection with the activities of non-bloodsucking forms. Fresh wounds, however, provide an opportunity for this phenomenon to occur.

EXCRETION

Mention has been made of the Malpighian tubes that open into the alimentary tract where mesenteron and hind-gut join together. They present a somewhat beaded appearance, and are of uniform width throughout. The two branches of each major duct are exceedingly long and convoluted, and are intimately involved with the abdominal fat body, from which it is difficult to separate them by dissection. The prevailing color of the Malpighian tubes is yellowish green. Their excretory function is no longer questioned, as both the cells and the lumen may be demonstrated to contain wastes of a urinary character. They are continually bathed by the blood in the body cavity, which gives ample opportunity for the extraction of these substances.

The Malpighian tubes of the larvae are similar in number and appearance to those found in the adult. Special studies on the larvae of *Lucilia* and *Calliphora* by Weinland (1906, 1909) showed that these forms, being meat eaters, excrete ammonia in large amounts. Wigglesworth (1939) points out that though some of this comes from bacterial action, a great deal comes from the tissues themselves, as shown by the fact that larvae reared under sterile conditions also produce large amounts (Hobson, 1932). It is apparently still to be determined whether the ammonia is produced in the Malpighian tubes or in the food canal. It is not present in the adult fly (Brown, 1936). Experiments by Aksinin (1929) with *Musca domestica* showed that the larvae of this species also produce ammonia in considerable amount, under certain conditions approaching the output of *Calliphora vomitoria.*

THE HAEMOCOEL AND VASCULAR SYSTEM

The heart or dorsal blood vessel is a more or less cylindrical structure lying in the body cavity just beneath the median dorsal line. It extends the length of the abdomen and is divided into a small anterior chamber and four larger

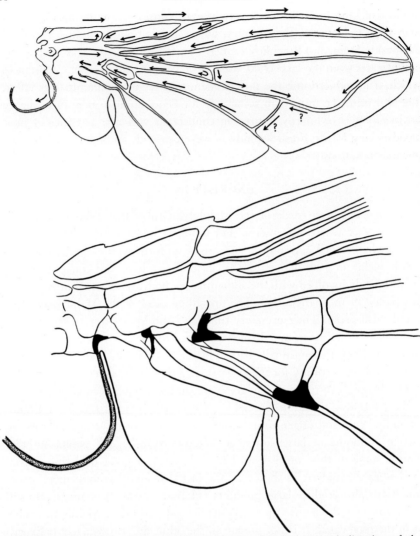

Figure 29. Circulation of blood in housefly wing. *Upper:* General direction of the flow, indicated by arrows. *Lower:* Pulsating organs. These four auxiliary hearts, located in the base of the wing, serve as aspirating organs, to draw the haemolymph between the tracheae and the walls of the veins. (Adapted from E. Thomsen, 1938.)

chambers all lineally arranged. Near its posterior extremity, each chamber has a pair of ostia, dorsolateral in position. At these points, the alar muscles arise. These run laterally in the floor of the pericardium, finally attaching to the sides of the dorsal abdominal plates. The remainder of the pericardium is composed of special large cells interspersed with fat cells. The pericardium has many tracheal connections. From the anterior end of the heart extends the dorsal aorta, a slender tube lying above the ventriculus. It terminates in a mass of cells believed to be lymphoid in character.

The blood, which is colorless and full of corpuscles, enters the ostia only when the heart is dilated. By rhythmic contractions of the chamber walls, it is driven forward through the dorsal vessel and spilled out in the anterior portion of the body cavity. The latter is much reduced by the cephalic tracheal sacs, air sacs in the abdomen, thoracic muscles, and variable fat bodies, the size of which depends upon the insect's nutritional state. The blood filters downward and backward, through whatever spaces are not occupied by viscera, carrying nourishment to all tissues and receiving wastes from them. The latter are removed chiefly by the Malpighian tubes. Eventually the blood finds its way once more into the ostia of the heart. The blood continually receives the products of digestion from the alimentary tract. Material not required immediately for the nourishment of the tissues is stored chiefly in the fat body.

The existence of pulsating organs or auxiliary hearts has been demonstrated in many insects, and it would be strange if the housefly lacked them. Wigglesworth (1939) points out that such structures are commonest in the thorax, where they appear to consist of a muscular plate that encloses a blood space beneath the dorsal wall of the thorax, often in the scutellum. Pulsating organs in the extremities are of obvious value. Of greatest use to a rapidly flying insect would be auxiliary hearts to serve the wings, and in this regard the housefly is well equipped.

According to E. Thomsen (1938), there are four auxiliary hearts (pulsating organs) in each wing of *Musca,* lying on the course of the efferent veins.

Many students are under the impression that the wing of the adult fly is essentially a dead structure, inasmuch as when the body fluids are withdrawn from the wing pad of the pupa and the wing assumes its definitive form, all parts appear to become dry and stiff. Such, however, is not the case. According to Wigglesworth, circulation of blood in the wings of insects was first noted by Baker in the grasshopper in 1744. In more recent times, Yeager and Hendrickson (1933, 1934) have reported at length on circulation in the wings of cockroaches. The phenomenon is now believed to be universal. The blood (haemolymph) enters the wing in the costal region, returning along the posterior margin. It is believed to travel between the tracheae and the walls of the veins. The pulsating organs, whether in the thorax or in the afferent veins, serve as an aspirating mechanism to draw the haemolymph through the venous network of the wing. This is accomplished by dilation, which occurs, apparently, when the thoracic muscles relax. Blood enters the costal region of the wing from adjacent intermuscular spaces of the thorax.

ADIPOSE TISSUE

The fat body or, more properly, fat bodies of the fly occupy a considerable portion of the coelom and are richly supplied with tracheae. Besides serving as a reservoir of food energy, they presumably function for the temporary storage of nitrogenous wastes. Scattered throughout the mass are large cells of the oenocyte type (Pérez, 1910), arranged in clusters. According to Janet (1907), the imaginal fat body arises during development from mesodermal leucocytes.

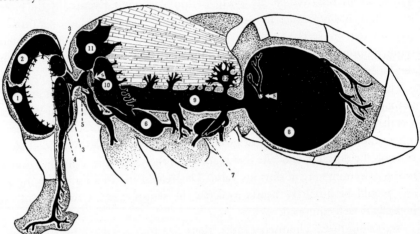

Figure 30. Tracheation in the adult fly. *1,* anterior cephalic sac; *2,* dorsal cephalic sac; *3,* posterior cephalic sacs; *4,* ventrolateral cephalic sac; *5,* cervical tracheal duct; *6,* anterior ventral thoracic sac; *7,* posterior ventral thoracic sac; *8,* abdominal air sac; *9,* longitudinal sac; *10,* air sac supplying sternodorsales muscles; *11,* air sac supplying dorsales muscles; *s,* spiracles. (Freely adapted from Hewitt, *The House-Fly* [Cambridge University Press, 1914].)

THE TRACHEAL SYSTEM

This is very well developed in muscoid flies. In a freshly dissected specimen, the tracheae are nowhere near as conspicuous as the large thin-walled air sacs that occur in almost every portion of the body cavity.

According to Wigglesworth (1939), these saccular dilatations frequently owe their great size to the fusion of the matrices of adjacent tracheal branches. In *Musca,* the walls of the sacs become bound to muscles and other adjacent tissue by a great number of small tracheal branches. In some parts of the body, the air sacs are subject to collapse, but in the head and in certain locations in the thorax, they remain permanently expanded. If, as sometimes occurs, a nerve or muscle traverses such a chamber, it is invested with ordinary tracheal coverings with the layers in reverse order, the cuticle being on the outside. At least Janet (1911) has so demonstrated in the bee.

It will be recalled that there are two pairs of thoracic spiracles and five pairs of abdominal ones in both males and females. It should be mentioned that the male fly has two additional pairs in the membrane that joins the rudimentary sixth and seventh abdominal sclerites. Each spiracle, regardless of location, leads to a shallow vestibule that is partially separated by a valvelike mechanism from the atrium within. In the abdominal segments, the atrium leads only to tracheae of the conventional type, which ramify among the visceral organs and divisions of the fat body. The air sacs, already mentioned, arise entirely from the thoracic spiracles. Each anterior thoracic spiracle is surrounded by a conspicuous peritreme, while the posterior pair, which are rather triangular in shape, are less conspicuous. All have their openings guarded by branched, dendritic processes that serve to exclude solid particles. All lead to vestibules with interior valves.

Each anterior spiracle serves two systems of tracheal sacs. One of these includes the anterior ventral thoracic sac that supplies the thoracic ganglion, a vertical sac that serves the anterior sternodorsales muscles, a flat sac that lies close to the dorsales muscles, and an elaborately branching, elongated sac that runs laterally to the alimentary canal. This last supplies several muscles and also the second and third legs, and finally gives rise to the great abdominal air sac, which, with its fellow of the opposite side, occupies nearly half of the abdominal cavity.

Early entomologists believed that the huge abdominal air sacs served chiefly for the purpose of giving buoyancy in flight. This may be true to a limited extent, since muscular contractions probably produce sufficient heat to cause some expansion of the air that they contain. More important, however, is the fact that they provide space that various expanding abdominal organs may occupy without materially affecting the fly's exterior proportions. It has been shown that in *Lucilia* the newly emerged adult has only small abdominal air sacs, while the gut is dilated with gas. Ten hours later, however, the condition is reversed. Also, as the fly continues to feed, the fat body and especially the ovaries come to occupy a greater portion of the available space. Although this results in marked reduction of the air sacs, gravid females appear to fly as well as ever. The obvious function of the abdominal air sacs as reservoirs of oxygen is apparently taken over by the thoracic and cephalic

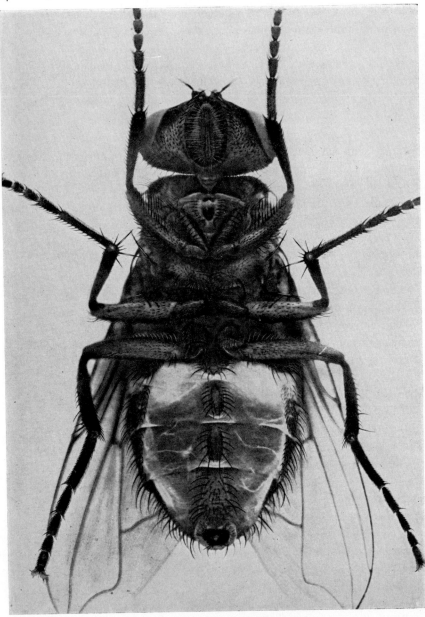

Figure 31. Ventral view of *Musca domestica* with abdomen distended. Note relatively tiny ventral sclerites and greatly expanded conjunctival areas with tracheal branches showing through. (Photograph by N. A. Cobb; copyright, National Geographic Society.)

chambers when pressure from other organs causes the abdominal units to collapse. The second system of chambers, which arises from the anterior side of the spiracle, includes first a flattened sac that serves the neck and anterior leg, then narrows to form a cervical tracheal duct extending into the head. After giving off lesser ducts, which serve the tentorium, each cervical duct unites with that from the opposite spiracle to form a common unit from which three elements, one median and two lateral, lead forth. The median duct enlarges into the bilobed dorsocephalic sac. Each lateral leads to a posterior cephalic sac consisting of an optic unit and a vertical, ventroposterior portion. From the tentorial tracheal ducts, a number of sacs arise which by secondary branching serve the anterior region of the head, including the antennae, rostrum, palpi, haustellum, and other parts.

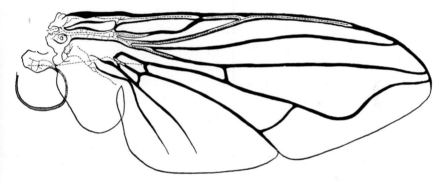

Figure 32. Tracheation in housefly wing. Certain tracheae persist in the wing of the adult fly. Their course is shown by dotted lines. (Adapted from E. Thomsen, 1938.)

The posterior thoracic spiracles give rise to sacs that supply those portions of the median and posterior thorax not adequately served by other elements. The large muscles of the body wall are the organs chiefly concerned. No branches extend either to the head or to the abdomen.

It should be remembered that the exchange of gases which makes possible true internal or tissue respiration takes place to little or no extent through the walls of the tracheae or air sacs, but rather through the thin-walled tracheoles in which all tracheal branches terminate. It is generally accepted that the tracheoles are of unicellular origin.

According to Weismann (1863), the tracheae of muscids fill with gas during development, while the insect is still bathed in fluid. He believed that this gas was liberated from solution in the tissue fluids.

REPRODUCTIVE ORGANS OF THE FEMALE

In mature females, the ovaries come to occupy the greater portion of the abdominal cavity. Each lies ventral and lateral to the food canal, which thus rests in the trough-shaped space between them. Seventy or more egg tubes go to make up each gonad. The ventral portion of each tube is normally distended by a single mature ovum, while two or three immature gametes are indicated by progressively smaller bulges in the distal portion. All the egg tubes of each ovary communicate with a thin-walled oviduct situated in the last abdominal segment. The two oviducts, which are very short, unite almost at once to form the common oviduct, which curves dorsally and forward to approach the ovipositor at a point somewhat ventral to the rectum. Here it dilates to form the sacculus, which is continuous with the still larger vagina. The latter opens into the ovipositor just behind the subanal plate of segment 9. Close to the junction of the sacculus and the vagina, a number of appendages are found. These consist of a pair of saclike accessory copulatory vesicles, a pair of elongated accessory glands, and three spermathecae, one on the right side and two on the left. Each spermatheca consists of a slender duct leading to a chitinous, oval capsule, black in color. Each capsule is partially enclosed in the cuplike distal expansion of the cellular wall of its duct. The intima of the duct is continuous with the chitinous wall of the capsule. The accessory glands are believed to secrete an adhesive fluid that covers each egg and causes it to adhere to the substratum or to other ova.

The foregoing description assumes the ovipositor to be in the retracted or withdrawn position. This structure, which consists of the four terminal segments of the abdomen, has been described in some detail in Chapter II. When retracted, the segments are telescoped, each within the other, an arrangement made possible by the extreme flexibility of the intersegmental membranes. The last (ninth abdominal) segment consists of a dorsal sclerite, also the principal subanal plate, already mentioned, and a second more ventral subanal plate, just in front of which may be found the female genital aperture. Visible externally, even when the ovipositor is withdrawn, are the two lateral tubercles of segment 9, each of which bears a number of stiff hairs.

It is of interest to note that though unmated females will deposit eggs, the number is nowhere near as great as with mated individuals (Glaser, 1923a). Fertile eggs occasionally hatch within the uterus, especially if oviposition is interfered with for any reason. This is rare in houseflies, but normal in *Musca larvipara,* where, according to Keilin (1916), only a single large egg passes into the uterus at one time. It invariably hatches at the time of oviposition, which thus becomes larviposition. *Musca larvipara* is, therefore, an ovoviviparous species.

Sikes and Wigglesworth (1931) state that all muscid larvae, in hatching, tear a hole in the vitelline membrane of the egg with their mouth hooks.

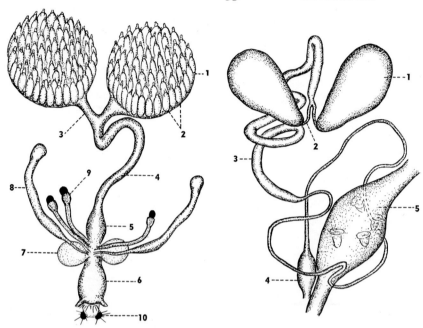

Figure 33. Reproductive organs. *Left:* Female. *1*, ovary; *2*, egg tubes; *3*, left oviduct; *4*, common oviduct; *5*, sacculus; *6*, vagina; *7*, copulatory vesicle; *8*, accessory glands; *9*, spermatheca; *10*, lateral tubercle (cercus) of ovipositor. *Right:* Male. *1*, testis; *2*, vas deferens; *3*, ejaculatory duct; *4*, ejaculatory sac; *5*, rectum, containing the four rectal glands. (Adapted from several authors.)

REPRODUCTIVE ORGANS OF THE MALE

The two brownish testes lie opposite one another in abdominal segment 5. Each is somewhat pear-shaped, with the small extremity pointing toward the median line. The short, slender vasa deferentia unite to form a single long, coiled ejaculatory duct, the first portion of which has a much greater diameter than the more distal part. The course of the ejaculatory duct is interesting. It first runs forward, then ventrally, followed by several convolutions on the left side of the body cavity. From here the duct, becoming more slender, arches dorsally above the rectum to run forward on the right side, curve downward, and complete its course by running caudally along the median ventral line. Before reaching the penis, the ejaculatory duct enlarges into an ejaculatory sac, the wall of which is fortified by an ejaculatory sclerite. This structure is subject to muscular control and is believed to assist in the ejaculation of the semen. There are no accessory glands. The chitinous structures concerned with copulation have been described at length in Chapter II.

THE MUSCULAR SYSTEM

The bulk of the body wall, especially in the vicinity of the wings, and likewise most of the nonchitinous portions of the legs prove to be made up of

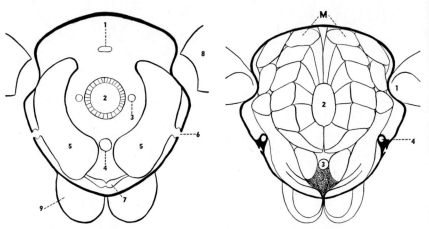

Figure 34. Cross section of thorax. *Left:* Schematic diagram at level of posterior thoracic spiracle. Muscles are purposely omitted. *1,* dorsal blood vessel; *2,* food canal; *3,* salivary duct; *4,* ventral diverticulum (crop); *5,* thoracic air sacs; *6,* spiracle; *7,* compound thoracic ganglion; *8,* portion of wing; *9,* coxa of mesothoracic leg. *Right:* Oblique section through wing base and third coxa, to show massive character of thoracic muscles. *1,* wing base; *2,* aperture for food canal; *3,* ventral diverticulum; *4,* trachea from spiracle; *M,* muscle bundles.

muscular tissue. As with many insects, man is impressed by the apparent strength of *M. domestica* in proportion to its size. A housefly, for example, can carry a match (Metcalf and Flint, 1928). The power of insect muscle is, however, apparent rather than real, as repeated investigations have shown it to be much less powerful in proportion to area of cross section than the muscles of vertebrate animals. Large vertebrates, it should be remembered, must first support and transport their own weight, regardless of whether or not they accomplish any additional work. It seems quite evident that a housefly enlarged to the size of a helicopter would not only fail to fly but would probably be quite unable to crawl or even to stand.

Histologically the muscles of insects do, however, remind us of the voluntary muscles of vertebrates (Sharpy-Schafer, 1938). Alternate light and dark bands at right angles to the long axis of the muscle fibers are characteristic of both. The color, however, is rarely the same. Insect muscles are whitish or transparent, while the color of vertebrate muscle is often pinkish or red.

Several thorough studies of the musculature of flies exist in available literature. Hammond published on the thorax of *Musca* (*Calliphora*) *vomitoria* in 1881, and in the same year Kunckel d'Herculais treated of the syrphid genus *Volucella*. It was a period in which great enthusiasm for morphological studies was being shown. Lowne's studies on blowflies (1870, 1895) also represented an important contribution.

Hewitt (1914a) grouped the important muscles under five heads:

1. Segmental muscles. Although the elaborate segmental muscles of the larva are lost for the most part in the adult fly, a few homologous elements remain. These are the cervical muscles, the minor muscles of the thorax, the thoracoabdominal muscles, the segmental abdominal muscles, the muscles of the ovipositor, and the muscles of the male gonapophyses.

2. Muscles of the thoracic appendages. These are the muscles of the root of the wing, the muscles of the halteres, the flexors of the coxae, and the internal muscles of the leg.

3. Special muscles. The muscles of the penis, the muscles of the spiracular valves, and various miscellaneous small muscles fall here.

4–5. The muscles of the cephalic region and the principal muscles of the thorax are of considerably greater importance than the foregoing groups. They are listed in Table 1.

THE NERVOUS SYSTEM

There is marked cephalization of the central nervous system in muscoid flies. The brain or supraoesophageal ganglion is so intimately fused with the suboesophageal mass that the two appear as one, perforated by a small central aperture or foramen for the passage of the food canal. In dorsal view, the brain appears to consist of three parts, the central cephalic ganglion proper, which is poorly divided by a median longitudinal fissure, and two large, lateral optic lobes, which serve the 8,000 or more ommatidia of the two compound eyes. The ocellar nerve that arises in the median line proceeds dorsally to the simple eyes. The two antennal nerves arise one on either side from the anterior portion of the central ganglionic mass. Histological sections show that the peduncles of the optic lobes arise from the procerebrum, the antennal nerves from the deutocerebrum or second brain segment. The tritocerebrum is represented by the most dorsal portion of the brain, the contiguous frontal lobes.

The suboesophageal portion of the cephalic ganglion gives off a pair of pharyngeal nerves that arise from the region of the almost obsolete circum-

Table 1

A. Muscles of the cephalic region

Name	Origin	Insertion	Function
Dilators of the pharynx	Anterolateral region of fulcrum	Dorsal plate of pharynx	Pump food into oesophagus
Retractors of the fulcrum	Internal margins of genae	Posterior cornu of fulcrum	Rotate fulcrum on epistome in retraction of proboscis
Retractors of the haustellum	Dorsolateral region of occiput	Dorsal margin of theca	Aid in folding and retraction of proboscis
Retractors of the rostrum	Sides of occipital foramen	Halfway down membranous rostrum, posterior side	Draw in rostrum during retraction of proboscis
Flexors of the haustellum	Sides of occipital foramen	Base of labral apodeme	Flex haustellum against rostrum
Extensors of the haustellum	Distal cornu of fulcrum	Head of labral apodeme	Straighten proboscis
Accessory flexors of haustellum	Lower anterior margin of fulcrum	Head of labral apodeme	Flex haustellum against rostrum
Flexors of the labrum-epipharynx	Anterior upper edge of fulcrum	Proximal end of labrum-epipharynx	One pair extends haustellum; two pairs flex it
Retractors of the furca	Upper portion of theca	Upper half of lateral process of furca	Diverge lateral processes of furca and open oral lobes
Retractors of discal sclerites	Lateral edges of upper portion of theca	Sides of discal sclerites	Diverge discal sclerites and open oral pit
Dilators of labium-hypopharynx	Middle region of theca, near middle line	Lateral edges of labio-hypopharyngeal sclerite	Widen channel of labium-hypopharynx
Dilators of labrum-epipharynx	Radially arranged in wall of labrum-epipharynx		Regulate size of pharyngeal channel

B. Principal muscles of the thorax

Name	Origin	Insertion	Function
Dorsales (6 pairs)	Postscutellum and mesophragma	Prescutum and anterior region of scutum	Loosen alar membrane and depress wing
Sternodorsales 2 pairs	Prescutum and scutum	Mesosternum	Tighten alar membrane and elevate wing
1 pair	Scutum	Postscutellum above spiracle	

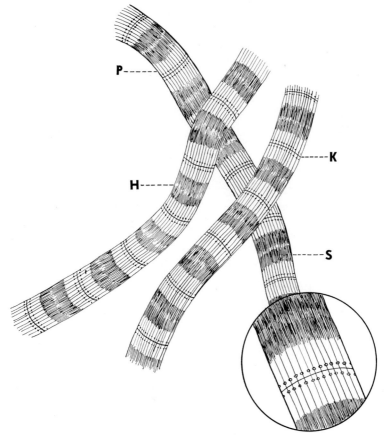

Figure 35. Fibers of insect muscle. *K*, Krause's membrane, dividing light band; *S*, sarcous elements, forming dark band; *H*, line of Hensen, dividing dark band; *P*, sarcoplasm, consisting of longitudinal lines, with dots. (Freely adapted from Sharpy-Schafer, 1938.)

oesophageal connectives. These extend forward to encounter the pharynx opposite the posterior cornu of the fulcrum. More ventral in origin are the labial nerves that extend the length of the proboscis. Their motor fibers innervate the muscles of that organ, while the sensory fibers branch freely in the oral lobes.

Extending backward from the suboesophageal ganglion is the cephalo-thoracic nerve cord, which appears to have lost all evidence of its original double character. Just before reaching the thoracic ganglion, this cord gives

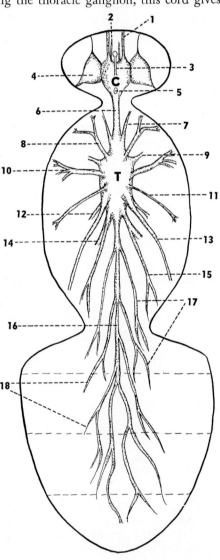

Figure 36. Plan of adult nervous system. *1*, antennary nerve; *2*, pharyngeal nerve; *3*, ocellar nerve; *4*, optic peduncle; *5*, space for oesophagus; *6*, cephalo-thoracic nerve cord; *7*, cervical nerve; *8*, prothoracic dorsal nerve; *9*, prothoracic crural nerve; *10*, mesothoracic dorsal nerve; *11*, accessory mesothoracic dorsal nerve; *12*, mesothoracic crural nerve; *13*, metathoracic dorsal nerve; *14*, metathoracic crural nerve; *15*, accessory metathoracic dorsal nerve; *16*, abdominal nerve cord; *17*, abdominal nerves of thoracic origin; *18*, abdominal nerves of local origin; *C*, cephalic ganglion; *T*, thoracic (compound) ganglion. (Adapted from Hewitt, *The House-Fly* [Cambridge University Press, 1914].)

rise to the two cervical nerves, which extend forward, one on either side, to innervate the muscles of the neck. The compound thoracic ganglion represents a fusion of the prothoracic, mesothoracic, and metathoracic ganglia with the so-called abdominal ganglion, from which extend backward the abdominal nerve and all its branches. The entire compound ganglion lies in the forward portion of the thorax. It is fully twice as long as broad, with the posterior portion somewhat narrowed. Dorsally it gives rises to the prothoracic, mesothoracic, and metathoracic dorsal nerves, which serve largely the thoracic muscles. Of these, the metathoracic are the largest, and supply the halteres. Also dorsal in origin are the accessory mesothoracic and methathoracic pairs, each caudal to the pair it supplements. More ventral in origin are the prothoracic, mesothoracic, and metathoracic crural nerves, which supply chiefly the three pairs of legs.

The ganglia are united dorsally by a continuation of the cephalothoracic nerve in the form of a median longitudinal band. In this portion of the cord, a median dorsal fissure is clearly evident. Both the cephalic ganglion and the compound thoracic ganglion are enclosed in a cortical sheath that must be removed if the constituent parts are to be clearly understood. This sheath is composed of two kinds of cells. The smaller cells have large nuclei, scant protoplasm, and anastomose freely with one another. The larger cells, which are fewer, may be described as ganglionic cells of unipolar, bipolar, and tripolar types.

The abdomen is served by two pairs of nerves that arise in the thorax plus a series of nerves that branch off alternately from the median abdominal extension of the cord. This median nerve terminates in the genital structures.

The sympathetic nervous system will not be described except to say that the cephalic ganglion gives rise to a slender nerve that extends backward above the food canal to the proventricular ganglion. From this ganglion, most of the visceral (sympathetic) fibers take their origin.

Our discussion of the nervous system would not be complete without reference to certain special sensory functions by which the fly is able to adapt itself to the environment in which it lives. These will be discussed under a number of separate heads.

CHEMICAL PERCEPTION

There is no absolutely satisfactory distinction between taste and smell. In man, the perception of the qualities of sweet, sour, salt, and bitter is regarded as belonging in the category of taste, and all other chemical perceptions as belonging to the sense of smell; but with flies it is doubtful if even this distinction can be made.

For the purpose of the following discussion, it may be considered that

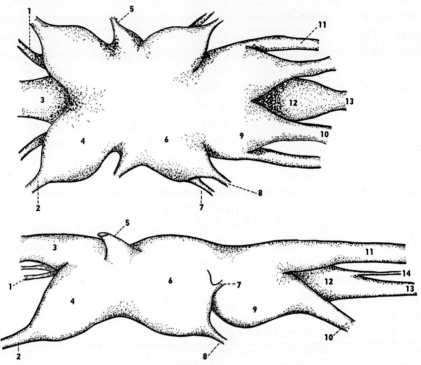

Figure 37. Compound thoracic ganglion with cortex removed. *Upper:* Ventral view. *Lower:* Lateral aspect. *1,* prothoracic dorsal nerve; *2,* prothoracic crural nerve; *3,* cephalothoracic nerve cord; *4,* prothoracic ganglion; *5,* mesothoracic dorsal nerve; *6,* mesothoracic ganglion; *7,* accessory dorsal mesothoracic nerve; *8,* mesothoracic crural nerve; *9,* metathoracic ganglion; *10,* metathoracic crural nerve; *11,* metathoracic dorsal nerve; *12,* abdominal ganglion; *13,* abdominal nerve cord; *14,* accessory metathoracic dorsal nerve. (Adapted from Hewitt, *The House-Fly* [Cambridge University Press, 1914].)

smell relates to perception of vaporous substances, and taste to an appreciation of contact with materials in the liquid or solid state.

As with *Calliphora, Drosophila,* and many nondipterous insects, the organs by which the housefly is able to perceive stimuli of a chemical nature are located in part at least on the distal extremity of the tibia and on the tarsal segments.

Hayes and Liu (1947), who studied the tarsal chemoreceptors of the housefly histologically, noted that chemoreceptive sensilla occur only on tarsal segments 2 to 5 and that they are always lateral in position. Each chemoreceptive organ consists of a group of more or less spindle-shaped sense cells, subepidermal in position and covered with a nucleated neurilemma. The latter is continuous with the neurilemma of the longitudinal nerve. The distal end of the sensilla is attached to a long, thin-walled chemoreceptive seta. Hayes and Liu failed to find comparable structures either in the cockroach or in the Mexican bean beetle, and suggest that the housefly's greater susceptibility to DDT may possibly depend upon its chemoreceptive organs. In this connection it should be noted that the cuticula of *M. domestica* measures only 12.5 to 25 microns in thickness, while that of *Epilachna* ranges from 25 to 45 (larvae 15 to 40) and that of *Blatella* from 60 to as great as 90.

Sarkaria and Patton (1949) studied the histology of the pulvillus of houseflies as compared with that of the honeybee, milkweed bug (*Oncopeltus*), and German cockroach, but could find no microscopic reason for the greater susceptibility of *Musca domestica* to DDT. They put forward three suggestions, namely, (1) that the fly travels in such a manner that its pulvilli are more constantly in contact with the surface than in the case of other species, (2) that the longer tenent hairs on the housefly pulvillus may trap crystals of DDT and hold them in contact with the foot, (3) that the pulvillar secretion is perhaps an effective solvent of DDT.

Deonier and Richardson (1935) tested the tarsal chemoreceptor response of *Musca domestica* to sucrose and levulose and found that an average of 90 per cent of the flies tested reacted positively. Flies permitted to feed first gave a lower percentage response than was the case with hungry flies, and starvation increased the percentage noticeably. Levulose was less effective than sucrose in all experiments. Further work by the senior author (1938) showed that poisonous concentrations of injurious substances elicited a negative response as shown by the behavior of the proboscis. Many nonvolatile substances were tested. A repellent concentration either failed to cause extension of the proboscis or, if the proboscis were already extended, caused it to be withdrawn. Deonier later (1939) extended his investigations to the blowflies, *Cochliomyia americana* and *Phormia regina*. In these, also, extension of the proboscis followed stimulation of tarsal chemoreceptors by sucrose or other attrahents. Both sexes appeared to react in the same manner. The results are in general agreement with those obtained by Minnich (1929), who studied the chemical sensitivity of the legs in the genus *Calliphora*.

For reception of stimuli of a vaporous character, the antennae are undoubtedly of value. According to Liebermann (1925), dung-feeding muscids have more sensory pits and sensilla than other species, and males are more

abundantly supplied than females. In this group, it is normal to find a number
of rods or cones arising close together at the bottom of a fairly deep pit. Each
is connected with its own sense cell, from which a nerve strand extends internally (Fig. 38). In flight, muscoid flies usually extend the antennae forward
by which means the olfactory pits are better exposed to the "head wind." Perhaps the tendency of houseflies to travel against the wind or crosswise, rather
than with the breeze, depends upon this reflex.

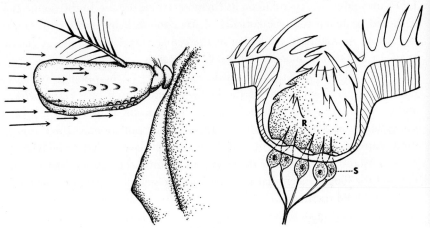

Figure 38. Special sensory structures. *Left:* Antennae, erected, as in flight. A con
tinuous stream of air encounters the olfactory pits. *Right:* Single olfactory pit, much
enlarged. *R,* sensory rod; *S,* sensory cell. (Adapted from Wigglesworth, *Principles of
Insect Physiology,* Fig. 133 [after Liebermann], by permission of Methuen & Co., Ltd.)

Until tested experimentally, the attractive or repellent qualities of particular
substances cannot usually be predicted. Laake, Parman, Bishopp, and Roark
(1931) studied the chemotropic responses of houseflies, greenbottles, and black
blowflies. Ethyl mercaptan, chloroform, butyraldehyde, arsenic solutions, and
formaldehyde all proved attractive to *Musca domestica.* Geraniol, bromo-
form, and certain other substances made meat more attractive to flies, but the
several species differed greatly in their response. No flies approached meat
treated with clove oil or powder carried in vegetable oils. Pine-tar oils proved
the most effective repellents.

Earlier work by Speyer (1920), who studied decomposition products of
banana and related compounds, is very illuminating. Unfermented carbohydrates, in general, attracted the flies very little. Valerianic acid, amyl acetate,
and amyl alcohol were attractive in the order named. Unripe bananas were less
attractive than all three; fermented banana was more so. Dried residue, following fermentation, attracted not at all. In generalizing for the amyl com-

pounds, Speyer states that the saturated alcohols, the aldehydes, and the acids elicit a positive chemotropism. Where the methyl group (CH_3) is introduced, these substances are still positive except where the molecular weight falls around 30 or below, 30 being the molecular weight of methyl alcohol. There is an aggravation of the chemotropic stimulus where the methyl group is augmented by combination with $(CH_2)x$. No positive response is given to compounds containing the benzene ring. Such substances, however, are not necessarily repellent. Speyer found no relation between the volatility of any substance and the intensity of the response. He suggested that saturated compounds which contain the molecular group $CH_3(CH_2)x$ may be the source of stimuli by which houseflies are guided to their food. Essential oils, with few exceptions, Speyer found repellent or at least unattractive. Each species tested responded somewhat differently to the compounds offered.

It has already been mentioned that certain substances which are attractive at a relatively low concentration may be repellent at a higher one. This was further demonstrated by Wieting and Hoskins (1939), who studied the olfactory response of M. domestica by means of an olfactometer of their own designing. Streams of air, heated to 41°C (105.8°F) were employed to attract flies to desired areas. The concentration of the vapors was controlled by flow meters connected with saturation chambers. Both males and females were attracted to ammonia in concentration of 0.012 per cent (by volume). They were strongly repelled, however, by any concentration greater than 0.03 per cent. Ethyl alcohol proved feebly attractive up to 0.012 per cent but acted as a repellent above 0.05. These workers were unable to detect any response to CO_2 in concentrations of 2 per cent or less. It is perhaps noteworthy that whereas ammonia proved more attractive to females than to males, with ethyl alcohol the situation was reversed.

Steiner (1945), working with Phormia regina, found that odors which were at first strongly repellent to the flies became much less so as the insects became accustomed to them.

In addition to serving as chemical receptors, the antennae are likewise sensitive to slight changes in external pressure, such as might affect a sensitive barometer. Wellington (1946b) tested seven species, including Musca domestica, and concluded that this pressure-sensitive apparatus, which, he states, is confined solely to the antennae, enables the fly both to evade attack and to escape crushing by a falling object.

In the normal fly, it is the aristae that perform this function, and one arista alone will serve the purpose, though the efficiency seems to be in proportion to its length. The degree of plumosity is of slight importance, apparently,

as Tachinidae with their essentially bare aristae startle as readily as Calliphoridae and Muscidae. Such pressure-sensitive aristae Wellington terms
"external baroreceptors." He discusses the reactions of flies to waves produced
merely by passing the hand near the normal insect. These reactions are definitely directional. With a portion of the arista removed, the responses are
more sluggish; with the arista absent, directional responses cease. Gaffron
(1933) points out that flies which would be instantly disturbed by a sudden
motion of the hand are not so disturbed when protected by a glass container.
Vision, evidently, is of slight or no importance in their reactions. For discussion of the erratic flight of houseflies prior to thunderstorms, see Chapter IX.

The transmission of the stimulus to the brain involves an additional apparatus present in the pedicels of the antennae. If the conjunctival plates of
the second segments be exposed, the insects retain only a partial sensitivity to
pressure, while the removal of the pedicels results in complete loss of wave
sensitivity. Covering these structures with collodion produces the same result. Imms (1938) states that Johnston's organ is probably auditory in function, and thus it is logical to suppose that pressure vibrations may also be transmitted by this apparatus, since sound itself is a pressure-wave phenomenon.

Frings (1941b) studied the olfactory sense in the blowfly *Cynomyia cadaverina*. He found the antennae and the labella to be the sole bearers of olfactory end organs in that species, and suggested that the function might be
somewhat differently specialized in the two locations. The antennal end organs, for example, probably function as chemoreceptors over a considerable
distance and provide for chemotropic orientation of a directional nature. The
labellar end organs, on the other hand, are believed to be nondirectional in
nature, serving to receive stimuli of a combined gustatory and olfactory character while the insect is feeding.

When one considers the various types of chemoreceptors on the fly's body,
it will be realized that those of the antennae are especially adapted for per-
ceiving the presence of vaporous substances, those of the oral lobes for tasting
solutions and suspensions, and those of the tarsi for initiating reflex behavior
that leads to the exercise of the tasting function. All may be sensitive to the
same substances, though in varying degree. Thus Minnich (1931), who
studied particularly the gustatory function of the marginal hairs of the oral
lobes in *Calliphora,* made some interesting comparisons in regard to their
sensitiveness to sugars of different types. He found saccharose and maltose to
be particularly stimulating, with glucose and lactose less so, in the order
named. The order of effectiveness was the same for the chemoreceptors of
the legs, but the latter were sixteen times as sensitive to saccharose as were

the oral lobes. For lactose the comparison was reversed; the labella were stimulated by sufficiently high concentrations, while the legs were wholly insensitive to this particular sugar.

CONSIDERATIONS RELATING TO VISION

Wigglesworth (1939) states that each compound eye of *Musca* contains approximately 4,000 facets. This genus has an ommatidial angle of 3 degrees, but the narrowest stripe that appears to be perceived subtends an angle of 5 degrees (Gaffron, 1933).

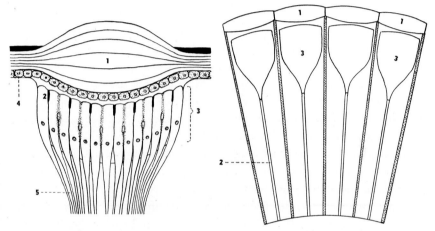

Figure 39. The eyes of insects. *Left:* Structure of an ocellus. *1,* cornea; *2,* rhabdom; *3,* retina; *4,* hypodermis; *5,* nerve. *Right:* Diagrammatic representation of compound eye. *1,* corneas; *2,* rhabdom; *3,* crystalline cones. (Redrawn from Comstock, 1936.)

Considerable interest thus attaches to the question as to how frequently two or more individual ommatidia may be coupled to a single nerve. Data are not available for the genus *Musca,* but histological studies on *Calliphora* have shown that coupling is much less pronounced in the anterior region of the eye, which would make this the region of greatest visual acuity.

The cones of the ommatidia in Muscidae are represented merely by a mass of liquid secreted by the crystalline cells. Such eyes are termed "pseudocone" eyes, the lens system being composed chiefly of the cornea. The images are formed by apposition. Thus they differ from those insects that possess a true crystalline cone (eucone type), and also from those in which a cone is formed by an invagination of the cornea, to which the term "exocone" eye has been applied.

Of considerable interest because of its relation to possible control procedures is the physiological response of flies to color. This has been studied recently by Waterhouse (1948), who released houseflies into a Peet-Grady chamber with a white lacquered interior. The corners were of various colors and were so arranged that they might be moved. Data consisted of interval counts of flies resting on the various colors. Red was most commonly preferred, with dusky blue a second choice. Yellow and medium-gray surfaces were equally popular as third-choice colors. Green came next, followed by light gray. Least used were surfaces painted sky blue or white. In general, it may be said that the surface which absorbs the most, that is, reflects the least total illumination, is the more attractive to domestic flies. Such discrimination, however, depends upon the relative constancy of other environmental factors. Houseflies always appear to be more sensitive to chemical stimuli than to quality of light, and will respond chemotropically even where it requires contact with surfaces of a color that they might ordinarily avoid.

Larvae probably lack specific organs of vision, but are rather sensitive to light intensity, nevertheless. It may be said that in general the maggots of Muscidae show a well-marked negative phototaxis. The light-sensitive areas are confined to the oral extremity, and although their structural nature is not understood, it is accepted that image formation does not occur. The stimulating effect depends on the brightness of the illumination. If only a single light is used, the larvae move in a straight line away from it. If two lights are displayed simultaneously, the larvae move along the line dividing the angle between the sources, while if the two lights differ in intensity, the line of travel deviates away from the stronger source.

Some workers consider that a pair of conical structures located at the tips of the bilobed oral lobes (maxillae) may be regarded as functional organs of light perception. These do, in fact, somewhat resemble ocelli, but are totally lacking in pigment. Experiments have been performed which tend to show that larvae lose their ability to respond to changes in light intensity when these structures are removed. Most workers, however, hold contrary opinions. One plausible suggestion, which takes into account the fact that sensitivity of larvae to light becomes greater with age, is that the imaginal discs of the adult compound eye function as the actual organs of light perception in the larval state.

COMBINED STUDIES OF CHEMICAL AND VISUAL REACTIONS

An interesting observation was made by Kuzina in 1940 on the relative importance of sight, taste, and smell in guiding females of *Musca domestica* to suitable media for oviposition. A number of specimens had glue applied to the proboscis, the latter being in a retracted position. This deprived them from using the labella as tasting organs. In another group, the eyes were covered with glue, while in a third series, the third antennal segments (which bear the aristae) were removed. Both pig and cow dung were made available, and the behavior of each group was compared with that of an equal number of unmutilated controls. Kuzina concluded that the flies are directed to a suitable medium almost entirely by smell, but that taste is a necessary stimulant for the deposition of eggs. The taste of milk proved sufficient when a barrier of muslin prevented them from reaching dung. Vision he found to be of slight importance in either connection.

GENETIC FACTORS IN RESPONSE

That differences in response to stimuli may be correlated with differences in structure, and are presumably conditioned by them, is well illustrated by the work of Wiesmann (1947). Wiesmann's findings also tend to show that such variations in all probability depend upon racial, i.e., genetic, factors. The investigation concerned two races of flies, one from Arnäs in northern Sweden, the other native to Basle, Switzerland. The Arnäs flies, it may be noted, had the legs much more pigmented, with stiffer tarsal bristles. The tarsal segments were broader, and the difference in size of successive tarsal segments was less pronounced. Of considerable significance is the fact that the cuticle covering the tarsal pads, as well as the articular membranes of the tarsal joints, is perhaps one-third thicker in the Arnäs strain than in the Basle race. This last characteristic appears to have largely to do with differences in susceptibility to DDT. The results of laboratory tests were striking.

The same exposure to DDT which caused knockdown of Basle flies in an average of 16 minutes had similar effect on Arnäs flies only after 54 to 143 minutes. The average was 93. Exposure to a DDT deposit of 0.001 mg. in a petri dish caused no reaction in Arnäs flies over a twenty-four-hour period but caused knockdown of the Basle specimens in an average time of six hours and ten minutes. The dabbing of specific parts of the body with 1 per cent DDT in acetone showed similar and consistent differences. It may be noted that there was least racial difference when the coxae were treated, and most contrast when the solution was brought into contact with the head.

Responses to temperature were studied also. At 45°C (113°F), heat torpor resulted in Basle flies after 34 minutes; in Arnäs flies, after 46. Corresponding differences were recorded for other high temperatures except that only 10 minutes was required for torpor to ensue in either group when the temperature reached 55°C (131°F). However, under such conditions, there was 100 per cent mortality in the Basle group, whereas 43 per cent of the Arnäs flies recovered.

At the opposite extreme, exposure to 12°C (53.6°F) made only 18 per cent of the Arnäs flies torpid at the end of three hours, while all Basle flies became torpid in not more than 42 minutes.

Studies of narcosis brought out racial differences, also. Arnäs flies were more slowly affected by methyl acetate than the Basle flies, but required a longer period for recovery, probably because a much larger amount of the narcotic had been taken in before collapse.

FLIGHT

How far can a fly travel? From a health standpoint, it is desirable to discriminate between the "potential" or "maximum" flight range and the "effective" or "average" range over which there may be frequent transmission of filthborne disease. If it were possible so to stimulate a fly that most of its time on the wing could be spent traveling in the same general direction, the distance

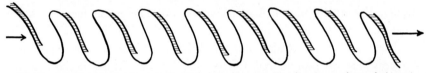

Figure 40. Course of wing tip in flight. In the downstroke the surface of the wing is used, whereas in the upstroke the costal margin cuts somewhat edgewise through the air. This tracing was made by a species of *Calliphora*. (Adapted from Wigglesworth, *Principles of Insect Physiology*, Fig. 77 [after Ritter], by permission of Methuen & Co., Ltd.)

would be relatively enormous—hundreds of miles, perhaps. Cobb (1910b) pointed out that the wing muscles of a fly, when weighed, were found to be heavier in proportion than those of any bird examined up to that time. For this reason, it is exceedingly difficult to tire a fly out. The same author (1910a) made accurate measurements on two species of *Sarcophaga*. He found that the two lateral batteries of wing muscle together averaged 5.88 mg., 12.2 per cent of the weight of the entire fly. The central battery was slightly heavier, averaging 6.75 mg. or 14.1 per cent of the total weight. Twenty-six and three-tenths per cent of the weight of the fly is thus seen to consist of muscles used in flight.

In *Musca* the muscles of flight comprise 11 per cent of the total body weight. As with other aerial forms, flight is accomplished largely by the indirect action of vertical and longitudinal muscle columns which alter the shape of the thoracic capsule by their contraction. The vertical muscles serve in elevating the wing, the longitudinal muscles in depressing it. Various methods have been used in studying wing movements. The most satisfactory for a fast-moving wing is the use of the cinematograph. In the act of hovering, the wing tips trace in the air an elongated figure 8, oblique to the long axis of the body, the lower extremity being anterior, the upper posterior, to the vertical. (Fig. 41.) When, however, the fly is in motion the wings describe a series of open loops in which a downward and forward motion alternates with a backward and upward movement (Fig. 40). There is also a noticeable rotation of the

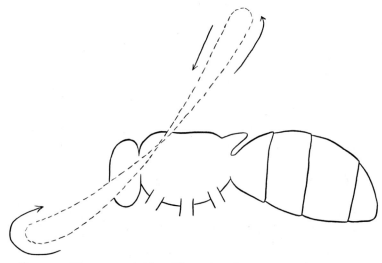

Figure 41. Movement of wing. Illustration shows course of wing tip in a syrphid fly (*Volucella*) when the specimen is held stationary. (Adapted from Wigglesworth, *Principles of Insect Physiology*, Fig. 76 [after Magnan], by permission of Methuen & Co., Ltd.)

wing on its long axis. This is due partly to the fact that the anterior margin is much less flexible than the posterior, and the latter tends to lag, but in some flies, at least (Bull, 1910), the action is essentially muscular, as shown by the fact that with most of the wing removed, a species of *Tipula* still inclined the remaining stub in opposite directions with each up stroke and down stroke as before. This reversal of inclination enables the flying insect to create a zone of high pressure directly behind, while a zone of relatively low pressure is formed above and in front. Direction is altered by unequal activity of the wings on the two sides. There is evidence that in steering, the frequency of vibration of the two wings remains the same but the amplitude of vibration is altered as required. Sudden sidewise movements are probably brought about by temporary cessation of action on one side altogether.

The rate of vibration has been estimated by (1) pitch of the sound produced, (2) tracing on a revolving kymograph, (3) motion-picture photography. In calculating motion from musical pitch, it should be remembered that each wing beat gives rise to two pressure waves so that a note equivalent to 600 cycles per second actually represents but 300 strokes of the wing.

Voss (1913) determined the number of vibrations for *Musca* as between 180 and 197 per second. The investigations of Marey (1901) had placed the count much higher, in the vicinity of 330. Weldon (1946) also quotes the higher figure, stating that the wing of the ordinary housefly beats "almost 20,000 times a minute." Chronographs of the wing vibrations of *Sarcophaga* give an average of 203 vibrations per second, with occasional rates as high as 400 for brief periods of time.

As for the speed that flies may attain when on the wing, it appears that the housefly is among the slower fliers of the insect world, since it travels usually at about two meters per second. This is roughly equivalent to 4.48 miles per hour, not a great deal faster than a horse can walk. Tabanid flies, on the other hand, have been clocked at 4 to 14 meters per second by various observers.

Hollick (1940, 1941) developed an ingenious device for studying the motions of flight in *Muscina stabulans*. The fly was held stationary and made to face air currents of measured velocity. In still air, the unmutilated fly moved the wing tip in the pattern of a modified ellipse, with one end attenuated and slightly hooked. With an air flow of 140 cm. per second, the stroke was definitely of the figure-8 type, the lower loop being perhaps twice as large as the upper. With air flowing into the face of the fly at the rate of 220 cm. per second, the figure-8 pattern became more symmetrical, with the upper loop, if anything, slightly the greater. The antennae were then removed and the tests repeated after an interval of 96 hours. The motion in still air was essentially the same as with the antennae intact. With an air flow of 140 cm. per second, the only change was a slight elongation of the ellipse, with the narrowed extremity more sharply hooked. With the air flowing at 220 cm. per second, a slight tendency to a figure-8 pattern was achieved; the upper loop, however, was exceedingly minute. Obviously the fly requires the sensory mechanism of the antennae in order to evaluate properly the fluctuations in air pressure and make appropriate modification in the motions of flight.

THE HALTERES AS ORGANS OF EQUILIBRIUM

The manner in which the halteres function in assisting equilibrium has been much disputed. Von Buddenbrock (1919, 1937) held that their function was purely of a stimulatory character. He considered that the chordotonal and campaniform sensillae which they carry are stimulated by their vibratory movements and that these stimuli facilitate the conduction of the reflexes concerned in flight. Fraenkel and Pringle, however (1938), consider that these

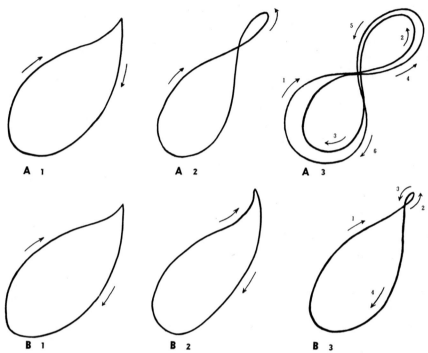

A 1   **A** 2   **A** 3

B 1   **B** 2   **B** 3

Figure 42. Wing stroke of fly held stationary. *A:* With antennae intact. *B:* Twenty-six hours after antennae were removed. *1,* in still air; *2,* facing an air flow of 140 cm. per second; *3,* facing an air flow of 220 cm. per second. (Modified from camera lucida drawings by Hollick, 1941.)

knobbed structures function as gyroscopic organs. They are set in motion whenever the insect walks or flies and stop when it stands still. The motion is up and down at right angles to the fly's body and involves from 160 to 210 vibrations per second. These motions alone do not affect the campaniform sensilla. Like any gyroscope the halter attempts to hold to the plane in which the fly is moving but, of course, is connected to the fly's body in such a way that it must turn as the fly turns. The halter offers a certain amount of resistance to such turning, and lateral shearing forces are set up in the cuticle at its base. These, in turn, affect the obliquely placed rows of elongated campaniform sense organs located there. By this means the fly is enabled to sense and control changes in direction. The fly can navigate rather well with only one halter, but is noticeably handicapped by loss of both. Fraenkel (1939) was able to offset this effect, however, by affixing a small piece of cotton to the tip of the abdomen. This seemed to stabilize the flight and to compensate more or less for the loss of equilibrium. Fraenkel considers that the loss in irritability and spontaneity evident in flies from which the halteres have just been removed is largely a shock effect.

A popular account of the gyroscopic action of a fly's halteres appeared in *Life* August 26, 1946. A more technical discussion will be found in the paper by Nageotte (1943), who suggests a functional parallel between the gyroscopic action of the halter and the semicircular canal system of vertebrate animals.

ALIGHTING ON INVERTED SURFACES

Early suggestions as to how the fly performs this feat fell under two heads. (1) The fly starts to loop the loop and, when inverted, finds its feet in contact with the ceiling. (2) The fly does a sidewise roll at the moment of contact. Blair (1942) offered a third explanation that differs from the first by assuming that the fly approaches the ceiling in the normal position with the front feet elevated. These, he believes, make the first contact and adhere to the surface by reason of their sticky pulvilli. Braking or perhaps merely closing of the wings then follows, the body being carried forward by residual momentum. This would bring the fly into the resting position, upside down and facing the direction from which it came. In approaching a vertical surface, a momentary hovering accompanied by clutching motions of the feet presumably suffices to effect a contact.

Ingenious as this explanation would seem, it is probably in error, as shown by recently successful slow-motion photography. E. D. Eyles (1945) of Kodak Research Laboratories, Harrow, England, made photographs at the rate of 1,500 exposures per second, at which speed the 100-foot length of 16-mm. film passed through the camera in a little more than two seconds. By projecting at the normal speed of sixteen frames per second, the motions were slowed down a hundredfold. The usual performance involved a "half-roll" with the fly coming to rest at an angle only slightly divergent from the original direction of flight.

Contact with solid objects is itself inhibitory to flight in many insects. Fraenkel (1932) observed that a suspended fly with wings vibrating immediately comes to rest if a little ball of cotton wool is placed between its feet. Contact with a single claw of one leg is sufficient to inhibit flight in *Musca*, but all such inhibition disappears if the tarsi are amputated.

MISCELLANEOUS CONSIDERATIONS RELATING
TO METABOLISM

Muscid larvae as they feed store energy both in the form of fat and in the form of glycogen. In some species, at least, the larvae are unable to utilize the glycogen as emergency food until they have attained the pupal state. In this connection Shelford (1929), citing Bernard (who studied *Musca lucilia*), points out that though their tissues contain glycogen, the larvae possess no enzyme that can hydrolyze it. However, as soon as they have transformed into chrysalids, a diastatic enzyme is produced. Thus the adult is provided with a quickly available form of food energy before its own feeding habits have become established. Flies, of course, are liquid feeders. According to the experiments of Wenyon and O'Connor (1917a, b), a fly can take in an average of 0.001 grams of fluid each half hour. Their method was to weigh a small quantity of feces on a cover glass and then allow starved flies to feed for half an hour upon it, after which the feces and cover glass were weighed again. Allowance was made for evaporation by two weighings of a control sample on which no flies were allowed to feed. Root (1921) used a different method. Flies in individual vials were starved from 17 to 21 hours, then transferred to a single vial and weighed. The flies were then returned to separate vials where they were allowed to feed on a diluted syrup. Finally all were transferred once more to the same single vial and weighed again. Subtraction gave the amount of syrup consumed and division by the number of flies gave the average. Houseflies starved 17 hours averaged an intake of 0.004 grams or 0.0039 cc.; those starved 21 hours, 0.007 grams or 0.0066 cc.

We thus see that the crop of the average fly actually holds very little, but due to the fact that the fly continually passes liquid feces, its water loss is enormous. This means that much fluid must be consumed, and the active fly seems to make a continuous effort to accomplish this. The liquid food first passes to the crop, from which it is transferred to the ventriculus as needed (Graham-Smith, 1934). Flies must drink frequently or die.

As for food materials other than water, Glaser (1923a) has pointed out that flies require both sugar and protein substances. Females fed on either without the other will not produce eggs. Roubaud (1922a) made similar observations.

All types of food must, of course, be either in solution or in the form of a finely divided suspension or emulsion. Bloodsucking species frequently produce a saliva that contains an anticoagulating principle, thus insuring a ready flow of liquid food. Although *M. domestica* will feed at open wounds, it is not a true bloodsucker and does not produce saliva of this sort. Cornwall and

Patton (1914) state that even among the bloodsucking Muscidae an anticoagulant may or may not occur. They found it absent in *Stomoxys* but definitely present in *Glossina*.

The behavior of flies is partially governed by the elapsed time since the insects were adequately fed. Thus Kerr (1948) demonstrated that the mortality of flies exposed to 0.1 and 0.2 per cent pyrethrins ran much higher among lots that had been starved for a few hours than among those that had enjoyed continuous access to food. Investigation showed this to be due to the fact that rapidity of flight increased with increasing starvation (at least up to two hours) and that this enabled the insects to acquire relatively greater amounts of the spray as they flew about in the Peet-Grady chamber, particularly since the proportion of flies in flight also increased with added starvation time. Consistent with these findings was the reduction of the mean interval for knockdown with the lengthening of the starvation period. Kerr pointed out that the generally practiced methods of handling flies preparatory to the testing of insecticides usually involve a variable period in which the insects receive no food. Since this could readily introduce variations in susceptibility of different samples, he suggested deliberate pretest starvation for controlled periods to increase (and make uniform) their susceptibility to official test insecticides.

OBSCURE EFFECTS OF TOXIC SUBSTANCES

Normal histological relations may be considerably altered by toxic substances. Such alterations have, in fact, been correlated with the action of certain insecticides, the practical value of which was recognized long before their physiological action came to be even slightly understood. Hartzell and Wexler, for example (1946), found that sesamin produced characteristic effects both in the brain and in the muscles of flies that had been affected beyond possibility of recovery. When stained with Delafield's hematoxylin and counterstained with eosin Y, the larger nerve cells of the brain showed marked vacuolation, while the muscle fibers showed accentuation of both nodes and Krause's membrane. Sesame oil in high concentration produced similar results. Pyrethrum also has a destructive effect upon nervous tissue, but affects the fiber tracts rather than the cell bodies. A proprietary compound, Improved Pyrin 20, affects tissues in much the same manner as sesamin and pyrethrum combined. It is known to contain both ingredients.

These results bear out the previous work of Hartzell and Scudder (1942) on pyrethrum and isobutyl undecylene amide. In these experiments pyrethrum was described as causing a widespread clumping of the chromatin of nerve-cell nuclei, while the activator caused a chromatolysis or dissolution of the chromatin. Hartzell and Strong (1944) record the alkaloid piperine as having a particularly destructive effect upon the fiber tracts along with vacuolization of the nerve tissue of the brain. A paper by Hartzell (1945) reported DDT as causing relatively slight changes of a histological character in proportion to the striking neurological effects it may produce.

Curiously enough, the larvae, in spite of their vulnerable appearance, are far more resistant to certain toxic substances than are the adult flies. Madden, Lindquist, and Jones (1947) ran a number of tests in which larvae of *M. domestica* were kept immersed in various solutions for periods of five seconds. Not one of thirty different solvents, for example, had their larvicidal properties increased by the addition of 5 per cent DDT! The latter substance was particularly noneffective in emulsified solutions. The larvae also proved exceedingly resistant to mercuric chloride, potassium hydroxide, ammonium hydroxide, and hydrochloric acid. It may be assumed that the integument of larvae furnishes mechanical protection against these substances.

Other physiological reactions of flies to repellents and insecticides, as well as to biological situations created by man with a view to species reduction, will be discussed in following chapters.

CHAPTER IV

Life History of the Fly

And the small gilded fly
Does lecher in my sight. Let copulation thrive!
—*Shakespeare,* King Lear

THE purpose of this chapter is to describe in sequence those changes that are passed through in the course of complete metamorphosis and to give such characteristics of the various stages as are not adequately treated in other chapters.

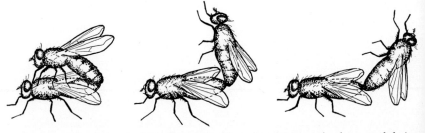

Figure 43. Copulation in houseflies. *Left:* Normal position; male above, and facing the same direction as female. *Center:* Rare position, occasionally seen when male is abnormally small. *Right:* Abnormal position due to loss of stability. (Modified from Hardy, 1944.)

MATING OF ADULTS

The mating of the housefly has been described by Réaumur (1738), Berlese (1902), and Hewitt (1914a). Actual copulation apparently never takes place in the air, though the seizure of the female by the male may occur in flight, after which the pair come rapidly to earth.

Houseflies copulate in the superimposed position with the male above the female and facing in the same direction. This method of coupling is required by the apparently rectilinear but actually "circumverted" terminalia characteristic of the muscoid group. (See Chapter II.) If the male is abnormally small, a position like that shown in Figure 43 (center) may sometimes be assumed. Only rarely and because of accidental loss of stability is a position similar to Figure 43 (right) occasionally observed. The superimposed position is referred to by Lamb (1922) as the "vertical pose." According to Hardy (1944), the simple "rectilinear" relation of the genitalia is normally associated in flies with "opposed" copulation, in which the sexes face in opposite directions. Only by an evolution of the male genital structures, in the nature of a rotation, has the superimposed position become natural or possible. A partially resolved rotation results in what may be called "curvilinear" genitalia, from which the completely reversed relationship, now found in higher muscoids, may be considered to have evolved. The accompanying diagrams adapted from Hardy show definitive relationships.

After seizure, the male caresses the head of the female with the fore tarsi. This may have a reflex effect, as the next step is normally the exsertion of her ovipositor to make contact with the genital atrium of the male. The accessory copulatory vesicles of the female then become turgid so that the female genital aperture is held in close contact with the terminal extremity of the penis, which extends downward from the roof of the genital atrium. Adjacent structures support the position of the essential organs until the spermatozoa have passed into the spermathecae of the female. The act requires from a few seconds to several minutes, during which time the male grasps the sides of the female with fore and middle legs. The tibiae and tarsi of the metathoracic pair are folded crosswise upon the ventral surface of the female's abdomen.

In nature, the sexes are usually about equal, but occasionally there is considerable departure from normal expectancy. It has been my observation that when the size of the average adult, in random sampling, runs small, the males will be more numerous, while if the average fly captured is of superior weight and size, such is never the case. This would appear to be in part an expression of the amount of food available during the larval state, especially so when nourishment is insufficient.

Thus Herms (1928), while studying *Lucilia sericata,* brought out the fact that an underfed larval population always yields a preponderance of males. He removed the larvae from food in lots of one hundred at six-hour intervals after allowing an initial feeding period of thirty hours. The longest feeding period allowed any lot was ninety-six hours. Those which enjoyed the longer feeding periods yielded a preponderance of female flies. As would be expected, the size became greater as the feeding period increased. Herms felt that larval females required more nourishment than males for their development and, therefore, perished in greater numbers when subjected to a starvation diet.

Deviations from a balanced sex ratio do not, however, constitute any significant impediment to species survival. An excess of males merely insures the fertilization of all females present. In the rare cases where females predominate, there is still a good chance that all will be fertilized, as an abundance of females is indicative of a vigorous population and it has been observed that well-nourished males show an inclination to copulate more than once. The great predominance of females at breeding grounds in the summer time, however (Herms 1911a), does not necessarily mean that all stand in need of fertilization. Many will have copulated elsewhere, later flying to the so-called breeding areas for oviposition. The males, not influenced by this chemotropism that impels their mates, tend to remain scattered wherever adult food materials are found. The somewhat greater longevity of the females may also be a factor in giving them a higher count.

OVIPOSITION

Egg laying begins from four to eight days after copulation. The instinct by which the female fly selects an appropriate substratum for the deposition of her ova, and by which the larval stages are guaranteed a developmental medium satisfactory for their nourishment, will be discussed in greater length in Chapter VII, which treats of the food requirements of flies. A few remarks, however, are desirable in this place.

Kalandadze and Chilingarova (1942b) studied the role of substrates in the oviposition and preimaginal development of *Musca* (*domestica*) *vicina,* in Georgia, U.S.S.R. Under insectary conditions, gravid females deposited more egg batches on sheep dung, provided it was fresh, than on any other type of manure available. After that, pig, horse, cow, and buffalo manure were chosen in the order named. (It is also of interest that the feeding preferences of the adults showed a similar order.) Liquid dung of any source was visited rarely, if at all. The experiments were carried out at an average temperature of 27°–29°C (80.6°–84°F) and a relative humidity of 51–61 per cent. Under these conditions, sheep dung and horse dung dried out rather rapidly and ceased to be attractive after about twenty-four hours. Buffalo and pig dung, however, continued to attract the flies for two or three days, and cow dung, being moister, for as long as five.

That the behavior of flies under insectary conditions is not always paralleled by their behavior in the field was brought out by a second series of experiments by the same workers in which open boxes containing the various media were set out at convenient points. Fresh material was added daily. Under these circumstances, the largest number of egg batches was found on pig manure, with sheep, horse, and buffalo dung following in the order named. Boxes containing yard sweepings attracted relatively few flies. It appears that under outdoor conditions, where the flies must come considerable distances to make use of isolated masses of breeding medium, odor is the principal factor in determining the direction of flight. Thus pig dung, which has the strongest odor, probably attracts ovipositing females from a larger area.

Insofar as temperature affects the ovipositional activity of flies, it is the temperature of the air rather than of the substratum which proves the deciding

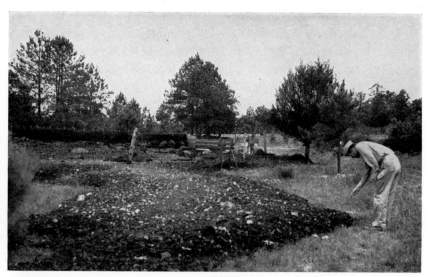

Figure 44. Oviposition in pig manure. Medical Corps officer is here shown demonstrating masses of fly eggs in a hogpen near Fort Jackson, South Carolina. (U.S. Army Photograph.)

factor. The above-mentioned workers state that all oviposition ceased at an atmospheric temperature of $10\,^{\circ}$C ($50\,^{\circ}$F) even though the upper layers of dung remained at $15\,^{\circ}$–$20\,^{\circ}$C ($59\,^{\circ}$–$68\,^{\circ}$F).

Related species do not always prefer identical media. Thus Golding (1946) found, by trapping, that *Musca domestica vicina* bred largely in latrines, trenching grounds, pits containing pig manure, and also in bedding, slaughterhouse refuse, and heaps of rotting food. *M. cuthbertsoni,* on the other hand, bred in cattle droppings, palm-kernel meal, and pig dung. *M. gabonensis* he records from heaps of cow manure.

By contrast, Thomson and Lamborn (1934) found that *Musca spectanda* laid its eggs solely on human excreta. In Egypt, Hafez (1939) reported

M. domestica vicina as utilizing horse dung in and near Cairo, and donkey dung in the country. Cow and buffalo dung were used rarely. He reports pig dung as more attractive than horse dung, but there were few pigs in that vicinity. Camel dung will be passed by if horse dung is available. The same author reports *M. sorbens* as breeding in horse dung, *M. vitripennis* in cow, *M. tempestiva* in cow (also possibly horse and camel), *M. crassirostris* in fresh cow dung, *M. larvipara* in cow (also possibly horse and donkey), and *M. vetustissima* chiefly in camel, with fresh cow dung a second choice.

The female fly is rather deliberate in depositing her eggs. She walks over the material that is to serve as food for her larvae, seeking crevices and cracks in which the ova may have a measure of protection. By action of certain muscles, she compresses her abdomen and the ovipositor shoots out. She then pushes or "worms" the ovipositor as far into the crevice as possible. One egg, or several, may be laid in a single spot, but all will be more or less hidden if opportunity permits. This habit is believed by Patton (1930) to give special protection against the ravages of certain ants, which devour the eggs whenever they can find them. When the physical nature of the medium permits, the fly crawls deep into the coarser crevices, so that she is quite out of sight while depositing her eggs. Eggs so located receive the maximum protection from desiccation and actinic light.

The number of eggs which mature in a fly's ovaries at one time varies between 100 and 150, with the average close to 120. It requires nearly a day for the female to deposit these, and if her ovipositional activities are disturbed, it may take longer. Occasionally all the eggs will be found deposited in a single mass, but more often they are distributed in a number of locations. In any one clump it is usual to find the eggs closely packed together and resting on their somewhat broader posterior ends. Each female, in her lifetime, is capable of developing from four to six batches of eggs, which she deposits at intervals of perhaps two weeks, the intensity of such activity depending on environmental factors.

Dissection of the female will reveal approximately how many batches of ova she has deposited. Kuzina (1942) reports that in the Muscidae a group of yellow bodies remains in the ovarioles (egg tubes), near the junction with the oviduct, after each batch has been extruded. The number of groups of yellow bodies are believed to correspond to the number of batches laid. This gives indirect information on the probable age of the fly, and may be significant in survey work. If all ovipositing females collected at a given time and place prove to be considerably aged, it is obvious that there must have been little or no production of new flies in that locality for several weeks.

DESCRIPTION OF THE EGG

The eggs are pearly white in color and measure approximately one milli-
meter in length. The greatest diameter, which is near the posterior end, measures a little more than one-fourth of the length. Both ends are bluntly rounded,
but the anterior is always more tapering. The chorion presents a polished
surface but on close examination shows a pattern of small hexagonal markings

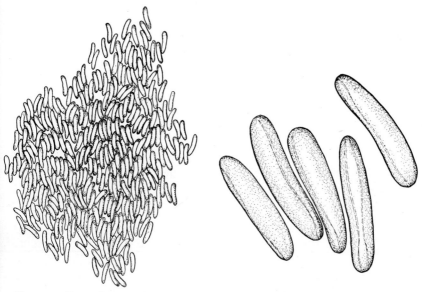

Figure 45. Eggs of *Musca domestica. Left:* Large mass, such as is sometimes deposited
by a single female. *Right:* A few eggs, greatly enlarged. Note reticulum formed by
anastomosing strands which make up the inner layer of the chorion.

reflecting presumably the cellular structure of the egg tube in which the ovum
developed. The dorsal side is easily recognized by the presence of two longitudinal, curved ridges that tend to diverge in the posterior portion but approach one another once more at the caudal end.

In *Lucilia,* Fish (1947–1948) states that the chorion consists of a smooth external layer and an internal layer composed of anastomosing strands. It is this
anastomosing structure that gives the impression of a network of polygons in
surface view. The vitelline membrane, which lies just beneath the chorion, is
in close contact with the latter except in the region of the two dorsal chorionic
folds. It is noncellular. Immediately beneath the vitelline membrane is found
the periplasm of the egg itself. This is protoplasmic in nature and slightly
thicker at the poles. It covers the reticular layer, which contains much yolk

material. Embedded in this and located approximately one-third of the distance from the anterior extremity is the egg nucleus, surrounded by a small amount of nuclear protoplasm. Recorded observations on the genus *Musca* seem to indicate essentially the same relationships.

EMBRYOLOGY

There is no modern monographic study of the early embryology of *Musca* comparable to the excellent work of Fish (1947–1948) on the Calliphorid species *Lucilia sericata* Meigen. The discussion that follows is drawn to a considerable extent from Fish's paper and should be considered a résumé of muscoid development in general rather than of *Musca* in particular. Statements concerning the later stages are adapted chiefly from *Embryology of Insects and Myriapods* by Johannsen and Butt (1941), who studied carefully all the important papers on muscoid embryology prior to that date.

Two features of the unfertilized egg should be mentioned before developmental changes are discussed. A special mass of protoplasm called the "oosome" is located in the dorsal portion of the periplasm near the posterior end. Its relation to the primordial germ cells will be treated later. The second feature relates to the character of the yolk in stained specimens. Such yolk consists of numerous spherical bodies interspersed with spheroid cavities from which the deutoplasm has presumably been dissolved out by the reagents used.

Sperm cells invade the eggs while the latter are still within the oviducts. It is believed that several sperm normally enter each egg through one or more micropyles situated near the anterior end. The actual union of gamete nuclei cannot, of course, take place until after maturation of the ovum, which normally occurs immediately following oviposition.

In maturation, the egg nucleus migrates dorsolaterally from its central position to fuse with the periplasm in the anterior third of the egg. After the reduction division, which appears to produce but a single polar body, the nucleus then migrates back toward the center of the egg where fertilization presumably occurs. The haploid number of chromosomes in *Musca domestica* is six; the diploid, twelve.

The zygote nucleus now proceeds to divide, producing two, four, and finally sixteen rather similar cells joined together by the egg reticulum. Synchronous division now gives way to random cleavage in which there is migration of cells anteriorly as well as posteriorly and laterally. There are still no cell walls and the arrangement is that of a syncytium. The more peripheral cells soon manifest a triangular outline and penetrate the periplasm, blunt edge foremost. The more interior cells, which remain rounded, return into the yolk.

Fish refers to these as *primary* yolk cells but points out later that this is perhaps a misnomer, as true primary yolk cells, such as occur in the honeybee, never migrate from their central position; in other words, they remain *in situ* where produced. In the posterior region, several of the migrating cells finally penetrate the oosome, causing this body to break up into a number of dark, circular masses. These protrude somewhat from the surface of the egg and constitute the anlage of the future fly's primordial germ cells. The time required for development up to this point is approximately two hours.

The peripheral cellular layer is at first called a *blastema*. Shallow clefts now appear extending inward from the outer surface and dividing the syncytium into a number of irregular cell compartments. The next nuclear divisions nearly obliterate these, but others soon appear, and by a succession of nuclear divisions and attempts at cell division, together with the appropriation of additional protoplasm and yolk material from the interior, a definite conspicuous layer of cells, the *blastoderm,* is finally established. The cells making up this primary epithelium at first have no walls on their interior surface. These are added later. There is no evidence (in *Lucilia*) of the anterior poles manifesting any more rapid development of blastoderm than the posterior. Fish states that the rate of germ cell formation closely parallels the rate of blastodermal cell development.

In muscoids, the blastoderm tends to close in somewhat beneath the germ cells, but the closure is incomplete, resulting in a funnel-shaped aperture from the margin of which a number of nuclei migrate inward to become yolk cells.

The primary epithelium of the lateral and dorsal surfaces next becomes thinner, forming the serosal envelope, while the ventral portion, which retains its full thickness, becomes transformed into the so-called "germ band." At either pole, the germ band continues more or less around the egg, but the middle section, which becomes divided transversely into six elements, is relatively narrow, being bounded by two curving longitudinal lines. The anterior piece is divided by a curving transverse furrow into two parts. The middle section then begins to sink below the level of the surface, where its more interior layer proceeds to differentiate as mesoderm. The anterior and posterior portions of the germ band soon give rise to the epithelial rudiments of the mid-gut. By deepening of a longitudinal ventral furrow, the mesodermal tissue becomes tubular.

Lengthening of the tubular mesoderm, together with the over-all growth of the embryo, results in the posterior portion of the mid-gut, together with the germ cells, being pushed around to the dorsal side. The same factors cause the transverse furrows, which have deepened somewhat, to assume an oblique direction. In Muscidae, this is the only indication of rotation. The anterior converging folds elongate and come closer together. The posterior transverse furrow, carried by the dorsally migrating posterior portion of the germ band, eventually becomes longitudinal, with the two branches fusing into one. It is just anterior to this that the ectoderm invaginates transversely, thus giving rise to the amniotic fold.

The further elongation of the mesoderm tube is accompanied by the pressing of the caudal extremity so far into the interior that the two ends of the tube lie nearly parallel. The lumen of the mesoderm tube will by this time have become obliterated. This is followed by the formation of lateral mesodermal clefts that represent the future body cavity. The somatic mesoderm eventually differentiates into the numerous muscles of the body wall. The splanchnic mesoderm becomes associated with the mid-gut and later differentiates into longitudinal and transverse muscle fibers. The latter process may not be completed until after hatching.

Parallel to the long axis of the egg (and at right angles to the amniotic cavity) the proctodaeum develops. At its inner extremity, the Malpighian tubules are represented by dorsal and ventral diverticula. This portion soon fuses with the posterior mesenteron.

By this time the germ band will have reached its greatest length; the head and tail of the embryo lie close together, and the amniotic invagination is just posterior to the head lobes as viewed from the dorsal side. In *Calliphora vomitoria,* six pairs of spiracles are visible in dorsal view, while a distinct segmentation marks the ventral surface. The stomodaeal invagination is also in evidence at this time. It soon impinges upon the anterior mesenteron rudiment, and the oesophageal valve is formed by the invagination of the smaller oesophagus into the larger mid-gut.

Meantime a general shortening of the embryo is taking place. When completed, this results in the anal structures once again coming to lie in the posterior extremity of the egg. Prior to this stage, anterior and posterior mesenteron rudiments will each have developed a pair of apical branches. In the shortened embryo, the branches of the posterior rudiment come to extend forward, and thus find themselves in position to fuse with the anterior pair. The "mesenteron ribbons," so formed, soon widen and fuse together to form the epithelium of the mid-gut, which thus encloses most of the yolk. All this takes place after the appearance of the mesodermal clefts.

It should be mentioned that some of the germ cells, which were carried dorsally by the early elongation of the germ band, migrate through the posterior mesenteron rudiment to a definitive location in the interior of the egg.

The nervous system is first indicated by the appearance of scattered neuroblasts, some of which arise from the inner surface of head lobe ectoderm while others make their appearance along either side of the median ventral neural groove. The arrangement is segmental. Brain, suboesophageal ganglion, and cord all differentiate more or less simultaneously from the ventral ectoderm. Cross commissures and intersegmental connectives are soon established. At first the cord extends nearly the full length of the body, but by the time hatching takes place, considerable cephalization will have occurred. This results in termination of the cord about halfway between the cephalic and caudal extremities of the embryo. Still further shortening occurs during the first larval stage.

HATCHING

The time required for the completion of embryonic development varies greatly with the temperature. Hewitt (1914a) states that two or three days may be required if the temperature remains as low as 10°C (50°F). Between

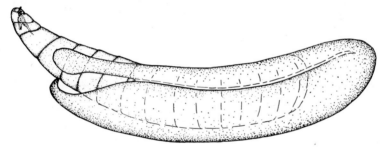

Figure 46. First-stage maggot emerging from egg. The rupture of the chorion follows the path of the curving ribs.

15°C and 20°C (59°–68°F), however, hatching takes place usually within twenty-four hours after oviposition, while at higher temperatures, such as 25°C to 35°C (77°–95°F), from eight to twelve hours may suffice. Béclard (1858) claimed that housefly eggs developed more rapidly under blue or violet light than under white, yellow, green, or red.

The actual process of hatching is rather simple. A slit appears on the dorsal side of the egg just lateral to the anterior extremity of one of the curving ribs mentioned earlier. This slit is extended posteriorly as the larva crawls out, anterior end foremost. Not infrequently the split continues around the anterior extremity and follows the second rib posteriorly. (See Figure 46.) After the emergence of the larva, the chorion usually undergoes collapse.

THE LARVA

The larva, or maggot, passes through three stages or instars. This means that it molts twice in the course of development, with distinctive changes of structure at each ecdysis. In the Muscidae, rate of growth agrees fairly well with Przibram's rule (Teissier, 1931), which holds that in most insects an increase of 25 per cent in the length of the rigid parts of the cuticle is achieved with each successive molt. There is no histological basis for this, however, as Pérez' (1910) studies on the blowfly and Alpatov's observations on *Drosophila* (1929) have shown that larval cells no longer divide after the embryonic period; they merely increase in size.

All stages have twelve easily recognized segments, of which the second, or postoral, segment is really double, giving a total of thirteen (Hewitt, 1914a). There are no eyes, legs, antennae, or other appendages. In the first-stage larva, only the two posterior spiracles are present. These are situated on the obliquely truncate posterior end. Each consists of a pair of small, slitlike apertures on a slight prominence. After the first molt, the slits become larger and more conspicuous. The posterior spiracles of the *third* stage each have three strongly sinuous slits surrounded by a heavily chitinized ring with a conspicuous, perforated button that extends inward from the mesial side. Second- and third-stage larvae have anterior spiracles as well.

First-stage larvae have been known to molt anywhere from twenty hours to four days after hatching, depending on environmental conditions. Not only is the general integument cast off, but the lining of the proctodaeum and stomodaeum as well, together with the cephalopharyngeal sclerites. The second instar requires from twenty-four hours to several days to complete development, while the third stage feeds from three to nine days before undergoing pupation.

Larsen and Thomsen (1940) made daily weighings during the preimaginal period and constructed weight curves to represent the rapidity of growth. *Musca domestica* grows rapidly as compared with other species, its weight being multiplied by fifty-four in the course of four days at 25°C (77°F). There is a conspicuous loss of weight after the larvae cease to feed, due, it is believed, to a particular water output from the larva.

A very careful study of the early larval stages of several muscoid flies was made by Tao (1927), whose descriptions of the first- and second-stage maggots of *Musca domestica* are reproduced herewith.

FIRST-STAGE LARVA

The first four segments of the larva are not provided with spines. From the fifth to the twelfth segment, there is a transverse, fusiform, swollen area provided with spines ventrally occupying the anterior third of the segment. At the posterior end of the sixth and seventh segments, there is one row of spines ventrally pressed against the spinose area of the following segment. These spines increase to three rows on segments eight through twelve. There are five short rows of spines dorsal to the anal opening. The spines are of various shapes—triangular, dome-shaped, and wedge-shaped. *Cephalopharyngeal sclerites:* Anterior to the median hook, between the median hook and the denticles, there are two pairs of poorly chitinized structures, a dorsal long, slender longitudinal pair and a ventral square pair. The lateral plates of the pharyngeal sclerites are narrow. The dorsal arch widens in the middle. The ventral prolongations are long and slender and end in points. The parastomal sclerites are long and slender. The hypostomal sclerite is composed of two parallel processes articulated to a transverse plate posteriorly. The pharyngeal sclerites are continuous ventrally with the floor of the pharynx.

SECOND-STAGE LARVA

The anterior spiracles are composed of six to eight branches. Spines are un-chitinized. At the anterior ends of segments two through five, there is a complete, spinose ring. From the sixth to twelfth segment at the anterior end, there is a ventral transverse swollen spinose area, which, continued laterally and dorsally by a single row of spines, forms a complete ring. The posterior ventral rows of spines in this stage are found on the fifth to the twelfth segments. *Cephalopharyngeal sclerites:* Three pairs of hooks replace the single median hook, a dorsal longitudinal pair, a ventral longitudinal pair, and a posterior transverse pair. The lateral plates of the pharyngeal sclerites become considerably broader. The dorsal arch becomes very broad near the middle and narrows toward both ends where they articulate with the lateral plates. The arch is deeply incised anteriorly at the middle. The anterior edge of the arch is uneven. The network structure of the arch serves to differentiate the family Muscidae from the Calliphoridae. The ventral prolongations are connected ventrally by a rectangular plate, the ventral crosspiece. The parastomal sclerites disappear entirely. The hypostomal sclerite is composed of two winglike plates, connected from the antero-ventral edges in the ventro-median line with two slender processes.

THIRD-STAGE LARVA

This is the maggot that even the casual observer is sure to see. It eventually comes to measure a good twelve millimeters or a little more. The broad posterior extremity is obliquely truncate and bears the two heavily chitinized posterior spiracles, which are separated from each other by a distance less than the diameter of either spiracle. The spiracles are D-shaped, with the straight margins that are innermost more closely approximated above than below. To an uninstructed observer, the spiracles look more like two black eyes! In posterior view, one notes the mid-ventral incision on the last segment, representing the anal aperture. The right and left anal lobes are useful in locomotion. Above and behind the anus is a pad or swelling corresponding to the spiniferous pads of more anterior segments.

In lateral view, the larva is found to consist of twelve apparent segments of which the second is somewhat constricted and proves, on study of internal musculature, to consist of two. The total number of segments is, therefore, considered as thirteen. The first larval segment, which Henneguy (1904)

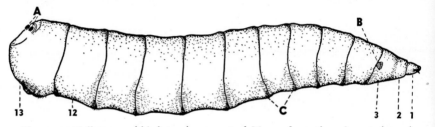

Figure 47. Full-grown (third-stage) maggot of *Musca domestica. A,* posterior spiracles; *B,* anterior spiracle; *C,* locomotor pads; *1, 2, etc.,* segments of the body.

called the "pseudo-cephalon," is very small. It bears ventrally the mouth aperture, which is so deeply situated that the segment itself may be said to consist of two oral lobes united posteriorly and on the dorsal side. Posterior to the mouth is a rectangular unit called the lingual process. Its anterior margin is slightly bilobed. In front of the mouth and extending forward and downward is the mandibular sclerite. This bears distally two mouth hooks, of which the right is strong and conspicuous while the left is small and obscure. Its reduced condition is characteristic of the genus *Musca.* The mandibular sclerite, which is capable of retraction, is but the visible extremity of the rather elaborate cephalopharyngeal skeleton that extends well into segment 4 and is composed of a number of closely united chitinous parts. Each oral lobe bears at its forward extremity (and dorsal to the mandibular sclerite) two short fleshy processes or tubercles, one above the other. These are undoubtedly sensory in function, though such a specific designation as "optic" tubercles (Hewitt, 1914a) might be questioned. Weismann (1863–1864a,b) called the lower tubercles "maxillentaster" and the upper pair "antennae." On the lateral surface of each oral lobe are many sinuously vertical, parallel lines, each of

which represents a food channel leading to the mouth. One side of each channel is raised slightly, thus overhanging the margin or flange of the opposite
side. By this the channels are made to resemble tubes rather than open troughs.
Many of the channels unite distally and all converge before emptying into the
mouth. Thus they perform a function equivalent to that of the pseudotracheae
of the adult fly.

The most plausible interpretation of the anterior structures, just discussed,

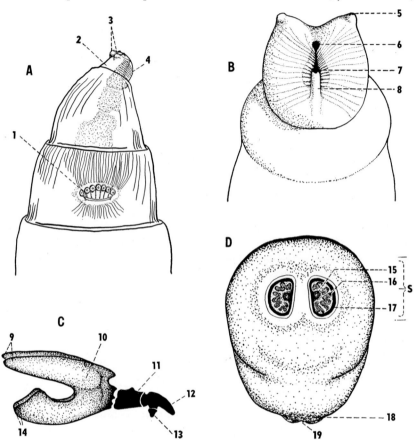

Figure 48. Special structures of third-stage larva. *A:* Anterior segments, lateral view.
B: Anterior segments, ventral view. *C:* Cephalopharyngeal skeleton, lateral view. *D:*
Thirteenth segment, posterior view. *1,* anterior spiracle; *2,* pseudocephalon; *3,* sensory
lobes (upper); *4,* food channel; *5,* sensory lobes (lower); *6,* mandibular sclerite (terminal
view); *7,* mouth; *8,* lingual process; *9,* dorsal cornua; *10,* pharyngeal sclerite; *11,* hypostomal sclerite: *12,* mandibular sclerite (lateral view); *13,* dental sclerite; *14,* ventral
cornua; *15,* button; *16,* slits; *17,* chitinous ring; *18,* supra-anal pad; *19,* anal opening;
S, parts of spiracle. (B, adapted from Hewitt, *The House-Fly* [Cambridge University
Press, 1914].)

is that the greater portion of the true cephalic segment has been retracted within the head. The cephalopharyngeal skeleton already mentioned is a residual part of this segment. It consists of seven recognizable sclerites of which the mandibular has already been mentioned. Somewhat ventral to its base are the much smaller dentate sclerites, one on either side. The hypostomal sclerite lies directly posterior to the mandibular and articulates with it. It consists of two irregular lateral masses of chitin united by a ventral bar. Most conspicuous are the two large pharyngeal sclerites, each of which articulates anteriorly with one wing of the hypostomal. The two pharyngeal sclerites are united dorsally in their anterior portions by the dorsopharyngeal sclerite, which may sometimes appear to be fused with them. Each pharyngeal sclerite can be described as a vertical triangular plate, narrowest in front and broadest behind. The posterior portion is deeply notched for the passage of the pharyngeal trachea and pharyngeal nerves. The ventral margins are continuous with the floor of the pharynx. The pharyngeal sclerites vary considerably in thickness at different points.

The second and third larval segments, which together constitute the "post-cephalic" segment of certain authors, comprise a conical unit approximately two and a half times the length of segment 1. The anterior portion (Newport's segment) is covered with minute, backwardly directed spines. The posterior portion (body segment 3) is most conspicuous for the spiracular processes, one on either side, which extend forward from the segment's posterior margin. These are termed "anterior spiracular processes" to distinguish them from the "posterior spiracles" on segment 13. Each process consists of a somewhat flat, fan-shaped structure bearing distally from six to eight terminal palpiform elements. Each of these palpiform processes is perforated by a pore. The channels that lead inward are lined with cuticular processes, the function of which is believed to be the arrest of solid particles. Air from the several palpiform processes passes next through a "felted chamber" in the body of the spiracular process to the longitudinal tracheal trunk. This so-called felted chamber derives its name from the fact that the lumen is traversed by a reticulum of chitinous threads, derived from the intima of its walls.

From segment 4 through segment 9, the gradual increase in diameter is well marked. The next three segments (10–12) show less of this, but the thirteenth is distinctly larger than all others. From the sixth to the twelfth segments, the forward portion of the ventral surface of each is characterized by the presence of a cresent-shaped locomotor pad, the surface of which is covered by minute recurved spines. The twelfth segment has in addition a similar pad near its posterior margin. The postanal pad on segment 13 has already been mentioned.

The larval integument consists of a layer of stellate hypodermal cells overlaid by a fairly thick dermis and a much thinner epidermis. The latter stains very readily with ordinary dyes. In nature, the entire cuticula is so transparent that many of the internal organs are visible from without. As the third-stage larva grows older, however, its fat body becomes larger and imparts to the maggot a creamy or yellowish appearance. For this reason, few or no internal structures can be recognized in a larva that is about to pupate.

INTERNAL ORGANIZATION OF THE LARVA

Space does not permit a full description of larval anatomy. Hewitt (1914a) has given a complete account of the internal structure with special emphasis on the musculature, which he worked out in great detail. The following summary is here included with the principal objective of aiding students who may have difficulty in gaining access to Hewitt's work, now long out of print.

Musculature and Locomotion

The muscles of the body walls may each extend over several segments, but are quite consistently attached to the body wall at the junctions of all segments concerned. The various groups are well shown in Figure 49. The cephalopharyngeal muscles, because of the retraction of the head structures, are rather complicated in their arrangement and require special study before their functions can be clearly understood. Figure 50 shows the position of the four essential groups. Tables 2 and 3 have been devised as a means of conveying a maximum amount of information with economy of space.

The recti muscles of the second and third segments are reduced to four pairs. The manner in which the lateral and external muscles are attached to the body walls of this region was accepted by Hewitt as evidence that two segments are here involved.

The locomotion of the footless larva can be surprisingly rapid, and is believed to be accomplished as described below.

The mandibular sclerite is thrust forward by action of the mandibular extensor muscles. At the same time, the entire anterior end of the larva is extended through contraction of the pharyngeal protractors. Next, the mandibular sclerite is anchored to the substratum by action of the mandibular depressors. A wave of contraction then passes the length of the maggot, from front to rear. The large cephalic retractor muscles initiate this, but its propulsion depends upon the co-operation of the ventral oblique muscles, ventrolateral obliques, internal lateral obliques, and chiefly the dorsolateral group.

As each segment moves into its new position, it establishes anchorage with the substratum by means of its ventral spiniferous pad.

As soon as the last segment has moved up, the mandibular sclerite reaches out once more, and a wave of extension passes backward, each segment in turn reducing its diameter and thereby increasing its length. This is accomplished by action of the lateral and intersegmental muscles. The combined elonga-

Table 2. Muscles of the body wall. The second and third segments are omitted.

Group	Special information	Function
Dorsolateral oblique recti	1. External 4 pairs—segments 6–12 5 pairs—segments 4–5 2. Internal 6 pairs—segments 4–5 4 pairs—segments 6–12	Contract larval body by bringing together the intersegmental rings
Longitudinal ventrolateral	1. Broad, ventral 2 pairs—segments 4–12 2. Narrow, lateral 2 pairs—segments 6–12 1 pair—segment 5 none—segment 4	
Ventrolateral oblique	1 pair—segments 6–12	
Internal lateral oblique	1 pair—segments 6–12	
Ventral oblique (number variable)	2 pairs—segment 4 4 pairs—segment 5 5 pairs—segment 7 7 pairs—segment 10 8 pairs—segment 11 6–7 pairs—segment 12	Bring forward the ventral spiniferous pads
Lateral	3 pairs—segments 4–12	Increase length of larva by drawing dorsal and ventral regions together
Lateral intersegmental	8 pairs—vertical, between segments 4–12	Increase length of larva by reducing size of intersegmental ring
Muscles of the last body segment (13)	Recti	Shorten segment
	Anal	Elevate anal lobes
	Dorsoventral	Lengthen segment

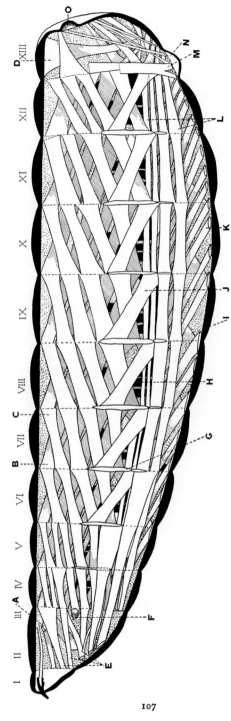

Figure 49. Body-wall muscles of mature larva. Right side, interior view. *A*, stomal dilator; *B*, external dorsolateral oblique rectus; *C*, internal dorsolateral oblique rectus; *D*, dorsoventral muscle; *E*, cephalic retractors; *F*, trachea serving anterior spiracle; *G*, lateral intersegmental muscle; *H*, laterals (in black); *I*, ventrolateral oblique; *J*, internal lateral oblique; *K*, ventral oblique; *L*, longitudinal ventrolateral; *M*, anal muscle; *N*, anal lobe; *O*, posterior spiracle. (Adapted from Hewitt, *The House-Fly* [Cambridge University Press, 1914].)

Table 3. Cephalopharyngeal muscles.

Group	Special information	Function
Cephalic retractors (all inserted on cephalic ring, anterior margin segment 2)	1 ventral pair, from posterior margin segment 6; 1 ventral pair (double) from posterior margin segment 5; 2 smaller pairs from posterior margin segment 3	Draw anterior end of larva (and pharyngeal mass) deeper into body
Protractors (inserted posterior extremity pharyngeal mass)	1 pair, dorsal, segment 3; 1 pair, ventral, segment 3	Extension of first segment
Depressors (dorsal to pharynx)	1 pair, from intersegmental ring (3–4) to pharyngeal mass	Depresses anterior sclerites by raising posterior extremity of pharyngeal mass
Mandibular extensors	1 pair from dorsal wall segment 3 to mandibular sclerite	Elevates and extends mandibular sclerite
Mandibular depressors	1 pair with 3 roots on posterior ventral process of pharyngeal sclerites; insertion, ventral process of dentate sclerite	Depresses mandibular sclerite by leverage of dentate
Stomal dilators (inserted on lateral surface of hypostomal sclerite)	2 dorsal pairs, from intersegmental ring (3–4) 2 ventral pairs: 1 from posterior dorsal process of pharyngeal sclerite; 1 from ventral process of pharyngeal sclerite	Regulate flow of food and saliva into pharynx by controlling anterior pharyngeal aperture
Oblique pharyngeal muscles	Several pairs in two bands; from lateral plates, ventrally and posteriorly to roof of pharynx	Draw liquid food into anterior portion of pharynx by raising and lowering the roof
Elongate oblique muscles	2 pairs from dorsal edges of lateral plates to roof of pharynx	Same as above; in more posterior region of the pharynx
Semicircular dorsal muscles	Several pairs; lie dorsolaterally upon pharyngeal wall	Favor peristalsis by rendering floor of pharynx more concave

tion of all the segments while the last remains stationary carries the mandibular sclerite far forward, where it proceeds to effect a second anchorage. By successive repetitions of this performance, the maggot makes continuous progress.

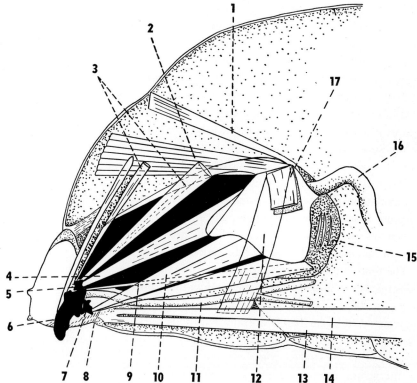

Figure 50. Muscles of the cephalopharyngeal sclerites of a mature larva. Left lateral aspect. *1*, right pharyngeal depressor; *2*, dorsal cephalic protractor; *3, 4,* stomal dilators; *5,* hypostomal sclerite; *6,* mandibular sclerite; *7,* dentate sclerite; *8,* cephalic ring; *9,* stomal dilator; *10,* mandibular depressor; *11,* salivary duct; *12,* ventral cephalic protractor; *13, 14,* ventral cephalic retractors; *15,* floor of posterior portion of pharynx; *16,* oesophagus; *17,* ventral cephalic protractors. (Redrawn from Hewitt, *The House-Fly* [Cambridge University Press, 1914].)

The Digestive Tract and Its Appendages

The alimentary canal of the third-stage larva is considerably longer than the larva itself. This is due chiefly to the excessive length of the mesenteron or mid-gut, which doubles back and forth upon itself in elaborate fashion.

Beginning at the anterior end is the mouth aperture, which opens on the ventral surface between the oral lobes. This is followed by the muscular pharynx, the greater anterior portion of which lies within the pharyngeal sclerites. The posterior extremity of the pharynx opens upward into the oesophagus, which passes through the nerve ring and extends backward to the posterior margin of segment 6. The next unit is the proventriculus, a short, thick-walled structure into which a portion of the oesophagus is invaginated. All parts listed thus far pertain to the stomodaeum and are lined with a chitinous intima, the reflected cuticle of the body wall. A small ring of deeply staining cells at the anterior extremity of the proventriculus is thought to represent the proventriculus of the adult fly. Two large salivary glands lie laterally in segments 5 and 6. The two slender salivary ducts pass forward and fuse in segment 3 to form a single channel. This opens into the pharynx from below, just posterior to the mouth. It is believed that the saliva not only aids in digestion but also serves to make the food more fluid. There is no crop in housefly larvae.

The mesenteron, or ventriculus, has no internal intima. Neither is there a peritrophic membrane. The anterior portion bears four tubular caeca, a feature not found in the adult. The point of juncture with the hind intestine, which lies in segment 10, is marked by the presence of the Malpighian tubes, four in number, which arise by bifurcation of the original two.

The hind intestine or proctodaeum consists of two parts. The first, or true intestine, which is of smaller diameter than the ventriculus, runs forward two segments, then turns and extends backward along the ventral body wall. In segment 10 it again bends dorsally and runs backward to the caudal extremity before turning downward toward the rectum. This second and last portion of the proctodaeum is short and muscular. It terminates in the anus on the ventral side of segment 13. Like the foreintestine, the entire proctodaeum is lined with a chitinous intima, continuous with the external cuticula. This is thickest in the rectal portion.

Respiratory Structures

From the posterior spiracles, there extend forward two longitudinal tracheal trunks, each of which finally terminates in the anterior spiracular process of its own side. At its origin, each of these trunks appears double due to the presence of a large lateral branch that soon bends ventrally, then passes beneath the principal trunk to serve the central visceral mass. These visceral branches come to an end in segment 7. The longitudinal trunks give off a dorsal and a ventral branch in practically every segment. The former supply the fat body; the latter, the visceral organs. Both send branches to the body wall. Two cross commissures connect the longitudinal trunks. The posterior of these lies just ahead of the posterior spiracles. The anterior, which passes above the oesophagus, is found in segment 4. Special branches in this vicinity supply air to the oral lobes, nerve ganglia, and pharyngeal mass.

Nervous System

The central nervous system of muscoid maggots shows an extreme degree of cephalization. A single large ganglionic mass, showing little evidence of segmentation, occupies portions of segments 5 and 6. The dorsal portion of the anterior part consists of two nearly spherical cerebral lobes. These are united above, but separate ventrally to create a foramen through which passes the oesophagus. The principal (ventral) mass of the ganglion gives rise to three groups of nerves. The first group consists of eleven pairs, two of which arise anteriorly, the other nine laterally. These represent the eleven pairs of original ganglia, which have become fused. The second group consists of three pairs that branch off from stalks leading to the imaginal discs of the pro- and mesothorax. The last group includes the so-called accessory nerves, which consist of one paired and two unpaired nerves arising from the median dorsal line.

The entire ganglionic mass is enclosed in a capsular sheath, richly supplied with tracheae and continuous with the outer sheath of the peripheral nerves.

The principal unit of the visceral nervous system is a small ganglion lying upon the oesophagus opposite the posterior portion of the cerebral lobes. From this ganglion, a fine nerve runs forward toward the pharynx. Another, after joining with a delicate nerve from each of the cerebral lobes, extends dorsally toward the anterior extremity of the aorta. A third follows the median dorsal line of the oesophagus to its posterior extremity, where it passes into a tiny ganglion from which fibers extend over the anterior portion of the proventriculus.

The Haemocoel

The body cavity is incompletely divided into two portions, the great ventral sinus and the dorsal pericardial sinus. The two communicate through a passage bounded by pericardial cells. In the pericardial sinus lies the cylindrical heart or dorsal vessel, which extends from the posterior tracheal commissure to a point opposite the cerebral lobes in segment 5. The posterior portion, or true heart, consists of three lineal chambers incompletely separated from one another by slight indentations that mark the location of the three pairs of valvular ostia. Through these blood enters from the pericardium. The heart is supported by three pairs of alar muscles. Leading forward from the heart is the tapering dorsal aorta. Both heart and aorta have transverse and longitudinal muscle fibers in their walls.

The aorta terminates in segment 5 in a somewhat circular structure known as Weismann's ring, which is connected with the principal imaginal cephalic discs.

The Imaginal Discs

The imaginal discs represent embryonic tissue that has been set aside, either before hatching or during larval development, to provide for structures peculiar to the adult fly. Most, if not all, arise as invaginations of the hypodermis, with which they sometimes remain connected by a stalk. Some have nervous connections and most of them are intimately served by tracheae. According to position, the discs are designated as cephalic, thoracic, and abdominal. The last are small and not easily distinguished, but the cephalic and thoracic are relatively easy to see in sectioned material. Each disc is enclosed in a sheath from which it everts during metamorphosis. The cephalic discs, of which there are several pairs, evert along a cord of cells attached to the dorsal wall of the anterior portion of the pharynx. They produce the head capsule with all its external features, including antennae and proboscis. The thoracic discs, which number five pairs (prothoracic, ventral mesothoracic, dorsal mesothoracic or alar, dorsal metathoracic, and ventral metathoracic), produce the entire skeletal structure of the thorax including the halteres, wings, and legs.

Pupation

The process of pupation consists of a general contraction of the larva within its own integument so that the latter comes to form a cylindrical puparium, in normal specimens about 6.3 mm. in length. The puparium shows a slight gradual increase in diameter from front to rear, except that both ends are bluntly rounded. The entire process may be completed in as brief a period as six hours, during which time the integument gradually darkens. Its definitive color is a rich, dark brown.

Since the pupal case is formed by the last larval skin, the pupa within is said to be *coarctate.*

There is undoubtedly a special stimulus of a hormone character which induces pupation in the third-stage larva. That this function is localized is indicated by the fact that extirpation of the cells of "Weismann's ring," which are believed to represent modified *corpora allata,* prevents pupation altogether. In testing this DeBach (1939) ligatured mature larvae anterior to the fifth segment (sense of Hewitt, 1914a). The segments posterior to the ligature underwent transformation; those anterior did not. When, however, the ligature was placed on segment 6, pupation took place anterior to this point. The hormone is apparently secreted from a very definite region of the body. Even the ligature on segment 5 did not prevent transformation of the anterior segments if delayed beyond a certain "critical" period, indicating that the hormone had, by that time, already been secreted into the blood. This critical period extends from 25 to 15 hours before pupation, the average being 20. The hormone nature of the stimulus for pupation is further substantiated by the work of Fraenkel (1935), who showed that cutting important nerve trunks does not prevent pupation, providing circulation of the haemolymph is properly maintained.

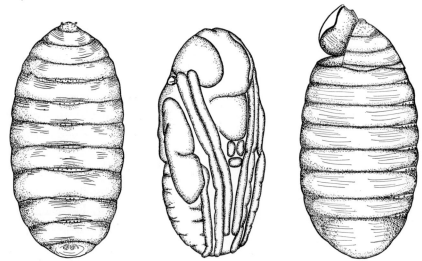

Figure 51. The pupal stage. *Left:* Puparium, dorsal surface. *Center:* Pupa, showing various structures of the adult fly. *Right:* Puparium open at anterior extremity after emergence of imago.

The hardening of the cuticle of the third-stage larva to form the protective puparium is a rather complex phenomenon that has only in recent years received adequate explanation. Pryor (1940), who had previously studied the hardening of the ootheca in the cockroach, followed the process in *Calliphora erythrocephala,* where he believes the steps to be as follows:

A dihydroxyphenol and a water-soluble protein are first secreted by the hypodermis into the outer layers of the cuticle. The protein then reacts with oxidation products of the dihydroxyphenol to form a rigid type of protein called *sclerotin,* very resistant to most enzymes and chemical reagents. This may be described as a "tanning" process. Essentially the same reaction takes place in the epicuticle, a layer that is first secreted as a protein membrane. In addition, the epicuticle later becomes impregnated with lipids that undergo the oxidation and polymerization necessary to render them insoluble in fat solvents. The phenol involved in sclerotin formation is very probably dihydroxyphenyl-acetic acid, produced in the hypodermis by deaminization of the blood phenol, dihydroxyphenyl-alanine.

External characters of the puparium are as follows: The posterior spiracles of the larva are represented by two flat, buttonlike prominences at the posterior end. Only twelve segments are recognizable due to the fact that the pseudocephalon is completely withdrawn. This causes the anterior spiracular processes to lie almost at the anterior end. The ventral surface may be recognized by the persistent spiny locomotor pads. An obscure pair of pupal spiracles make their appearance in the conjunctiva between the fifth and sixth visible segments, on the dorsal side. These appear to be the pupa's single source of air, as the larval spiracles connect only with the now-discarded tracheal system of the third-stage maggot. These larval tracheal trunks, which have been withdrawn from the interior of the pupa, lie pressed against the inner surface of the pupal case along with the lining of the proctodaeum and stomodaeum including the cephalopharyngeal sclerites.

DEVELOPMENT OF THE PUPA

Within forty-eight hours, under reasonably favorable conditions, most of the essential structures of the adult fly can be accounted for. The wing pads, legs, and proboscis are all distinct, and the segmentation of the abdomen is very clear. All parts are enclosed in a semitransparent nymphal sheath, through which may be observed the antennal rudiments and the large, hemispherical, compound eyes. The future prothoracic spiracles of the fly are represented by knoblike processes that connect with the thoracic spiracles of the puparium, already mentioned. As the hours pass, the three segments of the antennae, the facial ridges, the maxillary palpi, the tapering labium, and bulbous oral lobes become clearly differentiated. The portion of the nymphal sheath which encloses the wing does not increase in size beyond a certain point, requiring the wing to become folded, especially on the distal third.

Development in the pupal stage is usually a little slower than in the larval, as there is a tendency for the third-stage maggots to seek a somewhat cooler situation in which to transform. At a constant temperature of 35°C (95°F), adults have been known to emerge in as little as three and half days after pupation, but in nature, five days is more common, and under adverse conditions several weeks may be required. The possibility of hibernation in the pupal stage is discussed elsewhere.

In all insects with complete metamorphosis, it was formerly assumed that pupal transformation consists first of certain histolytic changes in which the parts most specialized for a larval existence are broken down. This is followed, theoretically, by the histogenesis of those structures that are of greatest significance in adult life. Pérez (1910), who studied the transformation of *Calliphora,* points out that in the muscoid group at least the latter process is actually under way before histolysis occurs. The two phases thus proceed side by side with progressive substitution of new parts for old. Phagocytosis has been shown to play an important part in the tissue reduction process. New structures are produced by the division of embryonic histoblasts, present in the specialized thickenings of the epidermis already referred to as the

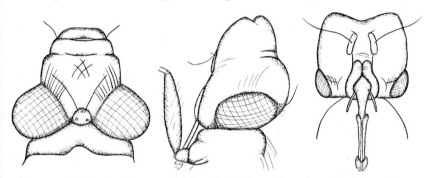

Figure 52. Ptilinum of a muscoid fly. These illustrations show how the ptilinum, when expanded, distorts the normal outline of the head. *Left:* Dorsal view. *Center:* Lateral view. *Right:* Ventral view. (Redrawn from Graham-Smith, *Flies in Relation to Disease* [Cambridge University Press, 1914].)

imaginal discs. It will be recalled that the imaginal discs are present before pupation, having been differentiated either during embryonic development or during larval growth. A number of anatomical features common to both larva and adult are not demolished, but undergo merely such reorganization as is necessary to adapt them for the insect's future needs. The Malpighian tubes and certain muscles are examples. It has been suggested that metamorphosis may perhaps be regarded as a return to embryonic development.

EMERGENCE OF THE ADULT

When transformation has been completed, the fly pushes off the anterior end of the pupal case. A circular slit appears in segment 6 (fifth visible segment), and the detached cap is split into two parts by longitudinal fissures more or less in line with the anterior spiracular processes. This is accomplished by the ptilinum, an inflated sac that protrudes from the frontal region of the head just dorsal to the base of the antennae. Once its head is free, the fly crawls out of the puparium, at the same time extricating itself from the nymphal sheath, which remains as a lining to the empty case.

In many instances the adult finds it necessary to work its way up through considerable debris, such as straw, leaves, sand, or manure, and in this the ptilinum proves most useful. Alternate expansion and contraction of this organ effect a passageway by which the fly eventually attains the surface of the heap. When expanded, the ptilinum is nearly as large as the head and renders the antennae quite invisible. When contracted, it appears merely as a dull area, fleshy-looking and free from hairs. Eversion is accomplished by

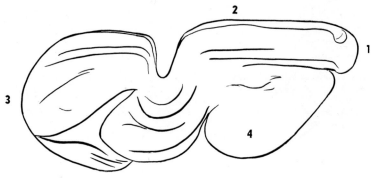

Figure 53. Wing of newly emerged fly. Left wing of fly that has just extricated itself from the pupal case. *1,* wing base; *2,* costal margin; *3,* apex; *4,* anal area. In a short time this teneral structure will expand and harden into the typical adult wing, with rigid veins and cross veins. (Redrawn from Graham-Smith, *Flies in Relation to Disease* [Cambridge University Press, 1914].)

changes in blood pressure (Réaumur, 1738), and retraction by special muscles that do not persist in aged adults (Laing, 1935).

The fly crawls rapidly about while its wings unfold and the exoskeleton proceeds to harden. By withdrawal of fluids, the wings become flat, thin, and transparent, rigidly supported by the longitudinal veins and cross veins. The chitin of the body becomes darker, each portion finally taking on its characteristic coloration. The ptilinum is at last withdrawn completely, leaving only the crescentic frontal "lunule," above the antennae, to mark its previous location.

DISPERSAL AND RANGE OF FLIGHT

Whether or not flies engage in general dispersal flights, as do some species of mosquitoes, is conjectural; nevertheless, there are interesting records of their traveling unusual distances. Hodge (1913a) found numerous specimens of *Musca, Stomoxys,* and *Calliphora* on cribs of waterworks located one and a quarter miles, five miles, and six miles from shore, in Lake Erie. There were no animals kept on the cribs, and all flies seemed very hungry. Perhaps they were blown from shore by strong winds and were merely fortunate in finding the cribs as resting places, but it is entirely conceivable that their own powers of flight brought them thither, regardless of the direction of prevailing winds.

Bishopp and Laake (1919) studied the dispersion of flies by releasing some 80,000 artificially colored specimens from a central point. Traps were set up at various distances in all directions. Marked specimens of *Musca domestica* were recovered from as far as thirteen miles away from the place of liberation. For *Cochliomyia macellaria* the maximum distance was fifteen miles; for *Phormia regina,* eleven; and for *Ophyra leucostoma,* seven. These authors observed that many favorable places for feeding and for breeding were apparently passed by in the course of these migrations.

The same authors (1921) report equivalent results from experiments in which the total number of flies involved was 234,000. It is noteworthy that *Musca domestica* was found six miles from the point of release in less than twenty-four hours. Males as well as females showed marked migratory tendencies.

Derbeneva-Ukhova (1942b), however, found the flight range of *Musca domestica* in the province of Archangel to be not usually more than 1,150 feet; and Hindle (1914b), who conducted some rather elaborate experiments, concluded that the usual maximum flight range in England was not more than a quarter of a mile, especially where houses were fairly numerous. He does record one case of flight across open fenland, a distance of 770 yards. Hindle's studies involved the use of fifty catching stations and the liberation of some 25,000 flies. His conclusions were that fine weather and a warm temperature were positive factors in the encouragement of dispersal and that flies tend to travel much farther in the country than in town, where, of course, food and shelter are available on every hand. Hindle also noted that the time of day affected the tendency of flies to engage in dispersal flights. Batches liberated during the morning hours scattered much more widely than flies liberated in the afternoon. In preparation for a flight of any distance, the insects were observed to mount vertically to a height of about forty-five feet.

Comparable experiments by Parker (1915, 1916c,d) gave rather similar results. A total of 387,877 flies were marked and released from four selected points. Seventy-eight collecting stations were established at distances ranging from 50 to 3,500 yards. Parker found that the average fly leads an extremely migratory existence and that a rather rapid spread over an area of five square miles about the point of release was fairly common, at least under city conditions. Odors, wind, temperature, and the general state of the weather all influenced dispersal. Individual flies not infrequently left the city environment and flew across open country to some distant point. This shows the obvious need for co-operation between communities in any program for effective fly control.

LONGEVITY

In the height of summer, it is doubtful if flies ordinarily live longer than two or three weeks. At lower temperatures, however, this may probably be extended to as much as three months. If there is true hibernation of adults, such individuals must, presumably, live even longer.

HIBERNATION

Authorities differ in their opinion as to how *Musca domestica* usually passes the winter in temperate zones. Mellor (1919) classifies such opinion under four heads:

(1) Newstead (1907, 1909) and Hewitt (1914a, 1915a) held rather strongly that the housefly passes the winter only in the adult stage. The latter favored the early suggestion of Copeman and Austen (1914), who stated that "the relative lateness of the season at which houseflies annually become abundant may be due to the smallness of the numbers of individuals that in an active or inactive condition survive the winter in houses or buildings."

(2) Copeman (1913) was inclined to the opinion that though the adults that survive the cold are the principal factor in carrying the species through the winter, it is possible that the pupal stage also hibernates. He did not furnish proof, however, that such took place.

(3) The third group, and the largest, holds that immature stages are more important than the adult stage in providing for the continuance of the species the following year. Williston (1908) stated that only in secluded places were the adult flies able to live through, and that normal survival was in the *pupal* stage. Howard (1911a) makes similar statements, pointing out that in manure heaps or at the surface of the ground beneath such heaps, pupae may survive very well. Howard thought that adult flies found active in warmed houses throughout the winter were of slight importance in starting the breeding program the following spring. Presumably such flies live out their normal life span and die off before opportunity for oviposition in a suitable medium is

forthcoming. More significant, according to Howard, are the few adults that remain dormant in cold, sheltered situations. These do not exhaust their energy with useless buzzing and meaningless flights from room to room and, therefore, with the approach of spring temperatures have many days of natural activity still before them.

Most serious investigators, however, warn of the danger of careless identification in interpreting observations on hibernating flies. Where careful examination has been made, the actual numbers of *Musca domestica* have usually been surprisingly low. Neither have supposed hibernating batches of flies shown any great preponderance of females over males, as might be expected if the survival of fertilized females constitutes the chief guarantee of species survival. Copeman and Austen finally reversed their stand and concluded that the customary explanation of the perpetuation of the housefly by overwintered adults must be abandoned.

The work of Bishopp, Dove, and Parman (1915) on the biology of houseflies in Texas showed that in that latitude hibernating adults are a rarity. Either breeding goes on throughout the winter in situations artificially warmed or, more commonly, the species survives in the immature stages. Larvae and pupae were observed by Dove (1916) to complete their development during the winter in manure piles kept warm by the fermentation of fresh manure added at frequent intervals, and adult flies emerged on mild days at temperatures as low as 45°–55°F (7.2°–12.8°C).

(4) The extreme viewpoint is represented by the work of Skinner (1913, 1915), who came to the conclusion that "houseflies pass the winter in the pupal stage and no other way."

A good portion of the confusion described above arises from the fact that conditions in Texas or southern Italy are scarcely to be compared with those in New York, for example, or in Scotland. Thus, in warmer latitudes it has been demonstrated repeatedly that though lower temperatures prolong the duration of the several stages and thus extend the life cycle, there is in fact no interruption to continuous breeding and that there is no necessity for hypothesizing a prolonged quiescent state.

The sub-zero temperatures of the northern United States and Canada, however, would seem to impose conditions incompatible with continuous development. Two possibilities suggest themselves: (1) hibernation of any or all stages, (2) migration from more southern latitudes as soon as weather conditions are suitable in the spring.

Recent observations by Matthysse (1945), on the other hand, tend to show that there is a very large amount of continuous breeding within dairy barns even in regions where outside temperatures often become extreme. In Clinton County, New York, which is the most northerly county of the state, huge numbers of houseflies were produced in midwinter in a normal type of dairy barn housing sixty head of cattle. The outside temperature was frequently

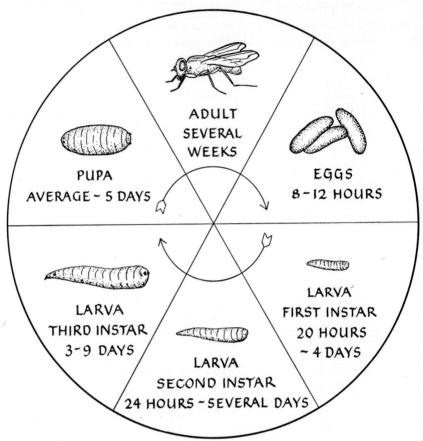

Figure 54. Life cycle of the housefly. It is possible for a generation to be completed in as little time as eight days, if all stages encounter favorable conditions. In nature the summer average is between ten days and two weeks for the temperate zone.

below 0°F (—17.8°C), but inside the men worked in shirt sleeves and the thermometer never registered below 32°F (0°C). Box stalls, which were only cleaned at fortnightly intervals, undoubtedly contributed the bulk of the fly population. Teneral adults were observed crawling up posts and stanchions, and the fly problem became actually greater in midwinter than it had been in late summer or early fall. With the advent of spring, these flies left the barn in large numbers, and it was observed that the fly population of the immediate vicinity notably exceeded that of regions some two hundred miles farther south. This observation, combined with the fact that freezing temperatures were still frequent in the month of March, argued strongly against the insects' being there as a result of a northward spring migration.

The same author points out that flies have been observed to breed freely during the winter in animal pens at the New York State Veterinary College in Ithaca, even to the extent that control measures became necessary in the month of January.

The obvious conclusion to this perplexing question is that since each geographical region is likely to have climatic peculiarities of its own, one is justified in making generalizations only after controlled investigations pertaining to the particular locality have been completed and analyzed.

FECUNDITY

Perhaps the most arresting thing about the housefly is its remarkable capacity to reproduce. The concentration of larvae in a suitable breeding medium is sometimes unbelievable. An ounce of manure taken from a few inches below the surface of the soil has been found to contain 868 pupae. In India no less than 4,042 flies were hatched from one-sixth of a cubic foot of soil taken from a trench used to bury night soil. When one realizes that these are *survival* figures representing the successful completion of development, the potential reproductive capacity of the species seems all the more astounding. Loss of eggs and larvae through desiccation, starvation, activities of parasites and predators, and other factors is inevitable, yet after all these have taken toll, adults may emerge in astronomical numbers.

Howard (1911a), allowing an average of ten days for completion of each generation in the summertime in the latitude of Washington, calculated that a single gravid female that laid 120 eggs on April 15 could, theoretically, be responsible for the emergence of 5,598,720,000,000 adult flies on or before September 10! These calculations also allow for a period of ten days after the emerging of all adult flies before sexual maturity is achieved. Many undoubtedly reproduce in less time than this; likewise, many females live to produce more than one batch of eggs, which would make the total infinitely greater. Devoe (1945) gives 325,923,200,000,000 as the possible number of summer descendants from a mated pair.

Of course no such actual increase takes place in nature, since only a limited number of individuals can hope to meet with conditions suitable for survival even in the most favored environmental situations. Kuzina (1936), for example, found that in ordinary rearing work, the eggs suffered a mortality of 2.23 per cent in the laboratory and of 11.33 per cent in the insectary that he used. For larvae, the figure was 17.33 per cent in the laboratory and 20.58 in the insectary. The pupae showed mortality rates in the two situations of 8.65 and 17.60 per cent.

Nevertheless, after all this is taken into account, the reproductive capacity of the fly is truly amazing.

GENETICS AND EVOLUTION

Studies on the heredity of the housefly comparable to those that have yielded so much valuable information concerning the fruit fly, *Drosophila melanogaster,* have yet to be undertaken. An example of what can be done, however, is suggested by the work of Barber (1948), who has succeeded in isolating two distinct strains, less vigorous than the normal, in which the distinguishing characters occur in the pupal stage. In one of these, called the "lethal line," the puparia are much more elongated than in the normal, and possess a pore at the anterior end. This pore results from the fact that the larvae are not able to retract their mouth parts in the ordinary manner when the puparium is formed. Both microorganisms and predatory arthropods may enter through it and attack the pupa, thus reducing the survival rate. Cannibalism may even occur, as when active housefly larvae enter the pore and proceed to destroy the pupal tissue. Added to these hazards is the fact that flies have great difficulty in emerging from the elongated puparia, and many of them perish in the attempt. The name "lethal line" appears to be well chosen. Barber succeeded in establishing a pure culture after three generations of selection; that is, the line was pure in the F_4.

The other strain, known as "flat," has puparia that are somewhat flattened and rectangular, with the segmentation unusually well marked. Anterior pores are not a feature in this strain. Barber's selected cultures contained normal puparia up to the twelfth generation, after which the line became pure. The percentage of emergence for the "flat" line is considerably higher than for the "lethal" but is always below the normal.

CHAPTER V

Taxonomy and Nomenclature

Some men are more vexed with a fly than with a wound.—*Jeremy Taylor,* The
Mysteriousness of Marriage

FITTING a species into its proper niche in the scheme of things is perhaps
as difficult a task as any with which the biologist may be concerned. According to the most conservative estimates there are at least 750,000 described
species of insects, of which perhaps 85,000 fall in the Order Diptera. Actual
numbers probably run much higher than these. How is the amateur to know
a housefly when he sees one?

In the first place the housefly is an animal, with all the attributes, structural
and physiological, which entitle it to a place in the animal kingdom. In general these attributes fall under two heads: (1) The possession of structures
suited to the ingestion and utilization of ready-made organic materials, specifically carbohydrates, proteins, and lipoids. These must have been previously
synthesized in the tissues of plants, or of other animals that depend directly
upon green plants for their sustenance. (2) The possession of structures permitting a greater degree of motility than is usual or possible among typical
plants. They are thus enabled to move from place to place, and are therefore
not dependent upon a fixed situation for food, shelter, or other environmental
features necessary to life.

Either of these attributes alone may not be sufficient to differentiate between
animals and plants. Certain of the latter, specifically the fungi, require complex, organic foods, even as animals do, and are quite as dependent upon the
synthetic activities of green plants. Again, motility is not unknown among the
unicellular green algae, where a number of forms such as *Volvox* make excellent progress through water by means of their flagellar processes.

But on this point the housefly presents no problem, since its animal characteristics are patent beyond any shadow of a doubt. We shall therefore proceed at once to the next step in classification, assignment to phylum or division.

THE PHYLUM ARTHROPODA

Animals fall into eleven major groups. The largest of these, both in number of species and number of individuals, is the phylum Arthropoda. Not only do arthropods exceed in number all other forms of animal life taken together, three to one, but they are exceedingly widespread geographically, and, except for very high latitudes (and altitudes), there are few places on or near the surface of the earth that do not boast an arthropod population. Three features characterize this large and varied group: (1) the presence of a number of pairs of jointed appendages, at least in certain stages of the life cycle; (2) an external skeleton of chitin, which must be shed at intervals to permit normal growth and development; and (3) an open circulation, which requires the coelom (body cavity) to function as a blood chamber or haemocoel.

Lobsters, crabs, crayfish, spiders, ticks, mites, scorpions, centipedes, millipedes and insects are familiar examples of arthropods.

THE CLASS HEXAPODA

Phyla are divided into classes, of which the phylum Arthropoda contains no less than thirteen. Only five or six of these, however, are very commonly encountered. The Crustacea, of which the crab is an example, are almost entirely aquatic, and breathe by means of true gills. All other classes are more or less terrestrial, and breathe by spiracles or by book lungs. The millipedes, which fall in the class Diplopoda, are slothful, wormlike creatures that, due to a fusion of their dorsal segments, appear to possess two pairs of tiny legs on each segment of the body. The centipedes, which constitute the class Chilopoda, move more rapidly, having conspicuously developed legs, of which one pair is borne by each typical segment. Centipedes have piercing jaws, and the larger forms can inflict a painful bite. The class Arachnida includes the spiders, scorpions, ticks, mites, and related forms. All typical adult arachnids possess four pairs of jointed legs, borne by the anterior portion of the body (cephalothorax). They are often found in situations similar to those inhabited by insects, and are sometimes confused with them.

All true insects on the other hand fall in the class Hexapoda, the most numerous and widespread of all the animal groups. Practically all adult forms possess six jointed legs (three pairs), borne by the thorax, or mid-section of the body. This is the only class of Arthropoda in which wings occur. Most orders display two pairs, of which the second and third thoracic segments each bear one. All insects have the body more or less clearly divided into three distinct parts: a head, which bears the antennae, eyes, and mouth parts; a

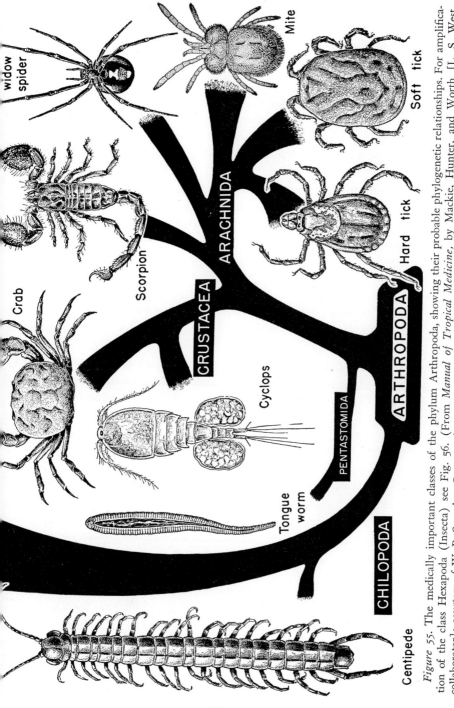

widow
spider

Mite

Soft tick

ARACHNIDA

Hard tick

Scorpion

CRUSTACEA

Crab

ARTHROPODA

Cyclops

PENTASTOMIDA

Tongue
worm

CHILOPODA

Centipede

Figure 55. The medically important classes of the phylum Arthropoda, showing their probable phylogenetic relationships. For amplification of the class Hexapoda (Insecta) see Fig. 56. (From *Manual of Tropical Medicine,* by Mackie, Hunter, and Worth [L. S. West, collaborator]; courtesy of W. B. Saunders Company.)

thorax of three segments, which bear the wings and legs; and an abdomen that may exhibit up to eleven distinct segments.

THE ORDER DIPTERA

Of the thirty or more orders of Hexapoda, the best known are the Coleoptera (beetles), Lepidoptera (butterflies and moths), Hymenoptera (ants, bees, and wasps), Orthoptera (crickets, cockroaches, locusts), and the Diptera (true flies). The Trichoptera (caddis flies), Odonata (dragonflies and damsel flies), Ephemeroptera (May flies), Plecoptera (stone flies), Mecoptera (scorpion flies), and certain other groups colloquially referred to as "flies" are not flies in the taxonomic sense, and need not concern us here.

The Diptera, to which order houseflies belong, may be characterized as follows:

Insects, in which the mouth parts are adapted for sucking and sometimes for piercing, but never for chewing solid food. The single pair of wings are borne by the second thoracic segment and are membranous in nature. The wings of the more highly specialized flies tend to have fewer veins and cross veins than the more primitive members of the order. A few degenerate forms are wingless. The second pair of wings is represented in all true flies by a pair of knobbed hairs, the halteres, which are believed to function as organs of equilibrium. Like most of the highly evolved orders of insects, Diptera show complete metamorphosis; that is, the life history consists of four phases: egg, larva, pupa, and adult.

This vast aggregation of two-winged insects may be divided into two suborders, on the basis of the manner in which the adult (imago) emerges from the pupal skin. In all primitive forms (some thirty families, including mosquitoes, black flies, horseflies, midges, and others) this is accomplished by means of a longitudinal or T-shaped slit, which appears on the dorsal surface and through which the adult fly makes its escape. These constitute the suborder Orthorrhapha.

The more specialized groups, however, escape from their oval or barrel-shaped puparia by means of a clean, circular slit, close to the anterior end. The cap or operculum is thrust off by the ptilinum, a special structure just above the antennae, which is later withdrawn into the head of the fly. These make up the suborder Cyclorrhapha, the group with which we shall be principally concerned.

It is customary to divide the Cyclorrhapha into two series, the Aschiza and the Schizophora. The Aschiza, composed of four families, are characterized by the absence or great reduction of the frontal suture. In this series the

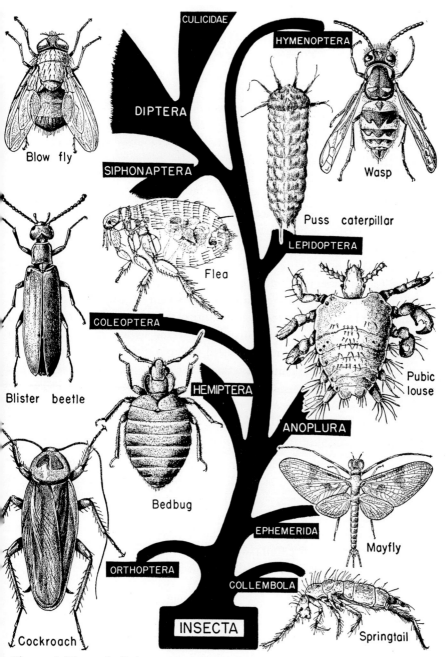

Figure 56. The medically important orders of the class Hexapoda (Insecta), showing their probable phylogenetic relationships. For further analysis of the order Diptera see Fig. 57. (From *Manual of Tropical Medicine,* by Mackie, Hunter, and Worth [L. S. West, collaborator]; courtesy of W. B. Saunders Company.)

ptilinum is usually small and fails to persist after the adult has emerged. The Schizophora, on the other hand, aggregating nearly forty families, possess a well-marked frontal suture behind which, within the head, the withdrawn ptilinum remains for the life of the fly.

Taxonomists recognize two sections of Schizophora. Species that constitute the smaller section, known as the Pupipara, are characterized by the fact that the larvae remain within the body of the female fly until ready for pupation. Four families of flies fall here. All are parasitic in the adult state, and many are wingless. The larger section, the Muscoidea (Myodaria), includes all of the better-known flies and probably represents more than half of the order Diptera. There are two subsections of Myodaria. Houseflies belong in that group known as the calyptrate Muscoidea or Calypteratae. All species here contained have squamae (alulae, calypters) which are large and well developed, and tend to conceal the halteres. The transverse suture of the thorax in the Calypteratae is distinct and easily recognized. These species stand in contrast with the acalyptrate Muscoidea, in which the calypters are small or vestigial and in which the transverse suture of the thorax is but rarely distinct. The family Scatophagidae (Cordyluridae), being somewhat intermediate in these respects, has sometimes been listed with one group and sometimes with the other, but present opinion associates these forms quite definitely with the Calypteratae.

THE FAMILY MUSCIDAE

The families of calyptrate Muscoidea have been variously classified by different authors, and the whole concept of their relationship has undergone much change as new and better characters have been discovered and put to use. Twenty five years ago the family was conceived of as including a limited number of genera, of which *Musca, Glossina,* and *Stomoxys* were among the best-known examples. Closely related families were the grayish Sarcophagidae (flesh flies), the metallic Calliphoridae (blowflies), the Anthomyiidae (which contained the genus *Fannia,* and was recognized chiefly by the absence of a sharp bend in the fourth longitudinal vein), the Oestridae (botflies, in part), Gasterophilidae (horse botflies) and the Tachinidae (the larvae of which are parasitic in insect hosts). A character much used in separating families was the arista, dorsal appendage of the third antennal segment. This structure is variously plumose in true Muscidae but bare in Tachinidae, except for the subfamily Dexiinae, in which it is at least pubescent to the tip (West, 1924, 1925b, 1948).

The presence or absence of hypopleural bristles is another character of great

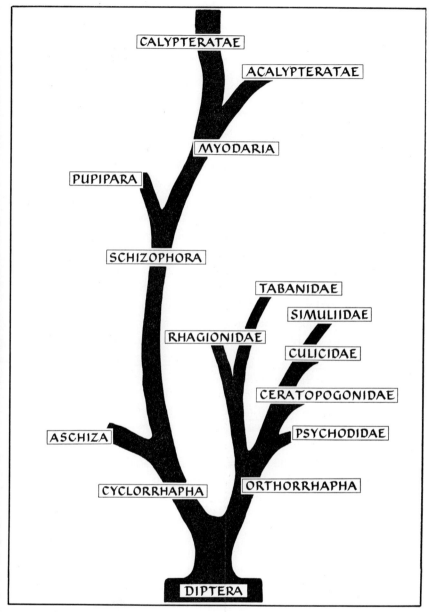

Figure 57. Basic classification of the order Diptera. In the suborder Orthorrhapha, only the medically important families are shown. There are many others. For a similar analysis of the calyptrate Cyclorrhapha, see Fig. 58.

importance, and its use in more recent years has considerably influenced family boundaries. Because both groups possess them, along with other unifying characters, Curran (1934) treated the Calliphoridae and Sarcophagidae of authors as one family, the Metopiidae, which he made to include part of the Tachinidae of Williston's *Manual* (1908). Hall (1948), however, prefers to consider the Calliphoridae distinct, separated from the Sarcophagidae by the absence, in the latter, of intrapostocular cilia. Also, in both sexes, the general structure of the genitalia tends to show the two families as quite distinct. Again, Curran defines the family Muscidae as including the Scatophagidae and Anthomyiidae of authors, plus all those Muscidae of Williston's *Manual* which lack hypopleural bristles. The union of the Scatophagidae with the Anthomyiidae seems to have been widely accepted, but writers of general texts seem loath to merge the latter family with the Muscidae. Thus Matheson (1944) uses the under surface of the scutellum, which is bare in Muscidae but hairy in Anthomyiidae, to differentiate between these groups. Also, the anal vein always reaches the margin of the wing in anthomyids, a condition rarely encountered in muscid species. The recently available *Manual of Myiology,* consisting of several volumes published by Townsend over a period of years, will undoubtedly influence muscoid classification for decades to come, but it will be some time before students become generally familiar with the groupings that Townsend has proposed. *Musca domestica* is treated in Part XII (1942), which bears the title "General Consideration of the Oestromuscaria." Dr. Townsend has undoubtedly amassed a greater amount of information concerning the muscoid flies than any other student of the group, and his work should not be underestimated.

Meanwhile it seems practical, for purposes of this volume, to consider the Muscidae as limited, in the sense of Matheson and others, to the nonanthomyiid genera which lack hypopleural bristles. It is convenient to separate the Muscidae into two subfamilies, the Stomoxyidinae, a true bloodsucking group, and the Muscinae, whose mouth parts are in most species for lapping only. The first includes the biting stable fly, *Stomoxys calcitrans,* the horn fly, *Haematobia irritans,* and the tsetse flies, which fall in the genus *Glossina.* The Muscinae include, besides the housefly, such forms as *Muscina assimilis, Muscina stabulans,* and *Cryptolucilia caesarion.*

THE GENUS *MUSCA*

In the broader sense this genus includes all those nonmetallic members of the subfamily Muscinae which possess a sharp angle in the fourth longitudinal

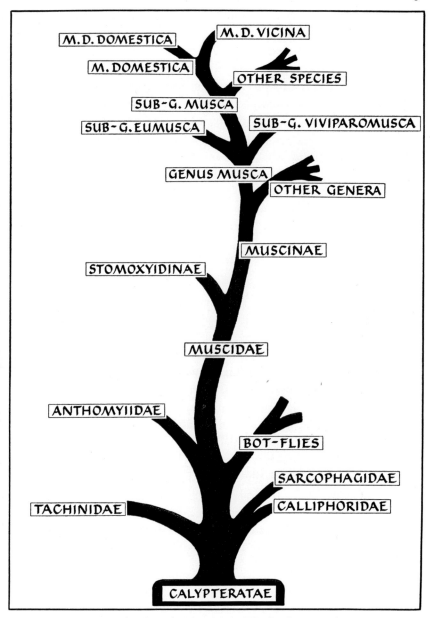

Figure 58. Important families of Calypteratae. The family Muscidae is further sub-divided to show the taxonomic position of *Musca domestica* and its subspecies.

vein. Townsend has erected a number of genera within this group, several of them monotypic, but economic and medical entomologists prefer to regard these as no more than subgenera, at most. An acceptable compromise appears to be the recognition of three subgenera, distinguished primarily on the basis of biological differences. By this arrangement the subgenus *Musca* Linnaeus, which includes at least twenty-three species besides *domestica,* may be described as an oviparous group in which the eggs lack any semblance of a stalk. The subgenus *Eumusca* Townsend is also oviparous, but the eggs possess distinct stalks by which they are attached to the substratum. At least twelve authentic species may be assigned here. The third subgenus, *Viviparomusca,* is believed to be entirely larviparous. At least fifteen species constitute this group. The type species of *Eumusca* is *M. antumnalis* De Geer; the type of *Viviparomusca* is *M. vivipara* Portchinsky.[1]

THE SPECIES *DOMESTICA*

This species is listed as number 54 under the genus *Musca* in the tenth edition of the *Systema Naturae,* published by Linnaeus in 1758. There seems to be no doubt whatever as to its identity or validity. The genus *Musca* as employed by Linnaeus was exceedingly broad in comparison with present-day concepts, and included certain species now assigned to the Syrphidae, Stratiomyidae, and Bombyliidae. This is not strange, however, when one considers that Linnaeus utilized only ten genera in his classification of all Diptera! Since that time enthusiastic taxonomists have proposed approximately forty new names for species which they believed to be distinct, but which according to present-day concepts of structure and taxonomy are regarded as synonymous with *domestica* of Linnaeus. The only form that has been generally recognized as biologically distinct is *vicina* of Macquart, a subspecies that tends to have a more tropical distribution than *domestica*. It differs from *domestica* chiefly in having the abdomen more extensively orange, especially on tergites 1 to 3. The males differ further in having the vertex somewhat more narrow, as compared with the width of the compound eyes.

[1] I am greatly indebted to Dr. Eugene G. Munroe for permission to make extensive use of his unpublished compilation of literature dealing with the genus *Musca*. The manuscript summarizes important taxonomic data gleaned from the careful study of more than a hundred technical papers and monographs published prior to 1940. The labor which Mr. Munroe's kindness has saved me is enormous.

CLASSIFICATION OF *MUSCA DOMESTICA*—RECAPITULATION

KINGDOM: Animalia
  PHYLUM: Arthropoda
    CLASS: Hexapoda
      ORDER: Diptera
        SUBORDER: Cyclorrhapha (Athericera)
          SERIES: Schizophora
            SECTION: Muscoidea (Myodaria)
              SUBSECTION: Calypteratae
                FAMILY: Muscidae
                  SUBFAMILY: Muscinae
                    GENUS: *Musca*
                      SUBGENUS: *Musca*
                        SPECIES: *M. domestica*
                          SUBSPECIES (two):
                            M. domestica domestica Linnaeus
                            M. domestica vicina Macquart

THE NAME

Musca domestica is one of the best-known and most-used scientific names, not only in the realm of pure and applied biology but in nonscientific circles as well. It therefore came somewhat as a shock in 1915 when C. H. T. Townsend, a very thorough student of taxonomic literature, challenged its authenticity by pointing out that Latreille, in 1810, had designated the large bluebottle fly today known as *Calliphora vomitoria* (Linn.) as the type of the genus *Musca*. By strict interpretation of the international rules of zoological nomenclature, the genus *Calliphora,* which was erected by Robineau-Desvoidy in 1830, should therefore fall to *Musca* of Linnaeus, which dates from 1758. Townsend, an analytical taxonomist, attempted to solve the problem by proposing a new genus, *Promusca,* for *Musca domestica* of authors.

To economic and medical entomologists, however, this was anathema, and the controversy between those practical workers who hesitated to abandon the well-known name and the theoretical taxonomists who seemed resolved to preserve the integrity of the International Rules at any cost became acute. The matter was further complicated by the disclosure that the larva of the housefly had in very remote times been erroneously described as a roundworm (*Ascaris conostoma*), and that this supposed helminth had been made the type of a distinct genus, *Conostoma,* about the year 1801. Thus, if *domestica* could no longer be assigned to the genus *Musca,* there would be quite as good a case for citing it in *Conostoma* as in *Promusca,* with the bulk of the evidence rather favoring the former, since it had been erected for a species that was the undisputed synonym of *M. domestica* and had a century or more of priority over Townsend's proposed name.

In 1917 C. W. Stiles published in *Entomological News* a notice to the zoological profession concerning possible suspension of the International Rules of Zoological Nomenclature in regard to *Musca* and *Calliphora,* so that both might continue to be used in accordance with the long-accepted concept of these groups. L. O. Howard, W. D. Pierce, and twenty-one other professional zoologists joined in this request to the International Commission. It was pointed out that *Musca domestica* had enjoyed consistent usage since 1758 and *Calliphora vomitoria* since 1830, in various literature pertaining to zoology, medicine, epidemiology, and veterinary science, and that a change in the nomenclature of either of these species would be most regrettable. The final notice appeared in 1923, stating that the committee would vote to exercise its plenary powers and, under suspension of the Rules, declare *M. domestica* the type species of the genus *Musca.* By the same action the genus *Calliphora* was validated, with *C. vomitoria* as type.

ON THE USE OF COMMON NAMES

The common name of *Musca domestica* has been "housefly" (house fly, house-fly) in English-speaking countries for centuries. A strenuous effort was made by L. O. Howard (1911a,b,c) and others of that time to establish the name "typhoid fly," since typhoid fever was the most serious and widespread fly-borne disease with which sanitarians of that period had to contend. "Cholera fly," "dysentery fly," "enteric fly" might have been quite as appropriate. It is probably desirable, however, not to refer to the species as linked with any particular infection or disease, as such usage tends to blind the average person to its possible vectorship of other pathogens. In many parts of the United States today *Musca domestica* is less a housefly than a "picnic fly," "park fly," "dairy fly," or "stable fly," but wherever found, it is almost certain to be the availability of human food or drink which brings it there.

This inevitable domesticity of the species thus continues to characterize its habits and migrations, regardless of changing social and sanitary practices. After prolonged intimacy with such a guest, humankind has in general come to accept the creature on at least a tolerated, if not a friendly, basis. For this reason it is not strange that the Portuguese-speaking inhabitants of São Paulo (Brazil) commonly refer to *Musca domestica* as "mosquito" (Pereira, 1947), a natural diminutive of "mosca," the Portuguese equivalent for "fly." An intimate touch is also conveyed by the traditional German designation "Stubenfliege" (Flu, 1911), while the widespread occurrence of the species is implied by the Italian expression "mosca commune" (Generali, 1886). Hodge's use (1910) of "filth fly" is certainly expressive, while his subsequent (1911a) modification "filth-disease fly" is even better, though apparently too cumbersome to have led to any very general acceptance.

The restless activity of the housefly is well expressed in Hutchinson's title (1911) "How doth the little *busy* Fly?" while the conventional French usage "mouche domestique" (Leboeuf, 1912) again emphasizes the insect's relation to the household. Newstead (1907) usually referred to the "Common Housefly" when *Musca domestica* was particularly intended, to distinguish it from other species frequently or sometimes found in houses, as did also Packard (1874) and Parkes (1911). The French translation of Portchinsky's studies (1910) on filth-breeding Diptera employs the term "mouches coprophagues."

OTHER SPECIES OF THE GENUS *MUSCA*

Two approaches have been employed in developing the classification of this genus. Malloch, in several papers, made use chiefly of the chaetotaxy, as did also Townsend in his numerous writings on the Myodaria. Patton, on the other hand, stressed the structure of the genitalia, along with various biological differences.

An example of Patton's biological groupings is his listing (1923a) of the Philippine species of *Musca* under three heads:

Group I is characterized as composed of nonbiting, occasionally haematophagous species, mainly associated with man. These breed in garbage as well as in excrement of many kinds. Examples are *M. domestica vicina, M. nebulo,* and *M. sorbens.* Group II comprises those nonbiting, haematophagous forms found only on or near animals. *Musca ventrosa, M. craggi,* and *M. bakeri* fall here. Group III is composed of the true biting forms. In the genus *Musca* these confine their attentions to animals, and breed normally in cow dung. Examples are *Musca conducens, M. planiceps, M. crassirostris,* and *M. inferior.*

Van Emden (1939) succeeded in harmonizing the two systems of classification and in resolving most of the points of controversy.

The Munroe manuscript recognizes fifty-one valid species, distributed over three subgenera, *Musca, Eumusca,* and *Viviparomusca.* One hundred and thirty synonyms (or wrong usages) are also indicated in his list, while seventeen species of uncertain affiliation are tabulated separately. Since their validity may not be refuted (even though it cannot be confirmed), we are confronted with a total of sixty-eight possibly valid species, distributed over various parts of the world.

Since I have seen only a small minority of these many forms, it would be presumptuous of me to attempt analytical keys for their identification. In North America, it is generally considered that *M. domestica* is the only recognizable species. South America and the West Indies can perhaps be credited with three or four additional valid forms (see Chapter VI). For identification of Palearctic species one should consult Patton's *Studies on the Higher Diptera of Medical and Veterinary Importance,* especially the series of papers published in the year 1933. Van Emden's 1939 paper, *Muscidae: Muscinae and Stomoxydinae,* is very satisfactory for the Ethiopian species, while for Oriental forms, the *Practical Guide to the Oriental Species of Musca,* by Patton (1937a), is quite indispensable. Puri (1943) gives a very satisfactory key to the house-frequenting species of *Musca* which occur in India.

The species and subspecies names of the genus *Musca,* with remarks on the taxonomic position of each, appear in Table 4.

Table 4.

The genus *Musca*

Species and subspecies names	Synonymy	Subgenus
1. *aethiops* Stein	Syn. of *M. gabonensis*	*Eumusca*
2. *africana* Bezzi	Syn. of *M. lucidula*	*Musca*
3. *alba* Patton nec Mall.	Syn. of *M. xanthomelas*	*Eumusca*
4. *albina albina* Wied.	Valid species and subspecies	*Musca*
5. *albina polita* Mall.	Valid species and subspecies	*Musca*
6. *albomaculata* Bezzi nec Macq.	Syn. of *M. cuthbertsoni*	*Musca*
7. *albomaculata* Auct. nec Macq.	Syn. of *M. xanthomelas*	*Eumusca*
8. *alpesa* Karsch nec Walk.	Syn. of *M. xanthomelas*	*Eumusca*
9. *alpesa* Walk.	Syn. of *M. lusoria*	*Viviparomusca*
10. *analis* Macq.	Syn. of *M. domestica vicina*(?)	*Musca*
11. *angustifrons* Thoms.	Syn. of *M. sorbens sorbens*	*Musca*
12. *antiquissima* Walk.	Syn. of *M. domestica vicina*	*Musca*
13. *aricioides* Walk.	Presumably valid	Uncertain

Species and subspecies names	Synonymy	Subgenus
14. *atrifrons* Big.	Syn. of *M. domestica vicina*(?)	*Musca*
15. *aucta* Walk.	Presumably valid	Uncertain
16. *aurifacies* Rond.	Syn. of *M. domestica domestica*(?)	*Musca*
17. *aurulans* R.-D.	Presumably valid	Uncertain
18. *australis* Macq. nec Bsd.	Syn. of *M. domestica domestica*	*Musca*
19. *autumnalis autumnalis* De Geer	Valid species and subspecies	*Eumusca*
20. *autumnalis pseudocorvina* van E.	Valid species and subspecies	*Eumusca*
21. *autumnalis somalorum* Bezzi	Valid species and subspecies	*Eumusca*
22. *autumnalis ugandae* van E.	Valid species and subspecies	*Eumusca*
23. *bakeri* Patt.	Valid species	*Viviparomusca*
24. *basilaris* Macq.	Syn. of *M. domestica vicina*(?)	*Musca*
25. *beckeri* Schnabl	Syn. of *M. albina albina*	*Musca*
26. *bezzii* P. & C.	Valid species	*Viviparomusca*
27. *biseta* Hough	Syn. of *M. sorbens sorbens*	*Musca*
28. *bivittata* Thoms.	Syn. of *M. sorbens sorbens*	*Musca*
29. *bovina* R.-D.	Syn. of *M. domestica domestica*	*Musca*
30. *calisia* Walk.	Presumably valid	Uncertain
31. *calleva* Walk.	Syn. of *M. domestica domestica*	*Musca*
32. *campestris* R.-D.	Syn. of *M. domestica domestica*(?)	*Musca*
33. *campicola* R.-D.	Syn. of *M. domestica domestica*(?)	*Musca*
34. *carnifex* R.-D.	Syn. of *M. tempestiva*	*Musca*
35. *chiliensis* Macq.	Syn. of *M. domestica domestica*(?)	*Musca*
36. *cingalaisina* Big.	Syn. of *M. planiceps*	*Viviparomusca*
37. *cluvia* Walk.	Presumably valid	Uncertain

Table 4 (continued)

Species and subspecies names	Synonymy	Subgenus
38. *conducens* Walk.	Valid species	*Musca*
39. *conducens* Patt. nec Walk.	Syn. of *M. sorbens alba*	*Musca*
40. *confiscata* Speiser	Syn. of *M. tempestatum*	*Musca*
41. *congolensis* Villen.	Syn. of *M. gabonensis*	*Eumusca*
42. *consanguinea* Rond.	Syn. of *M. domestica vicina*(?)	*Musca*
43. *continua* R.-D.	Syn. of *M. autumnalis autumnalis*	*Eumusca*
44. *convexifrons* Thoms.	Valid species	*Viviparomusca*
45. *convexifrons* Auct. nec Thoms.	Syn. of *M. xanthomelas*	*Eumusca*
46. *corvina* Fabr.	Syn. of *M. domestica domestica*(?)	*Musca*
47. *corvina* Frogg. nec Fabr.	Syn. of *M. sorbens sorbens*	*Musca*
48. *corvina* Port. nec Fabr.	Syn. of *M. autumnalis autumnalis*	*Eumusca*
49. *corvinoides* Patt.	Syn. of *M. larvipara*	*Viviparomusca*
50. *cuprea* Macq.	Syn. of *M. tempestiva*	*Musca*
51. *craggi* Patt.	Valid species	*Eumusca*
52. *crassirostris* Stein	Valid species	*Musca*
53. *cuthbertsoni* Patt.	Valid species	*Musca*
54. *dasyops* Patt. nec Stein	Syn. of *Musca* sp.	*Musca*
55. *determinata* Walk.	Syn. of *M. nebulo*	*Musca*
56. *determinata* Patt. nec Walk.	Syn. of *M. domestica vicina*	*Musca*
57. *dichotoma* Bezzi	Syn. of *M. sorbens sorbens*	*Musca*
58. *divaricata* Awati	Syn. of *M. domestica vicina*(?)	*Musca*
59. *domestica domestica* Linn.	Valid species and subspecies	*Musca*
60. *domestica vicina* Macq.	Valid species and subspecies	*Musca*
61. *dorsomaculata* Macq. nec Meig.	Syn. of *M. xanthomelas*	*Eumusca*
62. *elatior* Villen.	Valid species	*Viviparomusca*
63. *eleodivora* Walton	Presumably valid	Uncertain

Species and subspecies names	Synonymy	Subgenus
64. *ethiops* Patt. (error)	Syn. of *M. gabonensis*	*Eumusca*
65. *eutaeniata* Big.	Syn. of *M. sorbens sorbens*	*Musca*
66. *familiaris* Harris	Syn. of *M. domestica domestica*	*Musca*
67. *fasciata* Stein	Valid species	*Musca*
68. *fasciata* Mall. nec Stein	Syn. of *M. tempestatum*	*Musca*
69. *fergusoni* Patt. nec J. & B.	Syn. of *M. convexifrons*	*Viviparomusca*
70. *fergusoni* J. & B.	Valid species	*Viviparomusca*
71. *flavifacies* Big.	Syn. of *M. domestica vicina*	*Musca*
72. *flavinervis* Thoms.	Syn. of *M. domestica vicina*	*Musca*
73. *flavipennis* Big.	Syn. of *M. domestica vicina*	*Musca*
74. *floralis* R.-D.	Syn. of *M. autumnalis autumnalis*	*Eumusca*
75. *fletcheri* P. & S.	Valid species	*Eumusca*
76. *formosana* Mall.	Valid species	*Viviparomusca*
77. *formosana* Patt. nec Mall.	A subspecies of *M. planiceps*	*Viviparomusca*
78. *frontalis* Rond.	Syn. of *M. domestica domestica*(?)	*Musca*
79. *fulvescens* R.-D.	Presumably valid	Uncertain
80. *gabonensis* Macq.	Valid species	*Eumusca*
81. *gibsoni* P. & C.	Valid species	*Eumusca*
82. *greeni* Patt.	Valid species	*Viviparomusca*
83. *grisella* R.-D.	Syn. of *M. autumnalis autumnalis*	*Eumusca*
84. *gurnei* P. & C.	Syn. of *M. inferior*	*Eumusca*
85. *gymnosomea* Rond.	Valid species	*Musca*
86. *harpyia* Harris	Syn. of *M. domestica domestica*	*Musca*
87. *hervei* Villen.	Valid species	*Eumusca*
88. *hervei* Ho (in part)	Syn. of *M. bezzii*	*Viviparomusca*
89. *hilli* J. & B.	Valid species	*Musca*
90. *hilli* Patt. nec J. & B.	Syn. of *M. ventrosa*	*Musca*

Table 4 (continued)

Species and subspecies names	Synonymy	Subgenus
91. *hottentota* R.-D.	Syn. of *M. domestica domestica*(?)	*Musca*
92. *humilis* Wied.	Syn. of *M. sorbens sorbens*	*Musca*
93. *incerta* Patt. nec Walk.	Syn. of *M. pattoni*	*Musca*
94. *indica* Awati	Syn. of *M. planiceps*	*Viviparomusca*
95. *inferior* Stein	Valid species	*Eumusca*
96. *insignis* Austen	Syn. of *M. crassirostris*	*Musca*
97. *illingworthi* Patt.	Valid species	*Viviparomusca*
98. *interrupta* Mall. et al. nec Walk.	Syn. of *M. lasiophthalma*	*Musca*
99. *interrupta dasyops* Stein	Valid species and subspecies	*Musca*
100. *interrupta interrupta* Walk.	Valid species and subspecies	*Musca*
101. *jacobsoni* Mall.	Valid species	*Musca*
102. *kasauliensis* Awati	Syn. of *M. ventrosa*	*Musca*
103. *kweilinensis* Ouchi	Presumably valid	Uncertain
104. *larvipara* Port.	Valid species	*Viviparomusca*
105. *lasiopa* Villen.	Valid species	*Eumusca*
106. *lasiophthalma* Patt. nec Thoms.	Syn. of *M. interrupta interrupta*	*Musca*
107. *lasiophthalma* Thoms.	Valid species	*Musca*
108. *lateralis* Macq.	Syn. of *M. domestica domestica* or *vicina*(?)	*Musca*
109. *latifrons* Wied.	Syn. of *M. sorbens sorbens*	*Musca*
110. *latifrons* Awati	Syn. of *M. gibsoni*(?)	*Eumusca*
111. *latiparafrons* Awati	Syn. of *M. gibsoni*(?)	*Eumusca*
112. *lineata* Brunetti	Syn. of *M. conducens*	*Musca*
113. *lucens* Villen.	Valid species	*Musca*
114. *lucidula* Loew	Valid species	*Musca*
115. *ludicifacies* R.-D.	Syn. of *M. autumnalis autumnalis*	*Eumusca*
116. *ludifica* Fabr.	Syn. of *M. domestica domestica*	*Musca*
117. *lusoria* Wied.	Valid species	*Viviparomusca*

Species and subspecies names	Synonymy	Subgenus
118. *lusoria* Bezzi nec Wied.	Syn. of *M. convexifrons*	*Viviparomusca*
119. *mediana* Wied.	Syn. of *M. sorbens sorbens*	*Musca*
120. *mesopotamiensis* Patt.	Valid species	*Musca*
121. *minima* Rond.	Syn. of *M. tempestiva*	*Musca*
122. *minor* Macq.	Syn. of *M. domestica domestica*	*Musca*
123. *minor* Patt. nec Macq.	Syn. of *M. sorbens sorbens*	*Musca*
124. *modesta* de Meij.	Syn. of *M. crassirostris*	*Musca*
125. *multispina* Awati	Syn. of *M. nebulo*(?)	*Musca*
126. *munroi* Patt.	Valid species	*Eumusca*
127. *nana* Meig.	Syn. of *M. tempestiva*(?)	*Musca*
128. *natalensis* Villen.	Valid species	*Viviparomusca*
129. *nebulo* Fabr.	Valid species	*Musca*
130. *nigripes* Panz. nec Fabr.	Syn. of *M. autumnalis autumnalis*	*Eumusca*
131. *nigrithorax* Stein	Syn. of *M. ventrosa*	*Musca*
132. *niveisquama* Thoms.	Syn. of *M. sorbens sorbens*	*Musca*
133. *occidentis* Walk.	Description inadequate	Uncertain
134. *osiris* Wied.	Syn. of *M. vitripennis*	*Musca*
135. *ovipara* Port. (Keilin)	Syn. of *M. autumnalis autumnalis*	*Eumusca*
136. *pampaising* Big.	Syn. of *M. domestica domestica*	*Musca*
137. *pattoni* Austen	Valid species	*Musca*
138. *pattoni* Patt. nec Austen	Syn. of *M. spinosa*	*Eumusca*
139. *pellucens* Meig.	Syn. of *M. domestica domestica*	*Musca*
140. *perlata* Walk.	Presumably valid	Uncertain
141. *phasiaeformis* Meig.	Syn. of *M. vitripennis*(?)	*Musca*
142. *pilosa* Awati	Syn. of *M. bezzii*	*Viviparomusca*
143. *planiceps* Wied.	Valid species	*Viviparomusca*
144. *pollinosa* Stein	Syn. of *M. planiceps*	*Viviparomusca*
145. *praecox* Walk.	Syn. of *M. conducens*	*Musca*

Table 4 (continued)

Species and subspecies names	Synonymy	Subgenus
146. *prashadii* Patt.	Syn. of *M. autumnalis autumnalis*	*Eumusca*
147. *primitiva* Walk.	Presumably valid	Uncertain
148. *prisca* Walk.	Syn. of *M. terrae-reginae*(?)	*Musca*
149. *promiscua* Awati	Syn. of *M. sorbens sorbens*	*Musca*
150. *promusca* Patt. (error)	Syn. of *M. sorbens sorbens*	*Musca*
151. *pulla* Bezzi	Syn. of *M. conducens*	*Musca*
152. *pulla* Patt. nec Bezzi	Syn. of *M. craggi*	*Eumusca*
153. *pumila* Macq.	Syn. of *M. sorbens sorbens*	*Musca*
154. *pungoana* Karsch	Syn. of *M. ventrosa*	*Musca*
155. *pusilla* Macq.	Syn. of *M. xanthomelas*	*Eumusca*
156. *riparia* R.-D.	Syn. of *M. domestica domestica*(?)	*Musca*
157. *rivulans* R.-D.	Syn. of *M. domestica domestica*(?)	*Musca*
158. *rivularis* R.-D. (Seguy)	Syn. of *M. domestica domestica*(?)	*Musca*
159. *ruficornis* Walk.	Presumably valid	Uncertain
160. *rufifrons* Macq.	Presumably valid	Uncertain
161. *rufiventris* Macq.	Syn. of *M. xanthomelas*	*Eumusca*
162. *rustica* R.-D.	Syn. of *M. autumnalis autumnalis*	*Eumusca*
163. *sanctae-helenae* Macq.	Syn. of *M. domestica vicina*(?)	*Musca*
164. *scapularis* Rond.	Syn. of *M. sorbens sorbens*	*Musca*
165. *scatophaga* Mall.	Syn. of *M. gabonensis*	*Eumusca*
166. *senegalensis* Macq.	Syn. of *M. domestica vicina*(?)	*Musca*
167. *senior-whitei* Patt.	Valid species	*Eumusca*
168. *sensifera* Walk.	Presumably valid	Uncertain
169. *setigera* Awati	Syn. of *M. xanthomelas*	*Eumusca*
170. *shanghaiensis* Ouchi	Presumably valid	Uncertain

Species and subspecies names	Synonymy	Subgenus
171. *sorbens* Patt. nec Walk.	Syn. of *M. conducens*	*Musca*
172. *sorbens alba* Mall.	Valid species and subspecies	*Musca*
173. *sorbens sorbens* Weid.	Valid species and subspecies	*Musca*
174. *sordidissima* Walk.	Syn. of *M. sorbens sorbens*	*Musca*
175. *spectanda* Speiser nec Wied.	Syn. of *M. lusoria*	*Viviparomusca*
176. *spectanda* Wied.	Syn. of *M. sorbens sorbens*	*Musca*
177. *spectanda* Curran nec Wied.	Syn. of *M. cuthbertsoni*	*Musca*
178. *speculifera* Bezzi	Syn. of *M. albina albina*	*Musca*
179. *spinohumera* Awati	Valid species	*Viviparomusca*
180. *spinosa* Awati	Valid species	*Eumusca*
181. *squamata* Mall.	Valid species	*Viviparomusca*
182. *stimulans* R.-D.	Syn. of *M. tempestiva*	*Musca*
183. *stomoxidea* R.-D.	Syn. of *M. domestica domestica*(?)	*Musca*
184. *sugillatrix* R.-D.	Syn. of *M. vitripennis*(?)	*Musca*
185. *taitensis* Macq.	Presumably valid	Uncertain
186. *tau* Sch.	Syn. of *M. autumnalis autumnalis*	*Eumusca*
187. *tempestatum* Bezzi	Valid species	*Musca*
188. *tempestiva* Fall.	Valid species	*Musca*
189. *terrae-reginae* J. & B.	Valid species	*Musca*
190. *tibiseta* Mall.	Valid species	*Musca*
191. *umbraculata* Fabr.	Syn. of *M. domestica domestica*	*Musca*
192. *vaccina* R.-D.	Syn. of *M. domestica domestica*	*Musca*
193. *vagatoria* R.-D.	Syn. of *M. domestica domestica*(?)	*Musca*
194. *varensis* R.-D.	Presumably valid	Uncertain
195. *ventrosa* Wied.	Valid species	*Musca*
196. *vetustissima* Walk.	Syn. of *M. sorbens sorbens*	*Musca*
197. *vicaria* Walk.	Syn. of *M. domestica domestica*	*Musca*

Table 4 (continued)

Species and subspecies names	Synonymy	Subgenus
198. *villeneuvi* Patt.	Valid species	*Viviparomusca*
199. *violacea* R.-D.	Presumably valid	Uncertain
200. *vitripennis* Meig.	Valid species	*Musca*
201. *vivipara* Mall.	Syn. of *M. larvipara*	*Viviparomusca*
202. *xanthomela* Walk.	Syn. of *M. ventrosa*	*Musca*
203. *xanthomelas* Wied.	Valid species	*Eumusca*
204. *yerburyi* Patt.	Syn. of *M. pattoni*	*Musca*

OTHER FLIES THAT FREQUENT HOUSES

In North America particularly, the following species besides *Musca domestica* are more or less common visitors in houses and outbuildings. It has been stated that the common housefly makes up 95 per cent of all flies found in houses, but I have seen situations, particularly in the North in early summer, where the large bluebottle fly constituted about the only noticeable species, being sometimes sufficiently numerous to be remarked as a minor nuisance.

The order of listing is roughly that of their importance as household pests in the northern United States. A similar list was published by McDaniel (1942).

Stomoxys calcitrans	Biting housefly, dog fly
Fannia canicularis	Lesser housefly
Fannia scalaris	Latrine fly
Muscina stabulans	True stable fly
Pollenia rudis	Cluster fly
Scenopinus fenestralis	Window fly
Calliphora vomitoria	Large bluebottle fly
Lucilia illustris	Greenbottle fly
Sarcophaga (several species)	Flesh flies
Piophila casei	Cheese skipper
Drosophila (several species)	Pomace flies
Psychoda (several species)	Moth flies

Stomoxys calcitrans (Linn.) (Family Muscidae)

This is the fly which is so annoying to animals in barnyards and which tends to enter houses before a storm. It is a fierce biter, and can be extremely bothersome on porches as well as at picnics and similar gatherings. The larvae develop in rotting straw, manger leavings, heaps of lawn cuttings, piled sea-weed, and similar media. In size and general coloring *Stomoxys* resembles the housefly, but its awllike, piercing proboscis makes it easy to recognize. The relation of the third and fourth longitudinal veins to the apex of the wing is also distinctive, as shown in Figure 59.

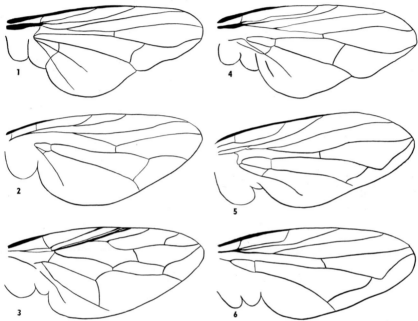

Figure 59. Wings of flies (other than *Musca domestica*) which frequently enter houses. *1: Stomoxys calcitrans. 2: Fannia canicularis. 3. Scenopinus fenestralis. 4: Muscina stabulans. 5: Pollenia rudis. 6: Calliphora vomitoria.*

Fannia canicularis (Linn.) (Family Anthomyiidae)

This grayish fly is 5 or 6 mm. in length and somewhat more slender than the housefly. It is easily distinguished from the latter by the somewhat divergent third and fourth longitudinal veins, both of which terminate posterior to the apex of the wing. The larvae develop in the same types of media as are used by the housefly, but are strikingly different, being characterized by the presence of many spinelike appendages. In houses the adults tend to hover or fly about, rather than settle upon, human food. (See Fig. 59.)

Fannia scalaris (Fabr.) (Family Anthomyiidae)

The latrine fly differs very little in general appearance from the lesser housefly. The middle tibia, however, possess a distinct tubercle, which *F. canicularis* lacks. Human and animal excrement are especially favored as breeding media. The larvae are flattened, like those of *canicularis,* but bear appendages that are quite different. The dorsal processes are scarcely larger than tubercles, while the lateral ones are fringed and so present a feathery appearance.

Muscina stabulans (Fall.) (Family Muscidae)

The nonbiting stable fly is slightly more robust than the housefly, which it resembles in having the four dark, longitudinal lines on the thorax. Both the third and fourth longitudinal veins swing forward slightly in approaching the apex, but at the same time remain nearly parallel, so that the venation is quite distinctive. (See Fig. 59.) The larvae develop in almost as wide a variety of organic substances as do those of the housefly. The maggots may be recognized by the character of the posterior spiracles, in which the peritreme is very broad and the three slits are relatively short.

Two closely related species are *Muscina assimilis* and *M. pascuorum,* the latter but recently introduced into America from Europe. The adults may be distinguished by the palpi, which are yellow in *stabulans,* reddish in *pascuorum,* and black in *assimilis.* In *pascuorum* the legs are entirely black. In *assimilis* the tibiae are mostly black, while in *stabulans* the tibiae and distal portion of the femora are yellow.

Pollenia rudis (Fabr.) (Family Calliphoridae)

This species is distinctly larger than the housefly and may be easily recognized by the abundance of yellowish, curly hair among the larger bristles of the thorax. These flies tend to congregate in buildings and especially in attics, during the first cold days of autumn. They are sometimes so numerous as to become a great nuisance. Clusters of them may be found behind picture frames, in the corners of ceilings, in closets, and in similar places. Many die as the winter progresses, but others survive until spring. They are sluggish insects, and fly with a buzzing sound. Their dead bodies give off a somewhat disagreeable odor. The larvae are parasitic in the bodies of several species of earthworms.

Scenopinus fenestralis (Linn.) (Family Scenopinidae)

These orthorrhaphous flies are found commonly on windowpanes, especially in the very early spring. The adults are black and measure about 6 mm. in length. The abdomen is of nearly the same width throughout, and terminates bluntly. In lateral view these flies have a somewhat humpbacked appearance. The whitish larvae are nearly three-fourths of an inch long, and very slender. They feed as predators upon other insects, chiefly the larvae of cereal moths and clothes moths. This is perhaps the only dipterous species common in houses which is actually beneficial to man.

Calliphora vomitoria (Linn.) (Family Calliphoridae)

This large, handsome fly may reach a length of 12 mm., with a wingspread of perhaps 25 mm. The eyes are red, the thorax is dark bluish gray, and the abdomen is metallic blue with a whitish pubescence on the anterior portion of each segment. No great number are ordinarily found in dwellings at any one time. They are much more abundant about slaughterhouses and similar places. The larvae develop normally on dead flesh, but the flies will also oviposit on sores and wounds of living animals, including man. Two very similar species are frequently confused with *vomitoria*. These are *Calliphora vicina* R.–D. (*erythrocephala Meig.*) and *C. livida* Hall (*viridescens* R.–D., of authors). The last named has three intra-alar bristles on each side, while the others each have but two. In *vomitoria* the beard is reddish; in *vicina,* black. Both *vicina* and *vomitoria* are Holarctic in distribution, but *livida* appears to be confined to the New World.

Lucilia illustris (Meig.) [2] (Family Calliphoridae)

This common pest is about the size of a housefly, but is easy to recognize since both thorax and abdomen are metallic green in color. It enters houses usually from the garbage can, where it often congregates in great numbers. Females prefer decaying flesh for oviposition, but the species also breeds in human excrement, animal manure, and living flesh. *Lucilia illustris* may be distinguished from *L. silvarum* and *L. sericata* by the fact that both these have three postacrostichal bristles, while *illustris* has only two. *Lucilia silvarum,* in turn, has black palpi, while those of *sericata* are yellow.

Sarcophaga spp. (Family Sarcophagidae)

These neat-appearing, grayish flies range from medium to large size. The males have a rather tapering abdomen; the females are more robust. The dorsal surface of the abdomen often presents a checkerboard pattern of dark and light gray, very clean-cut. Their presence in houses is rather accidental. A

[2] This is *Lucilia caesar* (Linn.) of American authors. The true *Lucilia caesar* is not a new world species.

common example is *Sarcophaga haemorrhoidalis* Fall., which is a wide-ranging scavenger. It frequents both carrion and human excrement and has been known to cause intestinal myiasis in man. The genus *Sarcophaga* is very large. Differentiation of the species depends chiefly on the distinctive features of the male genitalia. (See Aldrich, 1916.)

Piophila casei (Linn.) (Family Piophilidae)

This fly will rarely be found in the house unless food materials are kept in such a manner as to invite its breeding there. The adults are small and shining black. These lay their eggs on cheese, ham, dried beef, or similar material, in which the white, cylindrical larvae develop to a length of nearly half an inch. When food is abundant they are relatively quiet, but if conditions become unfavorable, they leap about conspicuously, by bringing the anterior and posterior extremities together and suddenly straightening the body. Horizontal leaps of ten inches are not uncommon, and have earned for this species the well-known designation "cheese skipper." The family falls in the acalyptrate Myodaria.

Drosophila spp. (Family Drosophilidae)

This genus, made famous by genetic studies of *Drosophila melanogaster*, includes a number of species of rather tiny flies that are attracted to overripe or rotting fruit, and breed therein. The pomace from cider mills is a favorite medium for their development. Certain more common species have bright red eyes and delicate wings. Since they can pass freely through the mesh of ordinary window screen, it is important that ripe fruit be exposed about the house as little as possible. These diminutive flies will often be found in very large numbers in garbage cans with lids so well fitted as to render them "fly-proof," in the ordinary sense of the word. Routine cleaning of cans with soap-suds, chemicals, or live steam is recommended. The family Drosophilidae is classified in the acalyptrate Myodaria.

Psychoda spp. (Family Psychodidae)

These are minute flies, with relatively large wings that are usually held rooflike over the body when at rest. The wings are covered with hairs, hence the common designation "moth-fly." Another name occasionally heard is "owlet midge." They frequently occur on windowpanes. Common species breed in excrement, decaying vegetables, or polluted water. The subfamily Phlebotominae is bloodsucking in habit, and various species of *Phlebotomus* (which is largely a tropical genus) transmit kala azar, Oriental sore, sand-fly fever, espundia, and verruga. All species of *Phlebotomus* are known as sand flies. They breed largely in the crevices of rubble and rock piles. All Psychodidae are rather feeble fliers and move about usually by a series of short, hopping flights. The family falls among the more primitive of the suborder Orthorrhapha.

SPECIAL NOTE ON BLACK FLIES FOUND IN HOUSES

Simulium salopiense Edwards (Family Simuliidae)

There is at least one record (Smart, 1942) of this species behaving as a swarming housefly, in England. They were observed to gather in large numbers at windows and mullions where panes were set. Males outnumbered females about fifteen to one. Although most female simuliids are bloodsucking, these did not attempt to bite. The flies had presumably been trapped by the unusual direction of the wind. All seemed intent on finding their way out. The Simuliidae are orthorrhaphous Diptera, somewhat more specialized than the Psychodidae.

CHAPTER VI

Geographical Distribution

The Lord shall hiss for the fly that is in the uttermost part of the rivers of Egypt.—
Isaiah 7:18

THE· geographical distribution of *Musca domestica* is usually given as world-wide. This statement, of course, requires some qualification, chiefly with regard to arctic regions and higher altitudes, where persistent cold excludes not only houseflies but practically all other types of poikilothermic animals. Another reason why we may choose to question its validity is that the opinion arose before the genus *Musca,* in the modern sense, was known to contain more than a very few species. Thus it is more than probable that a number of early records of houseflies in regions remote from civilization were based on mistaken identity, and actually concerned forms related to, but not identical with, *domestica.* Such mistakes, however, were soon rectified in most instances by the more or less prompt arrival of the latter, a species which has been a most constant companion to man in all his wanderings.

Apropos of the above, the following paragraph from Allee and Schmidt's revision of Hesse's *Ecological Animal Geography* seems particularly significant:

There is a whole group of commensals and parasites directly associated with man. Among these are the silverfish (*Lepisma*), cockroach (*Periplaneta*), house cricket (*Acheta domestica*), bedbug (*Cimex lectularius*), clothes moth (*Tineola biselliella*), house fly (*Musca domestica*), house mouse (*Mus musculus*) and house rat (*Rattus norvegicus*). These forms are dependent upon human culture, and are not to be found, for example, in ruins. They have followed man around the earth and become cosmopolitan; where man does not live, neither do they. They are accompanied by a host of less closely associated forms which vary with climate, vegetation, and surrounding animal life.

In the same vein, Graham-Smith (1914) makes the following arresting statement: "*Musca domestica* is probably the most widely distributed insect to be found; the animal most commonly associated with man, whom it appears to have followed over the entire earth. It extends from the sub-polar regions to the tropics, where it occurs in enormous numbers."

We see, therefore, that here is a most adaptable species—adaptable in the same sense that the human race is adaptable, and for many of the same reasons. Both are omnivorous in the extreme, being able to survive on food of animal origin, of plant origin, or on a combination of the two. Both are prolific, and tend to increase in numbers even under relatively adverse conditions. Both are given to the exploring habit, and need little encouragement to invade new territory when the opportunity presents itself. For the fly, however, new territory holds little that is inviting unless it contains the elements associated with human habitation, particularly human habitation in relation to animal husbandry. The more intimate the relationship between man and his domestic animals, the more favorable the environment for housefly multiplication. The almost complete replacement of horse-drawn vehicles by motor cars in certain urban locations has been more responsible than any other factor for the generally fly-free character of such areas.

But although man *may* live in such a manner that flies cease to find comfort in the relationship, the fact remains that vast numbers of human families in various countries of the world *still* live surrounded by conditions which the fly finds most hospitable, and which doubtless will remain so for decades, and probably for centuries, to come. When man migrates, without essentially altering his habits, he may logically expect his companion of the years to appear soon in the new location.

As an example of flies following men, we may cite Miller's report (1932) on the Muscidae of New Zealand. It appears that *Musca domestica* reached that country sometime prior to 1856, probably by way of Australian cattle ships. In the year mentioned, Walker described the New Zealand fly as *Musca vicaria,* a name now listed in synonymy with *M. domestica.* It seems to have been the opinion of the colonists that the rapid increase of the housefly had something to do with the abatement of blowflies, which had become great pests about human habitations in that part of the world, before *Musca domestica* put in its appearance. A rather quaint statement from an anonymous publication of 1872, entitled *New Homes for the Old Country,* reads as follows: "The little civilized house-fly, has, however, landed, and its refined and gentle presence is rapidly driving into the wilds this noisy spoiler of meat."

DISTRIBUTION OF THE GENUS *MUSCA* [1]

A very different picture is presented when one considers the genus *Musca* as a whole. Of the seventy or more valid forms, a few approach, to a greater or lesser extent the adaptability of *Musca domestica*. *Musca autumnalis,* for example, is common in Oriental, Ethiopian, and Palearctic life zones and utilizes a variety of breeding media. *Musca sorbens sorbens,* a house-

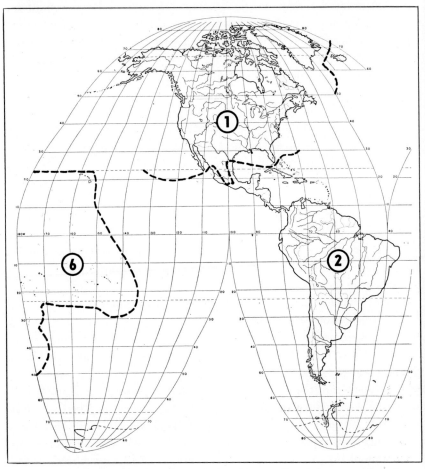

Figure 60. Zoogeographical regions of the Western Hemisphere. *1,* Nearctic; *2,* Neotropical; *6,* Australian (marginal). For detailed explanation see pages 156 and 160. (Based on Goode Base Map No. 101HC; copyright 1939 by The University of Chicago; used by permission of The University of Chicago Press.)

[1] As in the preceding chapter, certain portions of the data here presented are from the manuscript of Dr. E. G. Munroe.

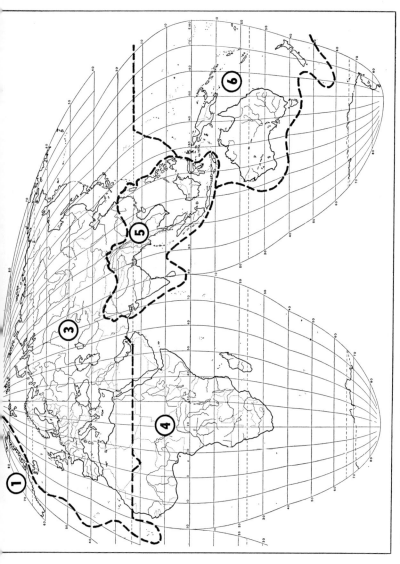

Figure 61. Zoogeographical regions of the Eastern Hemisphere. *3,* Palearctic; *4,* Ethiopian; *5,* Oriental; *6,* Australian. For detailed explanation see pages 161, 162, 165, and 166. (Based on Goode Base Map No. 101HC; copyright 1939 by The University of Chicago; used by permission of The University of Chicago Press.)

frequenting type, is widespread in Ethiopian and Oriental areas, and probably in the Australian life zone also. *Musca greeni,* on the other hand, is known only from Malaya, while *M. cuthbertsoni* is perhaps confined to Rhodesia, as is *M. gymnosomea* to Malta and North Africa.

In indicating the normal range for each of the several species it is useful to have in mind the major subdivisions of the earth's surface as recognized by biologists and geographers. Figures 60 and 61 show the generally accepted boundaries of the six principal zoogeographical regions: Nearctic, Neotropical, Palearctic, Ethiopian, Oriental, and Australian. The descriptions of these regions and their subdivisions, which appear on following pages, are essentially the same as given by Smart (1943).

It should be remembered, of course, that a great variety of habitat exists within any given geographical area. Altitude is the most influential factor in this connection. Mt. Kenya, for example, which is practically on the equator, boasts near its summit environmental conditions somewhat comparable to northern Lapland, near sea level. It is therefore conceivable that a species adapted for survival in one of these locations might readily survive in the other, if food and other essentials were available. The existence of natural barriers, such as oceans, deserts, and prevailing winds, prevents normal migration between the points in question, but when, by accident or human intention, transportation actually occurs, establishment in the new locality may not prove difficult. The increasing use of airplanes opens up great possibilities for the redistribution of the insect fauna of the world, as the time spent in flight is usually too brief to cause the death of the stowaway through denial of food and water, while variations in temperature and atmospheric pressure which can be tolerated by man will be survived by many species of arthropods.

Welch (1939) published a considerable list of insect species found on aircraft at Miami, Florida, during 1938. It is perhaps significant that *Musca domestica* proved to be the most prevalent insect, throughout the year.

Rainfall is another important factor in establishing essential differences in ecology. Desert and jungle may lie in relatively close proximity and may show similar average temperatures, but differ greatly in their hospitality toward particular species because of relative humidity, presence of vegetation (which is the basis of a food supply), and the availability of shade and other forms of shelter. Winds are significant also, as the evaporating power of continuing wind is probably as great as that of the sun, and can render arid a territory that might well be a green belt, if evaporation were less rapid.

The season of the year obviously affects the degree of influence which any of the above-mentioned factors may exercise on breeding activity. In temperate regions, for example, continued frozen conditions for a period of time may preclude all possibility of species survival. This accounts for the relatively small number of species in temperate-zone fauna as compared with the tropics. Only those species that have some method of hibernation, or confine their activities to man's domicile, or live as permanent parasites, or operate below frost line will escape destruction in the winter season. Forms may thus be recorded as having been collected in the region which are, in fact, nothing more than seasonal invaders. It should be pointed out, however, that hibernation in one stage only is sufficient, and that if the pupa, for example, can survive the winter, the seasonal death of eggs, larvae, and adults in no way detracts from the authenticity of the distributional record.

Seasons in the tropics vary less in regard to temperature than in regard to rainfall and direction of wind. Breeding of tropical forms rarely terminates completely as a result of seasonal change. When it does, the insect is said to aestivate. With muscoid Diptera, true aestivation is apparently rather rare. More common is a mere reduction in the intensity of reproductive activity. Breeding goes on, but more slowly, while the death rate remains normal or increases. The result is a falling off in population until the species becomes scarce and possibly unobtainable. With the return of favorable conditions the species reappears, increases in numbers, and may reach a seasonal peak. Two such seasonal peaks, associated with optimum moisture conditions, are not uncommon in the case of filth-feeding flies.

Larger subdivisions of the continents, in terms of physical geography, are indicated in Figures 62 and 63. A more complete analysis is represented by Figures 64 and 65.

Besides latitude, altitude, and seasonal differences, the "microclimate" is important in determining the success of a species in a given region. In an earlier publication (1946) I have pointed out the great significance of microclimate in determining the abundance of mosquitoes in restricted areas. As each species may have particular requirements for immature as well as adult stages, a large, mixed fauna usually means that a considerable number of essentially different microclimates coexist in the immediate vicinity. Strong fliers, such as muscoid flies, are usually less dependent on the microclimate in the adult state than are species with a fondness for resting, such as mosquitoes and Phlebotominae, but the larval requirements may be very demanding. Humidity, light, temperature, and food materials may be found in favorable combination only in the manure of a particular animal, only when that manure is deposited in certain situations, only when the manure is of a certain age (or freshness), and only in a certain portion of the mass, heap, or pat.

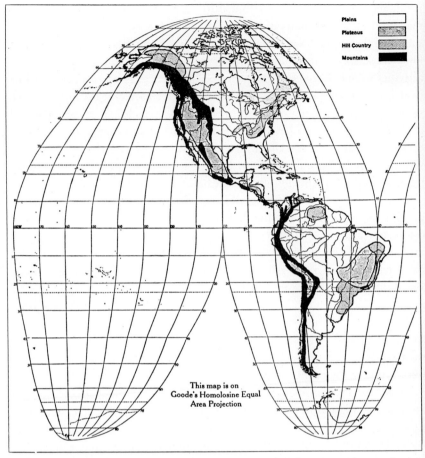

Figure 62. Major land forms of Nearctic and Neotropical regions. Topography has great influence on temperature, water supply, vegetation, and fauna, including insect life. Compare with Figure 64, which shows types of climate for similar areas. (Based on Jones and Whittlesey Map No. 7; copyright 1925 by The University of Chicago; used by permission of The University of Chicago Press.)

The Nearctic Region:

GREENLAND, ALASKA, CANADA, UNITED STATES, NORTHERN MEXICO

With the exception of one problematical species, there is no reliable evidence that the North American continent supports any representatives of the genus *Musca* other than *M. domestica*. Part IV of Walker's list (1849) does, indeed, record *M. corvina* Fabr. as occurring in Nova Scotia, but present-day workers seem united in considering this species a synonym of *Musca domestica domestica* Linn. Likewise *Musca flavipennis,* which was described by Bigot in

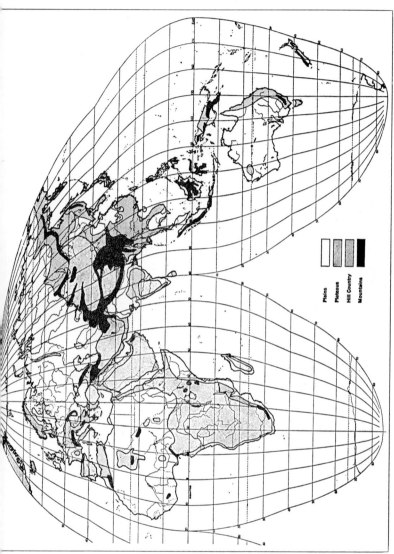

Plains
Plateaus
Hill Country
Mountains

Figure 63. Major land forms of Palearctic, Ethiopian, Oriental, and Australian regions. Compare with Figure 65, which shows types of climate for similar areas. (Based on Jones and Whittlesey Map No. 7; copyright 1925 by The University of Chicago; used by permission of The University of Chicago Press.)

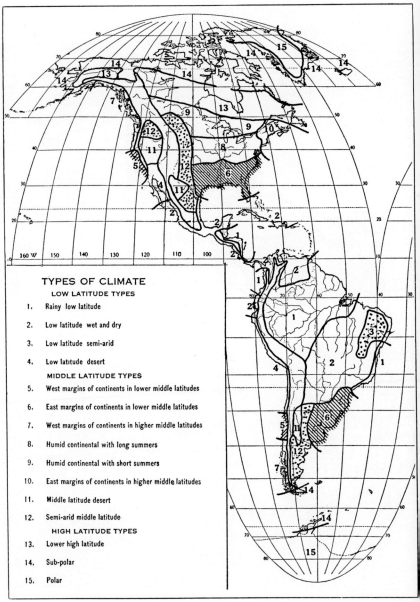

Figure 64. Types of climate found in Nearctic and Neotropical regions. Unnumbered areas are largely highlands, which may be quite dissimilar from one another climatically. (Based on Jones and Whittlesey Map No. 1; copyright 1925 by The University of Chicago; used by permission of The University of Chicago Press.)

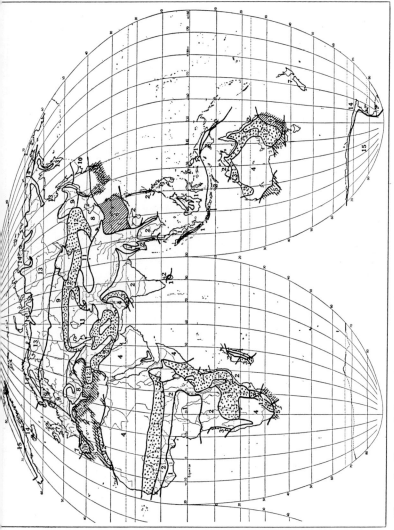

Figure 65. Types of climate found in Palearctic, Ethiopian, Oriental, and Australian regions. Numbering as in Figure 64. (Based on Jones and Whittlesey Map No. 1; copyright 1925 by The University of Chicago; used by permission of The University of Chicago Press.)

1887a,b from specimens taken in the Rocky Mountains, is today regarded as synonymous with *Musca domestica vicina* Macq. *Musca roralis* O. Fabricius, originally described from Greenland in 1780, has been pronounced "unrecognizable" by Lundbeck (1898–1900). Another Greenland species described by the same author, *Musca vivax,* has been shown by Lundbeck to belong to the family Syrphidae, while a third, *M. cloacaris,* is in all probability a synonym of *Scatophaga litorea* Fall. *Musca occidentis* of Walker is a valid species (on paper), but no modern worker attempts to identify it. Concerning Walker's work on the Diptera of the Saunders Collection, Aldrich (1905) writes: "Many new species, mostly described in a very brief and unsatisfactory manner."

We are thus reduced to the two authentic sub-species, *M. domestica domestica* and *M. domestica vicina,* which possibly hybridize.

This paucity of species in the New World is somewhat strange, in view of the ease with which foreign pests belonging in other families (and orders) have been able to establish themselves following accidental introduction. Within the family Muscidae we have the recent example of *Muscina pascuorum,* a late emigrant from Europe, and it would not be surprising if one or more additional representatives of the genus *Musca* should sooner or later put in their appearance on the American scene.

A summary of the Nearctic species is given in Table 5.

Table 5

Species and subspecies	Range or type locality	Miscellaneous remarks
M. domestica domestica	Practically world-wide, but best adapted to temperate zone	Oviparous; house frequenter; not bloodsucking
M. domestica vicina (as *flavipennis*)	Middle East, tropical Asia and Africa, South America, Rocky Mts. of U.S.(?)	Similar in habit to *M. domestica domestica*
M. occidentis(?)	Described by Walker from U.S.	Not recognized by modern workers

The Neotropical Region:

ALL WEST INDIAN ISLANDS, SOUTHERN MEXICO, CENTRAL AMERICA, SOUTH AMERICA

The record is almost as limited for South and Central America as for the northern portion of the Western Hemisphere. There is good evidence that *Musca atrifrons,* which was described by Bigot from Cuba and Mexico in 1887(a,b), should be considered a synonym of *M. domestica vicina* Macq. The same interpretation holds for *M. flavinervis,* originally described by Thomson from Honolulu, and later recorded from Mexico by Giglio-Tos. *Musca pusilla* Macq., which was originally described from "Hayti," has been placed in synonymy with *M. xanthomelas* Wied., which may therefore be listed, at least tentatively, as occurring both in the New World and the Old. *Musca sensifera* Walk., described from Mexico, is presumably a valid species, though its identity requires confirmation by modern workers. The same is true for Robineau-Desvoidy's two species, *M. fulvescens* (Central America) and *M. aurulans* (Brazil). We have therefore a maximum of six species, or seven distinct forms, if the two subspecies of *domestica* be counted separately, but of these at least three are of doubtful validity. (See Table 6.)

Table 6

Species and subspecies	Range or type locality	Miscellaneous remarks
M. aurulans	Brazil	Taxonomic position in doubt
M. domestica domestica	Practically world-wide; best adapted to temperate zone	Oviparous; house frequenter; not bloodsucking
M. domestica vicina	Middle East, tropical Asia and Africa, South America, U.S.(?)	Similar in habit to subspecies *domestica*
M. eleodivora	South America	Taxonomic position uncertain
M. fulvescens	Central America	Taxonomic position uncertain
M. sensifera	Mexico	Taxonomic position uncertain
M. xanthomelas (as *pusilla*)	Egypt to Canton and Hainan; Haiti(?)	Deposits stalked eggs; puparium whitish

The Palearctic Region

This large area is considerably richer in species than the New World. Space does not permit a searching discussion of its subdivisions, but it is well to bear in mind that four more or less overlapping areas are here involved:

European—British Isles, France, Switzerland, Austria, Hungary, Rumania, Russia north of the Caucasus and west of the Caspian Sea, together with all other countries north and west of these, including Iceland and Spitsbergen.

Mediterranean—Spain, south coast of France, Italy, Yugoslavia, Bulgaria, Turkey, Syria, Russia south of the Caucasus, Iran, Afghanistan, India west of the Thar desert, Mesopotamia (Iraq), Arabia north of the vicinity of the Tropic of Cancer, North Africa north of the Tropic of Cancer but including all of the Sahara desert, all other Mediterranean countries, Cape Verde Islands, Canaries, and Azores.

Asiatic—Asiatic republics of the U.S.S.R., Siberia, inland Asiatic states, Sakhalin.

Chinese—Japan, Korea, Manchuria, and all of China north of 30°N latitude or the vicinity thereof.

Modern dipterologists recognize sixteen determinable Palearctic forms, including the two subspecies of *domestica*. A seventeenth form, *M. shanghaiensis,* described by Ouchi from East China in 1938 is probably valid. In addition there are two of Desvoidy's species, *M. violacea* and *M. varensis,* both described from France, for which proper taxonomic assignment seems impossible. *Musca primitiva* Walk. also is probably undeterminable. A summary is given in Table 7.

The Ethiopian Region

Still more prolific in species is the African continent. Although the whole of the Sahara desert is included in the Palearctic region, the remaining area includes a wide variety of ecological conditions. Four more or less specialized zoogeographical areas are recognized within the Ethiopian realm:

Cape—All country south and east of the Kalahari desert, running up through and including the Transvaal, Southern Rhodesia, Mozambique, and the southern part of Southwest Africa.

Malagasy—Madagascar, the Seychelles Islands, Mauritius, Reunion, and other lesser islands around them.

African—The arid and savanna regions of countries inland from the Guinea coast, across the Sudan to and including Ethiopia; the Somalilands and southern Arabia. Through East Africa and the Congo, excluding the rain forest region of the latter, but including the Great Rift Valley until it meets the Cape area, thence to the Atlantic coast, skirting the southern border of the West African rain forest area.

West Africa—The rain forest areas of the Guinea coast, to and including the rain forest areas of French Equatorial Africa and the Congo basin. According to Smart, the rain forests of the lower valleys of the Senegal and Gambia rivers should be considered isolated patches of this region.

Table 8 includes a few species more Palearctic than Ethiopian, but which are usually treated in keys to the Ethiopian fauna. Thus interpreted, the re-

Table 7

Species and subspecies	Range or type locality	Miscellaneous remarks
M. albina albina	From North and East Africa to India and Ceylon	Favors desert and semi-desert; puparium whitish
M. autumnalis autumnalis	Europe, including Britain; Palestine, Kashmir,Shantung	Eggs stalked; puparium whitish; adult haematophagous
M. convexifrons	North China	Deposits larvae in second instar
M. crassirostris	Mediterranean, ranging into Oriental and Ethiopian regions	Bloodsucking; deposits large eggs, ready for hatching
M. domestica domestica	Practically world-wide; best adapted to temperate zone	Oviparous; house frequenter; not bloodsucking
M. domestica vicina	Middle East, tropical Asia and Africa, South America, U.S.(?)	Similar in habit to M. domestica domestica
M. gymnosomea	Malta and North Africa	Habits imperfectly known
M. hervei	North China to Burma and North India	Breeds in cow dung; adult haematophagous
M. larvipara	Palearctic generally; important in Russia	Bloodsucking; deposits living larvae
M. lucidula	North Africa	Habits imperfectly known
M. mesopotamiensis	Tigris and Euphrates valleys	Lays eggs singly in cow dung
M. nebulo	Mostly Old World tropics; Egypt	Similar in habit to M. domestica
M. primitiva	China	Taxonomic position uncertain
M. shanghaiensis	East China	Taxonomic position uncertain
M. sorbens sorbens	Largely Ethiopian and Oriental; perhaps Australian	House-frequenting; breeds in human and animal excrement
M. tempestiva	Mediterranean region to Kashmir	Adult haematophagous
M. varensis	France	Taxonomic position uncertain
M. ventrosa	North China; also Ethiopian; Oriental region to Australia	Adult bloodsucking; breeds in cow dung, in fields
M. violacea	France	Taxonomic position uncertain
M. vitripennis	Europe, Near East, Oriental region	Habits imperfectly known
M. xanthomelas	Hainan and Canton, to Egypt	Deposits stalked eggs; puparium whitish

gion boasts no less than thirty distinct forms, of which all but one (*Musca perlata* Walk.) are recognized by modern workers.

Table 8

Species and subspecies	Range or type locality	Miscellaneous remarks
M. albina albina	From North and East Africa to India and Ceylon	Favors desert and semidesert ecology; puparium whitish
M. albina polita	Southwest Africa	Habits imperfectly known
M. autumnalis autumnalis	Shantung and Kashmir to Palestine, Africa, and Britain	Egg stalked; puparium whitish; adults haematophagous
M. autumnalis pseudocorvina	Aberdare Range; heath zone of Mt. Elgon	Similar in habit to subspecies *autumnalis*
M. autumnalis somalorum	Somaliland	Similar in habit to subspecies *autumnalis*
M. autumnalis ugandae	Birunga, Uganda	Similar in habit to subspecies *autumnalis*
M. conducens	Widespread in Oriental and Ethiopian regions	Breeds in cow dung in fields; adults haematophagous
M. crassirostris	Mediterranean, ranging into Oriental and Ethiopian regions	Bloodsucking; deposits large egg, ready for hatching
M. cuthbertsoni	Rhodesia	Uses many breeding media; adult omnivorous
M. domestica domestica	Practically world-wide; best adapted to temperate zone	Oviparous; house frequenter; not bloodsucking
M. domestica vicina	Middle East, tropical Asia and Africa, South America, U.S.(?)	Similar in habit to subspecies *domestica*
M. elatior	Belgian Congo; Mt. Elgon (8,000 ft.)	Habits imperfectly known
M. fasciata	East Africa, Mauritius, Seychelles Islands	Haematophagous
M. gabonensis	Tropical Africa to Natal	Haematophagous
M. interrupta dasyops	Uganda and Kenya (7,500 to 13,000 ft.)	Habits imperfectly known
M. interrupta interrupta	South Africa	Habits imperfectly known
M. lasiopa	Africa	Male unknown
M. lasiophthalma	South Africa	Breeds in cow dung and other excrement

Species and subspecies	Range or type locality	Miscellaneous remarks
M. lucidula	North Africa	Habits imperfectly known
M. lusoria	Africa	Deposits second-stage larva in cow dung or other excrement
M. munroi	Natal	Habits imperfectly known
M. natalensis	Natal	Believed to be bloodsucking
M. nebulo (not truly Ethiopian?)	Egypt; Oriental region generally	Similar in habit to *M. domestica*
M. perlata	Natal	Taxonomic position uncertain
M. sorbens alba (not truly Ethiopian?)	North Africa	A desert form
M. sorbens sorbens	Largely Ethiopian and Oriental; perhaps Australian	House-frequenting; breeds in human and animal excrement
M. tempestatum	North Africa	Small species; haematophagous
M. tempestiva (not truly Ethiopian?)	Mediterranean region to Kashmir	Adult haematophagous
M. ventrosa	North China; also Ethiopian; Oriental region to Australia	Breeds in cow dung, in fields; adult is bloodsucking
M. xanthomelas	Hainan and Canton to Egypt	Deposits stalked eggs; puparium whitish

The Oriental Region

This is the most important zoogeographical region from the standpoint of species listed. Although the land masses involved total less than the Ethiopian, the number of possibly distinct forms is thirty-six, as compared with thirty for the latter. *Musca aucta* Walk. is probably unrecognizable, as is *M. rufifrons* Macq. *Musca fasciata* Stein, included here for completeness, is primarily Ethiopian.

Recognized subdivisions of the region are as follows:

Peninsular—All territory hitherto known as British India south of Deccan (Hyderabad), in addition to the Island of Ceylon.

India—All of India north of the peninsular area, including Bengal but excluding a narrow strip of semi-Alpine territory in the extreme north.

Indo-Chinese—Burma, Siam (other than territory on the Malay Peninsula), French Indo-China, southern China, Formosa, Hainan, Assam, and a strip of territory consisting of the Alpine and sub-Alpine regions of the southern slopes of the Himalaya Mountains.

Malayan—The Malay Peninsula, Sumatra, Java, Borneo, Philippines, Celebes, Timor, and the lesser Sunda Islands east to and including Roma.

The Oriental species are summarized in Table 9.

The Australian Region

Somewhat detached from other zoogeographical realms, the Australian tends to have a fauna and flora more or less unique. This is particularly true for Australia and Tasmania. Difference of opinion exists, however, as to the

Table 9

Species and subspecies	Range or type locality	Miscellaneous remarks
M. albina albina	From North and East Africa to India and Ceylon	Favors desert and semidesert ecology; puparium whitish
M. aucta	East Indies	Taxonomic position uncertain
M. autumnalis autumnalis	Shantung and Kashmir to Palestine, Africa, and Britain	Eggs stalked; puparium whitish; adults haematophagous
M. bakeri	Malaya and Philippine Islands	Adult bloodsucking
M. bezzii	India (above 1,500 feet)	Deposits second-stage larvae in cow dung
M. conducens	Widespread in Oriental and Ethiopian regions	Breeds in cow dung, in fields; adults haematophagous
M. craggi	South India, Malaya, Ceylon	Adult bloodsucking
M. crassirostris	Mediterranean, ranging into Oriental and Ethiopian regions	Bloodsucking; deposits large egg, ready for hatching
M. domestica domestica	Practically world-wide; best adapted to temperate zone	Oviparous; house-frequenter; not bloodsucking
M. domestica vicina	Middle East, tropical Asia and Africa, South America, United States(?)	Similar in habit to subspecies *domestica*
M. fasciata	East Africa, Mauritius, Seychelles Islands	Haematophagous
M. fletcheri	Assam and western Ghats	Believed to be bloodsucking
M. formosana	South China and Formosa	Habits imperfectly known
M. gibsoni	South India (above 4,000 feet), Assam, Sikkim	Lays stalked eggs, singly, in patches of cow dung
M. greeni	Malaya	Adult bloodsucking

Species and subspecies	Range or type locality	Miscellaneous remarks
M. hervei	North China to Burma and North India	Breeds in cow dung; adult is haematophagous
M. inferior	India to Java	Breeds in cow dung; adult is bloodsucking
M. illingworthi	Malaya to Philippine Islands	Adult haematophagous
M. jacobsoni	Sumatra	Habits imperfectly known
M. kweilinensis (perhaps Palearctic)	South China	Taxonomic position uncertain
M. lucens	Ceylon	Habits imperfectly known
M. nebulo	Egypt; Oriental region generally	Similar in habit to M. domestica
M. pattoni	Southern India, generally	House-frequenting; omnivorous
M. planiceps planiceps (another, unnamed subspecies occurs in Hainan)	Java, India, Ceylon	Deposits third-stage larvae on cow dung; adult favors cattle blood
M. rufifrons	Java	Taxonomic position uncertain
M. senior-whitei	From India and Sumatra to Philippine Islands	Believed to be bloodsucking
M. sorbens sorbens	Largely Ethiopian and Oriental; perhaps Australian	House-frequenting; breeds in human and animal excrement
M. spinohumera	Ganges plain and adjacent regions	Deposits second-stage larvae on cow dung
M. spinosa	India, Burma, and Ceylon	Deposits eggs singly in patches of cow dung
M. squamata	Celebes	Habits imperfectly known
M. tempestiva	Mediterranean region to Kashmir	Adult haematophagous
M. tibiseta	Sumatra	Habits imperfectly known
M. ventrosa	North China; also Ethiopian; Oriental region to Australia	Breeds in cow dung, in fields; Adult bloodsucking
M. villeneuvi	Southern India	Puparium whitish; found near elephant dung
M. vitripennis	Europe, Near East, Oriental region	Habits imperfectly known
M. xanthomelas	Hainan and Canton, to Egypt	Deposits stalked eggs; puparium whitish

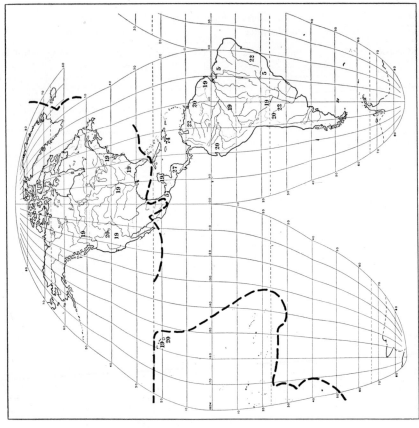

Figure 66. Geographical distribution of the species and subspecies of the genus *Musca*: Nearctic and Neotropical regions. Species of restricted range are represented by one number only. In the case of widespread forms, the number appears more than once. A list of species, by number, is given on page 170. (Based on Goode Base Map No. 101HC; copyright 1939 by The University of Chicago; used by permission of The University of Chicago Press.)

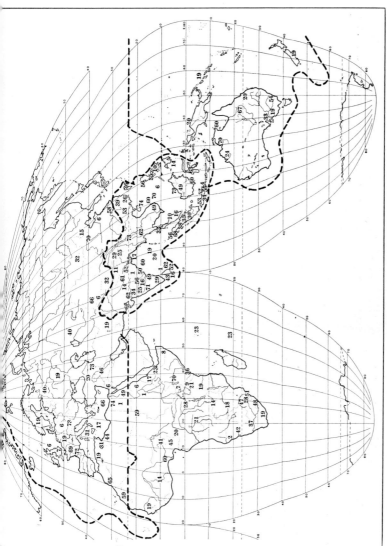

Figure 67. Geographical distribution of the species and subspecies of the genus *Musca*: Palearctic, Ethiopian, Oriental, and Australian regions. Species of restricted range are represented by one number only. In the case of widespread forms, the number appears more than once. A list of species, by number, is given on page 170. (Based on Goode Base Map No. 101HC; copyright 1939 by The University of Chicago; used by permission of The University of Chicago Press.)

Valid and presumably valid species and subspecies of the genus *Musca*—geographical distribution. Key to numbering on hemisphere maps (Figures 66 and 67). *Musca occidentis* Walk. is not included in the list. Numbers marked with an asterisk are omitted from maps because of uncertainty of record.

1. *albina albina* Wiedemann
2. *albina polita* Malloch
*3. *aricioides* Walker
4. *aucta* Walker
5. *aurulans* Robineau-Desvoidy
6. *autumnalis autumnalis* De Geer
7. *autumnalis pseudocorvina* van Emden
8. *autumnalis somalorum* Bezzi
9. *autumnalis ugandi* van Emden
10. *bakeri* Patton
11. *bezzii* Patton and Cragg
*12. *calisia* Walker
*13. *cluvia* Walker
14. *conducens* Walker
15. *convexifrons* Thomson
16. *craggi* Patton
17. *crassirostris* Stein
18. *cuthbertsoni* Patton

19. *domestica domestica* Linnaeus
20. *domestica vicina* Macquart
21. *elatior* Villeneuve
22. *eleodivora* Walton
23. *fasciata* Stein
24. *fergusoni* Johnson and Bancroft
25. *fletcheri* Patton and Senior-White
26. *formosana* Malloch
27. *fulvescens* Robineau-Desvoidy
28. *gabonensis* Macquart
29. *gibsoni* Patton and Cragg
30. *greeni* Patton
31. *gymnosomea* Rondani
32. *hervei* Villeneuve
33. *hilli* Johnson and Bancroft
34. *inferior* Stein
35. *illingworthi* Patton

36. *interrupta dasyops* Stein
37. *interrupta interrupta* Walker
38. *jacobsoni* Malloch
39. *kweilinensis* Ouchi
40. *larvipara* Portchinsky
41. *lasiopa* Villeneuve
42. *lasiophthalma* Thomson
43. *lucens* Villeneuve
44. *lucidula* Loew
45. *lusoria* Wiedemann
46. *mesopotamiensis* Patton
47. *munroi* Patton
48. *natalensis* Villeneuve
49. *nebulo* Fabricius
50. *pattoni* Austen
51. *perlata* Walker
52. *planiceps* Wiedemann
53. *primitiva* Walker
54. *ruficornis* Walker
55. *rufifrons* Macquart
56. *senior-whitei* Patton

57. *sensifera* Walker
58. *shanghaiensis* Ouchi
59. *sorbens alba* Malloch
60. *sorbens sorbens* Wiedemann
61. *spinohumera* Awati
62. *spinosa* Awati
63. *squamata* Malloch
*64. *taitensis* Macquart
65. *tempestatum* Bezzi
66. *tempestiva* Fallen
67. *terrae-reginae* Johnson and Bancroft
68. *tibiseta* Malloch
69. *varensis* Robineau-Desvoidy
70. *ventrosa* Wiedemann
71. *villeneuvi* Patton
72. *violacea* Robineau-Desvoidy
73. *vitripennis* Meigen
74. *xanthomelas* Weidemann

170

best location of the boundary line between the Australian and Oriental regions. Essig's well-known *College Entomology,* for example, shows this line passing to the west of the Celebes and just east of Java. Smart's interpretation, which is more generally used, excludes from the Australian realm not only the Celebes but also Roma and Timor. In other words, the boundary is imagined as following the Molucca Passage, rather than the Strait of Macassar. On the basis of this interpretation, four subdivisions of the Australian region have been defined:

Papuan—All of the island of New Guinea, the Moluccas, Sula, Peling, and the Lesser Sunda Islands east of Roma; also the Solomon Islands and the Bismarck Archipelago.

Australian—Australia and Tasmania.

Pacific—Micronesia, Polynesia, and the Hawaiian Islands.

New Zealand—New Zealand and all small islands closely adjacent.

It may be considered that *Musca domestica* was perhaps absent from most of this region prior to European exploration and colonization. At present, however, it seems proper to list both subspecies as established here. No exhaustive study of the genus *Musca* has been published for the Australian region comparable to Van Emden's keys to the Ethiopian species. When such a study is published, a considerable number of species now considered Oriental will doubtless be recorded from the Papuan subregion, at least. In the meantime, it seems best to adopt a conservative viewpoint and list in Table 10 only those species of undisputed Australian distribution.

Table 10

Species and subspecies	Range or type locality	Miscellaneous remarks
M. domestica domestica	Practically world-wide; best adapted to temperate zone	Oviparous; house frequenter; not bloodsucking
M. domestica vicina	Middle East, tropical Asia and Africa, South America, U.S.(?)	Similar in habit to subspecies domestica
M. fergusoni	Australia; Palm and Magnetic Islands	Adult bloodsucking
M. hilli	Australia	Habits imperfectly known
M. ruficornis	Australia	Taxonomic position uncertain
M. sorbens sorbens	Largely Ethiopian and Oriental; perhaps Australian	House-frequenting; breeds in human and animal excrement
M. terrae-reginae	Australia	Habits imperfectly known

CHAPTER VII

Food Requirements

Busy, curious, thirsty fly,
Drink with me, and drink as I.
—William Oldys, "On a Fly
Drinking out of a Cup of Ale"

MUSCA DOMESTICA is almost omnivorous. The adults delight in sputum, fecal matter, and discharges from wounds and open sores, preferring such material perhaps to sugar, milk, and other items regarded by
man as far more wholesome. Yet this preference is by no means sufficiently
strong to afford us any real protection against fly-borne disease. If the fly were
purely and simply a fecal feeder, it would not feel the impulse to spend so
much time exploring the human table. This is just what makes the species so
dangerous. All day long its restless nature causes it to fly back and forth between the privy and the kitchen, between a wound that is infected and a fresh
incision.

The only limitation regarding the type of material on which the fly may
feed is that it must be liquid, or at least capable of being rendered so. The
suitability of water, milk, cold tea, beer, and other beverages is obvious. Solid
materials, on the other hand, must be prepared for ingestion. For this the fly
has one master technique that it employs on all occasions. The reserve food
from the previous meal, which it stores in its well-developed ventral crop, is
capable of being regurgitated, without apparent effort, at all times. When a fly
explores a solid or semisolid surface, such as candy, sugar, mashed potatoes,
or a spot of grease, a drop of vomitus is extruded at the point of interest and
then sucked up again, a process that requires some time and gives ample opportunity for certain substances to pass into solution, if that is possible. Other
substances, such as starch, are taken up in the form of a suspension that, if
too heavy to pass easily through the apertures of the fly's pseudotracheae, is

merely thinned down by additional vomitus until it reaches the desired consistency.

The fly is not very thorough in cleaning up after this procedure, with the result that a portion of the vomitus almost always remains to form a vomit speck upon the surface explored. Windowpanes, as well as walls, are favorite surfaces for exploration, with the result that an almost unbelievable number of these telltale smears sometimes adorn an apparently clean surface. Graham-Smith (1910) counted 1,102 vomit specks on a pane of glass six inches square. It is of interest to note that in the same area only 9 fecal specks appeared, indicating that the fly probably distributes infectious organisms far more often by its vomitus than by its feces.

The present chapter deals, however, not with the fly as a distributor of microorganisms but with the fly as an animal species, a species with basic biological needs, the first and most important of which is food. The discussion falls naturally into two phases: food for the larva and food for the adult. The remaining stages of the life cycle, namely, egg and pupa, of course take no food and need not be considered here. Something has already been said concerning the feeding habits of adult flies. At the end of the chapter we shall pursue somewhat further the question of food in relation to the longevity of flies and also in relation to their reproductive capacity. For the present let us consider the food habits and requirements of the larvae.

LARVAL FOOD MATERIALS

When most writers speak of the "breeding" of the fly, they mean, in reality, the activity of the larvae within a medium suitable for larval nourishment. Thus Hewitt (1914a) records *Musca domestica* as "breeding" in horse, cow, human, pig, rabbit, chicken, and other manures; in carrion, spoiled meat, offal of slaughterhouses, old broth, a boiled egg, rotting fowl feathers; in spent hops, decaying grain, cooked peas, boiled rice, barley malt, excreta-soiled straw, bread, cake, bread and milk, rotten peaches, plums, cherries, bananas, apricots, potatoes, potato peelings, cabbage, carrots, cucumbers, cantaloupe, and watermelon. In addition the list includes such miscellaneous items as kitchen refuse, fermenting substances, sawdust and excrementous refuse, garbage-pile drainage, cesspool material, ensilage, paper and rags soiled with excrement, earth containing expectorated material, rubber, and snuff.

It must be remembered that though larvae have reasonable powers of migration, this activity is limited for the most part to the stage prior to pupation (Barber, 1919; Fay, 1939) and has much more to do with the selection of a site suitable for that phenomenon than with the seeking of materials for nourishment. Any discrimination, therefore, which may have been exercised in causing the larvae to be where we find them has been exercised by the mother fly rather than by her newly hatched offspring.

The ovipositing female is obviously not as particular as many species of insects, some of which limit their oviposition to a single species of host plant, the only species, in certain instances, on which the larvae can survive. That the fly is generalized rather than specialized in this respect is easy to see, though there must be some common factor, probably chemical in nature,

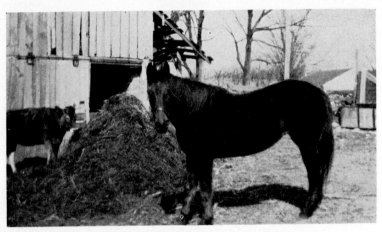

Figure 68. Barnyard manure pile. Such an environment produces many flies. This situation was considerably improved by the installation of a track and boom, which made possible direct dumping into spreader for prompt removal to fields. (Photo by Ruth West.)

which renders the various breeding media attractive to the gravid female. That the fly has preferences is well established. Crumb and Lyon (1917) state that the chief incitants to oviposition are the products of fermentation, important among which, according to their findings, is carbon dioxide. These authors report carbon dioxide as giving an 82.8 per cent higher stimulus to oviposition than ammonia, for instance, which is one of the common constituents of fermenting stable manure. Later experiments by the same workers (1921) showed sodium carbonate to be more attractive than either, which they explain by suggesting that the carbonic acid in the sodium carbonate becomes completely liberated during the fermentive process and is the substance which actually stimulates the flies. They found gravid houseflies completely indifferent to grain alcohol, to glycerine, to organic bases, and to lactic acid compounds, and concluded that decaying organic matter is stimulating to oviposition in proportion to the amount of carbonic and acetic acids liberated in fermentation.

This is somewhat at variance, however, with the work of Richardson (1916b), who secured positive results only with ammonium hydroxide and ammonium carbonate. Of the female flies tested, 90.7 per cent chose the latter. Neither water nor carbon dioxide proved attractive to gravid females in these experiments. Richardson found that the flies would even deposit eggs on acidulated manure if the latter were in close proximity to wet ammonium carbonate. The presence of the water in this case is considered to have prevented the deposition of ammonium acid carbonate, which is less volatile. Cotton or filter paper could also be made suitable for oviposition by treatment with water, ammonium carbonate, and either valerianic or butyric acids, both of which occur naturally in manures. In the attempt to rationalize such divergent findings, Richardson and Richardson (1922) prepared a bran medium that volatilized carbon dioxide only. In no case were the flies induced to oviposit. On the other hand, a bran that volatilized products of the decomposition of ammonium carbonate in aqueous solution attracted the gravid females and induced oviposition. Ammonia is obviously of some importance, though these authors were able to secure only a partial response by use of pure ammonium hydroxide. It should be remembered, of course, that ammonium hydroxide differs in several respects from an aqueous solution of ammonium carbonate.

Whatever the factors that control oviposition, there are a great many substances and materials which flies will utilize. Saunders (1916a) induced flies to lay eggs on a banana, either under loosened skin or in crevices in the pulp. Simmons and Dove (1942) found waste celery a great breeding medium for both *Musca domestica* and *Stomoxys calcitrans*. I can find no record of the housefly ovipositing in nature on a medium from which the larvae can derive no nourishment, though apparently the maggots sometimes have a difficult experience. For instance, Chapman (1944) found a number of larvae of *M. domestica* active in the bedding of an infant. It was assumed that development had taken place in the mattress filling, which had been more or less saturated with urine at various times. By way of confirmation, Chapman induced flies to oviposit on urine-soaked cotton and succeeded in rearing a number of undersized adults. It was necessary to add urine from time to time or the larvae would have died. In the case of the infested mattress, it may be supposed that oviposition took place in the daytime when the bedding was thrown back to allow the mattress to dry. The warmth of the infant's body at night doubtless maintained a proper temperature for development.

Lörincz and Makara (1935) found almost any decomposing material capable of supporting larvae, though less suitable media always resulted in a reduction in size. Nearly full-sized individuals were reared from tobacco powder, however. These authors found that the further advanced the fermentation in any substance, the longer was the period required for the completion of larval development. Thus four or five days sufficed for larval growth in fresh manure, but old dung proved so lacking in real food elements that 30 to 60 days were required. Overcrowding also resulted in smaller flies. The variation was sometimes remarkable. Large flies emerged from pupae weighing as much as 25 mg. At the other extreme, midget flies were reared from pupae less than one-sixth of this weight. Such flies, however, were incapable of reproduction.

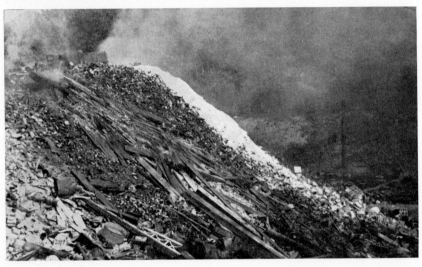

Figure 69. City garbage and refuse dump, such as can still be found on the outskirts of many small American cities and towns. An attendant keeps a slow fire burning which consumes the combustible refuse and more or less dries out the rest. Much remains, however, as a breeding medium for flies. The rat population of this particular dump is enormous. (Photo by Rollin Thoren.)

Eltringham (1916) observed that spent heaps, especially if removed from the vicinity of houses, produced no flies at all. Evidently females do not oviposit in such a medium if a better one can be found close by.

Mellor (1919) is another worker who observed that cold manure, which has completed its fermentation, is not a suitable medium for houseflies and that ovipositing females are rarely attracted to it. He mentions, however, that other species of Diptera have been successfully reared therefrom.

Some rather unusual choices of media might be mentioned. Milliken (1911) recorded houseflies as breeding in alfalfa ensilage in good feeding condition. Veitch and Greenwood (1924) found larvae of *M. domestica* feeding on the rotting seeds of *Vigna catiang,* a leguminose plant, in Fiji. De La Paz (1938b) found garbage the principal breeding material in the vicinity of Manila, where horse dung, though abundant, was not used. His interpretation was that the horse manure dried out too quickly in that climate to remain a suitable medium.

In British Guiana, Bodkin (1917) found thousands of larvae of *M. domestica* in decaying masses of lime-peel refuse from the lime factories. This created a control problem, as the refuse was used there extensively as a top dressing for young lime plants. In India, Cook-Young (1914) reported a serious outbreak of flies some ten days after the spring house-cleaning festival. The flies had oviposited in the large amount of household rubbish just thrown out.

That the fly sometimes prefers media not the best suited for complete nourishment of its offspring seems well established. In other words, the fly's instincts are not infallible. Leikina (1942) studied the value of various substrata as media for the development of *M. domestica* and observed that pig dung, human feces, sheep dung, calf dung, cow dung, and horse dung were favorable for larval development in the order named. The adults, however, were much attracted to horse manure for oviposition under the conditions of the experiment. Again, Smirnov (1937) found that *M. domestica* was never attracted to any of the meat baits which he used, but found that the larvae could be reared on such medium if transferred thereto. Of course, adults do oviposit on flesh under certain circumstances, as recorded by Mazza and Jörg (1939), who found carcasses, exposed to air, supporting small numbers of *M. domestica* larvae, along with greater populations of *Cochliomyia, Sarcophaga,* and *Lucilia,* in South America. Again, Bevan (1926), working in Southern Rhodesia, reared both *Musca domestica* and *M. humilis,* as well as *Chrysomyia* and *Lucilia,* from carcasses in various stages of decomposition. James (1928) records *M. domestica* from carrion.

The deposition of eggs in living tissue is probably a rare occurrence, and usually takes place only when the wound is infected and somewhat malodorous. When it occurs, the larvae in most cases seem quite adaptable and frequently complete their development. Fitch (1918) mentions *Musca domestica* among the larvae occasionally infesting wounds of horses and mules, and states that cleansing these wounds with disinfectants did not destroy them. Fitch found it necessary to remove the larvae with forceps.

The presence of *M. domestica* larvae in the lesions of flyblown sheep is certainly irregular, but Hardy records this condition in Australia (1934), pointing out, however, that the larvae were found in matted lumps of wool, rather than in the flesh itself, and that the flies were probably attracted by the feces present.

This interpretation is further emphasized by Mackerras and Fuller (1937), who state that the larvae of *M. domestica*, like those of *M. hilli* and *Peronia rostrata*, have never been found actually invading the skin. They are found rather in the matted, dead, and usually somewhat dry wool that has lifted from old "strikes."

Knipling and Rainwater (1937) studied 901 batches of larvae taken from human and animal wounds and found *M. domestica* seventh in point of incidence in a list of ten species (or genera) identified.

Patton and Cookson (1925) record the case of a man over eighty years of age who suffered from varicose veins of the feet and legs and also had some dermatitis. Maggots of *M. domestica* were removed in large numbers from the leg of the patient; all were small and undeveloped, though some were in the third instar. The authors considered the entire batch to have hatched from the eggs of a single female that had been attracted to an ulcerous cavity. Finding themselves in an unsuitable medium, the larvae had migrated to the surface. These larvae had been active in the tissues for weeks, with no inconvenience to the patient.

I have indicated that flies will make a definite choice of materials for oviposition when several desirable types of media are available. It is interesting to note that in different regions of the world the same species will select different breeding media and be quite consistent in doing so. Such behavior requires careful checking and experimental investigation, as several factors may be involved. First, the species may not actually be the same in two widely separated countries, even though the same name has been used for many decades. Second, species identification may be correct, but two or more physiologically distinct races may be involved. Geographical barriers prevent, or at least have prevented, the interbreeding of the two racial populations, and thus the behavior characters of each variety tend to become preserved. Behavior differences will be manifest in such commonplace tropisms as preference for human dwellings, oviposition in one type or another of animal manure, and tendency to visit carcasses, carrion, or open wounds. The third possibility, and one which is probably of paramount importance, lies in the fact that climatic and other factors greatly modify the rate and character of fermentation and/or putrefaction of organic substances. Thus conditions that render decomposing horse manure so attractive to ovipositing females in parts of Russia may not be duplicated in the Philippines, where garbage seems to be preferred. The manner in which the manure is stored, piled, or spread may be the deciding factor in many instances. Isolated droppings rarely remain suitable for long, save in a very moist climate.

It would seem well established that regardless of the suitability of substances for larval consumption, gravid flies will oviposit only in response to the presence of certain attrahents and incitants produced by particular types of organic decomposition. That these types are very widespread in nature is attested by the fact that such a wide variety of substances is utilized. Nevertheless, there are many situations which human judgment might deem suitable but which gravid females will ignore. A number of examples will serve to emphasize the very widespread diversity of habit in *Musca domestica* and closely related species throughout the world:

Austin and Mayne (1935) report *M. domestica* in Nyasaland breeding mostly in fermenting vegetable matter and human excrement. In the same country, however, *M. domestica vicina* and *M. ventrosa* prefer fowl manure. Awati (1920a) states that *M. divaricata,* an Indian species, always chooses goat dung. *M. promiscua* will utilize goat dung also, but not if fresh human feces are available. *M. divaricata* is sometimes to be found in stale human feces and human feces mixed with other materials (1920c). Patton (1922b) reared *Musca villeneuvei* from elephant dung in southern India, but reports *M. incerta* as utilizing heaps of undigested vegetable matter in slaughterhouses in Madras. Baxter (1940a) found cow dung the principal breeding medium for *M. domestica* and allied species in Fiji, an observation borne out by Lever (1944), who reared *M. domestica vicina* from both pig and cow dung, 64 per cent of his specimens being from the latter. In Mesopotamia Patton (1920a) found *M. humilis* breeding in cow dung and isolated patches of human excreta. *M. mesopotamiensis* has the peculiar habit of laying its eggs singly in patches of cow dung in the field. Bodkin (1923) found larvae and pupae of *M. domestica* in large numbers in both mule and cow pens in British Guiana.

Olson and Dahms (1946) found partly digested sewage sludge an ideal environment for the breeding of houseflies. This observation is similar to that of Hargreaves (1923), who mentions *M. domestica* as breeding in enormous numbers in the crust of septic tanks in Italy. Strangely enough, tanks containing fermenting mixtures of human excrement, animal manure, and other organic matter were observed by Illingworth (1926a) to produce very few *Musca domestica* in Yokohama, though *M. convexifrons* and species of *Lucilia* and *Calliphora* bred in this material in large numbers.

Derbeneva-Ukhova (1937) reports three times as many larvae of *M. domestica* in pig dung as in horse or cow manure or any other kind of refuse. In

Archangel (1942), however, he reports houseflies as breeding chiefly in calf manure; horse and pig dung were not available. Hafez (1939) states that in and about Cairo horse dung is most attractive to *M. domestica vicina,* with donkey dung taking its place in the open country. Cow and buffalo dung are rarely used, and camel dung is least attractive. Hill (1921) found *M. domestica* a very versatile breeder in Australia, where the list of environments includes the nests of the black-throated grebe, *Podiceps novae hollandiae.*

In the Hawaiian Islands Illingworth (1923a) found *M. domestica* develop-

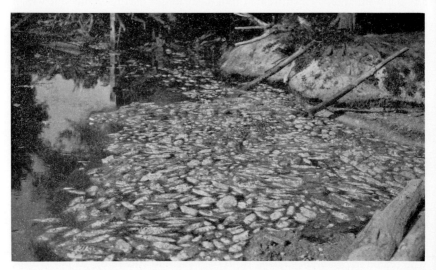

Figure 70. Pollution of streams, an indirect cause of fly production. These fish, killed by industrial pollution of the Huron River, constitute an inviting medium for the breeding of flies. (Courtesy of Michigan Department of Health.)

ing in large numbers in fowl manure stored in kerosene tins for use on gardens. Chicken manure is only used when moist, as pointed out by C. H. Richardson (1915), who studied fly control in New Jersey and reared flies from various animal manures. He mentions that cow manure was used only when mixed with straw.

The material with which the manure is combined appears to be of great importance in determining its attractiveness to ovipositing flies. Thus Robertson (1917), in testing various types of stable litter, reared 244 flies from a quantity of fresh straw litter, 18 from a similar amount of litter containing sawdust and shavings in place of straw, and none from a litter in which fresh peat was used.

The peculiar suitability of pig dung for *M. domestica* has been demonstrated repeatedly and has been emphasized by a number of workers. Rostrup (1922) states that pigsties are favorite breeding places in Denmark and that flies oviposit on the fresh excreta. Makara (1935) studied the breeding places of the housefly in Hungary and found pig dung the preferred breeding medium in that country. Kuzina (1938) noted that if all manures were fresh, the flies appeared to prefer horse dung; 70.70 per cent of their visits were to that medium, 23.83 per cent to pig dung, and 5.47 per cent to cow dung. But if the

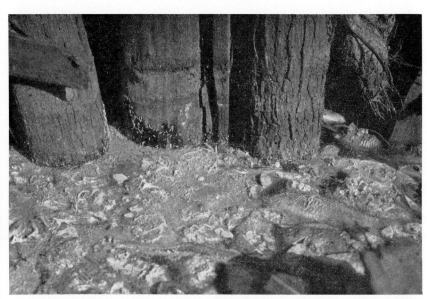

Figure 71. Flies breeding in dead fish. A closer view of the carcasses of fish killed by pollution of the Huron River. Note maggots climbing up piling, in search of a proper place to pupate. (Courtesy of Michigan Department of Health.)

pig dung was kept covered and allowed to become a little "old," it was chosen in preference to other fresh manures. Several papers by Thomsen (1934, 1935a, 1936) dealing with fly control in Denmark stress the preference of flies for pig manure. Horse, chicken, and rabbit dung are less attractive than pig dung in that country, and cow dung least of all. Calf dung is preferred to cow dung, the milk in the calves' diet being a factor here. Normal cow dung is so little used for oviposition that the spreading of a layer of cow dung over the pig manure has been found an effective method of control. Thomsen and Hammer (1936) point out that pig dung retains its suitability as a breeding medium much longer than the other manures and that this constitutes a serious control problem in Denmark, which in 1934 was estimated to have produced no less than 8.4 million tons of pig manure.

Some species are much more specialized than *M. domestica*. In Uganda, *M. sorbens* breeds chiefly in human feces, though Smirnov (1940) reports this species breeding both in feces and in pig dung in Tajikistan. According to Romanov (1940), both *M. larvipara* and *M. tempestiva* breed chiefly if not entirely in cow dung, which is also claimed to be the only medium used by *M. autumnalis* (*corvina*) in tropical Africa (Roubaud 1911). *Musca inferior*, a bloodsucking species of India, is recorded by Siddons and Roy (1940) as breeding in isolated pads of cow dung in the field.

SPECIAL FOOD REQUIREMENTS OF DIPTEROUS LARVAE

Are Bacteria Essential?

Bogdanow (1906, 1908) studied particularly the flesh fly, *Calliphora vomitoria*, but he also made observations on the housefly. He found that sterile larvae on sterile food never developed normally and concluded that the immature forms require for maturation a definite, rather simple bacterial flora. He succeeded in rearing *Musca domestica* on paste or gelatin, but only if certain molds or bacteria were also present. Meantime, however, Weinland (1907) had demonstrated that meat could be digested by the larvae of *Calliphora* without the assistance of bacteria.

Wollman (1911, 1921b) was probably the first to succeed in maintaining cultures of flies for an indefinite period on media free from microbes. Glaser (1924c) also took up the study and brought out the fact that bacteria and yeasts do produce essential accessory growth elements which must be present for the proper development of the larvae, but that these may be obtained from other sources and that the presence of the microorganisms themselves is not required. Some years later, in order to test certain theories regarding the origin of bacteriophage, Glaser developed his own sterile culture technique and published a short paper (1938a) in which are described the sterilization of the eggs, the preparation of the breeding receptacle and of the larval medium, and the procedure by which the eggs are introduced.

Anduze (1945), working with *Dermatobia*, *Sarcophaga*, and other genera, developed *four* different media for the sterile culture of various dipterous larvae.

Glaser found that the "essential food factors," normally supplied by the microorganisms that so abundantly contaminate the food of larvae under natural conditions, could be introduced into a sterile culture medium by the addition of dead bacteria or yeasts, of fresh, sterile animal extracts, or of fresh, sterile plant juices. Sterilizing the medium at high temperatures destroys these essential food elements.

Common Properties of Larval Food Materials

Bodenheimer (1931) states that the actual food of *M. domestica* larvae is virtually unknown. It is quite obvious that certain fermentive processes which attract the ovipositing females also contribute to providing food for the larvae, but a determination of just which products of decomposition are nourishing to the maggots is still to be made. It is conceivable that the requirements may be found to differ somewhat in the three larval stages.

In any event it seems well established that larvae can absorb only liquid food. Wollman (1922) calls attention to the fact that solid substances on which they are feeding always liquefy rapidly. He considers that the proteolytic action of certain bacteria may act in combination with soluble ferments secreted by the larvae. In some instances microorganisms may themselves serve as food material. Wollman obtained complete development of *M. domestica* by feeding the maggots on a gelose culture of typhoid bacilli, but remarks that the adult flies secured were of less than normal size. One of Wollman's findings is especially significant, namely, that fly larvae can thrive on food which has been heated to the point where destruction of vitamins renders it quite useless for the nutrition of vertebrates.

Quantitative Considerations

As indicated in preceding paragraphs, any deficiency either qualitative or quantitative in larval food supply results definitely in fewer adults, smaller flies, and/or a decrease in the fertility of those that survive. Kuzina (1936) studied mortality percentages in the egg, larval, and pupal stages and concluded that insufficient food for larvae always reduces the weight of the puparia and the size and fertility of the resulting flies. To test the effect of overcrowding, Vladimirova and Smirnov (1938) placed different numbers of newly hatched larvae of *M. domestica* and *Phormia groenlandica* (*terraenoveae*) on pieces of liver, each piece weighing five grams. For *M. domestica* there was no evidence of unfavorable results due to competition until the number exceeded 70. Between 70 and 200 the average pupal weight was noticeably reduced, though the total mass of larvae present (biomass) still continued to increase. With more than 200 larvae both the average weight and the biomass decreased. When this number was doubled or tripled, the mortality became very high. With 550 larvae the mortality percentage was 96.2; with 600, 98.1; with 700, 99.1.

With *Phormia*, the larvae of which are larger, the disastrous effects of competition became evident with much smaller numbers. It was clearly demonstrated that *M. domestica* can survive in larger numbers than *Phormia* when conditions are difficult, and that houseflies will develop in small numbers under conditions that preclude growth and transformation of *P. groenlandica* altogether. When the two species were tested in direct competition with one another, only *Musca domestica* survived.

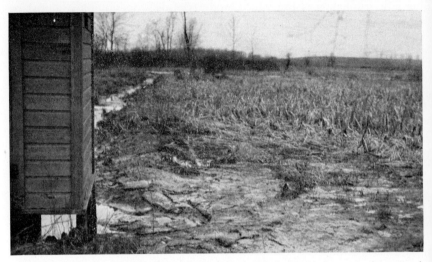

Figure 72. Faulty public-school sewer outlet. Dried sludge is shown in foreground, from which open ditch leads to sluggish creek. This condition has since been corrected by the installation of a modern sewage treatment plant. Partially digested sewage sludge is an ideal medium for the development of housefly maggots. (Courtesy of Michigan Department of Health.)

THE FOOD OF ADULT FLIES

As with all animals, the food of the adult flies is important in two ways: first, to maintain the body processes—that is, to sustain the life of the individual; and, secondly, to provide for the maturation of the sex organs and thus make possible reproduction of the species. Certain foods that serve adequately the former purpose may lack elements essential for the second. Glaser (1923a, 1924a) studied the physiology of *Musca domestica, Stomoxys calcitrans,* and *Lyperosia irritans.* For houseflies some form of sugar or assimilable starch proved necessary for normal longevity. In addition, a protein ingredient, such as might be obtained from bouillon or blood serum, was required for the production and deposition of eggs. This might be provided either by proteins in solution or by products of protein hydrolysis. Similar findings are reported for flesh flies by Dorman, Hale, and Hoskins (1938). These authors found carbohydrate essential for the continued life of the adult fly and protein for the growth of the ovaries. Several recognized sources of protein proved inadequate for this purpose. For example, casein, sodium or ammonium caseinate, blood albumin, and a commercial preparation of beef extract failed to promote ovarian development. Fish protein proved acceptable.

Derbeneva-Ukhova (1935a) made a careful study of the development of the ovaries of virgin flies (*Musca domestica*) maintained under constant conditions of temperature and relative humidity. The diet was varied in a number of ways. Regardless of this, ovarian development was the same for the first day of adult life. This was obviously at the expense of internal resources, as starved flies did quite as well as properly nourished females. Beyond the first day, the effect of qualitative differences in food was very noticeable. On a diet

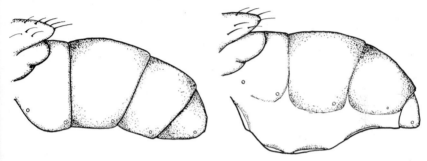

Figure 73. Adaptive expansion of the fly's abdomen. *Left:* Condition in an unfed specimen. *Right:* Abdomen distended by recent engorgement of liquid food. It will be recalled that the expanded portion of the crop lies in the abdomen. Note great expansion of conjunctival areas.

of water and egg albumen no further ovarian development took place and all flies were dead by the fourth day. When fed on a 20 per cent solution of sugar the flies survived, but the ova did not develop. On a high fat diet, consisting of water, butter, and vegetable oil, 86.2 per cent of the flies died in 24 hours, and the entire colony succumbed the following day. Death may have been due to the tracheae becoming plugged with fat. When carbohydrates were added to the albumen, full sexual development was completed by the seventh day. This is somewhat slower than normal development, as shown by the fact that on a diet of milk or other properly balanced food the same was achieved in five days, most of the development being completed by the fourth day, sometimes the third.

The above-described experiments support, in general, the findings of Kobayashi (1934a), who studied the influence of foods on the fecundity of *M. domestica* and concluded that saccharose or soluble starch is necessary for longevity, and protein or peptone for maturation of the ovary.

Experimental workers have successfully maintained breeding colonies of flies on a relatively simple diet. Grady (1928) fed his adults on milk, bread, sugar, and a little yeast. Tischler (1931b) believes that bread soaked in milk is entirely adequate. The bread, he states, serves merely as an absorptive medium. He does not consider it necessary to add yeast, meat broth, or sugar, and believes that essential vitamins are supplied by fermentation of the milk, which proceeds rapidly at the temperatures in which flies are usually reared (85°–90°F). The frequency with which flies are permitted to feed seems very important. Tischler records a very high mortality when he fed less often than two or three times a day.

Water is always necessary. Lodge (1918) found that without it houseflies could not live more than 48 hours. For further discussion of the handling of flies under laboratory conditions, the reader is referred to Chapter XV.

In nature, flies seek a wide variety of substances; their instincts thereby insure a complete and balanced food intake. Their preference for the swill barrel is one of the annoyances of sanitarians.[1]

Parker (1914) remarks that beer seems especially attractive to most species of fecal-feeding flies, and that this can create a health problem in taverns and saloons. Lodge (1916) found that she could make poison baits immediately attractive to flies by the addition of beer or stout. Blood is always attractive to flies, and technicians working outdoors or in unscreened quarters frequently have their blood films ruined by flies feeding on them when the slides are laid out to dry. Packchanian (1944) observed that flies infected with the flagellate parasite *Herpetomonas muscae domesticae* frequently passed these in their feces while visiting blood films. This can lead to serious errors in diagnosis, as inexperienced technicians may easily mistake *Herpetomonas* for trypanosomes.

Malodorous discharges from lesions of animals will attract flies from some distance. Morris (1919) in his studies on anthrax observed many flies feeding at the open carbuncular swellings of sick animals. He advised against the deliberate opening of such swellings as a dangerous and useless practice.

Flies do not ordinarily feed on plant juices unless these contain substances attractive to them in an olfactory way. They would undoubtedly take the nectar of many flowers if they were structurally adapted for getting at the nectaries. Exposed honey, as everyone knows, comes in for its full share of attention. Juices less attractive from a human standpoint are sometimes eagerly

[1] Jackson (1908) records over 1,000,000 bacteria from each fly taken on swill barrels. Morrill (1914a) reports an average of 4,000,000.

sought out by flies. Leidy (1871), for example, noticed flies sipping diffluent matter from the stinkhorn fungus, *Phallus* (*Ithyphallus*) *impudicus*.

Casual observers of flies have not always discriminated between activities related to feeding and activities related to oviposition. Graham-Smith (1916) points out that *M. domestica* may enter houses immediately after emergence and remain there until ready for oviposition, but that no eggs are ever deposited on food in kitchens. Dexler (1918), who observed the activities of flies in the markets of Vienna, found that though *M. domestica* and *M. meridiana* will feed on fresh meat, neither has been known to oviposit there. Certain species of *Calliphora, Fannia, Phormia, Muscina,* and *Lucilia* do, however, both feed and oviposit in such situations.

As for the actual ingredients of foods that excite the feeding instinct, we have the work of Richardson (1917a), who found glucose, fructose, maltose, and starch not very attractive to feeding flies. Lactose and dextrin were more stimulating. Sucrose proved to be a very poor attrahent. A 4 per cent solution of amylic alcohol was more attractive than the same concentration of ethyl alcohol, 4 per cent acetic acid, 10 per cent acetic acid, or 10 per cent amylic. Four per cent ethyl alcohol proved superior to 10 per cent, but in the case of acetic acid the percentages were reversed. Succinic acid and lactic acid were fairly attractive. The flies moved eagerly to the water-soluble portion of gelatin derived from wheat flour and were attracted by fat-free caseinogen, but showed no inclination to visit butterfat. Richardson found an aqueous preparation of wheat flour and molasses, plus sodium arsenite and some amylic alcohol, to be a very effective poison bait.

Awati and Swaminath (1920) studied the food habits of two houseflies of India, *M. divaricata* and *M. promiscua*. Rice, wheat, pulses, egg, meat, and fish were allowed to decompose and the chemical changes resulting from fermentation or putrefaction were noted at daily intervals. For each food there was a period of beginning attraction, followed by a period of maximum appeal. After this there was a noticeable falling off in the ability of the substance to attract flies, and a stage was finally reached in which there was no attraction whatsoever. These authors recorded that decomposing egg, meat, and fish were by far the most attractive foods. Pulses were less often chosen, while rice and wheat had very little attraction for the flies if other foods were available. They found the relative alkalinity or acidity of the mass to be of little or no importance. Awati and Swaminath reasoned that the presence of ammonia, hydrogen sulphide, phosphorous compounds, and other substances with distinctive odors is necessary before the fly is even stimulated to approach a food, though that food might be entirely satisfactory from a nutritive point of view.

FACULTATIVE BLOODSUCKERS

Several species of the genus *Musca* have been referred to as facultative blood-suckers, in recognition of their appetite for fresh animal blood, even though they themselves lack the buccal apparatus necessary to puncture the skin of

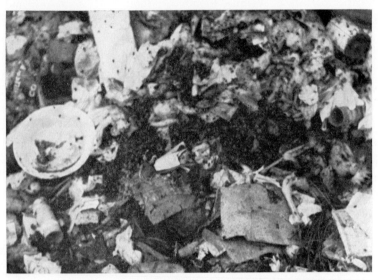

Figure 74. Flies feeding and breeding in neglected refuse dumped along highway and in open fields. It is easy to understand the vast fly populations of late summer, when such conditions are permitted to exist. (Courtesy of Michigan Department of Health.)

the vertebrate host. Hammer (1941) places *M. autumnalis* and *M. tempestiva* in this category. *Musca sorbens* is another species of similar habit. Lamborn (1937) studied this form with reference to its possible role in the transmission of leprosy. Although nonbiting, *M. sorbens* is attracted to the slightest break in the surface of the skin, and has been known to feed on the face without its presence being noticed. Lamborn goes so far as to suggest that the disappearance of leprosy from Europe may have depended, at least in part, on the control of *M. autumnalis,* brought about by general improvements in sanitary standards.

Mercier (1925) makes mention of both *M. autumnalis* and *M. vitripennis* as among those which, though not true bloodsuckers, feed on exudations from the skin. He found that both these species readily ingested blood which appeared at the wounds left by true bloodsucking flies. Both are common on cattle in Normandy.

Austen (1910b) and Patton and Cragg (1913a) record *M. pattoni* as feeding on blood that oozes from the bites inflicted on cattle by biting flies. The latter authors describe as many as six large *M. pattoni* assembled around one small *Philaematomyia insignis*, waiting for the true bloodsucker to finish its meal. *M. gibsoni* depends in a similar manner on species of *Stomoxys* and *Bdellolarynx*. Derbeneva-Ukhova (1942a) speaks of *M. larvipara* as feeding facultatively on drops of blood from wounds made by Tabanidae. Similar habits are recorded for *M. fasciata* in Southern Rhodesia by Cuthbertson (1934a), who found both sexes especially abundant during April and May. These flies fed freely on bleeding cuts and sores of cattle, horses, and human beings, and actively sought the exudations from bites of tabanids and other bloodsucking forms.

Musca domestica is not too commonly associated with the facultative haematophagous types, but being polyphagous, it utilizes this method of feeding when opportunity affords. Aders (1916) found this species and others feeding in close association with *Stomoxys calcitrans* and *S. nigra* in the Zanzibar Protectorate. He states that the secondary feeders usually alight close to the bloodsucker and when the latter moves there follows an immediate scramble for the droplet which remains. Lever (1934) reports a similar relation between *M. domestica vicina* and *Lyperosia exigua*, bloodsucking pest of cattle in the Solomon Islands.

The genus *Musca* also includes a few true bloodsuckers. *M. crassirostris*, a South African species, is a pest of horses on the veldt in March and April. It prefers the open country and rarely enters stables to bite the animals, though it frequently attacks them in the kraals (Du Toit and Nieschulz, 1933). *Musca inferior* feeds on bovine blood in India.

The feeding habits of adult muscoid flies of fifteen different species, including *M. domestica*, were studied by Derbeneva-Ukhova (1942b) in connection with investigations on ovarian development. Five classes or groups were recognized.

(1) Obligatory coprophagous species. These must obtain all their albuminous nutriment from dung, and cannot (or do not) use protein from other sources. By virtue of their habits they are of no medical or veterinary importance.

(2) Facultative coprophagous species, which, in addition to animal dung, feed also on human feces, kitchen refuse, and foodstuffs. *Muscina assimilis* and species of *Fannia* fall here.

(3) Obligatory blood feeders. These must have animal blood for normal development and reproduction. *Stomoxys, Lyperosia,* and *Glossina* are typical genera.

(4) Facultative haematophagous species. These seek blood when they can obtain it, but can and do make out on other food if circumstances require. *Musca larvipara, M. autumnalis,* and *M. tempestiva* are of this type.

(5) Polyphagous types. These feed on a wide variety of food materials and are less dependent on particular types of protein than any other group. *Musca domestica* is the classical example, though, as we have seen, it also has specific food requirements. *Muscina stabulans* is usually listed as polyphagous, also.

The chapter that follows treats of two important environmental factors that influence markedly the development and behavior of common flies, namely, temperature and relative humidity.

CHAPTER VIII

Temperature and Humidity

To a boiling pot flies come not.—Herbert, Jacula Prudentum

IN ADDITION to the presence or absence of suitable food materials, there are several important environmental factors which strongly influence the life processes in all stages of the life cycle and which may accelerate, retard, or at times prevent entirely the insect's growth, transformation, and reproduction.

The temperature, both of the atmosphere in which the fly carries on and of the medium in which the larvae develop, is one of the most important. Intimately involved with temperature is the relative humidity, a factor particularly influential in maintaining the condition of the medium in which the larvae grow and develop. Light conditions, the movement of air currents, altitude (which introduces changes in barometric pressure), and vibratory disturbances all have a bearing on the biology of the fly and help to form the ecological setting in which the species must survive or perish. Again the acidity (or alkalinity) of various substances may have a bearing on their attraction for ovipositing females. Likewise, the solid, liquid, or gaseous condition of a substance may not only influence its attractiveness to adult flies but may perhaps determine its suitability as larval or adult food. Last, the presence or absence of microorganisms, of parasites, and of predators may modify profoundly the environmental picture.

In the present chapter we shall inquire particularly into the influence of temperature and humidity on the life processes of the fly, reserving the remaining factors for discussion elsewhere.

EFFECTS OF TEMPERATURE ON THE EGG STAGE

The several stages of the life cycle will be discussed in turn. For each stage there is a maximum temperature above which development may not proceed, a minimum temperature at which activity also ceases, and an optimum tem-

perature, usually closer to the maximum than to the minimum, at which
growth, development, and normal activity proceed most satisfactorily. Lethal
temperatures, which cause the death of the organism, are encountered above
the maximum and below the minimum for bodily activity. These are not nec-

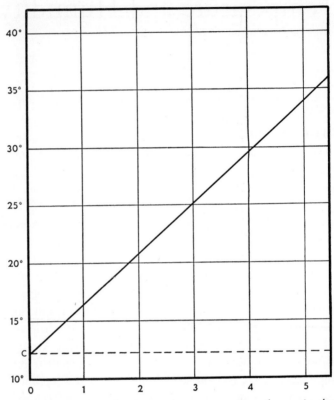

Figure 75. Effect of temperature on maturation of ova. As the
temperature rises, the number of days required for the preoviposition
period declines. This graph was plotted from the reciprocals of the
empirical values for the duration of the period. It is therefore a
curve of velocity. The threshold of development is considered to be
in the vicinity of 12.2°C. (From Larsen and Thomsen, 1940.)

essarily fixed at exact points for any species; the duration of exposure is an
important factor in determining whether or not a given temperature may
prove lethal. Individual differences are also encountered among houseflies, as
with other organisms, and natural selection is continually at work, eliminating
the poorly adapted and preserving strains capable of tolerating extreme conditions.

In nature, optimum conditions are rarely met with for any extended period of time. *Musca domestica,* however, has a very wide range of adaptability and tolerates a much greater deviation from its preferred ecology than most species of insects. It is this adaptability, of course, which has enabled it to achieve such success in utilizing the domestic environment of man.

Eggs of the housefly cannot, apparently, survive a temperature above 46.1°C (115°F). Roubaud (1915a) advocated their destruction by burying fresh manure in old heaps so that captive fermentation might raise the temperature of the mass above the death point. The actual lethal temperature is probably a little lower than this, especially if the exposure to high temperature is long sustained. Davidson (1944), for example, found that relatively few eggs hatched at 41.6°C (106.9°F) and none, in his experiments, at 42.8°C (109°F). The peak temperature he considered to be somewhere in the vicinity of 36°C (96.8°F). Davidson also demonstrated that variations in the temperature are of great importance in determining the rate of embryonic development. His observations for temperatures ranging from 15.0°C to 40.0°C (59.0°–104.0°F) are shown in Table 11.

Table 11. Incubation period in hours for eggs of *Musca domestica.*

Temp. °C	Temp. °F	Hours required before hatching
15.0	59.0	51.45
17.8	64.0	33.28
20.6	69.1	23.08
23.3	73.9	17.16
26.1	79.0	13.50
28.9	84.0	10.65
31.7	89.1	9.00
34.4	93.9	8.14
37.2	99.0	7.63 (optimum)
40.0	104.0	8.05

These results are in general agreement with those of Melvin (1934), who showed that both high and low temperatures tend to prolong the incubation period. Melvin found that the eggs of several species, including *Musca domestica,* will hatch at temperatures as high as 104°F (40.0°C), but that none will hatch at 109°F (42.8°C).

Lörincz and Makara (1935) found that incubation required seven days at temperatures ranging from 8° to 10°C (46.4°–50°F). At 20°C (68°F) the period dropped to 22 hours, and at 30°C (86°F) to 15 hours. At 40°C (104°F) the eggs hatched 12 hours after oviposition. It will be noted that these figures differ considerably from those of Davidson, particularly at the higher temperatures.

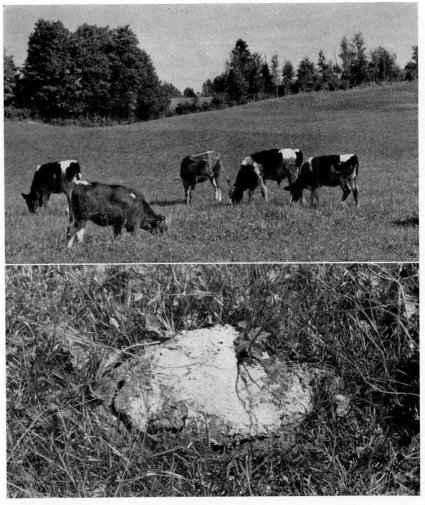

Figure 76. Manure in pasture rarely produces houseflies. *Upper:* Animals grazing. Cow pats are scattered and dry out quickly. *Lower:* Individual cow pat, dried by sun. Photograph shows a few emergence holes, probably made by Scatophagidae. Houseflies prefer a medium that remains moist for several days. (Photos by Rollin Thoren.)

Simmonds (1928), in writing of the housefly in Fiji, mentions that when temperatures range between 74° and 86°F (23.3°–30.0°C), hatching of the eggs takes place approximately 21 hours after they are laid.

Hafez (1941b), working in Egypt, records that the eggs of *M. domestica vicina* require 6 hours for hatching at 35°–38°C (95–100.4°F), 11 hours at 25°–30°C (77°–86°F), and 40 hours at 10°–15°C (50°–59°F).

In general it may be said that of all the developmental stages, the egg is the most sensitive to abnormally high temperatures, the larva next, and the pupal stage the least. Such were the findings of Larsen (1943), who also noted that death from exposure to heat may sometimes occur long after the exposure has taken place. Larsen obtained very similar results for *M. domestica, Stomoxys calcitrans, Haematobia stimulans,* and *Scatophaga stercoraria.*

At the opposite extreme, we have the observations of Kobayashi (1921) in Korea, on the exposure of flies to cold. As with high temperatures, it was the egg of *M. domestica* which proved to be the least resistant stage. Adults were

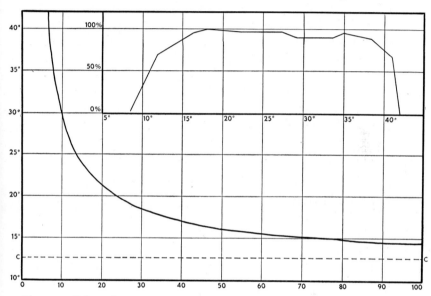

Figure 77. Effect of temperature on period required for hatching of eggs. This constructed hyperbola shows increase in number of hours at lower temperatures. Special plotting at top shows how the hatching percentage is affected by extremes of temperature. Below 10°C and above 42°C, very few ova survive. The optimum is near 18°C. (From Larsen and Thomsen, 1940.)

most able to survive. Larval and pupal stages fell somewhere in between. In a subsequent publication (1940b) the same author gives 10°C (50°F) as the temperature at which all eggs (as well as larvae) perished.[1]

From observations such as these it is apparent that the ovum is particularly vulnerable to extremes of temperature and that no hibernation or aestivation in the egg stage may be expected to occur.

[1] Feldman-Muhsam (1944b), working with *M. domestica vicina* in Palestine, found that though the eggs were very sensitive to prolonged cold, they were more resistant than other stages to intense cold for a short period.

EFFECTS OF TEMPERATURE ON LARVAE AND PUPAE

Observations incidental to conventional disposal practices give at least a rough idea of the conditions that larvae and pupae may tolerate. Joshi and Dnyansager (1945), for example, studied fly breeding in compost trenches in India. The trenches, which were twenty feet long, six feet deep, and three feet wide, were filled with alternate layers of town waste and night soil. Two inches of dirt covered the topmost layer of rubbish. From April to June, inclusive, the temperature of the upper layer of rubbish ranged between 60° and 65°C (140°–149°F). As this amount of heat is lethal to fly larvae, few maggots or pupae could be found. During the rainy season, however, the temperature of this layer fell to between 37° and 49°C (98.6°–120°F) and many maggots and pupae were observed. During this period there was, of course, a much higher relative humidity. This is favorable up to a point, but excessive moisture is a real deterrent to transformation. Thus under monsoon conditions many pupae perish. Joshi and Dnyansagar found that only 10 to 20 per cent of the pupae collected at this time proved viable when transferred to a favorable environment.

It should be remembered, however, that a relatively dry atmosphere is no guarantee of successful metamorphosis unless temperature conditions are also favorable. Thus in Australia 32 puparia of *Musca vetustissima* (1943) were observed to yield 30 adults at a temperature of 30°C (86°F), but 120 puparia yielded only 101 flies at 18°C (64.4°F). Temperature and humidity are inextricably involved with one another, and neither can be adequately evaluated as an environmental factor without giving due consideration to the other.

De La Paz (1938c), who advocates a zymothermic method of larval control, found that all stages of the flies, as well as many of the pathogenic organisms which they carry, could be destroyed by the temperature of his "fermentation chambers," which ranged from 60° to 70°C (140°–158°F).

Bridwell (1918) states that in the Hawaiian Islands horse manure alone ferments so rapidly that housefly larvae cannot exist in the high temperatures produced. Baber (1918), who devised the so-called *Baber* trap for destroying housefly larvae, found that the latter are driven to migrate from manure when the temperature of fermentation reaches a certain level. These temperatures reach 130°F (54.4°C) and even 160°F (71.1°C).

In this connection it should be pointed out that susceptibility of larvae to extremely high temperatures depends, in part, on factors other than the temperature itself. Thus Roubaud (1915b), who also advocated the *méthode biothermique* for larval control, records that larvae die in three minutes at

50°C (122°F) if protected from the gases of fermentation, but die in one minute at 51°C (123.8°F) if such gases are present. At 60°C (140°F) with exposure to gases of fermentation, larvae die in four to five seconds.

Regarding the question of larval survival at low temperatures, there is some difference of opinion. Bodenheimer (1931) places the critical cold point for larvae of *Musca domestica* at 5°C (41°F), but Petrishcheva (1932) found that mature larvae of *M. domestica* might survive 14 days at temperatures

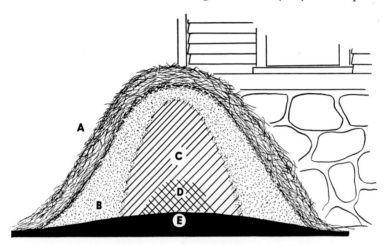

Figure 78. Five microclimates in one manure pile. *A,* superficial zone. This is usually too much dried out to support fly maggots. It may also be too cool, though in desert areas it can become too hot. *B,* breeding zone. Moisture is available and heat of fermentation is usually not too great to be tolerated. *C,* hot zone. Humidity is ample, but heat of fermentation is usually so great that larvae either die or migrate elsewhere. *D,* cooler zone; maggots sometimes present. *E,* cold zone, in contact with earth. Pupae may be present, but not active larvae.

ranging from —1° to —2°C (30.2–28.4°F). Even very young larvae withstood —2°C for three and a half hours, but died at any lower temperature. In no case would mature larvae pupate at a temperature lower than 10°C (50°F). The apparent discrepancy between the findings of Bodenheimer and those of Petrishcheva may possibly be explained by the assumption that the Palestinian race is less adapted genetically to reduced temperatures than that found in Samara on the Volga.

The effect of *changing* temperatures on larval activity is equally significant. I am unable to find precise data for *M. domestica,* but Miller (1929) studied the effect of altered temperature on the larvae of *Lucilia sericata* and noted that below 10°C (50°F) locomotor activities are abruptly reduced. There is a slow increase in the rate of motion between 10°C (50°F) and 30°C (86°F), with a slow decrease again above 42°C (107.6°F).

Larvae not only display varying degrees of activity with fluctuating temperatures but if given a choice will actively seek conditions suitable for their best development. Derbeneva-Ukhova (1940a) observed that outdoor heaps of horse manure, when heated by fermentation, frequently harbored larvae of *M. domestica* within an inch of the surface, if the day was warm, but that on cold days they tended to concentrate at a depth of from two to four and a half inches, where the temperature ranged from 102.2° to 107.6°F (39°–42°C). These findings confirm in general the earlier work of the same author (1937), who determined that the most desirable temperatures for the larvae lie between 42° and 45°C (107.6°–113°F). He found none at a depth of six inches, where temperatures ranged from 50° to 63°C (122°–145.4°F). At a depth of twelve inches, however, where temperatures ranged from 35° to 44°C (95°–111.2°F), larvae again were present. Only pupae were found at a depth of two feet. One should remember that pupation always takes place at lower temperatures than those favored by the larvae. Cotterel (1940) never found larvae or pupae deeper than three inches from the surface of manure piles in West Africa. The temperature at this depth was, he states, somewhat less than 50°C (122°F).

Thomsen and Thomsen (1937) undertook to study the thermotropisms of larvae. They did this by means of a long trough, one end of which was heated and the other cooled, thereby establishing a temperature gradient. A special humidifying device was installed at the heated end to prevent excessive dryness. The trough was then filled with horse dung or other suitable material, and the larvae were introduced at various points. Very young larvae of *M. domestica* sought a temperature between 30° and 37°C (86°–98.6°F). As they became older, the larvae migrated to regions of successively lower temperature until, just prior to pupation, the preferred temperature became 15°C (59°F). That the larvae do not absolutely require these particular temperatures at successive stages was demonstrated by the fact that the same experimenters successfully maintained a stock colony at a constant temperature of 25°C (77°F).

Haematobia stimulans larvae chose temperatures between 19° and 23°C (69°–73.4°F), *Lyperosia irritans* between 27° and 33°C (80.6°–91.4°F). The latter is a summer breeder, while the former reproduces more effectively in the spring and autumn months.

Puri (1943) states that in general high temperatures are conducive to fly production by shortening the developmental period of the larvae, by hastening sexual maturity, and by stimulating mating and oviposition. The general truth of this cannot be challenged; however, the highest temperatures are not always associated with the largest numbers of flies. Bodenheimer (1931) noted a decrease in fly population during midsummer in Palestine, due, apparently, to the fact that the surface layers of manure piles frequently became heated above the maximum temperature which the larvae could tolerate. This, he states, is about 60°C (140°F). Such conditions sometimes prevail to a depth of as much as eight inches.

Some workers place the critical high temperature much lower than this. Thus Cotterel (1940) states that flies cannot develop in manure with a temperature of 114.8°F (46°C), while Elton (1927) quotes Austen (1926) to the effect that larvae of *M. domestica* will die at temperatures of 105°F (40.6°C) or over. This would appear to be questionable, as Hase (1935), who cultured *Musca domestica* as well as species of *Fannia* and *Drosophila*, observed the larvae to be very flourishing in media that had attained a temperature of 42°C (107.6°F). This temperature exceeded that of the surrounding air by 18.5°C (33.3°F) and may be supposed to have been largely produced by fermentation, though the presence of the larvae themselves doubtless contributed in part to the generation of heat.

Ecological relations are somewhat different in the case of blowflies, but it is interesting to note, in this connection, that very striking increases in temperature may sometimes be achieved by the activities of larvae in decomposing animal tissue. Deonier, for example, who published his observations in 1940, noticed that in the American southwest, flyblown carcasses, at least at certain points, were sometimes as much as 70°F (38.9°C) higher in temperature than the surrounding air. Masses of larvae were found active at points 50°F (27.8°C) above atmospheric temperature. A little of this was undoubtedly due to sunshine, but Deonier considers the phenomenon traceable largely to the heat generated by the larvae themselves. Such adaptation enables the maggots to continue active under winter conditions, when the weather is usually quite unsuitable for normal activity on the part of the adults.

INFLUENCE OF TEMPERATURE ON DURATION
OF IMMATURE STAGES

For complete development from egg to adult fly, great variations are possible. Kvasnikova (1931) records that development may be completed in 13 days when the temperature is 23°–24°C (73.4°–75.2°F). Dropping the temperature to 20°C (68°F) increased the developmental period to somewhere between 20 and 31 days. This author states that when prevailing temperatures reached 10°–12°C (50°–53.6°F), adult flies disappeared entirely from the fauna.

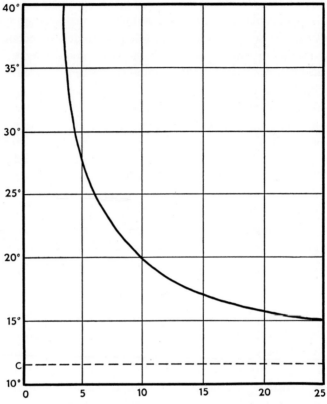

Figure 79. Relation of temperature to duration of pupal state. As the temperature declines, the number of days required for transformation is increased. The curve shown above is a constructed hyperbola. (From Larsen and Thomsen, 1940.)

Kramer (1915), who made a careful attempt to eliminate all factors except the temperature, was able to show, with light and humidity constant, that development required only half as long at 30°C (86°F) as at 20°C (68°F). Elevation to 35°C (95°F) shortened the period still more.

Kobayashi (1940b) found that oviposition and larval development occurred in Japan at temperatures down to 15°–16°C (59°–60.8°F). The same author (1935,) working in Korea, showed that total development could take place in as brief a time as 6 days with the temperature at 28°C (82.4°F), but that this was extended to 41 days when temperatures ranged between 13°C (55.4°F) and 19°C (62.2°F). Optimum conditions existed between 25°C (77°F) and

30°C (86°F), at which level development normally required from 7 to 12 days.

In Bermuda (Allnutt, 1926), with a prevailing temperature of 90°F (32.2°C) and a relative humidity of 90 to 100 per cent, flies emerge with reasonable consistency 12 days after the eggs are laid. Bodenheimer (1931) gives 10 days as the normal time required for the completion of the life cycle under midsummer conditions in Palestine. Controlled experiments by Petrishcheva (1932) in Russia show the accelerating effect of increased temperature. In a rearing chamber maintained thermostatically at 95°F (35°C) development was completed in from 6 to 8 days. This fell to 5 at temperatures between 100.4° and 104°F (38°–40°C).

A government notice from British Guiana (1916) states that larvae of *Musca domestica* require 6 days for completion of development at 84.6°F (29.2°C) in that country, and 4 at 90°–98°F (32.2°–36.7°C). This last was considered the most favorable temperature range for the larvae by these workers. The same paper states that incubation of the egg of *M. domestica* required 13 hours at a temperature of 78.8°F (26°C).

Mention has already been made of the fact that larvae about to pupate usually seek a site for transformation where the temperature is somewhat less than that utilized for larval growth and development. Not only is a lower temperature more suitable for this stage of the life cycle, but pupae actually appear to tolerate lower temperature extremes than larvae without suffering an arrest of development. Kobayashi (1921) observed that pupae survived and gave rise to flies in rooms too cold for larval activity. Dove (1916) records that during a twelve-hour period 85 flies emerged from puparia exposed to a maximum of 55°F (12.8°C) and a minimum of 43°F (6.1°C). These were the actual temperatures of the media, which consisted of cow manure with some straw. Derbeneva-Ukhova (1935b) reports flies emerging in Moscow down to 51.62°F (10.9°C). When the average temperature reached this point, however, emergence ceased. It is specifically stated in this report that the relative humidity was approximately 78 per cent.

Among the many investigations carried out to throw light on the relation of temperatures to development, those of Derbeneva-Ukhova (1940b,c) are especially illuminating. Newly hatched maggots of *Musca domestica* were placed in tumblers on fresh dung, which was renewed daily. The relative humidity was kept between 70 and 80 per cent. At 43°C (109.4°F), in either pig or horse dung, larval development required approximately 5 days. In horse dung, at 36°C (97.8°F) the average was 4. In pig dung, 34°C (93.2°F) larval development averaged only 3.1 days, with a minimum of 2.5. At still lower temperatures the time was again increased, becoming 7.5 days in pig dung and 6.5 days in horse dung at 25°C (77°F). The differential effect of the two types of media is very interesting. Except at extremes of high and low temperature, development in pig dung was always quicker than in horse or cow manure, and larvae reared on pig dung attained greater size. Derbeneva-Ukhova considers this to be due to the more favorable humidity of pig dung, which left to itself tends to be intermediate between that of the other two.[2]

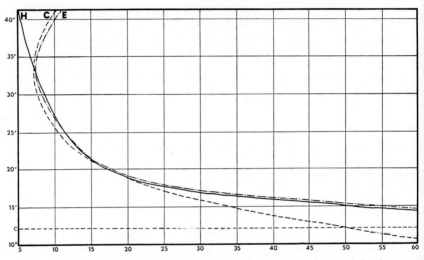

Figure 80. Effect of temperature on total time required for preimaginal development. Abscissa represents duration of development in days. Empirical plottings are approximated by curve *E*. It will be noted that the catenary curve, *C*, tends to follow the empirical most closely at higher temperatures, while the hyperbola, *H*, runs closer in the intermediate range. (Adapted from Larsen and Thomsen, 1940.)

Second-instar larvae were observed to be active between 10° and 42°C (50°–107.6°F). The optimum was 35°C (95°F). Tolerance was greater in the case of third-instar maggots; the range of activity for them extended between 8° and 45°C (46.4°–113°F). Optimum for third-instar larvae was 36°C (97.8°F). However, when fully grown and about to pupate, the larvae were most active at 29°C (84.2°F) and the range of their activity fell to between 5°C and 43°C (41°–109.4°F). This, of course, is in accordance with the well-known

[2] Hafez (1941b) found that, under identical conditions, larvae of *M. domestica vicina* completed their development in pig and horse manure in 8 days, in sheep dung within 10 days, in human excrement in 14, and in kitchen refuse in 20. He also states that pig dung (in Egypt) retained its suitability as a breeding medium much longer than cow, horse, or donkey dung.

tendency of mature larvae to migrate to a cooler environment for pupation. It was found that larvae in this condition endeavored to leave the breeding medium at 36°C or above. All that were transferred to a temperature of 25°C (77°F) pupated and gave rise to normal flies. Those allowed to remain at temperatures ranging from 36° to 43°C (97.8°–109.4°F) suffered mortality in direct proportion to the temperature.

It was noticed that the activity of both second- and third-instar larvae decreased markedly at temperatures above the optimum. This was more pronounced for the second instar than for the third.

Temperatures that proved too high for larval development in the laboratory are apparently sometimes tolerated in nature, especially if the maggots have an opportunity to adapt themselves somewhat gradually. This opportunity frequently exists, as manure piles that may have a temperature below 35°C (95°F) at the time the eggs are laid can, through fermentation, become heated to around 40° or even 45°C (104°–113°F), at least near the surface, by the time the larvae reach the third instar. Experiments were performed in which the eggs were first placed in situations with temperatures ranging from 32° to 33°C (89.6°–91.4°F). The temperature was then increased gradually during the course of development, so that the third-stage larvae were exposed to temperatures ranging from 44° to 48°C (111.2°–118.4°F). When tested, these larvae showed a temperature range for activity extending from 12° to 48°C (53.6°–118.4°F), with the optimum at 41°C (104.9°F). Larvae of the same degree of development which had been reared at 25°C (77°F) showed a range of activity from 8° to 45°C (46.4°–113°F). Their optimum was 36°C (96.8°F). Mortality tests showed that fatal temperatures varied directly with those at which the larvae had been kept. Even the most heat-tolerant, however, died at 51°C (123.8°F).

Special interest attaches to the so-called *Levant* housefly, *Musca domestica vicina,* the domestic fly of Egypt and of Palestine. Hafez (1941b) made extensive studies of this species in the vicinity of Cairo, where it occurs throughout the year, being notably abundant in the spring months and again in September. Favorable atmospheric temperatures for this fly range from 28° to 35°C (82.4°–95°F). The higher temperatures of summer prevent oviposition and development. In the winter breeding is confined to stables and similar situations. Hafez found that the three larval stages lasted about 15 hours, 20 hours, and 2 days, respectively, at approximately 30°C (86°F). Under the same conditions pupal transformation required 3 days. With the temperature ranging from 20°–26°C (68°–78.8°F), the figures became 20 hours, 30 hours, and 3 days, with the pupal stage lasting 4 days. Under controlled conditions, development was completed in 5 days and 6 hours at 38°C (100.4°F), whereas at 13°C (55.4°F) 19 days and 8 hours were required. At 40°C (104°F) larval mortality was very high.

Feldman-Muhsam (1944b) studied the same species in Palestine. He brought out the interesting fact that though the sexes emerged in equal numbers in the laboratory, in nature females predominated during the winter months, males during the summer. Possibly related to this is the prevailing temperature of the dung in which pupation occurs. This ranges from 21° to 50°C (69.8°–122°F) in summer, but in winter becomes 10°–23°C (50°–73.4°F). It may be that these temperatures are selective for survival of the sexes. In reporting on larval development Feldman-Muhsam makes use of Blunck's improved rule of temperature sums, namely, that the "effective" temperature (in degrees) multiplied by the duration of development (in days) is a constant, within the limits of a certain biological temperature range. The "effective" temperature is the difference between average prevailing temperatures and that low temperature which represents the threshold of development. Thus the thermal constant for the egg stage proved to be 7.4 hour-degrees C (13.32 hour-degrees F). The constant for the larval period was 132 day-degrees C (237.6 day-degrees F), for the pupal period 87 day-degrees C (156.6 day-degrees F), and for preovipositional development of the ova 45 day-degrees C (81 day-degrees F). The threshold temperatures were found to be 12.6°C (54.68°F) for the egg, 8°C (46.4°F) for the larvae, 11.3°C (52.34°F) for the pupae, and 14°C (57.2°F) for preoviposition stages.

The thermal constant of total development, if such an expression is desired, may be obtained by adding the thermal constants for the different stages, determined experimentally. Such a procedure was utilized by Zwölfer (1934) in his studies of forest insects.

There is often an appreciable difference in reaction to temperature on the part of the various species within a genus. For example, Romanov (1940) observed that whereas *Musca larvipara* completed its development in cow dung within two days at temperatures ranging from 18° to 46.5°C (64°–115.7°F), *Musca tempestiva* required from two and a half to three days under the same conditions.

USE OF MATHEMATICAL SYMBOLS

It seems impossible, at the present time, to reduce to mathematical certainty the relationships between fluctuating temperatures, humidities, and the time required for the completion of the various stages of development. A number of workers have, however, used mathematical devices to express relationships more definitely than can be accomplished by mere tabulation of data. As yet the majority of medical and entomological workers are not sufficiently trained in higher mathematics to make ready use of this type of report, but as techniques are improved and more exact data becomes available in greater amount, the increased use of mathematical formulas to symbolize the effects of environmental factors on duration of development seems inevitable.

A few examples of the use of mathematics in the study of housefly biology are given below.

Kobayashi and Mizushima (1937)[3] studied the relation between laboratory temperatures and the development of flies from oviposition to adult emergence. These authors reared 1,533 individuals of *M. domestica*. It was found that a hyperbola of the formula $y = a \div (x - a)^b$ expressed temperature relationships very well. In the above equation, $y =$ the length of development in days; x, the mean laboratory temperature; and a, the threshold temperature. The symbols a and b stand, respectively, for 126.795 and 0.96921, constants that these authors worked out for *Musca domestica*. Such constants differ for each species studied. By threshold temperature is meant that temperature below which development may not, theoretically at least, take place. It is not a biologically well-defined temperature point but is very useful in comparing one species with another. Equivalent terms are "critical lower temperature point" and "developmental zero."

One of the most important papers in recent years is that by Larsen and Thomsen (1940). These authors question the reliability of Kobayashi's data chiefly because of the temperature fluctuations in the larval medium that he used ("pressed draff of bean-curds"). This material ferments actively and on warm days may rise 3°–7°C (5.4°–12.6°F) above the temperature of the surrounding air. Since the mean "experimental temperature" of Kobayashi and Mizushima was calculated for each experiment by means of the average daily temperatures, it would appear that their figures, especially at high temperatures, probably deviated considerably from those at which the larvae actually developed.

Larsen and Thomsen review the work of Kramer (1915), Hutchison (1916), Peairs (1927), Melvin (1934), Füsthy (1937), Bodenheimer (1924) and Cousin (1932). In their own studies they made use of electric incubators and a

[3] This report is a more detailed account of preliminary observations published by Kobayashi in 1935.

constant-temperature room, by means of which a fairly accurate record of actual developmental temperatures was obtained. Other special techniques are discussed in Chapter XV. These authors plotted their results (Fig. 80) against constructed hyperbolas and catenary curves. The formula for the equilateral hyperbola differs but slightly from that of Kobayashi and Mizushima:

$$t = \frac{const.}{T - c}$$

In this expression t = duration of development

T = registered temperature

c = threshold of development

constant = temperature sum or "thermal constant."

For substitution values Larsen and Thomsen tried several points, finally fixing on $21.5°C$ ($70.7°F$), with development in 15.67 days, and $30.3°C$ ($86.5°F$), with development in 8.04 days. Substituting in the formula $t (T - c) = t_1 (T_1 - c) = $ const., c is found to be $12.2°C$ ($53.96°F$). This value may then be substituted in either equation, giving a thermal constant of 145.5, which is thus seen to be the product of the duration in development and the effective temperature. This particular constant is given in "day degrees." Thermal constants may of course be given in "hour degrees," "minute degrees," or in any unit of time.

The formula for the symmetrical catenary curve is that of Janisch and others (1928, 1933).

$$y = \frac{m}{2} (a^{w-x} + a^{-w+x})$$

In this expression y = the time

m = shortest duration of development

w = optimum temperature

x = registered temperature

a = a constant

The values used were as follows:

$$y = \frac{6.92}{2} (1.133^{33.2-x} + 1.133^{-33.2+x})$$

This is based on the duration of development at optimum temperature (6.92 days at $33.2°C = 91.76°F$).

The hyperbola gives a lower threshold of development than other types of curves, and the required calculations are far simpler for the hyperbola than for the catenary.

It is doubtful if either type of curve can be used to symbolize accurately the effect of temperature on development at all levels. It will be noted (Fig. 80) that the plottings for the total preimaginal development tend to follow the catenary curve for the higher temperatures, and tend again in the same direction for the lower temperature readings, at which development is naturally prolonged. The empirical curve agrees well with the hyperbola, however, over a fairly long stretch. The work of Peairs (1927) does not show the same deviations as that of Larsen and Thomsen, but he used beef as food for the larvae, whereas they used manure, and it may well be that poisonous gases from the beef slowed down development at higher temperatures. Cousin (1932), who worked on *Lucilia sericata,* obtained results closely in accord with those of Larsen and Thomsen in many respects. The findings of Bodenheimer (1924, 1931), which were really in the nature of pioneer work, deviate rather widely from the more exact incubator experiments of later investigators, but this is not surprising considering the conditions under which he worked.

A truly symbolic curve could be exceedingly useful, as it would permit the prediction of developmental cycles, as Bodenheimer (1925) attempted. He considered that the time of development, in relation to the surrounding temperature, forms an exact equilateral hyperbola. Assuming this, if the duration of development is known for but two points of temperature, the entire hyperbola may be constructed.

SPECIAL REMARKS ON HUMIDITY AS AN ENVIRONMENTAL FACTOR

We have little but general data concerning the effects of humidity alone on housefly development. Certain observations, however, are sufficiently interesting to deserve mention. Feldman-Muhsam (1944a), who studied *M. domestica vicina* in Palestine, noted that in that country the cow manure dried very quickly, forming a crust. Both larvae and pupae could be found beneath, usually about four inches below the surface. This drying of the surface of the manure pile obviously inhibits the prepupal migration, and is believed to delay and possibly prevent development in many cases. The same author (1944b) points out, however, that in winter conditions are very different. Many larvae and pupae then die because of excessive humidity. The same factor is believed to inhibit oviposition. It should be remembered that winter in Palestine is rarely cold enough to cause the death of adults or to interfere with the development of the immature stages.

Fay (1939), who worked on methods of controlling larvae in Illinois, found that though a temperature of 120°F (48.9°C) was always lethal to the maggots, the latter could develop at 110°–116°F (43.3°–46.7°C) if the medium remained moist. Like other workers, Fay found that larvae survived only in the outer four inches of manure piles, due to the internal heat. This is greater in heavier manures than in light.

Hutchison (1914) showed that the presence or absence of moisture greatly influenced the behavior of larvae about to pupate. He found that 98–99 per cent of the third-stage larvae could be made to leave the manure if the latter was kept moist, but that only 70 per cent migrated when the manure was more or less dry.

An excessive amount of moisture may be fatal to the larvae in any stage. Derbeneva-Ukhova (1943) found that only 60 per cent survived when the moisture content of the soil was 10 per cent.

Copeman (1916) pointed out that though 115°F (46.1°C) was lethal for all fly larvae which he observed (regardless of the amount of moisture present), the time required to accomplish death was much less with wet heat than with dry.

Bruce (1939) performed experiments with the pupae of *Lyperosia irritans, Cochliomyia hominivorax,* and *Musca domestica,* including 1,600 specimens of the last. Maintaining a constant temperature of 80°F (26.7°C), Bruce placed the puparia in jars of fine sand in which the water content ranged from 0 to 17 per cent. Adults emerged from sand with a water content up to 14 per cent, but rarely from anything higher. The upper limit was around 16.1 per cent. *Lyperosia,* which did best with a water content of around 7 per cent, failed entirely to survive at a percentage less than 0.25.

EFFECTS OF TEMPERATURE AND HUMIDITY ON THE ACTIVITY OF ADULT FLIES

The work of Dakshinamurty (1948), in which *Musca domestica* was exposed to four different combinations of temperature and humidity, shows that adult flies tend to be most active when temperature is high and humidity low. They remain reasonably active at tolerably low temperatures, regardless of humidity, but tend to become extremely sluggish when both readings are high. These findings tend to bear out the impressions of most casual observers under natural conditions.

Nieschulz (1935) studied the behavior of both *M. domestica* and *Fannia canicularis* when exposed to controlled temperatures. He found that activity for *M. domestica* began at an average temperature of 6.7°C (44°F). The optimum temperature was not quite the same for the two sexes, being 33.1°C (91.6°F) on the average for females and 34.2°C (93.6°F) for the males. When the temperature was raised to 44.6°C (112.2°F), symptoms of heat paralysis became evident; complete cessation of movement was obtained, on the average, at 46.5°C (115.7°F). *Fannia* was affected by lower average temperatures all the way through. For that species, activity began at 4.2°C (40.1°F). Heat paralysis began at 39.1°C (102.3°F) and was complete at 40.9°C (105.5°F). The optimum temperature for both sexes was 23.7°C (74.6°F). After comparing these results with previous work done on *Stomoxys calcitrans* (1933b, 1934), Nieschulz came to the conclusion that each species has its own optimum temperature and range of normal activity.

In conducting these experiments Nieschulz placed the flies in test tubes, in a water bath. The temperature was raised 1°C (1.8°F) every three minutes. He states (for *Stomoxys*) that results are not affected by age, sex, humidity, amount of food taken, or degree of maturation of the eggs in the body of the female.

Another piece of apparatus used by Nieschulz (1933b) is worthy of mention. This consisted of a long metal tank, one end of which was inserted in a chamber with a constant temperature of 50°C. The other end was inserted in an icebox. After a few hours' operation, the tank reached a condition that might be termed thermal equilibrium, each point remaining constant. The flies were liberated into the tank and their behavior was observed through glass. *Stomoxys,* for example, came to rest within a half hour and thereafter remained between 27°C and 32°C. It will be recalled that Thomsen and Thomsen (1937) used a similar device for the study of larval tropisms.

Nieschulz and Du Toit (1933) also made comparative studies of *Stomoxys calcitrans, Musca vicina,* and *M. crassirostris* in South Africa. For *M. (domestica) vicina,* heat paralysis did not begin until the temperature reached 45.4°C (113.72°F). It was complete at the same point as for the European housefly (46.5°C). For *Musca (Philaematomyia) crassirostris,* the lowest temperatures at which movement was noted averaged 10.4°C (50.72°F); heat paralysis began at 44.9°C (112.82°F) and was complete at 46.3°C (115.34°F).

Temperatures that permit the general activity of flies result of course in reproduction and increase in fly population. Thus Katagai (1935), working in Formosa, reported flies scarce from January to April, with a sudden increase in May, a decrease in June, and a second peak in September. These peaks were invariably associated with temperatures above 77°F (25°C). Katagai noted a regular irregularity in sex ratios. Females were in the ascendancy between November and April, but males predominated during the remaining months of the year. This would seem to be due in part to the greater ability of the females to survive during that portion of the year which approached winter conditions.

In Manchuria, Ono (1939) records *Musca domestica* as first appearing in April at temperatures around 42.8°F (6°C). The flies became abundant in mid-June, and decreased in November. Dove (1916) found that at Dallas, Texas, flies which were inactive at 45°F (7.2°C) crawled slightly at 48°F (8.9°C) and flew voluntarily at 53°F (11.6°C). No flies, according to his observations, survived freezing temperatures for more than three days.

Oviposition appears to require a slightly higher temperature than that which permits general physical activity. Kalandadze and Chilingarova (1942b) found that the number of egg batches deposited by *M. domestica vicina* in Georgia (U.S.S.R.) decreased sharply with any sudden drop in atmospheric temperature, and ceased entirely at 10°C (50°F). It is noteworthy that no oviposition took place even though the temperature in the upper layers of manure heaps remained between 15° and 20°C (59°–68°F). Dorman, Hale, and Hoskins (1938) consider the developmental zero for egg formation to be in the vicinity of 14°C (57.2°F.) The *rate* at which ovarian development proceeds is likewise dependent on prevailing temperatures. Uvarov (1931), citing Bishopp, Dove, and Parman (1915), states that the length of the preoviposition period for houseflies may vary from four days at a temperature of 30.6°C (87°F) to twenty days at a temperature of 20°C (68°F).

The same author, citing Rödel (1886) and Dönhoff (1872), gives data to show that flies are killed at temperatures not many degrees below the freezing point of water. Thus, death resulted from a five-minute exposure at —12°C (10.4°F), a twenty-minute exposure at —8°C (17.6°F), a forty-minute exposure at —5°C (23.1°F) and, in another experiment, a three-hour exposure at —10°C (14°F), later raised to —6°C (21.3°F).

Hafez (1941b) found that *M. domestica vicina* could withstand as low a temperature as —7°C (19.4°F) for six hours, but that death occurred when the flies were exposed to —11°C (12.2°F) for three hours.

Within tolerable temperatures, however, longevity is definitely greater at thermometer readings somewhat below those at which adult activities are usually carried on. Dove (1916) found the most favorable temperatures for survival to be under 60°F (15.6°C). *Musca domestica* maintained at such temperatures lived as long as 91 days, an observation that has a strong bearing on the question of hibernation, especially in more southern latitudes (see Chapter IV). It is worthy of note that houseflies always seek temperatures above 60°F, when given an opportunity to do so.

The interaction of temperature and humidity in determining both activity and survival is a subject that deserves additional investigation. Beattie (1928), who studied the simultaneous effect of these two factors on the blowfly, *Calliphora erythrocephala,* found that the ability of this species to withstand exposure to high temperatures was especially poor between humidities of 60 and 80 per cent. The optimum within this range was 70; that is, the flies died at lower and at higher humidities, when the temperature was even lower than that which they survived at a relative humidity of 70 per cent. It has been suggested that flies die at high temperatures because of loss of water, but Beattie determined that there was no loss of weight at a relative humidity of 90 per cent. This would seem to indicate that insects die in saturated air because they do not have the ability to control their body temperatures by evaporation. Why the flies should die at humidities of less than 70 per cent, however, is not easy to understand, as there is no greater loss of weight below this level than at 70 per cent.

Observations on one or two other species and varieties may be mentioned:

Musca domestica vicina, as studied by Feldman-Muhsam (1944b), lived as long as 106 days in captivity at favorable temperatures; they died more quickly as temperatures rose. The lethal effect of high temperatures was much less marked, however, with a relatively high humidity than with a low. Above 20°C (68°F) the flies lived longest at a relative humidity of 42 to 55 per cent. Below 20°C, 30 to 40 per cent humidity permitted them to be active and enjoy a life span of reasonable length, while 80 per cent humidity made them weak, sluggish, and short-lived. Zimin (1939–1941b) records that the lowest temperatures at which *M. sorbens, Chrysomyia albiceps, Sarcophaga* spp., and other southern forms enter houses in Tajikistan range from 24° to 27°C (75.2°–80.6°F) at a relative humidity of 32 to 35 per cent. For certain cosmopolitan species and those of a more northerly distribution the figures are 8°–16°C (46.4°–60.8°F) with a relative humidity of 47–58 per cent.

It should be remembered that in nature, all or at least many environmental factors are subject to fluctuation at the same time. Even under experimental conditions, investigators frequently fail to control all factors affecting their results. Mellanby (1934), who worked chiefly on lice and mosquitoes, points out that published figures on the thermal death point of the genus *Musca* differ as much as 5°C. This is obviously due to variations in several interacting factors. The duration of exposure is one of these, as is the relative humidity during the exposure period. Furthermore, at different temperature levels, time of exposure and relative humidity may differ both in their separate and in their combined effects. It is reasonable to suppose that the rate of metabolism increases with higher temperatures, particularly in a poikilothermic animal. Thus at high temperatures death may be due chiefly to exhaustion of the reserve food supply. Mellanby's experiments make it evident that well-fed insects survive much longer at high temperatures than do starved ones.

PREFERRED TEMPERATURES OF FOODS

For food to be attractive to adult houseflies its temperature should be somewhere between 12° and 56°C. Olive Lodge (1918) tested houseflies in regard to this and found that the optimum temperature for food lay between 38° and 48°C (99°–118°F). The maximum at which food was taken by flies was 55°–58°C (132°–136°F), while the minimum was 10°–13°C (50°–55°F). That flies prefer food materials somewhat warmer than the average of the atmosphere in which they fly is perhaps a reflection of their long association with human kind.

CHAPTER IX

Miscellaneous Ecological Factors

It is easier to catch flies with honey than with vinegar.—English proverb

THE ecological factors other than food, temperature, and humidity which influence the development, activity, and reproduction of animal organisms are many. We have data, however, on but relatively few. The following discussion will be confined largely to certain effects of light, air currents, and barometric pressure on the biology of flies. In time, it is to be hoped that additional research will throw light on many areas now obscure. Studies on the interaction of two or more environmental factors are especially to be desired. There is probably no phase of muscoid biology which is more inviting to the young investigator or more deserving of attention at the present time. With modern physiological equipment, avenues of approach are now open which did not exist for the student of a generation ago. The incorporation of ecological problems in the planned programs of our experiment stations and graduate schools is most desirable.

LIGHT AS AN ENVIRONMENTAL FACTOR

Casual observations make it evident that flies in general are positively phototropic. Many species tend, for instance, to congregate on sunny walls. When taken in the collector's net practically all Diptera fly upward, a habit of which the entomologist takes advantage when he holds the net mouth down, in transferring his specimens to the killing jar. For beetles, with their tendency to "play possum" and drop to earth, such technique would be disastrous. Other conditions being similar, flies also prefer to feed in well-lighted places, though their favorite foods often remain moist and attractive for a longer time in somewhat shady situations; when the two stimuli are pitted against one another, the gustatory usually takes precedence.

Breeding activities likewise are favored by ample illumination of the environment. In this connection may be mentioned the experimental work of

E. P. Felt (1910c), who pointed out that flies do not breed freely if confined in darkness. They show a rather decided preference for sloppy filth in light places. Gravid females, however, will and do crawl into dark crevices to deposit their eggs, a concession to the larva's dependence on a relatively high humidity (see Chapter VIII).

Of course, light may be so intense as to drive flies to rest elsewhere. Thus Zimin (1939–1941b) records *Musca domestica vicina,* which is very abundant in Tadzhikistan during July and August, as avoiding both excessive shade and bright sunshine. *Calliphora erythrocephala* he mentions as preferring weak light and being most active in the late hours of the day. Such observations, however, in no way nullify the generalization that *Musca* and allied genera are essentially diurnal groups which, in the adult state, carry on most of their activities in reasonably well-lighted situations.

LARVAE NEGATIVELY PHOTOTROPIC

The larvae, in contrast to the adults, are more or less negatively phototropic, a provision that serves the species in causing them to avoid exposure to strong light with the desiccation that such exposure frequently involves. Whether strong light is of itself toxic to the larvae may be disputed, but it is generally accepted that with animals of such delicate integument, any prolonged exposure to ultraviolet light must have a deleterious effect. The ultraviolet content of unobstructed sunlight is, of course, considerable. In this connection it is of interest to note that Uvarov (1931), citing Weidling, mentions intensive exposure to electric light as retarding the development of the larvae of *Calliphora* for about a week.

QUALITY OF LIGHT IMPORTANT

The foregoing general observations, though interesting, have but relatively little scientific value, since light is of many qualities and insects sometimes react differently to one portion of the spectrum than to another. A few pertinent experiments will be discussed.

In his work on fly control in dairy barns, Parrott (1927) used lights of various colors to attract flies to electric traps. He records that a clear bulb, or a white frosted bulb, attracted more flies than blue, green, or yellow of the same power. Red light proved least attractive of all the colors used.

Somewhat similar observations by Awati (1920d) show that the houseflies of India do not differ greatly in their phototropisms from those of the new world. Awati exposed the flies to various qualities of artificial light and also to Tanglefoot papers of different colors. Yellow proved the most attractive, red and violet the least. Blue, green, and orange were intermediate in this regard. He found the response to be the same in daylight as by night and noted that males and females did not differ in their response. Certain species of Calliphoridae showed similar color preferences.

Somewhat different results were obtained by Harsham (1946), who counted the flyspecks on packages wrapped in covers of selected colors. His findings do agree, however, with those of Awati in showing that yellow is never repellent to the flies. Nine packages were suspended in an illuminated Peet-Grady chamber and exposed to approximately 500 flies for a period of 48 hours. The results were as follows:

Type of Wrapper	Number of Flyspecks
Purple	175
Light yellow	180
Lime green	180
Dark yellow	192
Orange	225
Strawberry red	230
Light red	260
Foil No. 1	375
Foil No. 2	700

Casual observation of the number of flies resting on the various packages during the course of the experiment was in general conformity with the counts. Such findings tend to cast doubt on the desirability of shipping foods in foil wrappers in territory where flies abound. There is at least an esthetic objection to the heavily specked package, even though the wrapper be flyproof, and purchasers tend to pass over such an item for a package that is relatively speck-free.

A similar demonstration was carried out by Freeborn and Berry (1935) to test the validity of a fairly common practice among California dairymen. Before this it had been generally believed that aluminum paint on the walls of such establishments acted as a repellent to flies. Freeborn and Berry found that the flies merely preferred dark colors and rough surfaces. Plain white paint was considerably more repellent than aluminum. The practice was certainly not justified.

Cameron (1938, 1939) studied the reactions of *Musca domestica* to light of different wave lengths. He used several methods, the more usual procedure being to remove the flies from the breeding cage and keep them in darkness for about ten hours. Each fly was then required to make ten test trips toward two test lights of different wave length, and a record was kept of the choice made by the insect. Cameron found the flies much more strongly stimulated by ultraviolet light of 3,656 Ångstrom units [1] than by any other portion of the spectrum used in his experiments. The effect decreased, at first rapidly and then more slowly, as longer wave lengths were employed. On the *short* side of the peak, attraction also declined. The shortest wave length available for testing was 3,022 Å., which proved by comparison slightly more attractive than did yellow light or green. It should be remembered that the wave lengths of the visible spectrum range from near 3,800 at the violet end to approximately 8,000 at the red, with yellow and green intermediate between the two.

Galaine and Houlbert (1916) made the interesting observation that flies confined under blue light first showed restlessness and then became inactive, as in the dark. From this they reasoned that food stored in cupboards with blue glass windows would probably be unattractive to flies. This is improbable, as Ingle (1943) actually used blue light to *attract* flies to screens for testing their reaction to various chemical substances. While blue light is perhaps not as attractive as some other colors, it clearly is not repellent.

LIGHT AND TEMPERATURE

When confronted with two variables, temperature and light, not all species of flies show the same adaptive discrimination. In this connection, Jack and Williams (1937) compared the behavior of *Musca domestica vicina* with that of *Glossina morsitans* and *Stomoxys calcitrans*. Regardless of light conditions, *M. d. vicina* showed far greater ability than the other two to find a comfortable temperature by trial and error. Other things being equal, however, *Musca* always prefers a lighted environment. When the temperature was raised to a point that was lethal for all three, most specimens of *Musca* died in the light portion of the cage, most specimens of *Glossina* in the dark. With *Stomoxys,* about half chose the darker section, half the light.

Considering this strong preference for light, *Musca,* when confined in darkness, sometimes manifests much more activity than would be expected. Smirnov (1937), citing the work of Kuzina, records *M. domestica* active by night as well as by day if the temperature is sufficiently high. No difficulty was experienced in catching flies in traps in the dark if the rooms were

[1] An Ångstrom unit is equal to one ten-thousandth of a micron, i.e., one hundred-millionth of a centimeter.

warm. Very few flies, however, were observed to enter voluntarily buildings that were dark. The foregoing observations were made in a special laboratory at the Tropical Institute in Moscow.

There is practically no modern data on the effect of exposure of larvae to light of selected wave lengths. The very early observations of Béclard (1858) may be mentioned briefly. Béclard, who worked with flesh flies, found that the maggots grew largest when exposed to violet light, and next largest under blue, red, white, and green, in the order named. Those reared under green were but one-third of the length and thickness of those reared under violet. Since this follows no particular system as regards length of light rays, it seems impossible to generalize on the basis of these findings. Experiments of this sort would bear repeating, with other ecological factors properly controlled and quality of light recorded by wave length rather than by color.

TIME OF DAY

Possibly related to quantity and quality of light are the reactions of flies to the position of the sun. Shinoda and Ando (1935) noticed a sort of diurnal rhythm in the activities of *Musca domestica* and other species in Japan. Temperature may or may not have been the deciding factor, but in mid-May most of the flies collected were taken at or about 11:00 A.M. From May to September, however, 9:00 A.M. and 3:00 P.M. were the more productive collecting hours, with relatively few flies in evidence at 1:00 P.M. With the exception of *Lucilia,* all muscoids were found more numerous during the morning than during the afternoon hours. The authors definitely state that houseflies, which were most abundant during August and September, were found chiefly active at or about a temperature of 28°C (82.4°F).

GEOTROPISM

The universal tendency of flies to swarm upward is not due entirely to a positive phototactic response. When walking, at least, a negative geotactic reaction is involved. Strickland (1945) calls attention to a simple method for reducing the number of blowflies in barracks and houses by use of this principle. A pencil hole is made at the upper right-hand corner of the window screen or screen door and through this the flies eventually find their way out. Other insects may enter, of course, but this does not take place very frequently. Mosquitoes may be excluded during the night hours by use of a small cork. There seems to be no way of accounting for the blowfly's tendency to prefer the right in crawling upward.

AIR IN MOTION

The effect of winds on the migratory movements of flies has been much discussed. Two very different relationships are involved, depending on the velocity of the air currents in question. Storms, hurricanes, and all winds strong enough to more than offset the fly's own efforts at self-propulsion, undoubtedly cause the species to be carried willy-nilly over stretches of desert, ocean, and even mountain barriers. All such unwilling migration may be regarded as accidental, since flies are extremely sensitive to wind and seldom venture into the open on windy days, even when very favorable temperatures prevail (Uvarov, 1931).

That such dispersal does occur, however, is borne out by the observations of Ball (1918). This author studied insects taken at the Rebecca Shoal Light Station in the Tortugas Islands. Ball collected houseflies and mosquitoes which he considers to have been carried there by winds from Cuba over 90 miles of water and also from Florida, 105 miles distant.

The second, and more common, relation of wind to the activities of houseflies is in connection with the more gentle movements of air, not strong enough to discourage ordinary flight. For example, flight-range experiments by Carment (1922) with stained specimens of *Musca domestica* in Fiji showed that flies, when not forcibly diverted from their course, tend to travel against the wind. At least no flies released by him were retaken to leeward of the starting point. Carment considered that the flies were attracted largely by odors which were wind-borne. Hindle (1914b), also Hindle and Merriman (1914), likewise noted that flies tend to travel either against or across the wind and speculated as to the reasons for it. They concluded that odors from upwind are certainly important but also suggested that a positive anemotropism, such as is manifested by certain birds, may be involved.

The foregoing observations are quite at variance with those of Copeman, Howlett, and Merriman (1911), who reported that flies tend to move with the wind. Hindle points out, however, that these investigators worked entirely in open country (where there is always a greater tendency for general dispersal) and that all their catching stations happened to be to leeward from the point of release.

BAROMETRIC PRESSURE

Atmospheric pressure has been defined as the force exerted per unit area by the total column of air above the level considered. It is usually measured in terms of the number of inches or centimeters of mercury which the atmosphere will support vertically within a vacuum. Other factors remaining stable, atmospheric pressure varies inversely with the altitude. Insects are usually tolerant of all variations in pressure found within altitudes characteristic of their range; their activities, however, may be markedly affected by changes in barometric conditions, especially if these changes are relatively abrupt. The housefly is a rather good example of this.

For instance, it is well known that muscoid flies usually follow most erratic flight paths just prior to a thunderstorm (Sterzinger, 1929). When the storm actually breaks, however, many of them become comatose. The suggestion of Gourdon (1929) that this coma may be due to the production of ozone in the atmosphere at such times seems scarcely tenable. More probable is the belief of Parman (1920) that the varying atmospheric pressures are directly or indirectly responsible. Parman observed that during the comatose state, flies are especially subject to the action of destructive agencies such as wind and spray. Fifteen days after the storm, flies are usually again abundant, sufficient time having elapsed for the production of a new generation. Parman likewise noticed that species normally attracted to lights are most active during periods of high barometric pressure, and especially when the barometer is rising.

The opposite behavior, however, is recorded by Underhill (1940, 1944) regarding black flies (Simuliidae), in which feeding activities are considerably stimulated at times of low or rapidly falling barometric pressure. Casual observations of sportsmen and campers certainly appear to bear this out.

Wellington (1945) was apparently the first to suggest that such increased activity is actually the result of a positive response to decreased pressure. In an earlier paper (1944) the same author points out that whereas only slight decreases in pressure may result in a marked increase in flight activity, at still lower pressures behavior may again be normal. Under the conditions of the study, positive reaction was most pronounced between sea level and an elevation of 1.5 kilometers. Wellington insists that this activity is in no sense a distress reaction.

Barometric observations show that as a storm approaches there is a rapid, steady fall in atmospheric pressure. To this the flies react by a general increase in bodily activity. In the last few minutes before the storm, however, the drop is much sharper and is complicated by a "pumping" behavior of the mercury column, with fluctuations in pressure of as much as plus or minus two millibars [2] about the median point. This is the result of the ever-changing pattern of air currents in advance of a storm. To this fluctuating condition the flies react more "wildly," changing direction with great frequency and seemingly for no reason at all. In this connection, Wellington has shown that flies react violently to continuous "pumping" in the laboratory and even dodge away from hand-pressure waves equivalent to not more than 0.3 mb. His conclusion, therefore, is that normal flies exhibiting erratic prestorm flight in nature are actually responding to localized pressure waves occurring here and there ahead of the storm. This is brought about by nothing other than the stimulation of the fly's *baroreceptors* and is superimposed upon the generally increased activity already present. In the laboratory Wellington (1946b) was unable to fatigue the flies, and failed to produce anything resembling the comatose state previously mentioned as sometimes observable in nature. He suggests that such a condition, when it does occur, may possibly bear a relation to changes in the rate of evaporation within the storm area proper.

To summarize, the general increase in activity exhibited when barometric pressure falls slightly is not a true "taxis," since it lacks a directional element. It may more properly be designated merely as a kinetic reaction. The seemingly erratic flight that follows, and is associated with localized pressure fluctuations, *is* definitely directional and therefore a true "taxis" or "tropism." The reorientation is instantaneous. Such a response, according to Wellington, may be considered tactic in a baronegative sense.

The rather striking ability of insects to withstand pressure changes of an extreme character is believed to be due to their mode of respiration; the spiracles, tracheae, and tracheoles serve to accomplish a very rapid adjustment of all tissues to the changed conditions. Rapid decompression, especially, seems to have no deleterious effects. A very rapid return to normal, however, may be attended by peculiar symptoms, such as have been recorded by Wellington (1945) for Calliphoridae. Immediately upon return of normal pressure, the flies buzzed violently for a few seconds. This was followed by a fifteen-minute period of insensibility. Both may be explained by assuming a mechanical pressure on important nerve centers through the distensible walls of the many tracheal sacs. The flies invariably recovered, and no aftereffects of any kind could be detected.

Wellington (1946a) offers the following classification of variations in at-

---

[2] A millibar (mb) is equal to 1,000 dynes of force per square centimeter. For purposes of conversion this is equivalent to a force capable of supporting 0.75 millimeters (0.0295 inches) of mercury (Wellington, 1946a).

mospheric pressure. As will be seen, not all types are likely to have significant effects on insect life.

(1) Rhythmic variations. These are slight and frequently masked by other fluctuations, but are determinable by long-term analysis. The cycle is a twelve-hour one, the peaks occurring approximately at 10:00 A.M. and 10:00 P.M., the low points at 4:00 A.M. and 4:00 P.M. This cycle is most observable near the equator. Only in the tropics is it believed that insect activities are affected thereby.

(2) Irregular variations. These are due to the movements of cyclonic and anticyclonic systems. There may be sharp fluctuations within a period of hours, or more gradual changes involving two or three days. The magnitude of change may range from 1 to 50 millibars. These irregular changes, often associated with storms, are the most important in their effects on insect biology.

(3) Seasonal variations. Over land masses generally, the sea-level pressure is greater during winter than in summer. This is due to the fact that the atmosphere contracts and becomes drier over a cooling region. With the approach of summer the atmosphere expands, gains humidity, and becomes lighter, the average barometric readings being reduced. Any relation of seasonal pressure to insect activity still remains to be worked out.

(4) Vertical variations. These are the normal decreases in atmospheric pressure with increasing altitude. Up to about 1,000 feet elevation, each 30 feet of ascent represents a drop of approximately one millibar; above this, greater intervals of height are required to produce equivalent effects. The vertical distribution of species is undoubtedly influenced by atmospheric pressure as related to altitude.

(5) Horizontal variations. Surface variation in the horizontal direction is only about one ten-thousandth as great as in the vertical. For this reason it might seem insignificant in ecological studies. It does contribute, however, to the character of the "microclimate" or limited ecological situation in which certain species spend all or a portion of their lives. By applying a correction for altitude, the ecologist may utilize standard weather-station data directly in studying the microclimate.

Of these five classes of pressure variation, the first three may be considered *temporal;* the last two, *spatial.*

THE PLACE OF ECOLOGY IN APPLIED SCIENCE

Although the statement was published many years ago, we can still agree with Dr. W. B. Herms (1909c), who wrote that in medical entomology there is great need for additional knowledge of the sensory reactions of insects: their responses to chemical stimuli, to light, to temperature changes, and to vibratory stimuli. Much knowledge has been gained over the past thirty years, but a great field is still open to the skillful investigator. It should be borne in mind that control procedures deal largely with the manipulation of environment, for the intelligent execution of which the best possible knowledge of ecological principles is not only a desirable but really an essential tool. An understanding of the insects' reaction to a changing environment rests, in turn, upon a thorough appreciation of the physiology of the species and how the processes of digestion, respiration, reproduction, etc., are affected by the responses of the organism to the various environmental stimuli that man provides. Lastly, all functions in any living body can only be performed by structural units, that is, by cells, tissues, organs, and systems of organs, which must be present in normal morphological relationship if proper functional activity is to be maintained. Thus practical control depends on ecology, ecology on physiology, and physiology on morphology, the most fundamental of all the biological sciences. Here, as in other branches of scientific work, the practical rests upon the theoretical, and the applied science upon academic fact.

One more phase of ecology remains to be discussed: the relation of the living fly to other organisms that share the same environment. The chapter that follows attempts to evaluate the importance of both microscopic and larger forms in determining the success of *Musca domestica* as a species.

CHAPTER X

Parasites, Predators, Symbionts, and Commensals

INCLUDING CERTAIN SPECIES OF VETERINARY IMPORTANCE

I killed a fly this morning—it buzzed, and I wouldn't have it.—W. S. Gilbert, Ruddigore

THE HOUSEFLY, like any other species, is hampered or assisted in its struggle for survival by the activities of a great array of other organisms which, directly or indirectly, influence its well-being. Those which are definitely restrictive to the growth, development, or reproduction of the species may be classed either as predators or parasites, depending on whether they actually consume the fly as food or merely gain nourishment by living on or in the tissues of the host. Each stage of the fly's life cycle is subject to attack by representatives of one or both groups, and the total destruction is unquestionably very great. We have only to picture the potential fecundity of the housefly, as brought out in Chapter IV, to realize that many agencies must obviously be at work at all times to keep the fly population at the relatively low level which normally prevails. Temperature, humidity, wind, and other ecological factors combine to limit the occurrence of the species to fixed geographical areas and its activities to particular seasons of the year. But superimposed on this is the influence of living organisms, large and small, which in the aggregate, are responsible for the elimination of countless numbers of individual flies.

The natural enemies of *Musca domestica* and related species may be grouped, taxonomically, under seven heads:

(1) Fungus and bacterial infections, including rickettsiae, viruses, and spirochetes.

(2) Protozoan organisms.

(3) Roundworms and flatworms.

(4) Insects and other arthropods.

(5) Reptiles and amphibians.

(6) Birds.

(7) Insectivorous mammals.

In addition to the many species that affect the fly adversely, there are, especially among the microorganisms, a considerable number, intimately associated with flies, which apparently have no detrimental effect upon their hosts. Certain bacteria, for example, common on the body or in the alimentary tract appear to do the fly no harm. These are perfectly adjusted, it would seem, to a relationship in which they live and multiply without significant injury to host tissue and without secreting any toxins to which the fly is specifically susceptible. *Proteus morganii* and *Pseudomonas fluorescens* are probably of such a type. Both, when taken in by maggots, survive through the pupal stage and may be recovered from the adult fly after the latter has emerged. In the majority of cases, such flies probably have as long a life span as those not contaminated with these organisms, and probably possess normal reproductive powers, though it should be mentioned that Glaser (1924c) considered nonpathogenic bacteria able to shorten the life span and reduce the number of ovipositions, when ingested by adult flies.

A third group of organisms, biologically speaking, is made up of those which merely enjoy a "free ride" during their brief stay in the body of the fly and which must eventually reach some other destination if they are to continue their existence and reproduce in normal fashion. *Bacterium conjunctivitidis, Corynebacterium diphtheriae,* and *Hemophilus duplex,* for example, remain alive on or in the fly only a few hours, in most instances. *Salmonella schottmülleri,* on the other hand, has been recovered eleven days after the flies were exposed to contamination. *Brucella abortus* is somewhat intermediate, in that flies retain infection 24 to 96 hours after becoming contaminated. *Eberthella typhosa,* the organism that has perhaps done more than any other to give the housefly its evil reputation ("typhoid fly"), is extreme in remaining viable in the fly's body for perhaps as long as 23 days! (Ficker, 1903).

From these and similar figures, it will be obvious that whenever such an organism is pathogenic to man or his domestic animals, the importance of the fly as a disease vector increases in proportion to the number of hours or days that it is able to retain the infective organism. A fly that has fed on typhoid ejecta only once may remain a menace to the community for perhaps three weeks or more, while one laden with the germs of undulant fever (*Brucella abortus*), for example, must make repeated trips to the source of infection if it is to distribute organisms for a period much longer than 96 hours.

The disappearance of all such organisms from the body of the fly in the course of time may be due to a variety of causes:

In some cases bacteriophage may be involved. Shope in 1927 prepared a salt solution extract of houseflies and found therein a bacteriophage destructive to *Staphylococcus muscae, Escherichia coli, Salmonella paratyphi,* and *Eberthella typhosa.* Glaser (1938b) found that wild-caught flies always contained bacteriophage. He was not able to bring about the production of bacteriophage by introducing a strain of staphylococcus into the alimentary tract of sterile flies, and concluded that the interaction of host and bacteria does not constitute an adequate explanation of bacteriophage formation. Bacteriophage survived alone (without the staphylococcus) in sterile flies for one generation; with staphylococcus present, bacteriophage was active for at least eight generations of flies.

Sometimes confused with the above is the action of certain so-called bactericidal substances natural to the fly and operative against specific microorganisms. Duncan (1926) investigated the existence of this principle in eight species of arthropods, including *Musca domestica.* He found the substance present in the gut content of all forms studied, and in the feces of the insects but not of the Acarina (ticks). There seems to be but one active principle in each species of arthropod, but different bacteria manifest differing degrees of susceptibility to it. Spore-forming aerobes such as *Bacillus anthracis, B. mesentericus,* and *B. subtilis* are easily affected. *Staphylococcus* spp. require a higher concentration for their destruction, and some bacteria are resistant altogether. The bactericidal action is greater at 37°C (98.6°F) than at room temperature. The principle retains its full power when dried for six months, and is not destroyed by temperatures ranging up to 120°C (248°F). It is not destroyed by trypsin and is not soluble in common fats. It may be precipitated from solution with proteins by alcohol or acetone, but is not itself affected thereby. It is rather definitely established that this substance is formed in the stomach, but it is not known whether this is by secretion of the gastric cells or whether it results from the process of digestion. The action on bacteria resembles that of antiseptics. There is no visible bacteriolysis, and Duncan states that it exhibits *none* of the properties of bacteriophage.

The action neither of these bactericidal substances nor of the bacteriophage itself is sufficiently well understood to permit generalization covering all cases. *Eberthella typhosa,* against which bacteriophage has been demonstrated, is known to survive through metamorphosis in the fly, and the same is true for *Bacillus anthracis,* which Duncan found susceptible to bactericidal substance. It may be that neither agent is active in the immature stages, at least for those forms which, when taken up by the larvae, can be recovered from the adult fly.

A third factor relates to the speed with which flies empty the alimentary tract, both by defecation and by regurgitation from the mouth. A very large percentage of the organisms taken in while feeding are thus eliminated in a few minutes with little or no opportunity for multiplication within the fly. Such was the interpretation of Rendtorff and Francis (1943) in their study of poliomyelitis virus, which decreased sharply in detectable amount in the abdomen two to seven hours after ingestion by the fly. Both fecal and vomit specks yielded virus of an active character up to six hours after feeding.

In the same connection it is interesting to note that cysts of *Endamoeba histolytica* may be passed within one minute after ingestion.

Remembering that some microorganisms actually destroy the fly, it is important to point out that individuals at times recover from such infection, and that the etiologic agent may die out or at least becomes more benign, as with many infections in man. In such instances, it is safe to suppose that immune mechanisms either of the phagocytic or humoral nature have been at work to attenuate the toxic effect or the mechanical injury to tissue.

Last, there remains the possibility of the organism neither affecting the fly adversely nor being eliminated by it, but being nevertheless changed perceptibly during its adventitious association with the carrier host. This development has been observed in *Vibrio comma,* etiologic agent of human cholera. Lal, Ghosal, and Mukherji (1939) found changes of a morphological, metabolic, and chemical nature in many strains recovered from the housefly. Whether these changes might become so extreme as to render the species unrecognizable during an interepidemic period was not determined. Such a possibility might conceivably become an important point in epidemiology.

Combining all organisms, detrimental and otherwise, which may be associated with the fly's biology in an intimate manner, we have then an enormous aggregate that can only be discussed adequately by division into groups. For convenience, we shall consider them as falling under two heads: (1) the microorganisms and (2) the macroscopic forms.

MICROORGANISMS BIOLOGICALLY RELATED TO FLIES

The microorganisms associated with flies include the bacteria, rickettsiae, viruses, fungi, protozoa, and the microscopic stages of certain worms. Data concerning these organisms are presented here largely in tabular form, as it is felt that by this means the greatest possible amount of information may be conveyed in a minimum of space. Special acknowledgment is due to Dr. Edward A. Steinhaus, who, in his excellent volume *Insect Microbiology* (1946) has brought together most of the factual material on which Table 12 is based.[1]

In a few cases, the identification of *Musca domestica* is implied, rather than definite. In the interest of completeness, however, it seems desirable to include these references with the others. They are indicated by the following designation: (det. assumed).

Table 12. Bacteria recorded in literature as associated with *Musca domestica*.

Name of organism	Nature of association	Authority
Aerobacter aerogenes (B. lactis aerogenes) (*B. oxytocus perniciosus*)	Isolated from intestine and intestinal content	Nicoll (1911a); Cox, Lewis, and Glynn (1912); Torrey (1912)
Aerobacter cloacae (*B. cloacae*)	Isolated from alimentary tract	Nicoll (1911a)
Alcaligenes faecalis (*B. faecalis alkaligenes*)	Isolated from intestinal tract of city-caught flies (det. assumed)	Torrey (1912)
Bacillus A Ledingham	Present on ova, in larvae, and in adults; survived through metamorphosis	Tebbutt (1913)
Bacillus anthracis (Causes anthrax in animals and in man)	Spores survive after ingestion by larvae; organisms survive through metamorphosis; bacilli isolated from stomachs and intestines of flies captured on animals dead from infection; much experimental work on record	Davaine (1868, 1870a, 1870b); Raimbert (1869); Bollinger (1874); Nuttall (1899a); Cao (1906b); Graham-Smith (1909, 1912b); Pierce (1921); Sen and Minett (1944)
Bacillus colosimile	Organism fed to larvae and later recovered from feces	Cao (1906b)
Bacillus gasoformans nonliquefaciens	Isolated from body surface and from intestinal tract	Nicoll (1911a)

[1] This chapter was written before Steinhaus' *Principles of Insect Pathology* was available. Steinhaus' work presents considerable information on the histological and physiological effects of various infections upon flies.

Table 12 (continued)

Name of organism	Nature of association	Authority
Bacillus grünthal (B. gruenthali ?)	Isolated from body surface and from intestinal tract	Nicoll (1911a)
Bacillus lutzae (Flavobacterium lutzae)	Pathogenic for housefly; dying insects yielded pure cultures	Brown (1927)
Bacillus piocianemus (B. pyocyaneus ?)	Found living in body of fly eight days after feeding	Cao (1898)
Bacillus radiciformis	Survived passage through alimentary tract; isolated from feces	Cao (1898, 1906a)
Bacillus similcarbonchio	Passes through alimentary tract in virulent condition; deposited on external surface of eggs	Cao (1898)
Bacillus tifosimile (B. typhosimile ?)	Several strains isolated from flies	Cao (1898, 1906a)
Bacillus vesiculosis (Bacterium vesiculosum ?)	Isolated from surface of flies	Nicoll (1911a)
Bacterium agrigenum (Bacillus septicus agrigenus)	Flies fed on cultures, made into inoculum 12 hours later; caused death of mice	Marpmann (1897)
Bacterium conjunctivitidis (Bacillus aegypticus) (associated with conjunctivitis)	Flies remain infective less than three and one-half hours after exposure to cultures	Patton (1930)
Bacterium delendae-muscae	Causes specific infection of houseflies and other Diptera; larvae ingest organism; death (Musca) at end of pupal stage	Roubaud and Descazeaux (1923)
Bacterium mathisi	Kills M. domestica 3 hours or more after ingestion	Roubaud and Treillard (1935)
Brucella abortus (causative agent of undulant fever)	Flies retain infection 24 to 96 hours after exposure to cultures; organism also found associated with Muscina stabulans, Calliphora, and Stomoxys	Patton (1930); Ruhland and Huddleson (1941)

Name of organism	Nature of association	Authority
Corynebacterium diphtheriae (causative agent of diphtheria in man)	Recovered from feces 51 hours after flies had fed on bacilli; remains alive a few hours on legs and wings	Graham-Smith (1910, 1914)
Eberthella belfastiensis (*Bacterium coli anaerogenes*)	Isolated from adult fly	Scott (1917a, b)
Eberthella typhosa (causative agent of typhoid fever in man)	May contaminate body, legs, or wings, or be present in content of alimentary tract; fly contaminates food and drink by contact, by vomitus, and by fecal specks; organism rarely persists through metamorphosis, but contaminated adults continue to yield viable bacteria for perhaps 23 days; outbreaks of typhoid fever traced definitely to *Musca domestica*	Celli (1888); Veeder (1898a); Ficker (1903); Hamilton (1903); Reed, Vaughan, and Shakespeare (1904); Klein (1908); Graham-Smith (1909); Faichnie (1909a,b); Bertarelle (1910); Ledingham (1911); Howard (1911a); Cockrane (1912); Tebbutt (1913); Bahr (1914); Manson-Bahr (1919)
Erwinia amylovora (*Micrococcus amylovorus*) (causes fire blight of plants)	May live for several days in intestinal tract; eggs may be contaminated when laid; infection acquired by larva survives through metamorphosis; also found associated with *Muscina assimilis* and *Muscina stabulans*	Ark and Thomas (1936)
Escherichia coli (*Bacterium coli*) (*Bacillus coli communis*) (*Bacillus schafferi*) (*Bacillus coli var. communior*) (*Bacillus acidi lactici*) (*Bacillus neapolitanus*) (*Bacillus coli mutabilis*)	Present in feces of most flies examined; larvae hatched from contaminated eggs carry infection through metamorphosis to adult state; much laboratory work done with this species	Cao (1898, 1906b); Nicoll (1911a); Cox, Lewis, and Glynn (1912); Torrey (1912); Scott (1917a,b); Ostrolenk *et al.* (1939, 1942b)
Gaffkya tetragena (*Micrococcus tetragenus*)	Isolated from adult fly	Scott (1917a,b)

Table 12 (continued)

Name of organism	Nature of association	Authority
Hemophilus duplex (causes subacute conjunctivitis)	Flies infective less than three and one-half hours after exposure to culture	Patton (1930)
Micrococcus flavus (Air and milk organism)	Isolated from body surface and from intestinal contents	Torrey (1912)
Mycobacterium leprae (causative organism of leprosy)	Flies caught on face of leper, found infected; organism survives several days in fly after meal of contaminated material; *Chlorops (Musca) leprae* also a possible vector	Nuttall (1899a); Currie (1910); Honeij and Parker (1914); Rosenau (1927)
Mycobacterium tuberculosis	Organism recovered from intestinal contents and feces of flies fed on tubercular sputum; housefly believed to play definite role in the dissemination of tuberculosis	Spielman and Haushalter (1887); Celli (1888); Hoffmann (1888); Graham-Smith (1914); Riley and Johannsen (1938)
Neisseria gonorrhoeae (*Diplococcus gonorrhoeae*)	Carried on feet of fly three hours after contamination with human secretions	Welander (1896)
Neisseria intracellularis (*Diplococcus intracellularis*)	Believed to be carried by *M. domestica* (det. assumed)	MacGregor (1917)
Neisseria luciliarum	Found in *Lucilia sericata;* pathogenic to *M. domestica*	Brown (1927)
*Pasteurella cuniculicida (*Bacillus cuniculicida*) and/or *Pasteurella avicida* (*Bacterium cholerae gallinarum*)	Isolated from fly taken in animal room; both organisms produce fatal septicemia in rabbits	Scott (1917a, b); Steinhaus (1946)

* *Pasteurella bollingeri*, though not recorded from *M. domestica*, has been found virulent in *M. inferior* 24 hours after the latter had bitten an infected rabbit. The same is true for other blood-sucking Muscidae.

Name of organism	Nature of association	Authority
Pasteurella pestis (causative organism of plague)	Evidence of fly transmission wholly experimental	Russo (1930); Steinhaus (1946)
Pasteurella tularense (*Brucella tularensis*)	Transmission by housefly possible, but not important	Steinhaus (1946)
Proteus morganii (Morgan's No. 1 Bacillus)	Various strains isolated from captured flies; infection in larvae survives metamorphosis	Morgan and Ledingham (1909); Nicoll (1911a); Graham-Smith (1912a, b, 1913); Cox, Lewis, and Glynn (1912)
Proteus vulgaris (*Bacillus proteus vulgaris*)	Isolated from captured adults; fed to larvae and recovered from feces	Cao (1906b); Scott (1917a, b)
Pseudomonas aeruginosa (*Bacillus pyocyaneus*)	Organisms taken up by larvae in food material remain in gut during metamorphosis; also isolated from outside of eggs of flies	Cao (1906b); Bacot (1911a,b); Ledingham (1911)
Pseudomonas fluorescens (*Bacillus fluorescens liquefaciens*)	Organisms fed to larvae and recovered from feces; survived through metamorphosis and were isolated from adult feces and from exterior of eggs	Cao (1906b)
Pseudomonas jaegeri (*Bacillus proteus fluorescens*)	Isolated from intestines of larvae (pathogenic for guinea pigs)	Cao (1906b)
Pseudomonas non-liquefaciens (*Bacillus fluorescens non-liquefaciens*)	Fed to larvae and isolated from feces	Cao (1898, 1906b)
Salmonella choleraesuis (*Bacillus cholerae suis?*) (*B. suipestifer*)	Isolated from adult flies	Scott (1917a,b)
Salmonella enteritidis	Isolated from body surface and from intestine of adult flies; survival through metamorphosis rare; *M. domestica* definitely a transmitter of gastroenteritis	Ficker (1903); Hamilton (1903); Graham-Smith (1909, 1912a,b); Ledingham (1911); Cox, Lewis, and Glynn (1912); Bahr

Table 12 (continued)

Name of organism	Nature of association	Authority
		(1914); Ostrolenk and Welch (1942a, b)
Salmonella paratyphi (*B. paratyphus Type A*) (*Bacterium paratyphi*)	Isolated from intestinal tract of flies	Torrey (1912)
Salmonella schottmülleri (*B. paratyphosus*)	Isolated from body and intestinal tract; flies carried organisms at least 11 days	Nicoll (1911a)
Sarcina aurantiaca	Fed to flies and recovered from feces; survives metamorphosis	Cao (1906a)
Serratia kielensis (*Bacterium kiliense?*) ("Red bacillus of Kiel")	Recovered in feces of larvae hatched from eggs in contact with polluted flesh; recovered from flies resulting from larvae fed on polluted flesh	Cao (1906b)
Serratia marcescens (*Bacterium prodigiosus*)	Cultivated from crop and intestine 4–5 days after inoculation; survived metamorphosis; lives in fly's intestine up to 18 days	Cao (1906b); Graham-Smith (1911, 1914); Buichkov (1932)
Shigella dysenteriae	Rarely survives metamorphosis	Graham-Smith (1914)
Shigella paradysenteriae	Isolated from flies in military kitchens and latrines; epidemic of bacillary dysentery fly-borne (det. assumed)	Graham-Smith (1909); Kuhns and Anderson (1944)
Shigella spp.	Isolated from intestinal tract	Ficker (1903); Hamilton (1903); Graham-Smith (1909); Ledingham (1911); Nicoll (1911a)
Staphylococcus albus (*Albococcus pyogenes*) (*S. pyogenes albus*)	Isolated from exterior of eggs and from surface of city-caught flies; gut contents of *M. domestica* not bactericidal to this species	Cao (1906b); Torrey (1912); Scott (1917a,b); Duncan (1926)
Staphylococcus aureus (*Micrococcus pyogenes aureus*)	Isolated from feet and other parts; retains virulence when passed through gut; gut contents of *M. domestica* not bactericidal	Celli (1888); Cox, Lewis, and Glynn (1912); Scott (1917a,b); Duncan (1926)

Name of organism	Nature of association	Authority
Staphylococcus citreus (*S. pyogenes citreus*)	Isolated from bodies of flies; survives metamorphosis	Cao (1906b); Scott (1917a,b)
Staphylococcus flaccicifex	Causes bacterial disease of fly	Sweetman (1936)
Staphylococcus muscae	Causes fatal infection in housefly; males more susceptible	Glaser (1924b, 1926a)
Staphylococcus spp. (*Albococcus, Aurococcus*)	Several strains isolated from surface of city-caught flies	Torrey (1912); Cox, Lewis, and Glynn (1912)
Streptococcus agalactiae	*M. domestica* vector of bovine mastitis?	Sanders (1940); Ewing (1942)
Streptococcus equinus	Isolated from flies, June through August	Torrey (1912)
Streptococcus faecalis	Isolated from intestinal tract; indicates that flies have fed on human feces	Torrey (1912); Cox, Lewis, and Glynn (1912); Scott (1917a,b)
Streptococcus lactis (?) (*B. lactis acidi*)	Isolated from surface of city-caught flies	Torrey (1912)
Streptococcus pyogenes	Isolated from city-caught flies and from flies in hospital wards	Scott (1917a,b); Shooter and Waterworth (1944)
Streptococcus salivarius	Isolated from intestinal contents and from body surface	Torrey (1912); Cox, Lewis, and Glynn (1912)
Vibrio comma (*Vibrio cholerae*) (causative organism of cholera)	Changes morphologically and physiologically when passed through fly; may be one phase of life cycle; relation of flies to cholera epidemics established beyond question	Nicholas (1873); Cattani (1886); Tizzoni and Cattani (1886); Simmonds (1892); Macrae (1894); Nuttall (1899a); Hamilton (1903); Faichnie (1909a); Ledingham (1911); Nicoll (1911a); Graham-Smith (1914); Howard (1911a); Gill and Lal (1931); Lal, Ghosal, and Mukherji (1939); Herms (1944)

Table 12 shows that in a majority of cases the fly is merely a transient host to the various species of bacteria and is not particularly affected by them. Striking are the exceptions, however, as in the case of *Bacillus lutzae*, which is decidedly pathogenic for *Musca*, and *Bacterium delendae-muscae*, which is fatal in the pupal stage. *Staphylococcus muscae*, which also causes a fatal infection in flies, is more destructive to males than to females. Further study may show this principle to be quite general, as the male is often more susceptible to sprays and poisons than is the female.

One cannot resist the temptation to speculate briefly regarding the evolution of a species which, above all others, is now so successfully adapted to both the sugar bowl and the latrine. It is not inconceivable that many species have attempted the colonization of the latter environment, only to find that the bacterial flora was destructive to them or to their larvae, eggs, or pupae. Not so with *Musca domestica*. Endowed with a natural immunity to the vast majority of microscopic infections, or at least with the ability to develop some sort of tolerance to their presence, the housefly and a few related species have thrived where many would have perished, to become "queens of filth" and a sinister factor in the environment of man.

Selection must have played a part in the adaptive process, with many falling by the way, but the so-called *plastic* species is in reality one possessed of great variability, and such variability *M. domestica* has, not structurally, perhaps, but physiologically, beyond a doubt. It is not sharply specialized either in its adult dietary or in choice of breeding medium, though it has its preferences, as we know full well; in those preferences lies our chief interest in the species. Other aspects of the evolution of the genus have been discussed in Chapter V.

Considerable interest attaches also to the fact that many more bacteria are carried within the fly's body than upon it. Torrey (1912) found the intestine of the housefly to contain 8.6 times as many bacteria as were borne by the external surface, and Yao, Huan, and Huie (1929) record similar observations made on flies in the city of Peiping. The external flora depends considerably, according to this study, on whether the fly is collected in a clean or dirty environment. These authors found that slum-collected flies averaged 3,683,000 bacteria on the external surface, while specimens from the cleanest district in the city averaged scarcely more than half this number. Many of the bacteria carried by the housefly are, therefore, as Steinhaus (1946) remarks, *adventitious*, their presence depending on locality, time of year, and especially the habits of the individual fly (or maggot from which the adult was derived).

Bacteria carried internally are not necessarily confined to the alimentary

canal or to solid tissues. Lilly (1931) considers it quite normal for the blood of
the housefly to contain one or more bacterial forms.

The transmission of the larval flora through the pupal stage to the imago
has been recognized by Cao (1906a,b) and Bacot (1911b). That this rarely
occurs, however, in the case of certain important pathogens was pointed out
by Graham-Smith (1914), who showed that *Eberthella typhosa, Salmonella
enteritidis, Shigella dysenteriae,* and similar nonsporeformers, when fed to
normal larvae, usually fail to survive metamorphosis.

Torrey (1912) made a study of the bacterial flora of flies collected under city
conditions of that period. He found that up to the latter part of June the flies
carried no bacteria of fecal origin. Fecal bacteria of the colon type first became
abundant in early July. These constituted 13.1 per cent of the organisms recovered from the body surface and 37.5 per cent of those found in the intestine.
As to total numbers, Torrey found periods in July and August during which
the count ran to several millions per fly. These alternated with times at which
the average fly carried but a few hundred bacteria. Torrey felt that these flies
must represent newly hatched swarms which had not yet had time to become
heavily contaminated. This interpretation seems subject to question, as newly
hatched flies are sometimes heavily contaminated from the breeding medium
and, again, breeding usually goes on more or less continuously throughout the
season. More plausible, perhaps, would be the assumption that the action of
bacteriophage or other bactericidal substances in the body of the fly serves
to attenuate multiplication of newly acquired bacteria after a number of days,
and only when new species or strains are picked up by the flies does the count
again reach astronomic proportions.

Torrey identified a number of the lactose fermenters and found that 79.5
per cent were of the colon-aerogenes group, while 20.5 per cent were of the
acidi-lactici type. There was a change in type according to the season. In
August, he found particularly abundant a bacterium of the paracolon type,
causing final intense alkaline reaction in litmus milk, and fermenting only
certain monosaccharides.

Rickettsiae

Only a single species of rickettsia is definitely associated, in the literature,
with houseflies. This is *Rickettsia conjunctivae* Coles, the causative agent of
an acute purulent conjunctivitis found in South African sheep. Similar infections in Germany, Algeria, France, Australia, and New Zealand are presumably caused by the same organism, which is sometimes referred to the
genus *Chlamydozoon.* This is the type of infection for which one would ex-

pect a vector of the arthropod type, probably a bloodsucker. So far no essential intermediate host has been discovered, but both *Musca domestica* and *Stomoxys calcitrans* are believed capable of transmitting the organisms in a mechanical way (Mitscherlich, 1943). Varieties of *R. conjunctivae* cause similar infections in the eyes of cattle and domestic fowl.

Mitscherlich was able to infect the eyes of calves with *Rickettsia conjunctivae* by placing thereon individuals of both species of flies which had themselves been infected up to eight hours earlier. This author demonstrated definitely that the rickettsia were not transmitted through the egg of either fly. This is important, as certain diseases of rickettsial origin, such as scrub typhus, for example, are dependent on transovarial transmission for their continuance. In the Mitscherlich experiments it was found that quarters which have housed infected calves will become noninfective in twenty-four hours if no special measures are taken.

Viruses

The possible role of filth-feeding Diptera in the dissemination of poliomyelitis has led to many investigations, and there continue to be divergent opinions in regard to the relationship. That the fly may be a mechanical vector seems generally accepted. Whether it serves as a genuine host is still to be determined. The virus has been isolated repeatedly from wild-caught flies, and Bang and Glaser (1943) were able to recover Theiler's mouse strain twelve days after the flies had fed on culture. The Lansing strain, however, survived only two days, and with neither strain did these authors succeed in producing infected flies from infected larvae. Rendtorff and Francis (1943) found that it was in the abdomen of the fly that the virus chiefly persisted. Active virus was found in both fecal and vomit specks, and these authors suggest that the decrease in detectable virus in the abdomen, noticeable a few hours after ingestion, is due more to rapid excretion than to the virus dying in the fly.

Mohler (1919) reported that *Musca domestica* may harbor the virus of hog cholera for a number of days, and can possibly infect animals by feeding on fresh wounds or about the eyes. He considers it very doubtful, however, that *M. domestica* serves as a vector under ordinary conditions.

As yet there has been no discovery of a virus to which *Musca domestica* is itself susceptible. Another of the muscoids, however, *Calliphora vomitoria,* is listed by Steinhaus (1946) as among the insects known to suffer from virus disease.

Spirochetes

Treponema pertenue, the causative organism of yaws, may be transmitted mechanically by houseflies, as shown by the experiments of Castellani (1907); though *M. domestica* is certainly far less important in this connection than certain species of *Hippelates,* which, being smaller, may actually penetrate beneath the scabs to feed. The usual transmission of yaws is probably not by the activity of insects.

There is a single reference in the literature (Kerr, 1906) to the possibility of syphilis being conveyed by flies, in Morocco, but this is of doubtful validity.

Fungi

Important among fungi associated with insects are the yeasts (order Saccharomycetales). Many mycologists prefer to group yeasts with the Ascomycetes, a well-known class of fungi reproducing by asci and ascospores. Only certain yeasts, however, have these characteristics; the majority multiply largely by budding or by fission.

Only occasionally have yeasts been isolated from houseflies. Probably in no case is the yeast detrimental to the fly—a rather astonishing fact, considering the very considerable number of yeasts and yeastlike fungi which occur intracellularly in insects. The more important relationship of flies to yeasts is undoubtedly the utilization of the latter as food, which the flies ingest along with other elements of the substratum on which they feed. For use of yeasts in preparation of culture media and also in studying dispersion of flies, see Chapter XV.

With reference to fungi other than yeasts, Charles (1941) lists *Musca domestica* as host to the following forms: *Aspergillus* sp., *Beauveria globulifera, Empusa americana, Empusa grylli, Empusa muscae, Empusa sphaerosperma,* and *Fusarium poae.*

The territory represented by Charles's survey includes the North American continent, the West Indies, and the countries of Central America.

Of these fungi the only form encountered very commonly is *Empusa muscae.* This species falls in the family Empusaceae, order Entomophthorales, class Phycomycetes. It occurs both north and south of the equator and is well known as a parasite of houseflies, blowflies, and other Diptera. In the fall of the year the infection frequently assumes epidemic proportions, and affected flies may be seem attached permanently to walls and ceilings, in a rather lifelike position.

The spores of the fungus, which have in one way or another become attached to the body surface, send out slender hyphae that either penetrate through the softer portions of the cuticula or enter the body by way of the spiracles. Hyphal bodies become detached from the general mycelium and are distributed by the haemolymph. After a few days the fungus will have invaded all tissues, and the fly dies, completely "plugged" with fungus. Germ

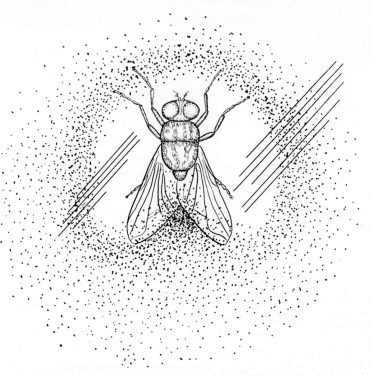

Figure 81. Fly on windowpane, killed by *Empusa muscae*. The discharged spores form an irregular circle about the dead insect. (Adapted from Steinhaus, 1946.)

tubes from the numerous hyphal bodies then grow out through the softer portions of the body wall and produce conidiophores at their tips. These bear conidiospores which are discharged in more or less of a circle and in a few days form a conspicuous halo about the body of the dead fly. This is especially striking when the fly is attached to a windowpane.

Hesse (1913) successfully cultured *Empusa muscae* and fed the living cultures to adult flies. *Musca domestica, Stomoxys calcitrans,* and *Fannia canicularis* all succumbed. Larvae which he fed on infected manure underwent pupation, but died in that condition. Hesse's experiments are interesting in indicating that infection need not be by way of the integument, but can also be by mouth.

Other species of *Empusa* and of the related genus *Entomophthora* attack a vast number of insect forms in many orders, and undoubtedly constitute an important factor in the natural control of these species. Diptera seem to be the favorite hosts (Thaxter, 1888).

Several writers have stressed the possible importance of *Empusa* in effecting a degree of natural control over *M. domestica* and related forms. Graham-Smith (1919) recorded the fungus as destructive to *Musca corvina*, while Kuhn (1922) considered the seasonal decrease of *M. domestica* after September (in Alsace and Baden) as due very probably to the effects of *Empusa muscae*. It was the finding of Gussow (1917), however, that only about one death in a thousand could be traced to *E. muscae*, and he therefore concluded that the general dying off of houseflies in autumn could scarcely be due to this. Interest in the relationship, however, has continued through the years. Paillot (1933) figured the mycelium and conidiophores of the fungus, while De Salles and Hathaway (1944) made a histological study of *Empusa* infection in *M. domestica*.

Confusion of species has sometimes led to controversy. Bernstein (1914) reported that when two groups of flies were fed on syrup containing *Mucor heimalus* and *Mucor racemosus* spores, respectively, all died with the usual manifestations of *Empusa muscae* infection. Cultures from the dead flies yielded only *Mucor racemosus*. Such findings indicate a degree of polymorphism in fungi, as suggested by the earlier work of Hesse. On the other hand, Ramsbottom (1914) found that a single *Empusa* spore, on germination, never gave rise to either the mycelium or the fruiting body of *Mucor racemosus*. When this appears to occur it can apparently be traced to a cluster of spores, which might very easily have contained the smaller spores of *Mucor* in their midst. There is still room for investigation in this field.

The so-called "black spores" observed in the bodies of flies of the genus *Musca* as well as in malaria-carrying mosquitoes are probably not parasitic in nature. Mayne (1929) considers them to be chitinogenous thickenings of the tracheal tubes. Whether they appear in response to the presence of an invasive organism, fungus or protozoan, remains to be shown.

Marchionatto (1945) records *Aspergillus parasiticus* from *Musca domestica* in Entre Rios, and *Empusa americana* from *Lucilia caesar* in Buenos Aires. He found infested adults of *Lucilia* hanging from branches in masses of thirty or more.

Protozoa

All classes of Protozoa have been found associated with insects, and it is more than probable that *Musca domestica* plays transient host to a large number of species. Actual records in the literature, however, all stem from researches undertaken from the viewpoint of the parasitologist or medical scientist. Interest has been concentrated in the amebae parasitic in man, in certain flagellates resembling the trypanosomes of man and animals, and in a microsporidian, *Octosporea muscae-domesticae,* also parasitic in *Drosophila* flies. It will be noted that these three are representative of three separate classes of Protozoa; the Sarcodina, Mastigophora, and Sporozoa, respectively. No Ciliata or Suctoria appear to be recorded from muscoid flies. Available information is recorded in Table 13.

Table 13. Protozoa associated with *Musca domestica.*

Organism	Nature of association	Authority
Sarcodina		
Endamoeba histolytica (causative agent of amoebic dysentery and other forms of amoebiasis)	Cysts pass unaltered through alimentary canal of flies and are viable in feces; may be passed one minute after feeding; ingested motile forms die within an hour; cysts found in feces of wild flies	Wenyon and O'Connor (1917a,b); Sieyro (1942); Root (1921); Roubaud (1918); Connal (1922)
Endamoeba coli	Half the ingested cysts dead after 14 hours; last living cysts observed after 52 hours; cysts found in feces of wild flies; ingested motile forms die within an hour	Wenyon and O'Connor (1917c); Roubaud (1918); Root (1921); Connal (1922)
Endolimax nana	Half of the ingested cysts dead after 18 hours; last living cysts observed after 39 hours	Root (1921)
Mastigophora		
Giardia intestinalis	Half of the ingested cysts dead after 8 hours; last living cysts observed after 16 hours; cysts found in feces of wild flies; ingested motile forms die within an hour	Wenyon and O'Connor (1917c); Roubaud 1918); Root (1921)
Chilomastix mesnili	Motile forms in feces 7 minutes after ingestion; half of the cysts dead after 36 hours; last living cysts observed after 80 hours	Root (1921)

Organism	Nature of association	Authority
Trichomonas hominis (?)	Motile forms in feces 5 minutes after ingestion; killed in less than an hour, if retained	Wenyon and O'Connor (1917c)
Trichomonas foetus	Living forms recovered from digestive tract one half hour to 17 hours after ingestion	Morgan (1942)
Herpetomonas muscarum (*Bodo muscarum*) (*Cerocomonas muscae-domesticae*) (*H. muscae-domesticae*) (*Schedoacercomonas muscae-domesticae*) (*Monomita muscarum*)	Very common in intestine, especially in tropics; normally found posterior to proventriculus; *Leptomonas* form predominates; usually passed in feces, in cystic form, which is taken up by other flies; believed also to occur, though confusion of species is probable, in *M. nebulo, M. humilis,* and other muscoids; adult flagellates and precystic forms also infective; has been cultured artificially	Burnett (1851, 1852); Leidy (1856); Stein (1878); Kent (1880–1882); Grassi (1879, 1882); Becker (1923a, b); Drbohlav (1925); Glaser (1922); Patton (1921a); Hoare (1924); Packchanian (1944); Root (1921)
Herpetomonas luciliae	*M. domestica* infected in laboratory by feeding on gut contents of *Lucilia sericata,* a natural host	Fantham and Robertson (1927)
Trypanosoma evansi	Positive transmission when *M. domestica* fed at bites of *Stomoxys calcitrans,* then visited wounds of healthy animals	Mitzmain (1916)
Trypanosoma hippicum	Transmitted to healthy mules by flies fed on sores of infected animals	Darling (1912a,b, 1913)
Sporozoa		
Octosporea muscae-domesticae	Found in gut and germ cells of flies	Steinhaus (1946)

Special Remarks on the Genus *Herpetomonas*

As indicated above, *Herpetomonas muscarum* appears in the literature more often than any other protozoan parasite of flies. Macfie (1917) found 42.5 per cent of *Musca domestica* collected from butchers' stalls to be heavily infested with *H. muscae domesticae,* as the species was then called. Workers of that day were much concerned with the possible relationships between these flagellates and leishmaniasis in man, an hypothesis later abandoned when *Phlebotomus* was established as the true vector of *Leishmania.* It should be mentioned that counts are not always as high as reported by Macfie. De Mello and Jacques (1919) found the parasite present in less than 1 per cent of the flies which they examined. These authors remarked the extreme polymorphism of the species and the great length of the flagellum. Fantham (1922) found *Herpetomonas* in only 4 out of 286 flies examined over a two-year period.

Ross and Hussain (1924) put forward some rather revolutionary ideas on the biology of *Herpetomonas*. In these experiments 7,000 flies were examined, of which 50 per cent proved to be infected. These authors demonstrated that the flagellate stage is ephemeral, continuing for perhaps not more than six hours. They state that reproduction takes place chiefly in the loose areolar tissue beneath the lining membrane of the intestine, which makes the organism less an intestinal parasite than a tissue invader. As described by Ross and

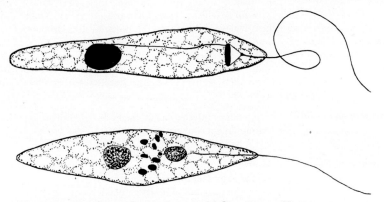

Figure 82. Flagellates parasitic in muscoid flies. *Upper: Herpetomonas muscarum* (*muscae-domesticae*). (After Calkins, *Biology of the Protozoa,* courtesy of Lea & Febiger.) *Lower: Herpetomonas calliphorae.* (Redrawn from Graham-Smith, *Flies in Relation to Disease* [Cambridge University Press, 1914], after Swellengrebel.)

Hussain, the life cycle is a rather elaborate one, with sexual phases. These findings are somewhat at variance with those of Drbohlav (1926), who examined 250 infected specimens of *Lucilia sericata*. He considered the parasites to be limited to the lumen of the alimentary tract, as he was unable to find them in the cells of the intestine, in the ova, in the ovary, or in other organs, even by culture methods. According to Drbohlav's observations, flagellated forms predominated in the foreintestine, and round forms in the posterior intestine and rectum.

Glaser (1926b) succeeded in culturing *Herpetomonas* free from bacteria, using as a medium the larval blood of the silkworm, *Bombyx mori*. After forty-five days the mobile forms were fewer, while the leishmania type, which he considered a resting stage, began to predominate. An inoculation of blood agar with such material resulted in the production of flagellated types within a period of one or two days. Nogouchi and Tilden (1926) developed serological and fermentation tests for differentiating the true herpetomonads of insects from developmental stages of the genus *Leishmania*. Among other characteristics, the leishmanias developed more slowly at 37°C (98.6°F) than did *Herpetomonas*. In the same year Nogouchi described three new species, based on biological tests. *Herpetomonas muscidarum*, from houseflies, ferments fourteen different carbohydrates; *H. media*, from *Calliphora*, seven; *H. parva*, also from *Calliphora*, six. It appears to be well established that certain species occur both in insects and in plants.

In 1937 Bellosillo studied *H. muscarum* as entozoic in *Lucilia*, in which genus he found 99 per cent of both spring- and fall-collected flies infected. He had no difficulty in demonstrating infection through the ingestion of flagellates excreted by flies on food. Larvae, in general, he found uninfected in nature, and he concluded that no hereditary transmission occurred. Confusion of *Herpetomonas* with *Trypanosoma* was reported by Packchanian (1944), who showed that human blood films contaminated with *H. muscae domesticae* through exposure to flies may be wrongly diagnosed as positive for *Trypanosoma cruzi* by technicians not thoroughly familiar with flagellate morphology.

Platyhelminthes and Nemathelminthes

Hall (1929) lists the following species of helminth parasites as definitely dependent on the genus *Musca* for development and transmission:

Species of Fly	Helminth Parasites
Musca bezzi (*sic*)	*Habronema* spp.
Musca domestica	*Choanotaenia infundibulum*
	Davainea tetragona
	Davainea cesticillus
	Habronema microstoma
	Habronema megastoma
	Habronema muscae
Musca fergusoni	*Habronema megastoma*
	Habronema muscae
Musca humilis	*Habronema megastoma*
	Habronema muscae
Musca lusoria	*Habronema megastoma*
	Habronema muscae

Species of Fly	Helminth Parasites
Musca terrae-reginae	*Habronema megastoma*
(*sic*)	*Habronema muscae*
	Agamospirura muscarum
Musca ventrosa	*Habronema megastoma*
	Habronema muscae
Musca vetustissima	*Habronema megastoma*
	Habronema muscae

Of the three tapeworms, two—*Davinea tetragona* and *D. cesticillus,* parasites of chicken, turkey, and guinea fowl—fall in the family Davainiidae. The other, *Choanotaenia infundibulum,* a chicken parasite, belongs in the Hymenolepididae.

The nematodes of the genus *Habronema,* which in the adult state are parasites of horses, asses, and mules, classify in the Spiruridae, a group dependent very largely on Coleoptera for the continuation of their life cycles, though fourteen species of flies do serve as vectors of the genus. The remaining species, *Agamospirura muscarum,* is of uncertain taxonomic position, falling somewhere close to the Dracunculidae. Its primary host is likewise very much in doubt.

The literature on habronemiasis is rather extensive.

The first satisfactory account of the life history of these parasites of horses and mules was given by Ransom in two publications (1911, 1913). The larvae of the roundworms fall to the ground with the feces of the vertebrate host, and later enter the bodies of fly maggots which develop from eggs laid on the manure. The parasites grow as metamorphosis proceeds. In the adult fly, they are found largely in the head and proboscis, but may also occur in the thorax and in the alimentary canal. The mature larvae escape from the fly's proboscis when the latter visits the horse's mouth. Johnston (1913) recorded what he believed to be the same species affecting sheep in Australia, and noted that both *Musca domestica* and *Stomoxys calcitrans* carried the parasite. He also found a similar larva in the head of *Musca vetustissima,* which is a great frequenter of the eyes of cattle. A similar record was published by Beal (1915), who studied an epidemic of verminous enteritis among sheep in Senegál. He identified the parasites as *Spiroptera microstoma* or *S. macrostoma.* Contemporary workers differed as to whether these forms might be considered cospecific with *Habronema muscae.*

Hill (1918), working in Australia, added considerable information relative to the life cycle of *Habronema.* He revealed that the larvae remain infective for eight days after leaving the rectum of the horse. There is a preliminary development in the manure before the parasite invades the maggot host, which apparently must be at least 48 hours old. Hill suggested that the horse acquires the stomach worms by ingesting either living or dead flies, perhaps at watering troughs or in fodder. *Habronema megastoma* and *H. microstoma* he considered separate species, the first spread probably by *M. domestica,* the latter certainly by *Stomoxys calcitrans.* Transmission by the swallowing of flies, plausible as it seems, must take place rarely, if at all, as no fly has ever been found in a horse's stomach. An alternative suggestion by Place (1915) that horses acquire infection by devouring chaff into which the larvae have been discharged also lacks convincing proof. Saceghem's work (1917, 1918) established that all three species are carried by *M. domestica* in the lower Congo. Both horses and donkeys may harbor *H. megastoma,* but *microstoma* and *muscae* he found in horses alone. Saceghem found that only horses in stables contracted the condition known as dermal granulosis. This is due to the great concentration of flies, by which a heavy nematode infection is brought about. The larvae, on entering a previously existing wound or scratch, cause inflammation which leads to enlargement of the wound, with opportunity for entrance of numerous additional larvae at the same point. In a later publication (1919), Saceghem advocated a paste to protect such wounds from further visitation by flies. This consists of 100 parts plaster of Paris, 20 parts alum, 10 parts naphthaline, and 10 parts quinine or some other bitter powder. The preparation is curative, if applied until all signs of exudation have disappeared. Bull (1919), in discussing habronemic granuloma, advocated excision, where location of the lesion permits.

Johnston's further work (1920b) found many species of flies to be capable of harboring *Habronema* larvae and acting as intermediate hosts. He pointed out that infested flies do not live long, which accounts for the low percentage of parasitism among flies collected in nature. When the larvae escape into the horse's mouth, they are swallowed and, having reached the stomach, develop into mature worms. Those larvae which invade wounds or scratches, thereby causing some form of granuloma, eventually die off, as there is no way for them to continue their life cycle. Under range conditions, habronemic granuloma, also called swamp cancer, is believed to be transmitted chiefly by *Stomoxys calcitrans, Musca vetustissima,* and *M. fergusoni,* with the latter more important north of 25° S latitude. The following year Johnston and Bancroft listed *M. domestica, M. humilis, M. lusoria, M. terrae-reginae, M. hilli,* and *Sarcophaga misera,* also a species of *Pseudopyrellia,* as hosts to *Habronema muscae* and *H. megastoma,* with *Stomoxys calcitrans* and possibly *Lyperosia exigua* as transmitters of *microstoma.* They also discuss habronemic conjunctivitis, which results when the larvae escape into the eye. Roubaud and Descazeaux (1921, 1922a,b) distinguished between *cutaneous habronemiasis,* produced when flies alight on wounds, and *pulmonary habronemiasis,* which results when the larvae escape into the nostrils. In neither case does the larva complete its development. The same authors throw considerable light on the behavior of the parasite in the insect host. *Habronema megastoma* is a parasite of the Malpighian tubes and causes a tumor in that location. *Habronema muscae* and *H. microstoma,* on the other hand, parasitize the adipose tissue.

Roubaud and Descazeaux believed seasonal conjunctivitis of man in hot regions to be due to *Habronema* infection. In the same year (1922), Bull suggested that the fairly common "bung eye" of Australia should be investigated with a view to establishing *Habronema* as the etiological agent.

More recent publications record habronemiasis from various parts of the world. Ware (1924) reports *H. microstoma* from the stomach of a horse in England. *Habronema megastoma* was reported by Phéloukis and Knithakis (1932) as probably the only species occurring in Greece. Twelve per cent of the houseflies caught in the vicinity of stable manure proved to be infected. Iwanoff (1934) described sores on cattle in Bulgaria as being due to nematode larvae carried by *Stomoxys calcitrans* and *Musca domestica.* In his collections, 5 per cent of the flies were infected. Cattle so affected yielded inferior hides. Schwartz and Cram (1925) collected all three species of parasites from horses in the Philippines. They noted that *H. megastoma* may be distinguished from the others by its smaller size and also by its residence in tumors in the gastric mucosa of the host. *Habronema muscae* and *H. microstoma* occur either attached to the mucosa or free in the lumen of the horse's stomach. South American studies were carried on by Margarinos Torres (de Magarinos Torres), who found 7.8 per cent of the horses examined in Rio to be infected (1923). Of 164 adult specimens of *Musca domestica,* 18.9 per cent carried the larvae of *H. muscae* in their heads. This author considers *M. domestica* to be the principal, if not the sole, vector of habronemiasis in Brazil. His later publications (1925a,b) deal with attempts to discover the factors that cause the mature larvae to leave the proboscis of the fly. Temperature and relative humidity were already known to be important. Margarinos Torres showed that horse blood, even if cold, will stimulate the ejection of larvae if the humidity is proper. He used this means of obtaining larvae for study without killing the insect host. Blood samples from rabbit, guinea pig, and man all proved negative, an observation which led him to conclude that bleeding wounds of man are in no danger of becoming contaminated with *H. muscae* in nature.

Further information on the spontaneous ejection of the larvae has been brought forward by De Mello and Pereira (1946), who carried out a number of experiments with infected flies, which they allowed to feed on a variety of liquids at controlled temperatures. They found that larvae escaped only when the temperature of the air was at or above 22°C (71.6°F) and that of the liquid at or above 23°C (73.4°F). Even a very favorable temperature, however, failed to induce their emergence when the flies fed on the blood, plasma, or serum of man, rabbit, guinea pig, cow, or swine, or solutions of milk (natural or condensed), dextrin, sugar, or honey. The larvae left the proboscis, however, when the proboscis was deeply immersed in warm saline, or in the blood, plasma, or serum of horses and asses. The sweat of horses failed to stimulate the larvae; in fact, the flies showed little appetite for it. Neither did saliva, human or equine, provide the necessary stimulus.

The only generalization which these authors suggest is that escape is dependent on the fly's remaining motionless for a considerable period of time, with the proboscis deeply immersed in the food material. It was noted that in all cases where larvae failed to emerge, the feeding was intermittent, with the proboscis barely touching the surface in most instances. De Mello and Cuocolo (1943a,b) also developed an improved technique for "xenodiagnosis," which will be briefly described:

Fly eggs are placed on horse dung in the bottom of a cylinder. At the top is placed an inverted funnel, with the stem capped by a test tube. The emerging flies, which make their way to the test tube, are then dissected for parasites. All flies in a batch are usually infected, if any are. As many as 60 larvae have been found in one fly's head. By such a procedure these workers found 87 out of 150 horses to be parasitized. Fifty-one donkeys proved to be 100 per cent infected. Care must be exercised to distinguish larvae of *Habronema* from those of other nematodes. The senior author (1946) recommended treatment of infected horses and asses with 30–40 gm. of phenothiazine or careful administration of arsenious acid. Simultaneous treatment of the environment to reduce the fly population is obviously desirable.

De Mello and Cuocolo proved definitely that the spirurid larvae never penetrate the chorion of the fly's egg. It is their opinion that the maggots usually *ingest* the parasites, sometime between the first and third day after hatching. The localization of *H. muscae* larvae in the fat body of the maggot causes necrosis, followed by the formation of cystlike bodies, in which the parasites remain until the pupal stage is past. The cysts then break open, and the larvae migrate to the head region of the fly. This migration is normally completed by the third or fourth day of the fly's adult existence.

Modern authors prefer to regard *H. megastoma* as falling in a separate genus, *Draschia* (Nicol, 1946).

Gapeworms of Poultry

Clapham (1939) has shown that flies may function as intermediate hosts of *Syngamus trachea,* parasite of the respiratory passages of barnyard fowl. While it is recognized that there can be direct transmission from bird to bird by ingestion of the eggs, snails, slugs, earthworms, and insects are frequently involved. In the experiments concerned, larvae of both *Musca domestica* and *Lucilia sericata* were reared on meat that had been spread with eggs of *Syngamus.* Twelve maggots were sacrificed and proved to contain one parasite larva each. After transformation, twelve flies were dissected, of which ten were found positive. Six chicks were fed 20 maggots each, and all developed gapes. A similar number were each given reared adults, and five developed the disease. Clapham states that infected maggots showed no reduction in activity as a result of being parasitized, but that the adult flies were rendered sluggish and therefore became much easier for the birds to catch.

Cestode Parasites

In 1892 Grassi and Rovelli found in the body of *Musca domestica* larvae whose scolices resembled those of the chicken tapeworm, *Choanotaenia infundibuliformis* (Goeze). Various observers subsequently confirmed the relationship. Gutberlet gave important data on the morphology of the parasite and stressed its transmission through *Musca domestica.* Ackert (1918) demonstrated that the housefly may transmit another fowl cestode, *Davainea cesticillus* (Molin). In these experiments flies were placed in lantern globe cages and given living onchospheres and portions of teased proglottids. When these flies died, some were sectioned, to prove the presence of larvae, while others were fed to birds. Nine of twelve chickens developed the cestodes, while control birds remained parasite-free. The following year, Ackert obtained similar data for the related species *Davainea tetragona* (Molin). A practical treatise on diseases of poultry by Bushnell and Hinshaw (1924) lists houseflies and stable flies as important intermediate hosts of bird tapeworms.

Modern confirmatory experiments have been performed in Kansas by Reid and Ackert (1937) and by Case and Ackert (1939). The latter authors point out that though houseflies serve as important intermediate hosts of *C. infundibulum* (Block) and other fowl cestodes, various species of beetles, flies, ants, snails, slugs, grasshoppers, and earthworms also serve in that capacity. In modern publications *Davainea cesticillus* is referred to the genus *Raillietina.*

Helminths Affecting Man

The relation of flies to human infection will be treated at greater length in the chapter that follows, but a few remarks seem in order at this point. In no case is the fly a cyclical host of any of the helminths affecting man. The transmission is purely mechanical. Nevertheless, a considerable number of species may be involved. Vaillard (1913) called attention to the fact that flies may transmit the ova of *Oxyuris* (*Enterobius*), *Trichocephalus*, *Taenia echinococcus*, and *Taenia* (*Hymenolepis*) *nana*. Shircore (1916) reported finding ova of *Trichocephalus dispar*, *Taenia saginata*, or *Ancylostoma duodenale* in 10 out of 100 houseflies collected in a native hospital. Two flies out of 25 taken in a meat market were also positive. One specimen contained ova of *Schistosoma mansoni*. Shircore notes that the ova *of Trichocephalus* can withstand putrefaction in the bodies of dead flies for perhaps 60 days. He also found that female flies carry helminth ova more commonly than do males.

Podyapolskaya and Gnedina (1934) studied transmission by both *Musca domestica* and *Calliphora erythrocephala*. The flies were permitted to feed on feces known to contain ova of *Ascaris, Enterobius, Trichuris* (*Trichocephalus*), and *Diphyllobothrium* and were later examined microscopically. No eggs were recovered from the proboscis, but all except *Trichuris* were found adhering to legs and wings. Many ova appeared in the droppings of *Calliphora* but not of *Musca*, indicating that the mouth aperture of the latter is rarely large enough to admit the eggs of helminths. Eggs of the liver fluke, *Dicrocoelium lanceolatum*, were found in droppings collected on glass slides in an abattoir. An egg of *Trichuris trichiura* appeared in a fly speck collected in a similar manner from a dining room.

Pokrovskii and Zima (1938) obtained similar evidence for transmission of *Hymenolepis, Enterobius, Diphyllobothrium*, and other species. Carriage on the body surface proved much more important than ingestion, at least for *Musca domestica*. Of 2,531 houseflies dissected, only 11 contained helminth ova. The percentage of flies carrying ova externally was higher in food shops than elsewhere, showing the need for protection of foodstuffs from contamination by flies.

MACROSCOPIC ORGANISMS BIOLOGICALLY RELATED TO FLIES

Arthropoda

Of the thirteen classes of Arthropoda, three are represented among the organisms so associated with *M. domestica* as to be worthy of mention in this place. These are the Chilopoda, Arachnida, and Hexapoda (Insecta).

Chilopoda. The relation of centipedes to common flies centers largely in the genus *Scutigera.* In most parts of the United States except the West, *Scutigera forceps* is a frequent inhabitant of human houses. It is an agile, somewhat delicate centipede, with legs which are very long and slender, especially the more posterior pairs. This species feeds on small household insects such as young cockroaches, clothes moths, and houseflies. Its numerous, jointed legs are useful in the capture of prey.

In France *Scutigera coleoptera* is a common centipede that frequents privies and is especially active at night, feeding on the muscoid fly *Fannia scalaris,* which breeds in human filth.

Scutigera smithii is an Australian species that feeds on houseflies by night.

Howard and Hutchison (1917) listed a number of known enemies of the housefly, including *Scutigera forceps,* which they credited with destroying large numbers of adult flies.

Arachnida. The arachnids that bear a biological relationship to flies fall in three orders, the Acarina, the Pseudoscorpionida, and the Araneida.

THE ACARINA. The Acarina, or mites, are represented by a number of forms that are found, more or less frequently, attached to the bodies of adult flies.

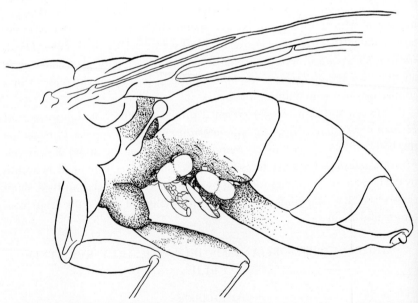

Figure 83. Mites, probably Gamasidae, attached to muscoid fly. The six-legged larvae attach by their mouth parts and suck up the juices of the fly. Adults of these forms are free-living. (From Hewitt, *The House-Fly* [Cambridge University Press, 1914]; also observed in nature.)

It is usually the six-legged larva which parasitizes the flies, the adult mites being free-living. Such larvae suck up the juices of the host by means of their threadlike mouth parts. A number of species also appear to use flies merely for transport. The passengers are usually the hypopus or hard-shell stage of various species which feed normally on cheeses, hams, and other food-stuffs.

A partial list of the mites recorded in literature as attached to hosts of the housefly type is given in Table 14.

Table 14. Mites taken on houseflies.

Species or group	Relationship and comments	Authority
Acarus reflexus	Larval form on body of fly	Attimonelli (1940)
Acarus muscarum	On head and neck of *Musca domestica*	Linnaeus (1758)
"Brown fly-mite"	On *Musca domestica*	Geoffroy (1764)
Trombidium parasiticum	Blood-red larvae, on housefly	Murray (1877)
Atoma (Astoma) parasiticum	Believed the same species as *Trombidium parasiticum*	Latreille (1795)
Atomus parasiticum	Nomenclature credited to Latreille	Howard (1911a)
Trombidium muscarum	Reared and named by Riley from numerous harvest-mite larvae found clinging at base of wing	Howard (1911a)
Trombidium muscae	Named by Oudemans from larvae found on houseflies in Holland	Howard (1911a)
Trombidium spp.	Larvae attached to body and wings of *Musca domestica*	Hewitt (1914a)
Pigmeophorus spp. (Tarsonemidae)	Cling to abdomen of fly; not certain whether fly is true or transport host	Howard (1911a)
Tyroglyphus spp.	Hypopus (migratory nymph) stage attaches to body of fly	Howard (1911a)
Histostoma muscarum	Proper generic position for adults of *Acarus muscarum* L., reared from *Muscina stabulans*	Berlese (1912)
Gamasidae	Immature forms swarm on flies emerging from rubbish heaps	Banks (1905)
Gamasidae (similar to *Dinychella asperata* Berlese)	Immature forms attached by mouth beneath abdomen of *Fannia canicularis* (lesser housefly)	Hewitt (1914a)

Table 14. Mites taken on houseflies. (continued)

Species or group	Relationship and comments	Authority
Macrocheles muscae (Gamasidae)	Larva always attaches at base of abdomen, ventral side, facing forward; true parasite	Ewing (1913)
Gamasidae	Affects *Muscina stabulans* in early June	Hamer (1910)
Trombidium sp.	Larva attached to right anterior tibia of *Musca domestica*	Berlese (1912)
Holostaspis marginatus Herm.	Migratory form attached to left hind tibia of *M. domestica*	Berlese (1912)
Thrombidium muscarum Riley	Confined to single host, *M. domestica;* never known to attach to man	Ewing and Hartzell (1918)
Unidentified red mite	Frequent on *M. domestica* in Amoy, South China	Feng (Lan-chou) (1933)
Holostaspis badius (Koch) (Gamasidae)	*M. domestica* heavily infested in autumn, in Venetia and Lombardy	Zanini (1930)
Macrocheles muscaedomesticae Scopoli	Immature stages attack ova of *M. domestica*	Pereira and De Castro (1945)

Pereira and De Castro (1945) consider *Macrocheles muscae* Ewing and *Holostaspis badius* Koch as synonyms of *M. muscaedomesticae* Scopoli, which they record as a fairly common arthropod enemy of the housefly in Brazil. The females gain transportation by attaching to the bodies of the adult flies. According to these authors, the mites must have food in order to deposit their eggs, which are produced at the rate of one a day. Incubation requires five to six hours. The larva, which takes no food, molts at the end of six hours to produce the protonymphal form, which feeds freely. This stage and the deutonymphal stage which follows require one day each. Eggs of *M. domestica* constitute the principal food of all the feeding stages. Occasionally a first-stage maggot is attacked, but adult flies are used for transportation only. A considerable number of Coleoptera and Diptera have been recorded as carrying the adult mites. Obviously the life cycle can go on only in an environment suitable for the deposition of fly eggs, as in horse dung. Female mites are stated to live longer and feed more voraciously than males. The species is believed to destroy large numbers of ova. The mites often leave them half-devoured.

PSEUDOSCORPIONIDA. Donovan (1797) was perhaps the first to record the attachment of false scorpions to muscoid flies. Kirby and Spence (1826), Moniez (1874), and Pickard-Cambridge (1892) stressed the significance of the relationship in effecting dispersal of the chelifers from one breeding habitat to another. An early specific reference to houseflies was published by

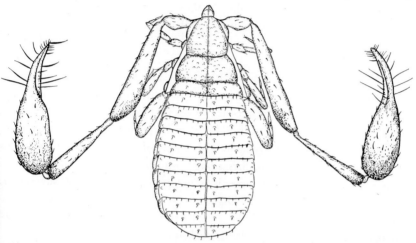

Figure 84. A pseudoscorpion. These forms frequently gain transportation by attaching to flies. They are not known to pierce the integument of the living fly, but have been observed to devour dead specimens.

De Borre (1873b), in which he recorded *Chelifer panzeri* Koch as attached parasitically to *Musca domestica*. Kew (1901) summarized existing knowledge of the occurrence of pseudoscorpions on various insect hosts, and commented on their habits and behavior in Lincolnshire, England.

Pseudoscorpions differ from true scorpions in having the abdomen robust for its entire length and in the absence of a caudal sting. They are also relatively minute, which makes it rather easy for them to attach to other arthropods for transportation. As found on flies, they are always attached by their claw-like pedipalps. Godfrey (1909) studied the habits of the false scorpions of Scotland, and records that the common *Chernes nodosus* lives mostly in refuse, manure heaps, and decaying vegetation. When flies visit such situations for oviposition, the *Chernes* has a good opportunity to seize their legs. An even better opportunity is afforded as teneral flies emerge from the pupal case.

Although pseudoscorpions feed freely on small insects, there is no evidence that they ordinarily succeed in piercing the integument of flies. The chief benefit to the chelifer is therefore dispersal of its species. On the other hand, they are known to remain attached to the transport host until the death of the latter, after which they not infrequently feed upon the dead fly. By this they become scavengers, rather than parasites. Hewitt (1914a) points out that since as many as ten may be attached to a single fly, the life of the latter may well be shortened by the burden, through interference with normal activity. It has not yet been demonstrated that pseudoscorpions feed upon the mites which may attach to flies, as they do upon the Acarina that infest beetles. Hickson (1905) has pointed out that if this should occur, it would place the pseudoscorpion in the list of species favoring the survival of the fly!

ARANEIDA. The use of flies as food by many families of spiders is common knowledge. Especially well known are the garden spiders of the family Epeiridae, which spin the beautiful orb webs. *Epeira sericata,* for example, usually chooses a site on or near buildings, and is frequently found on porches. But other groups are great flycatchers also. Any of the species that spin webs are likely to take their toll of flies along with other species of insects which become entangled in their snares. It is not possible to say that any spider, given a choice, actually prefers Diptera to other prey, but doubtless house-flies are among the more desirable items, as their integument is easily penetrated and the body juices are readily sucked out.

Non-web-spinners, such as the jumping spiders (family Attidae), also capture flies in great numbers. Their agility and skill are sometimes remarkable. Hewitt (1914a) specifically mentions that *Salticus scenicus,* a small species, has successfully captured flies almost twice its size.

Howard (1911a), quoting Banks, makes particular mention of *Theridium tepidariorum,* which locates its webs in the upper corners of rooms; *Steatoda borealis* and *Teutana triangulosa,* which prefer recesses behind furniture; and *Agalaena naevia,* which usually spins its web in outhouses or summer kitchens. All of these capture flies, those which build in most exposed places taking the larger toll. It is not possible to consider spiders as a very significant factor in the control of fly populations under civilized conditions, for the better the housekeeping, the fewer the webs remaining to capture flies.

Of special interest in Mexico is *Coenotele gregalis* E. Simon, a tiny spider which, living socially, produces a nest sometimes forty cubic feet in bulk and of a consistency resembling sponge. Shade, high relative humidity, and a living tree provide ideal conditions for nest building. The toll in prey is said to be enormous. A larger spider, *Poecilochroa convictrix* E. Simon, is associated as a commensal, while a small clavicorn beetle, *Corticaria nidicola*

Grouv., keeps the nest clean by consuming the dead flies after the spiders have sucked out the juices of their victims. Diguet (1915a,b) notes that if the beetles are absent, the cleaning function is performed by migratory ants. *Poecilochroa* appears to perform a real service by attacking prey too large for *Coenotele* to handle.

Hexapoda. Of the thirty or more orders of insects now recognized, relatively few include species that can be classed as parasites or predators of houseflies. The following discussion makes mention of the Orthoptera, Odonata, Anoplura, Hemiptera, Dermaptera, Coleoptera, Diptera, and Hymenoptera, of which the last fills by far the most important place.

ORTHOPTERA. One family of this order, the Mantidae, is predaceous in its habits and, when opportunity affords, attacks flies as well as other suitable prey. In certain parts of India it has long been the custom to employ a species of praying mantis to reduce houseflies about human dwellings (Hewitt, 1914a). It is doubtful if this method of control was ever very effective, but combined with other factors it may be significant.

ODONATA. Dragonflies are well known as destroyers of insect life. Since they appear somewhat partial to both mosquitoes and flies, the medical entomologist may well count them as friends of man. According to David and Marian Fairchild (1914), a single dragonfly may consume as many as forty flies in the space of two hours. When one considers the many long days of summer during which vast numbers of Anisoptera are on the prowl, the total destruction of common flies must truly be significant. Dragonflies habitually capture their prey while on the wing.

ANOPLURA. Records of true lice attaching to flies are few and of scant significance. For completeness' sake, however, it should be mentioned that Leon (1920) proved it possible for human body lice to be transported by houseflies, and that Bedford (1929) recorded immature individuals of *Linognathus vituli* L. as attached to *Musca interrupta* Walker (*lasiopthalma* Thoms.) at Capetown. In neither case does it appear that the flies were in any way inconvenienced or affected by the parasites.

HEMIPTERA. To date I have encountered but a single reference indicating that Hemiptera feed on houseflies. The record pertains to laboratory experiments carried on by Uribe (1926) concerning the transmission of *Trypanosoma cruzi*, causative agent of Chagas' disease. Uribe found that *Musca domestica* was acceptable food for *Apiomerus pilipes*, the reduviid host under investigation. Whether this or any other reduviid feeds regularly on houseflies in nature is exceedingly doubtful.

DERMAPTERA (EUPLEXOPTERA). The natural habits of these forms take them frequently into situations where dipterous larvae may be found. Hewitt cites Compere (1912) as recording the destruction of stable fly maggots by earwigs in southern China. It was Compere's opinion that earwigs were important in controlling the housefly population in Hong Kong, but most entomologists do not consider that Dermaptera exercise a very strong influence in this direction, in the Far East or elsewhere.

COLEOPTERA. Predaceous beetles apparently do much to reduce housefly populations under favorable circumstances. Venables (1914) studied the habits of *Tenthredo variegatus* and found that this species fed voraciously on houseflies, at least under laboratory conditions. The beetle first makes a wound in the body of the fly and then extracts the internal tissues, leaving the chitinous exterior.

Lever (1938) reported on the predatory habits of *Hister chinensis,* a coleopteran that was introduced into Fiji from Java to assist in the control of *Musca domestica vicina. H. chinensis* feeds particularly on the maggots. The predators burrow continually in dung in pursuit of the fly larvae, a habit that works to their advantage, as otherwise they would be devoured in large numbers by giant toads *(Bufo marinus).* The importation into Fiji appears to have come out of a suggestion by Simmonds (1932), who cited the successful use of dung beetles against *Lyperosia irritans* in the Hawaiian Islands. Simmonds himself (1940) reports that a single individual of *Hister chinensis* will devour from ten to twenty full-grown maggots within twenty-four hours, but can, if necessary, survive without food for fifteen days. Whereas this species is quite effective against houseflies in Java, the climate does not seem to be too satisfactory for its establishment and increase in Fiji.

Carrion-breeding Diptera are also held in check by Coleoptera. Kryzhanovskii (1944) records three species of *Saprinus* (Histeridae) as destroying the larvae of *Lucilia, Sarcophaga,* and *Chrysomyia.*

Howard (1911a) mentions certain Carabidae, of the genera *Harpalus, Platymus,* and *Agonoderus,* as feeding on fly larvae; both larvae and adults of Staphylinidae were similarly engaged. An interesting early record by Packard (1874) reports a beetle pupa within the puparium of a housefly.

A dung beetle, *Copris incertus* var. *prociduus* Say, introduced into Fiji in 1929 does not seem to have proved of much value in fly control.

DIPTERA. Portschinsky, in two interesting papers (1913a,b) describes the activities of certain dipterous larvae that destroy the maggots of other species. Most important is *Hydrotaea dentipes,* the larvae of which become predaceous in the third instar. They were observed to attack the maggots of *Stomoxys* and

Lucilia, as well as those of *Musca domestica,* and Portschinsky believes that this species constitutes a very important check on the natural increase of the latter. The larvae of *Hydrotaea* develop slowly. In one experiment a generation of third-stage larvae devoured three consecutive broods of *Musca domestica* before transforming. They have never been known to destroy one another. The adult flies do not enter human dwellings and are not annoying to man in any way.

The second paper deals with the biology of *Muscina stabulans,* which also has predatory habits in the third larval stage. *Muscina* larvae pursue and attack the larvae of *Musca domestica* (and other species), exterminating all that they can find. The technique employed by the attacker is rather interesting. The *Muscina* larva, having made contact with the victim, twists itself around the latter, holding fast by means of small hooklets situated on its ventral surface. The *Muscina* larva then strikes the victim several powerful blows with its mouth hooks. This punctures the integument of the housefly larva, which ceases to struggle, as its body fluids are lost. The victor is then joined by a number of its own species, which share in devouring the spoil. As with the larvae of *Hydrotaea,* no larva of *Muscina* ever devours one of its own species.

Less definite information is available concerning *Calliphora erythrocephala,* which sometimes breeds in the same situation as *M. domestica.* Kvasnikova (1931) noticed that both species were ovipositing on exposed meat but that later only larvae of *Calliphora* could be found; he suggests that the larvae of *Musca* were devoured by those of *Calliphora.* Lacking definite observation, we must consider destruction by *Calliphora* as only one of several factors that might have prevented development of the houseflies. It is possible that the medium was not physiologically suitable.

Adult houseflies, also, have their dipterous enemies. Hewitt (1914c) comments on the predaceous habits of *Scatophaga stercoraria* L. (Cordyluridae). These aggressive flies were seen capturing seven or eight species of Diptera, including *Musca domestica.* They apparently have a great preference for muscoid flies. After seizing the victim, the predator wraps its legs around the prey and then pierces the neck of the latter by blows struck with the proboscis. After feeding a short time in this position, the aggressor turns the victim's body over and inserts the proboscis in the conjunctiva between adjacent abdominal segments. Feeding goes on here for a long time, presumably until the prey has been sucked dry or until the feeder is replete.

Both Howard (1911a) and Graham-Smith (1914) make mention of robber flies (Asilidae) as including houseflies in their bill of fare. Hewitt (1914a) specifically records *Laphria canis* Will. as catching and devouring *Musca domestica*.

HYMENOPTERA. Both predators and parasites are found here. Among the first, predaceous ants are probably of greatest importance. Howard (1911a) refers to certain Army Medical Corps experiments in the Philippines in which it was impossible to rear flies for study unless eggs, larvae, and pupae were carefully protected from ants. In the United States Howard lists the fire ant, *Solenopsis gemminata diabola,* the little black ant, *Monomorium minimum,* and the Argentine ant, *Iridomyrmex humilis,* as capable of feeding on the immature stages of flies. Rather outstanding is the genus *Pheidole,* species of which have been studied by workers in widely separated regions. Bridwell (1918) reported *Pheidole megacephala,* in Hawaii, as penetrating the isolated droppings of both horses and cows, where they destroyed not only the eggs, larvae, and pupae of *Musca domestica,* but likewise the newly emerged adults. Jepson (1915), reporting from Fiji, called attention to Ill- ingworth's observation that houseflies are sometimes controlled by "small brown ants," and Simmonds (1925) gave it as his opinion that the small num- ber of flies in Fiji (at that time) could be attributed chiefly to the activities of *Pheidole megacephala,* which had been accidentally introduced from Hawaii in 1910. Previous to that date *Musca domestica* had been very abun- dant in Fiji, and much enteric and ophthalmic disease had been attributed to its vectorship. The same author (1928) pointed out that these ants are par- ticularly effective in removing eggs and larvae from horse droppings, in one locality accounting for the destruction of 50 per cent of the immature forms. With cow droppings, however, at least in that climate, the situation is differ- ent, as the surface does not harden quickly enough for the ants to swarm over it and remove the eggs before the larvae have hatched and gone deeper. In 1940 Simmonds reported that the housefly menace in Fiji had again become serious, due to the increased number of cattle, and that new means should be sought to effect a natural control.

A significant observation on the role played by ants in reducing screwworm flies is recorded by Lindquist (1942), who found that in Texas *Cochliomyia hominivorax* (*americana*) might be largely prevented from development by the activities of ants which become attracted to carcasses where the maggots are feeding. Only 4.1 per cent of the larvae survived under such conditions, as compared with 93.1 per cent when ants were intentionally excluded.

In Tajikistan, Kryzhanovskii (1944) records *Pheidole pallidula* as effective, along with certain Coleoptera, in destroying the larvae of flesh flies and blow-flies.

Also predatory in their behavior are certain wasps. Vaillard (1914) mentions *Bembex* as a natural enemy of flies. Jepson (1915) attributed the reduction of flies in the province of Bera, Fiji, to the activity of *Polistes hebraeus,* which is predaceous on both larval and adult forms. Parker (1917), in his revision of the Bembicine wasps, records *Musca domestica* as one of eleven species of flies found in three nests of *Bembex spinolae.* According to G. W. and E. G. Peckham (1905), a partially grown larva of this wasp succeeded in devouring forty-two houseflies and one large *Tabanus* in the short space of five days.

Froggatt (1917) reported fossorial wasps of the genera *Stizus* and *Nysson* as especially active in capturing *Musca autumnalis* (*corvina*) and other small flies.

Vespa germanica Fabr. and *Mellinus arvensis* L. are both recorded by Herold (1922) as preying on houseflies in Europe, while *Vespa orientalis* is considered by Zmeev (1939–1941) as a distributor of dysentery through its habit of feeding on filth-frequenting flies.

In the United States and Canada various species of *Vespa* have been observed to cut off the wings of captured flies before eating them or carrying them away. I have seen this occur repeatedly in camps and cabins, until a noticeably large number of wings littered the floor or table.

HYMENOPTEROUS PARASITES. The hymenopterous parasites that attack *Musca domestica* and related forms belong for the most part either to the Cynipidae or the Chalcidoidea. Most species of Cynipidae form galls on plants, but the Figitines are parasites and of these a number attack flies, especially those which breed in excrement. It is the larval stage of the host which is parasitized. The minute adult wasps may frequently be seen on or near excreta, seeking for maggots on which to deposit their eggs. Parasitized maggots fail to survive.

The Chalcidoidea that parasitize muscoids are pupal parasites. The small female wasps deposit their eggs in the puparia of flies, and the parasitic larvae develop at the expense of the dipterous pupae, which eventually shrivel and die. Oviposition is usually a rather laborious task, involving perforation of the integument followed by enlargement of the aperture, before oviposition can take place. One common species hibernates as a full-grown larva in the puparia of flies, transforming to a pupa in the spring. The literature on hymenopterous parasites of muscoids is fairly extensive. To save space, certain information is summarized in Table 15.

Table 15

Genus and species	Explanatory remarks	References
	Chalcidoidea	
Dirhinus pachycerus	Attacks pupae of *Musca, Chrysomyia,* and *Sarcophaga;* ignores *Stomoxys* and *Drosophila;* can locate pupae under loose earth	Roy and Siddons (1939); Roy *et al.* (1940)
Hemilexomyia abrupta	Scarce parasite of *M. domestica* in Australia	Johnston and Tiegs (1922)
Mormoniella vitripennis (See also *Nasonia brevicornis,* which is a synonym)	From pupae of several muscoid genera, including *Musca;* contaminates environment so that other parasites remain away; prefers *C. erythrocephala, Lucilia caesar,* and *Phormia terra-novae* to *M. domestica;* cannot locate pupae 1 mm. under sand	Parker and Thompson (1928); James (1928); Seguy, W. (1929); Smirnov and Kuzina (1933); Smirnov and Wladimirow (1934); Wladimirow and Smirnov (1934); De Bach (1944); Moursi (1946)
Mormoniella sp.	Attacks *Lucilia* and related forms in Australia; pupal stage immune to parasites on first day and last two days	Hardy (1924)
Muscidifurax raptor	Reared from puparia of *Musca domestica* in Illinois; not as prolific as *Nasonia*	Girault and Sanders (1910); Howard (1911a); Hewitt (1914a); Graham-Smith (1914)
Nasonia brevicornis (*Mormoniella vitripennis,* which see)	Reared from puparia of various filth-breeding Diptera in Illinois; parasitizes various flies in Australia; may be secondary parasite on *Alysia*	Girault and Sanders (1909); Howard (1911a); Hewitt (1914a); Graham-Smith (1914); Alston (1920); Froggatt (1921)
Pachycrepoideus dubius	True primary parasite of housefly and *Sarcophaga* spp.; emerges through jagged hole in pupal case; destroys houseflies in N. Queensland, Australia; active in Puerto Rico	Girault and Sanders (1910); Howard (1911a); Hewitt (1914a); Graham-Smith (1914); Johnston (1921); Johnston and Tiegs (1922); Puerto Rico Report (1938); Lever (1945)

Genus and species	Explanatory remarks	References
Prospalangia platensis	Parasitic on pupae of *M. domestica, Stomoxys calcitrans,* and other flies near Buenos Aires	Brèthes (1915)
Pteromalus sp.	Bred repeatedly from pupae of *Calliphora erythrocephala*	Graham-Smith (1914)
Spalangia cameroni .	Introduced from Hawaii to combat flies in Fiji	Simmonds (1929a,b)
Spalangia hirta	Parasite of *M. domestica;* reduces puparium to flattened cuticle	Richardson (1913b)
Spalangia muscae	According to Sanford, deposits ova in puparia of houseflies in United States	Howard (1911a); Graham-Smith (1914)
Spalangia muscidarum (also var. *stomoxysiae*)	Bred from pupae of *M. domestica, Stomoxys calcitrans,* and *Haematobia serrata;* consumes blood plasma of host; occurs in Puerto Rico	Richardson (1913a,b); Bishopp (1913a); Pinkus (1913); Hewitt (1914a); Lindquist (1936); Puerto Rico Report (1938); Simmonds (1940)
Spalangia niger	According to Bouché deposits ova in puparia of houseflies in Europe	Howard (1911a)
Spalangia nigra	Parasite of *M. domestica;* reduces puparium to flattened cuticle	Richardson (1913b)
Spalangia philippinensis	Introduced into Hawaii; bred from puparia of housefly and other Muscidae; also introduced into Puerto Rico	Fullaway (1917); Puerto Rico Report (1938)
Spalangia spp.	From pupae of *M. domestica* and *Sarcophaga,* in France; employed to control *M. domestica* and *Stomoxys calcitrans* in Guam; introduced into Fiji from Queensland or Hawaii; bred from *M. domestica vicina* in Calcutta	Simmonds (1922); Parker and Thompson (1928); Vandenberg (1930, 1931a,b); Roy and Siddons (1939)
Stenomalus muscarum	Parasite of housefly pupae; found in houses with hibernating flies	Howard (1911a); Graham-Smith (1914); Waterston (1916)

Encyrtidae

Tachinaephagus giraulti	Reared from *Lyperosia exigua* and *Musca domestica*	Ferrière (1933)

Table 15 (continued)

Genus and species	Explanatory remarks	References
Eulophidae		
Syntomosphyrum glossinae	Normal parasite of tsetse fly; reared experimentally from *M. domestica*	Roubaud and Colas-Belcour (1936)
Diapriidae		
Ashmeadopria sp.	Ten per cent of *M. domestica* parasitized in some collections	Puerto Rico Report (1938)
Cynipidae		
Eucoila impatiens	Suspected by T. D. A. Cockerell of parasitizing *M. domestica*	Howard (1911a)
Eucoila sp.	Parasite of *M. domestica* in Fiji	Simmonds (1940)
Figites anthomyiarum	Reared from housefly maggots by Reinhard, in Germany; attacks any maggots in carrion	Howard (1911a); Hewitt (1914a); Graham-Smith (1914); James (1928)
Figites scutellaris	Reared from housefly maggots by Förster, in Europe	Howard (1911a); Hewitt (1914a); Graham-Smith (1914)
Figites striolatus	Reared from *M. domestica*	Hewitt (1914a)
Kleidotoma marshalli	Attacks almost any dipterous larvae found in carrion	James (1928)
Kleidotoma sp.	Attacks nearly all maggots found in carrion	James (1928)
Braconidae		
Alysia manducator	European species; parasitizes all flies; attacks full-grown maggots	Froggatt (1921); James (1928)

Vertebrate Enemies of Houseflies

The consumption of flies or larvae by fishes is purely accidental and cannot be considered to have a bearing on natural control. Manure, containing maggots, occasionally falls from a manure spreader or cart as it crosses a bridge or ford, and fish may consume the floating insects, but such incidents are too rare to be significant.

Amphibians and reptiles, on the other hand, are great devourers of flies. The aquatic or semiaquatic habitat of most species of frogs operates against their including any great number of houseflies in the dietary, but the common garden toad, *Bufo americana,* is often found near the doorstep or stable and feeds eagerly on *Musca domestica* whenever it can. Under tropical conditions it is not uncommon to find small lizards in and about the native houses, where they destroy large numbers of flies. Both amphibians and reptiles rely chiefly on their sticky, extensible tongues to make contact with the insect prey.

Most insectivorous birds seem not to prefer houseflies, but this is due largely to the fact that *Musca domestica* is rarely present in numbers in those areas in which the birds prefer to feed. Houseflies have been found in the stomachs of the palm warbler, white-eyed vireo, wood pewee, and cedar bird. The so-called "flycatchers," as a group, however, feed largely on winged Hymenoptera. Maggots are apparently palatable to many birds, but only those of certain feeding habits have an opportunity to discover them. Domestic poultry, for example, if admitted to barnyards, will consume enormous numbers of larvae, and can be an important factor in reducing the fly population. Howard (1911a) mentions a single record of thirty-three dipterous larvae being taken from the stomach of a horned lark, but it is highly probable that they were of some species other than *Musca domestica.*

Mammals closely associated with human habitations sometimes learn to be flycatchers. Adult flies are frequently destroyed by mice on window sills during the hours of night when the insects are sluggish, inactive, and more or less at the mercy of the nocturnal rodents. Rats are known to catch and eat flies in broad daylight, with spectators present. Reliable authority records a single rat as taking over one hundred flies from a window sill at a single meal. The fly is either raked with one front paw against the other or is caught between the two paws as they are brought together. The animals sometimes stand on their hind legs, extending their bodies to full length in order to reach the prey.

Cats, also, will occasionally capture flies, apparently more for amusement than for food. When an individual animal has adopted the practice and become proficient, a very large number of flies may be accounted for. I am indebted to my colleague, Miss Mary McCarthy, for information concerning a cat which formed the habit of capturing flies in a window seat and became "very dextrous" in the sport.

CHAPTER XI

Flies and Human Disease

Put cream and sugar on a fly, and it tastes very much like a black raspberry.—
E. W. Howe, Country Town Sayings

IN THE YEAR 1912, a current educational pamphlet referred to the housefly as "the most dangerous insect known." In spite of great improvements
in methods of fly control, world sanitarians today are still unable to dispute
the general truth of this assertion. For the individual who has grown to maturity in a well-sanitated area, there can be no conception of the hazards to
health which still exist wherever flies have unrestrained access both to human
feces and to human food.

It should be remembered that the adult fly can transmit infectious organisms in at least four separate ways: (1) by the hairs of its body; (2) by the
sticky tenent hairs of its feet (which also permit the fly to cling to vertical
and even inverted surfaces); (3) by regurgitation of its vomitus; (4) by
passage through its alimentary tract. The last is perhaps the most significant,
as it often provides opportunity for multiplication of the organisms concerned. Many types of bacteria, protozoan cysts, certain helminth ova, and
probably a number of viruses owe their dissemination, at least in part, to
fecal specks deposited by flies. This is not strange when one considers that
a well-fed fly has been observed to defecate at intervals of approximately four
and a half minutes all day long (Cobb, 1910b). In the same reference we find
this pithy observation, "The fly does far worse things than get into the oint-
ment, for unless we take care he gets into or onto pretty much everything
we eat or drink." This alone would not be so significant were it not for the
fact that the fly also gets into or onto every conceivable form of excreta and
other filth that has not been disposed of in a flyproof manner.

According to Ara and Marengo (1932), 44 per cent of the flies captured in
rooms of typhoid patients proved to be infected with typhoid. The bacillus
continued to be present in the fly's alimentary tract for as long as six days

after capture. This is but one example among many in which infections more or less pathogenic to man are carried on or in the bodies of flies, in many instances with no adverse effect upon the carrier host.

In this connection, however, it is well to recall that organisms harbored by the fly or its immature stages may differ strikingly in their ability to affect the fly's well-being, to curb its powers of reproduction, or to alter its potential longevity. From the fly's standpoint, in other words, such organisms may be either quite harmless, relatively benign, or definitely pathogenic. But when the same organisms gain transference to the human body, their potential

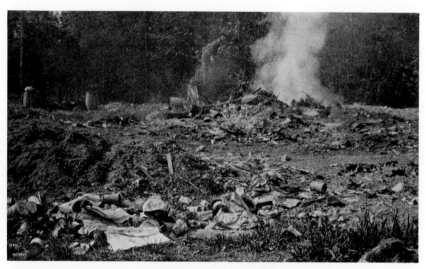

Figure 85. An unnecessary nuisance in the vicinity of an adequate incinerator. Note dumping of rubbish, which should have been processed but which serves instead as breeding medium for flies. Health authorities recommended that this area be cleared up and sown with grass seed. (Courtesy of Michigan Department of Health.)

pathogenicity requires complete reclassification. The *Empusa* fungus, for example, which is so destructive to flies, does not even have the capacity to establish itself on human tissue. The typhoid bacillus, on the other hand, the causative agent of a serious human disease, appears to affect the housefly not at all. Intermediate between these extremes is the *Staphylococcus* group, two species of which cause fatal diseases in flies, while within the same genus are forms known to produce annoying and, at times, alarming symptoms in man. A more specific example is the plague bacillus (*Pasteurella pestis*). This organism, which is usually fatal to man, can be carried for perhaps eight days by flies, after which the insects themselves die of the disease (Nuttall, 1897).

The pages that follow are concerned primarily with those infections which cause pathological conditions in man whether or not the fly is in any way inconvenienced by the passage. There is at the present time acceptable laboratory proof for the transmission of approximately thirty diseases (or parasitic organisms) by *Musca domestica* and related forms. The more important of these are characterized below. Certain infections of primary interest to students of veterinary medicine have already been discussed in Chapter X.

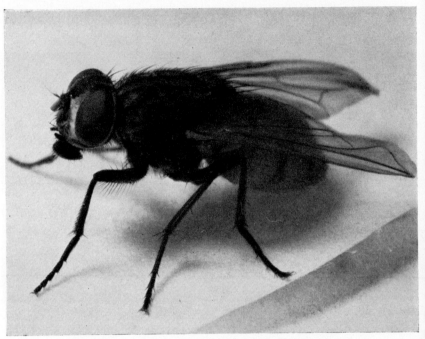

Figure 86. The fly in an exploratory mood. Note claws, pulvilli, labella, and numerous body bristles. These are the structures that make it easy for the fly to function as a distributor of filth and filth-borne disease. (Courtesy of Rohm and Haas Company, Philadelphia, Pa.)

BACTERIAL DISEASES

Typhoid Fever

Also known as enteric fever or abdominal typhus. A specific, eruptive, communicable fever marked by inflammation and ulceration of Peyer's patches, by enlargement of the spleen and of the mesenteric nodes, and by catarrhal inflammation of the intestinal mucous membrane. Convulsive and haemorrhagic forms of the disease may occur. The causative organism is *Eberthella typhosa*. Transmission is by fecal contamination of food and drink.

The Paratyphoids

Fevers, usually less severe, resembling in most respects typhoid fever and caused by organisms which infect the same tissues as are involved in that disease. Two types exist. The correct name of the organism formerly known as *Bacillus paratyphosus* A is *Salmonella paratyphi*. *Salmonella schottmülleri* is the accepted designation for *Bacillus paratyphosus* B of authors.

Cholera

Also called malignant or Asiatic cholera. An acute infectious disease marked by copious, watery discharges from the bowels, cramps, prostration, and suppression of the urine. Usually fatal. Death results either from congestion of the lungs or from convulsions and exhaustion. The cadaver usually shows extreme dehydration. Causative organism is *Vibrio comma*, also known in literature as *Spirillum cholerae*. Transmission is usually by fecal contamination of drinking water.

Bacillary Dysentery

An infectious disease marked by intestinal pain, straining at stool (tenesmus), and diarrhea, with blood and mucus in the intestinal discharges. There is always more or less toxemia. Distribution is largely, though not wholly, tropical. Causative organisms are *Shigella dysenteriae* and *S. paradysenteriae*. Transmission is by contamination of food and drink.

Infantile Diarrhea

Also known as summer diarrhea. An acute intestinal disturbance, chiefly of children, during the great heat of summer. Symptoms may develop comparable to milder types of bacillary dysentery. Believed to be caused by a variety of bacterial (or virus) organisms including several of the genus *Shigella*. Transmission is similar to other types of enteritis. Flies are considered to play an important part.

Anthrax

Usual reference is to *malignant anthrax,* a fatal infectious disease of cattle and sheep, also transmissible to man. Hard edema or ulcers formed at point of inoculation. Lesion may be in the form of a carbuncle or malignant pustule. Symptoms of collapse usually follow. Cerebral anthrax is also known. Causative agent is *Bacillus anthracis*. Infection is usually by inoculation of spores or active bacilli into a superficial abrasion of the skin.

Conjunctivitis (Not Including Trachoma)

Nonspecific inflammation of the conjunctiva marked by acute redness and swelling in one or both eyes, with mucopurulent and purulent discharges. If round, pinkish bodies appear in the retrotarsal fold, the type is said to be follicular. Causative agent, any of a number of pyogenic organisms, including the hemoglobinophilic bacilli. *Gonococcus* is sometimes responsible. Transmission is by direct contact or indirectly through soiled articles or by activity of insects. Eye gnats of the genus *Hippelates* (family Chloropidae) are of much greater importance than *Musca* in transmitting conjunctivitis in the southern United States.

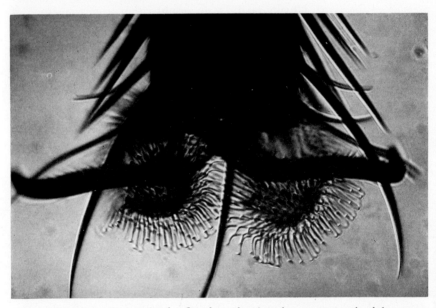

Figure 87. Photomicrograph of a fly's foot, showing the numerous glandular tenent hairs borne by the pulvilli. It is the sticky secretion of these hairs which gathers bacteria, spores, and cysts, and is thus responsible for their distribution as the fly walks about. (Courtesy of A. C. Lonert, General Biological Supply House, Chicago.)

Tuberculosis

An infectious disease, the symptoms of which vary with the tissue affected. Local activity of the organism results in the formation of tubercles in the tissues. These later undergo caseous necrosis. Infection may be spread through blood and lymph vessels. General symtoms include hectic fever, emaciation, and night sweats. Causative agent, *Mycobacterium tuberculosis.* Infection usually acquired by mouth, but also in other ways.

Leprosy

Preferably called Hansen's disease. A transmissible disorder characterized by lesions of the skin and mucous membranes and by neurological manifestations. Lesions may be in the form of patches of macular erythema, which develop into anesthetic patches of scar tissue, or in the form of tubercles and nodules, which may either absorb or ulcerate. Deformity and mutilation of the digits is common. Causative agent, *Mycobacterium leprae*. Not easily communicable, but discharges from lesions are considered dangerous.

Plague

Also known as malignant polyadenitis. An acute febrile and usually fatal disease characterized by chills and fever, followed by prostration. Headache, vomiting, delirium, and diarrhea may occur. The bubonic form is marked by swelling of the lymphatic nodes, with resultant buboes in femoral, inguinal, axillary, and cervical regions. The pneumonic form, which is most often fatal, resembles septic pneumonia. Causative organism is *Pasteurella pestis,* which may be recovered from buboes or sputum according to the type of disease. Transmission is normally by the bites of fleas, but may be direct in the pneumonic form in which connection flies may be involved.

VIRUS DISEASES

Trachoma

A specific, destructive, chronic inflammation of the conjunctiva, marked by follicular or papillary granulations, leading ultimately to scar tissue, deformity of the eyelids, and possible blindness. Susceptibility is increased by malnutrition and prolonged exposure to dust, sun, and wind. The causative organism has not been determined. Transmission is by direct contact with lesions or indirectly by contact with contaminated objects or insects.

Poliomyelitis (Especially Acute Anterior Poliomyelitis)

Also known as infantile paralysis, Heine-Medin disease, and acute atrophic paralysis. An inflammation of the gray substance of the spinal cord, characterized in early stages by fever and, in many cases, producing motor paralysis, with resultant atrophy of muscles, and deformity. Causative agent, a specific filterable virus. Transmission by introduction of virus into brain by way of nasal membranes and olfactory nerves.

SPIROCHAETE INFECTION

Yaws

Also called treponematosis, frambesia, pian, and bubas. Usually marked by raspberrylike elevations on face, hands, feet, and sometimes the genitals. Lesions may run together in funguslike masses. Pustules and ulcers not uncommon. Deformity of countenance due to gangosa, sometimes extreme. Causative agent, *Treponema pertenue*. Transmission is by direct contact with lesions or indirectly by both biting and nonbiting flies.

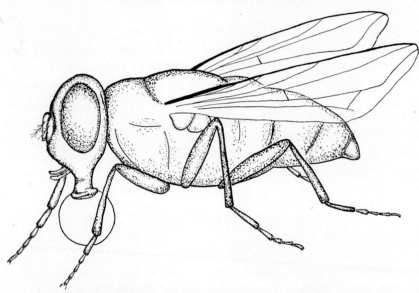

Figure 88. Fly regurgitating. Most of the flyspecks on walls and windowpanes are composed of vomitus rather than fecal matter. Human food and drink exposed to flies may become heavily contaminated in this manner. (Adapted from Matheson, after Hewitt.)

PROTOZOAN DISEASES

Amoebic Dysentery

Also called intestinal amoebiasis, or amoebic enteritis. A disease with a wide variety of clinical symptoms, including usually cramping diarrhea with little fever or tenesmus. Stools often contain flecks of blood-stained mucus. "Sea anemone" and "Dyak hair" ulcers of colon are typical. Extensions of the infection may lead to liver or brain abscess, to cystitis, vaginitis, and other complications. Causative agent, a tissue-invading protozoan, *Endamoeba histolytica*. Transmission, by food, drinking water, fingers, and flies.

Giardiasis

Inflammation of the biliary system and intestinal tract, with symptoms resembling a mild, chronic, catarrhal cholecystitis. Chronic, recurring diarrhea with some flatulence and distention characterizes heavier infections. Causative agent a flagellate protozoan, *Giardia lamblia*. Transmission as in amoebiasis. Cysts are passed through the intestinal tract of flies.

MISCELLANEOUS ORGANISMS

In addition to the above, the following parasites known to occur in man are undoubtedly capable of having their transmission assisted by flies:

(1) *Endamoeba coli* (intestinal amoeba)—flies carry cysts.
(2) *Endolimax nana* (intestinal amoeba)—flies carry cysts.
(3) *Chilomastix mesnili* (intestinal flagellate)—flies carry cysts.
(4) *Enterobius vermicularis* (pinworm)—flies carry ova.
(5) *Ascaris lumbricoides* (roundworm)—flies carry ova.
(6) *Trichuris trichiura* (whipworm)—flies carry ova.
(7) *Ancylostoma duodenale* (hookworm)—flies carry ova.
(8) *Taenia solium* (pork tapeworm)—flies carry ova.
(9) *Dipylidium caninum* (dog tapeworm)—flies carry ova.
(10) *Hymenolepis nana* (dwarf tapeworm)—flies carry ova.
(11) *Hymenolepis diminuta* (rat tapeworm)—flies carry ova.
(12) *Echinococcus granulosus* (hydatid cyst)—flies carry ova.
(13) *Dermatobia hominis* (human botfly)—houseflies may carry eggs.

Although specific records appear to be lacking, it seems likely that the eggs of *Taenia saginata* would be as easily carried as those of *Taenia solium,* and that ova of the American hookworm, *Necator americanus,* are carried about quite as often as those of *Ancylostoma.*

It has been noted by several observers that flies feeding on feces seem particularly attracted to helminth eggs and make a definite effort to ingest them.

As discussed in Chapter III, individual flies differ greatly in their ability to so distend the mouth aperture that ova can be taken in, but the smaller eggs never seem to present much difficulty. There are several species, no doubt, which few, if any, flies can transmit other than externally on their bodies. Thus Nicoll (1911b) considered houseflies incapable of ingesting the large, round eggs of *Hymenolepis diminuta,* though large blowflies may do so.

In the foregoing lists, no mention is made of smallpox, diphtheria, syphilis, or Oriental sore. Hewitt (1914a) summarized suggestive evidence for transmission of these infections by filth-feeding flies, but since there is a dearth of modern, confirmatory data, it seems best to omit discussion of these.

EVIDENCE FOR DISEASE TRANSMISSION BY FLIES

A moderate viewpoint on the medical importance of filth-feeding Diptera should always be maintained. Flies are rarely the *sole* transmitting agency in

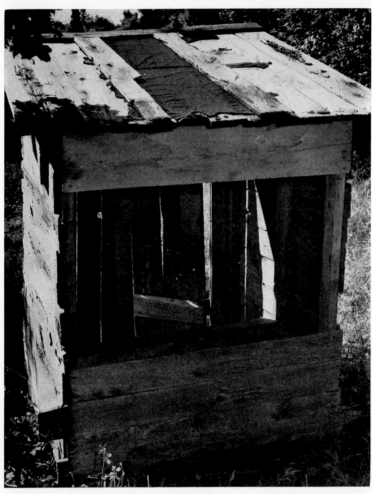

Figure 89. Makeshift privy near campsite. Absence of rear wall has permitted photographer to show primitive type of seat. There is no way to keep flies from pit, which means an unsanitary camp. In harmony with these conditions, the well was located about twenty feet downhill from the privy. (Photo by Rollin Thoren.)

any epidemic, and in most cases their role, however important, must logically be considered subordinate.

Thus Nicoll (1917a,b), while admitting that organisms producing bacillary enteritis may often be found in flies under natural conditions, remarks that in no case has *Musca domestica* been demonstrated to be the exclusive vector of any disease. He especially emphasizes that though the housefly serves as a cyclical host for *Habronema* of horses, it is not the true intermediate host of *any* organism causing disease in man. The fly is rather a mechanical carrier of pathogens, which in some cases may not even multiply in the fly's body. Nicoll found no evidence, for example, that typhoid bacilli can reproduce in the housefly; nor, indeed, can they live there for any great period of time. He also points out that many bacteria in the fly's intestine bear a very close resemblance to important pathogens and that very stringent tests must be employed to differentiate between benign and pathogenic types.

Again, Roubaud (1918) expresses the view that *Musca domestica* cannot act as a vector of the principal intestinal protozoans of man except under very limited conditions. He points out that the excreta of flies must ordinarily be deposited directly upon liquid or moist food, if the contained cysts are to reach the human organism with sufficient vitality to cause infection. Since cysts which are deposited on a dry substratum perish almost immediately, it may even be that the flies contribute extensively to their destruction by withdrawing them from the media in which they are able to exist. Woodcock (1918, 1919) did not consider flies a very great factor in the epidemiology of amoebic dysentery. Likewise, Jausion and Dekester (1923), who experimented with four species of muscoid flies, including *M. domestica,* considered their role in the transmission of *Endamoeba "dysenteriae"* to be very limited. Morison and Keyworth (1916) felt that flies played but a minor part in the distribution of epidemic diarrhea and dysentery in Poona, as treatment of the water supply resulted in no epidemic the following season.

Lebailly (1924) concluded that neither *Muscina stabulans* nor *Musca domestica* is able to transmit foot and mouth disease of animals. Malmgren (1935), who studied an extensive outbreak of tularemia in Sweden consistently found *M. domestica* negative for *Pasteurella tularensis* (*Bacterium tularense*). It is now generally accepted that bloodsucking forms are much more likely to be involved in the transmission of this disease.

We should also remember that flies undoubtedly serve as temporary carriers of potentially pathogenic organisms under circumstances which rarely favor their transmission to a second mammalian host. Thus Ewing (1942) found *Streptococcus agalactiae* in decreasing numbers for seven days on the body surface of flies that had been permitted contact with a skim-milk culture of the organism over a four-day period. Although the *Streptococcus* remained viable in the tissues of the fly for three days longer, as shown by examination of ground-up flies, Ewing considers it rather doubtful if flies transmit any great amount of bovine mastitis while feeding at the teats of cows.

Experiments conducted by Stewart (1944) on the viability of dysentery bacilli in Algiers demonstrated that Flexner and Schmitz bacilli might be carried by flies for as long as twelve days. This seems important in view of the fact that the bacilli rarely survived more than two days in feces which were allowed to dry naturally. Yet the incidence of dysentery dropped sharply, in this instance, during August and September, with plenty of flies still present. As it is well known that Flexner bacilli survive thirty days or more in plain water, one should never overlook the possibility of water-borne infection under circumstances such as these.

Patton (1930) gives it as his opinion that flies play no very active part in the dissemination of cholera.

Over and against such findings, there exists, however, a substantial body of evidence tending to incriminate the fly. Some of this is circumstantial, some epidemiological, but the bulk comes out of laboratory experiments under more or less controlled conditions and cannot be discounted or ignored. A résumé of data and opinion from various sources is given herewith.

EARLY CONTRIBUTIONS REGARDING FLY-BORNE DISEASE

In 1871, Professor J. Leidy, who had observed the spread of hospital gangrene during the American civil war, presented a strong argument in support of the theory that flies may carry disease. He pointed out that flies which have taken up diffluent matter from a certain fungus (*Phallus impudicus*) may later exude two or three drops from the proboscis. Microscopic examination showed both these drops and the stomach content of such flies to be swarming with fungus spores. Leidy held that similar dissemination of disease germs might logically occur. In the same year, Sir John Lubbock, while speaking in the British House of Commons, deplored the misconceptions which school children might acquire concerning sanitation from the textbooks of that day. He took particular exception to the statement, "The fly keeps the warm air pure and wholesome by its swift and zigzag flight." Veeder (1898a) especially criticized the prevalence of fevers and dysenteries in military camps and called attention to the great numbers of flies passing between feces in trenches and the cook tents.

The following year, Haeser (1899) called attention to the possible dissemination of plague by common flies. More than ten years previous, Hofmann (1888) had done the same for tuberculosis.

Also in the year 1899, Dr. Victor C. Vaughan, a distinguished physician, read a paper before the American Medical Association in which he stressed that typhoid fever spreads only by the transference of the excretions of an infected individual to the alimentary canals of others. He further pointed out that an infected soldier may scatter infection in every latrine or regiment before the disease is evident in himself, and that infective organisms may be present in his excrement a long time after apparent recovery. Great interest in the transmission of typhoid was stimulated in that period by the fact that approximately one-fifth of the U.S. soldiers serving in encampments during the year 1898 developed typhoid, and that this disease was responsible for 80 per cent of all deaths in service regardless of cause. It is further recorded that flies, swarming in and about the mess tents and crawling over food, frequently showed traces of lime which had clung to their bodies since their last visit to the latrines.

Walter Reed (1899) especially stressed flies as a principal cause of the outbreak of typhoid in the army during the Spanish-American War, and with Vaughan and Shakespeare (1904) published an extensive report on the subject.

Dr. L. O. Howard (1900) was particularly vociferous in publicizing the part played by flies in the spread of intestinal infection; he showed that since *Musca domestica* totaled 98.8 per cent of all insects captured in houses throughout the whole country in that day, this species must be considered the principal offender. It was Dr. Howard (1909b) who suggested that the name "housefly" be replaced by the designation "typhoid fly" as more descriptive of the fly's habits and its potential danger to man. Howard's publications were numerous and his work had great influence upon both medical practitioners and entomologists, who cited him frequently (Fletcher, 1901). It soon became known that typhoid organisms may continue to be discharged in both the urine and feces of recovered patients, and that some of these become "carriers" for life. The opportunity for continued contamination of soil and water is thus much greater than was originally supposed, and the opportunity for flies to contact the pathogen, even with no active disease in the community, is very real.

An early but very effective exposition of the role played by the fly in distributing enteric disease was published by Hamilton (1903) subsequent to an epidemic of typhoid fever in Chicago. She pointed out that the outbreak was not to be explained alone by contaminated water, contaminated food, or the ignorance of the population concerning these things. Miss Hamilton noted that only 48 per cent of the houses in that area had sanitary plumbing and concluded that when discharges from typhoid patients are left exposed in privies or in yards, flies become important agents in the dissemination of infection. Subsequent publications by the same author (1904, 1906) reiterated and fortified this point of view. A. W. Martin (1903), F. W. Thomson (1912), and Sweet (1916) also made important contributions to the literature on typhoid as a fly-borne disease.

Interest in tuberculosis, also, was being actively maintained. Hayward (1904) pointed out that tubercle bacilli may pass through the alimentary tract of flies and remain virulent. In the same year, Lord demonstrated that flies which have ingested positive sputum may excrete tubercule bacilli which remain virulent for at least fifteen days. He suggested that human infection might occur by ingestion of flyspecks deposited on food. In 1907 Miss Hamilton succeeded in isolating the tubercle bacillus from privy-caught flies.

Hunter in 1907 was quoted in the *Nursing Times* as having observed the occurrence of plague bacilli in the digestive tract of flies that had fed on infected material in Hong Kong. A year later, Robertson concluded that the housefly was capable of carrying the organism of yaws.

THE PERIOD UP TO AND INCLUDING WORLD WAR I

The next thirteen years were exceedingly prolific of publications concerning fly-borne disease, many of which, because of their popular or semipopular character, will not be mentioned here. A few, however, deserve brief comment.

W. D. Hunter, in a presidential address before the American Association of Economic Entomologists (1913), discussed various phases of medical entomology and concluded that American losses due to insects concerned in the carriage of dysentery alone amounted to at least $2,800,000 per year. Doane (1914), in discussing the disease-bearing insects of Samoa, considered *M. domestica* to be a factor in the transmission of typhoid, yaws, and a type of ophthalmia common in children and sometimes leading to blindness. Beresoff (1914) reported in detail upon experiments which tended to show that not only hibernating flies but also their dead bodies may harbor infection of various types.

Besides such general contributions, studies on specific diseases were also numerous. Morris (1919) pointed out that flies may carry anthrax infection to wounds on healthy animals after feeding on the discharges from open carbuncles or on anthrax-infected flesh. He found that flies bred out of un-opened anthrax carcasses did not carry infection, though flies bred in the pres-ence of spores might do so. Morris believed that the vegetative form of the organism in unopened carcasses was destroyed by the process of decomposition. His 1920 paper reiterates these conclusions.

The dysenteries likewise came in for the usual attention. Orton and Dodd (1910) recorded the recovery of pathogenic bacilli from flies several days after their exposure to infection. In the same year Converse pointed out the possibility of flies transmitting amoebiasis by flying from the feces of infected cases to the food of healthy persons. By 1917 this possibility had been definitely con-firmed. Wenyon and O'Connor (1917a,b) established *Musca domestica* and other muscoids as carriers beyond a doubt. Cysts from human hosts can sur-vive long periods if kept moist, and if taken up by flies (which feed every few minutes) will be passed continually in their feces. The cysts may remain in the fly's gut forty-two hours if the fly is prevented from feeding, but may pass in the feces from five minutes to twenty hours after ingestion when feed-ing is normal. These authors pointed out that the cysts are not distributed by regurgitation and that, due to the sun's heat and to the fly's habit of "cleaning" itself, mechanical distribution by way of the body surface is not too likely. Gabbi (1917) mentioned both *M. domestica* and *Calliphora erythrocephala* as among the vectors of amoebiasis. Craig, in the same year, reported a light epidemic of amoebic dysentery among troops serving in the El Paso (Texas) district as being largely fly-borne. At least, no new cases developed during the time of year when flies were absent or very few. Taylor (1919), who studied bacillary dysentery in the Salonica command, found that high inci-dence of the disease corresponded with the prevalence of flies, which was greatest from spring to early summer and again from late summer to early fall. He found the flies capable of carrying both Flexner and Shiga bacilli, although after twenty-four hours the prospect of recovering the organisms diminished rapidly. A rather small percentage of caught flies were found natu-rally infected. In the same year, Patton reported *Musca domestica determinata* Walker and *Musca humilis* Wied. (*angustifrons* Thomp.) as transmitting bacillary dysentery in Mesopotamia. The first-named species also transmitted a form of ophthalmia. Patton considered that these two flies constituted the most serious insect menace in that region of the world, and stated that fu-ture success in the colonization of Mesopotamia might depend largely upon their successful control. Both breed freely the year around in that country.

Manson-Bahr (1919) studied the activities of *M. domestica* in Egypt, espe-cially in relation to the occurrence of bacillary dysentery. He found the bacillus in the intestinal tract of flies caught in the desert two miles and more from the nearest camp, and a great distance from deposits of human feces. Manson-Bahr found that the organism might live as long as four days in the intestinal tract of the fly, but that it dies in a few hours when exposed to the desert sun. It is, therefore, obvious that the flies must feed on the blood and mucus of dysentery stools almost immediately after passage if they are to carry infection under such conditions of climate and temperature. Such, of course, would be impossible where good sanitary practices prevail, but as long as such a great proportion of the world's population live under conditions definitely lacking such protection, the danger remains both very real and very great.

Considerable light was cast by C. J. Martin (1913) on the relation of flies to summer diarrhea. Martin concluded that, though they may not be the dominant factor, they are truly important in its spread. Two papers by D. B. Armstrong (1914a,b) stressed the point that in equally congested areas fly protection is usually associated with a low incidence of the disease; neglect of flies, with increasing prevalence of diarrhea during the summer season.[1]

During this period, serious attention was given for the first time to the possible relation between flies and leprosy. Currie (1910) studied the habits of *Musca domestica,* and species of *Sarcophaga* and *Lucilia,* and found that flies which have fed on leprous fluids usually contain the bacilli in the intestinal tract for several days. He also noted that individuals which have access to a leprous ulcer will frequently convey very large numbers of leper bacilli directly or indirectly to the skin, nasal mucosa, or alimentary canal of healthy persons. Currie had no way of proving whether such bacteria are infective, but he considered that flies should be viewed with suspicion until proved guiltless. Leboeuf (1912, 1914) found *Musca domestica* capable of absorbing enormous quantities of Hansen's bacillus and demonstrated great numbers in the feces of infected flies. He did not find evidence of multiplication within the fly, but neither did the organisms appear to degenerate. Leboeuf suggested that infected flies might infect human beings by depositing excrement upon raw cutaneous surfaces. He found Hansen's bacillus in nineteen out of thirty-six flies captured in a lepers' infirmary, and considered patients with open lesions to have been the source of contamination. Leboeuf's work, along with that of others, has been critically evaluated by Bayon (1915). Marchoux (1916) showed that leprosy bacilli can live in the alimentary tract of flies for four days, but was unable to produce infection by flies removed from septic

[1] A modern study by Watt and Lindsay (1948) reports reduction of diarrheal diseases in areas of high morbidity through control of flies by DDT.

material for twenty-four hours. Sugai and Kawabada (1918) worked with both leprosy and tubercle bacilli. Flies fed a suspension of the latter organisms passed bacilli five hours later which were infective to guinea pigs. Their experiments with Hansen's bacillus were confined to fish.

In the meantime, tularemia had been recognized as a human disease. Wayson (1914), using guinea pigs, studied its transmission by both *Musca domestica* and *Stomoxys calcitrans*. Houseflies were first permitted to crawl and feed on the viscera of animals that had died of the disease. They were then transferred to the conjunctiva of healthy guinea pigs, which had been prepared in advance by scarification of the conjunctival membrane. This was accomplished by use of cocaine, followed by rubbing with a grain of sterile sand beneath the palpebra. The animals developed a severe purulent conjunctivitis after forty-eight hours and died in from five to nine days, which is the normal incubation period for tularemia.

Trachoma also began to receive attention. Nicolle, Cuenod, and Blanc (1919) asserted that flies may transmit the infection for at least twenty-four hours after contact with infected eyes or with bandages up to six hours after the latter have been removed from an active case. Nicolle's later paper (1922) summarizes the earlier work and brings it up to date.

Somewhat speculative writings appeared concerning poliomyelitis. Flexner and Clark (1911) reported that flies might harbor the virus for forty-eight hours, but made no attempt to discriminate between superficial contamination and infection of the alimentary tract. Kling and Levaditi (1913) criticized this work as probably too artificial to have real scientific value. They admitted, however, the possibility of the propagation of infantile paralysis by flies in a purely mechanical manner. Meanwhile, C. W. Howard and Clark (1912) had brought forward additional data showing that though the virus survives only a number of hours in the food canal, it may be carried in an active state on the body surface of *Musca domestica* for several days. Cleland and associates (1919) reviewed the possibilities of insect vectorship in connection with the Australian epidemics and mentioned both *Musca domestica* and *M. vetustissima* as being under suspicion.

THE PERIOD BETWEEN WORLD WARS

Investigations continued in regard to enteric disorders. Paraf (1920a) studied an epidemic of bacillary dysentery during which he found the bacillus in 12 of 30 flies captured near latrines, in 7 of 36 taken in hospital wards, and in 3 of 38 captured at the dining table. Milk for surgical cases was found to contain dysentery bacillus 6 times out of 26 samplings; bread, once out of 12 times. The bacillus remained in the fly's intestine five days after initial infection.

Ledingham (1920) analyzed further the situation in Mesopotamia, where the greatest number of flies occur in April, May, and November. During the hotter days of summer, the flies almost completely disappear; during this time dysentery and enteric disease also fall off, but not proportionately. His interpretation was that a mass of fresh infections is established in the spring, largely due to flies, and this leaves a large amount of chronic and carrier infection during the season when weather conditions naturally favor enteric disturbances. This combination maintains a moderate incidence of dysentery and diarrhea until the fall rise in fly population, which precipitates a mass of fresh infections. Buxton (1920), in speaking of Lower Mesopotamia, dwelt especially on the importance of flies in the spread of amoebiasis. He reports that over 60 per cent of the flies caught carried human feces, that 4 per cent carried human entozoa, and that 0.5 per cent bore cysts of *Endamoeba histolytica.*

The work of Root (1921) on the carriage of intestinal protozoa by flies brought out the fact that cysts of both *Giardia* and *Endamoeba* survive much longer in "drowned" flies than in the living insect. Because of the moisture requirements of protozoan cysts, Root concluded (1) that fly feces are only dangerous to man if deposited on moist or liquid foods; (2) that the earlier hours after the fly's feeding on cysts are the most dangerous, as a larger proportion of the cysts are still alive; and (3) that human beings may contract the infection by swallowing liquids in which flies have drowned. Frye and Meleney (1932) found 38 per cent of the population of a certain rural community to be carrying *E. histolytica.* Of 7,948 flies collected in and about eighteen houses, 6 contained characteristic cysts. They concluded that where the incidence of infection is high, and the deposition of human feces promiscuous, flies probably spread the infection from house to house.

An unusual observation in regard to bacillary dysentery is recorded by Zmeev (1939–1941), who found adults of the large hornet, *Vespa orientalis,* naturally infected with the pathogen. He offered proof that these Hymenoptera acquire this and other intestinal organisms by feeding on common flies.

The possible relation of flies to cholera transmission had long been recognized. M. Simmonds (1892) succeeded in obtaining cholera organisms from the bodies of flies captured in a room where post-mortems were being carried out on patients who had died of the disease. Graham-Smith, in a series of publications (1909–1913), discussed all possible ways in which flies may carry and distribute pathogenic (and other) bacteria, and in regard to cholera stated that he had recovered the vibrios from the food canal of flies forty-eight hours after contamination, and from legs and body up to thirty hours. The most significant contribution in this field, however, is probably the work of Gill and Lal (1931), who have shown that the vibrios may disappear from the fly's alimentary tract the second day after ingestion only to reappear about the fifth day. The flies are then capable of contaminating human food by their fecal discharges. There is perhaps a "cyclical" relation here. Direct contamination of food and drink by way of the fly's proboscis up to twenty-four hours after infection of the fly was also demonstrated.

Interest in the leprosy problem was sustained largely by Lamborn (1935b), who brought evidence to show that *Musca sorbens* might well be a vector in Nyasaland. Acid-fast bacilli were found in the excreta thirteen days after the flies had fed on leprous sores. The vomit spots were positive from eight hours to five days after feeding. Five hours after feeding on infective material, the flies were permitted access to fresh drops of blood. Seven out of nineteen such drops were later found to be positive. Control flies fed on ulcers that contained no leprosy bacilli at no time passed acid-fast bacilli. Lamborn's subsequent publications (1936a,b, 1937) dealt further with the leprosy problem and also proved *Musca sorbens* a transmitter of yaws. Though *M. sorbens* does not have a piercing proboscis, it feeds readily on all sores and accomplishes transmission of the spirochetes through contamination of the mouth parts by regurgitation. Lamborn and Howat (1936) also succeeded in fatally infecting a dog with *Trypanosoma rhodesiense* by allowing *Musca sorbens* which had fed on the blood of a human patient to have access to an incision on the animal's ear.

Lamborn's 1939 report records *M. sorbens* as harboring and passing tubercle bacilli for many days after feeding on both fresh and dried sputum. The numbers apparently increased within the fly. Coccoid forms were most persistent. Similar experiments with leprosy bacilli using dried material showed that flies could deposit the organisms up to the twelfth day and occasionally to the nineteenth.

Other students of leprosy transmission included De Mello and Cabral (1926), who found infection in four out of ten specimens of *Musca bezzi* P. and C. which had been captured in a leper hospital. Flies intentionally fed on leprous patients and then transferred to fruit juice and water all proved positive for a limited time. Two hours later, four out of six remained infected; forty-eight hours later, one out of three. Wings and legs were removed before examination to eliminate contamination from that source. Shuzo (1933) contributed further data. Of 447 flies collected in wards housing advanced cases of leprosy, 118 proved to contain the organism. In lepers' rooms, the count was 41 out of 1,786. In a leprous settlement, 9 out of 192 flies were found positive; in a nonleprous house nearby, one out of 76. Of 53 specimens of *Musca domestica* which fed on infected material, 16 became infected. A somewhat higher proportion was realized with *Lucilia cuprina* and *Calliphora lata*. Hansen's bacillus remained alive in various species of flies for twenty-four hours, and sometimes as long as ninety-six. The figures of Arizumi (1934) are rather similar. One hundred and ninety-five flies out of 689 from wards for advanced cases, and 177 out of 723 captured in the wards for milder cases, proved positive. Arizumi concluded that though the bacilli do not multiply in the fly, they are not affected by the bactericidal action of the fly's secretions. He observed that larvae which had fed on the bacilli expel them just before pupation. This was borne out by the fact that examination showed no infection in 300 pupae from infected maggots.

Miscellaneous contributions during this period are also of interest. Nieschulz (1928) succeeded in transmitting anthrax to guinea pigs through the vectorship of *Musca inferior* Stein. He showed that both tabanids and muscids had a higher transmission capacity for this organism than for surra, trypanosome disease of horses and mules. Ross (1929) showed that flies ingest the eggs of *Echinococcus granulosus* in Australia and may thus carry them from the feces of dogs to human food. Since hydatid disease is a serious problem in that country, he suggests the use of fly traps in the vicinity of dog yards, sheep killing pens, and stables, all of which should be maintained in a clean condition. Removal or burning of dog feces each day might be a good practice, as it would lessen the danger of contaminating the dog's coat.

Simitch and Kostitch (1937) showed that *Musca domestica* can carry *Trichomonas intestinalis* in a mechanical way from human or animal feces to moist food or drink. The organism can survive in the intestine of the fly eight hours, but does not multiply there.

Lins de Almeida (1933) corrected Pinto's determination of *Sarcophaga terminalis* Wied. (really *Musca [Sarcopromusca] arcuata* Townsend) as a carrier of the eggs of *Dermatobia hominis* L. He also refers to Neiva and Gomes' incrimination of *Musca domestica* in 1917.

Thomson and Lamborn (1934) discussed the mechanical transmission of trypanosomiasis, leishmaniasis, and yaws by several species of nonbiting hematophagous flies. They especially call attention to *Musca spectanda* Wied., an abundant species in Nyasaland, which prefers man as a host and breeds freely in human feces.

Metelkin (1935) investigated the role of several species of muscoid flies, including *Musca domestica,* in the dissemination of coccidiosis of animals. He found that all flies could ingest the oocysts, which remain alive in the insect's alimentary tract for at least twenty-four hours and continue viable in the fly's discharges until the latter become desiccated. The flies can also carry the oocysts externally, especially on their legs.

At least two reviews of current information appeared during this period. Andrews (1925) published a general account of the medically important Diptera, the third portion of which is devoted entirely to disease transmission through the agency of filth-feeding flies. Ferrière (1920), *Insectes et Epidémies,* discusses a number of lessons learned from World War I and devotes a separate section to the relation of flies to typhoid, dysentery, cholera, diphtheria, ophthalmia, infantile paralysis, tuberculosis, and leprosy.

In regard to tuberculosis, MacGregor (1917) wrote as follows: "With the high vitality and resistance to drying possessed by *B. tuberculosis,* the possibly long incubation period within the body, and the insidious onset of the disease, the danger from *Musca domestica* in this connection is not sufficiently recognized." In spite of this challenging and rather stimulating declaration, no very conclusive work was accomplished for a number of years which might further incriminate houseflies. Lamborn (1940), however, working with *Musca sorbens* in Nyasaland, obtained data of considerable interest. He found that the tubercle bacilli might remain viable in the body of this species for over a week. As an experimental procedure Lamborn injected a guinea pig intraperitoneally with the gut contents of three flies that had fed eight days previously on positive sputum. The animal died four months later of generalized tuberculosis, as did a second animal injected five days after the flies had fed.

CONTRIBUTIONS OF THE PAST DECADE

The most striking development during and after World War II has been the interest that both entomologists and clinicians have shown in the relation of flies to anterior poliomyelitis. No other disease capable of transmission by filth-feeding insects has received so much attention in recent years.

Paul, Trask, and associates reported in 1941 on the detection of the virus in flies captured during epidemics in Connecticut and Alabama. In the first of these, *Lucilia, Phormia, Musca,* and *Muscina* were involved, along with other genera, the first two being in the ascendency. Two types of inoculum were prepared, one from an emulsion of macerated flies, the other from washing 400 to 600 flies in 50 cc. of water. A Cynomologus monkey, inoculated in several ways from such sources, developed poliomyelitis after an incubation period of fifteen days. In the Alabama studies, a fly trap was placed in the vicinity of a privy used by three households where cases had occurred. The catch was not identified as to species, but is stated to have included houseflies, blowflies, and greenbottles. The monkey host developed poliomyelitis nine days after inoculation.

In the same year, Sabin and Ward announced the recovery of poliomyelitis virus by similar methods from flies trapped in urban areas close to houses in which the disease had recently occurred. Their studies were carried on in Atlanta, Georgia, and in Cleveland, Ohio. Again, Cynomolgus monkeys were the test animals used. By this time, poliomyelitis was coming to be regarded as primarily an infection of the food canal, with secondary localization in nervous tissue. In a second publication (1942), the same authors stressed the resemblance of poliomyelitis to typhoid and dysentery, and pointed out that the disease can occur the year round, though its incidence usually rises in summer and autumn, when its transmission is favored by certain factors which are negligible during the remainder of the year. Among these factors, insects, particularly flies, should be considered important. The experiments of Sabin and Ward involved chiefly *Musca domestica* and *Lucilia sericata*. Their work was criticized by Brues (1942) on the ground that an inoculum prepared from a mixture of trapped insects leaves much to be desired. If only one species should be the true culprit, its identity is obviously lost by the technique employed. Brues's criticism would appear to be justified.

Toomey, Takacs, and Tischer (1941) paralleled the work of Sabin and Ward by preparing a suspension from 2,000 flies collected near the mouth of a brook that carried raw sewage into Lake Erie from a portion of the city of Cleveland. Many large blowflies and a lesser number of houseflies were involved. Monkeys injected with the suspension developed typical poliomyelitis. Trask, Paul, and Melnick, in two publications (1943), recorded similar findings and stressed the point that positive results were obtained only with *Macacus cynomolgus* monkeys. Cercopithicus and Rhesus monkeys could not be infected by the techniques that they used. In their positive fly samples, *Phormia* and *Lucilia* were always present, while *Musca domestica* occurred only in two out of four batches, and then in relatively small numbers. It is perhaps significant that these workers found positive flies only in lots collected within ten days of the onset of a local case. The collecting areas used ranged from fifteen to twenty acres in extent. It was believed that most of the flies taken had had an opportunity to feed upon fresh human feces which might have contained poliomyelitis virus.

Bang and Glaser (1943) did careful work both with Theiler's mouse polio-myelitis and Armstrong's mouse-adapted human strain. They found that the virus could be recovered from the adult fly only when the adult itself had been infected by feeding. They never found virus in flies that had been reared from infected larvae. Theiler's virus survived in *Musca domestica* for as long as twelve days, but the mouse-adapted human strain could not be re-covered beyond forty-eight hours. Flies were infected by being allowed to feed on infected brain emulsion diluted with distilled water. The virus was found present in both fecal and vomit specks of flies kept in bottles. An inoculum from fly tissue was later used to infect healthy mice. The latter developed the disease more quickly when inoculated with flies but recently infected than when the inoculum consisted of flies that had carried the infec- tion for a longer time. This would seem to indicate that little or no multiplica-tion of the virus takes place in the fly. The injection of a preparation of fly intestine into healthy mice and their subsequent development of disease symptoms seemed clear proof that the virus was not limited in location to the exterior portions of the fly. Bang and Glaser also studied transmission by *Muscina, Sarcophaga, Calliphora,* and *Lucilia,* but in none of these did the virus survive so long as in houseflies.

More significant from a practical standpoint than the infection of animals by injection of macerated flies is the type of experiment reported by Miss Horstmann (1945). In this work, food exposed to flies in nature, during an active epidemic, proved infective when later fed to chimpanzees. She men-tions that the virus survived experimentally in *Musca domestica* up to forty-eight hours, sufficient time, obviously, for the flies to make distribution to human food and drink. A full report by Ward, Melnick, and Horstmann the same year records that the excreta of the two chimpanzees which they used had been proved free from virus just prior to the experiment, but became positive after the animals had swallowed fly-contaminated food. Both chim-panzees showed a rise in temperature, but did not develop paralysis. It was considered that poliomyelitis of a subclinical grade had been induced. In one animal, the excreta remained infective for fourteen days; in the other, for twenty. In the epidemic studied, which occurred in North Carolina, *Musca domestica* made up 349 of a trapped sample of 428.

Melnick and Penner (1947) fed human poliomyelitis virus from stools of polio patients to blowflies (*Phormia regina*). The virus was recovered from the bodies of the flies for two weeks following, and from their feces for three. It is interesting to note that when Theiler's TO strain or murine-adapted strains were used, they were eliminated in five days, after the manner of biologically inert material. This was true for species of *Phaenicia* and *Sarcophaga*, as well as for *Phormia regina*.

Melnick (1949) trapped 93,000 flies during the poliomyelitis epidemic in Rockford, Illinois, in 1945. Cynomolgus monkeys were used as test animals to determine the presence of virus in the flies. *Phormia regina* and *Phaenicia sericata* were the only species found positive during the peak of this epidemic, which occurred late in August. Two weeks later *Phaenicia sericata* ceased to be positive, but *P. regina* continued to yield virus, with *Musca domestica* and several species of *Sarcophaga* joining the list. During the third two-week period no positives were obtained. Two weeks later, however, when the epidemic had virtually ceased, a species that had not been present earlier in the season, *Cynomopsis cadaverina*, yielded positive results. This author points out that numerical prevalence of a given species is no indication that it will be found a vector. *Phaenicia sericata* proved negative at a time when it constituted 24 per cent of the total catch, while *Musca domestica*, though making up only 4 per cent of the fly population, yielded virus of poliomyelitis.

Francis, Brown, and Penner (1948) tested the ability of flies of various genera to acquire the virus by feeding on infected human stools. The presence of the virus in the fly was proved by inoculation into Rhesus and Philippine monkeys. *Phaenicia, Phormia, Sarcophaga, Muscina,* and *Calliphora* came to the stool-baited traps in much larger numbers than did *Musca* or *Fannia* under the conditions of the experiment. The results tend to show that practically any species of filth-feeding fly may acquire the organism.

A sudden arrest of five outbreaks of poliomyelitis was reported by Deeny and MacCormack (1946) following the spraying of houses and grounds in the vicinity of infected patients with a kerosene solution of DDT. Bedroom and kitchen utensils were also carefully disinfected, and personnel were instructed in the avoidance of droplet infection. It is, therefore, difficult to say how important fly control really was in accomplishing these results, but certainly no modern prophylactic program would be considered complete without it.

A brief but stimulating summary of American research concerning housefly transmission of poliomyelitis was published (in French) by Leclercq in 1948(a).

AMOEBIASIS AND CERTAIN HELMINTH INFECTIONS

Recent data on the transmission of *Endamoeba histolytica* by *M. domestica* have been brought forward by Roberts (1947), who fed 107 houseflies on a standard emulsion containing *histolytica* cysts. The cysts were passed in the feces from five minutes to thirty-one hours after feeding. Roberts identified 1,792 cysts in 147 fecal drops, passed by 68 flies. He also recovered cysts from vomit drops over a period of nine hours.

According to Sieyro (1942), *Musca domestica* may pass cysts of *Endamoeba histolytica* anywhere from one minute to thirty-five hours after feeding. According to the eosin test (which Sieyro does not think wholly reliable), viable cysts could be found in the fly's excreta up to twenty-four hours after ingestion. Sieyro found also that cysts of *Giardia* might be transmitted, as well as active trichomonads, which do not form cysts.

Chang (1943) dissected 153 specimens of *Musca domestica vicina* captured in Chengtu without finding a single trophozoite, cyst, or ovum. He did, however, find 60 out of 146 *Chrysomyia megacephala*, 4 out of 68 *Lucilia sericata*, and 2 out of 42 undetermined specimens of *Sarcophaga* to be carrying human parasites.

Harris and Down (1946) studied the dissemination of cysts and ova of human intestinal parasites by flies in the island of Guam. Flies that had been trapped near latrines in native villages were permitted to deposit specks on gauze moistened with saline. The fluid was then wrung from the gauze and centrifuged. The cysts (or ova) of no less than ten human parasites were identified microscopically. *Endamoeba histolytica* was cultured both from the sediment and from serum specked by flies on a native kitchen table.

These workers also allowed flies to have access to fish placed on autoclaved earth near a native dwelling. Natural rainfall kept the earth in a moist condition. After five days, examination of the ground surface by dissecting microscope revealed the presence of active nematode larvae resembling in all respects the filariform larvae of hookworms. Larvae isolated later by the Baermann technique possessed typical hookworm morphology. Harris and Down consider it not improbable that these larvae were brought into the area by flies. The evidence, of course, is but circumstantial.

Among modern investigations, the work of Pipkin (1949) is especially worthy of mention. Pipkin holds that the external carriage of either cysts or trophozoites on the body of the fly probably plays no significant role in the transmission of amoebiasis except in situations where sanitary rules are generally ignored. Transmission by way of the alimentary tract, however, he has found to be important. Neither cysts nor trophozoites had their viability reduced by storage in the fly's crop, as shown by modern culture techniques. There is some deterioration in the gut and rectum, however. Pipkin concludes that, since viable cysts of *E. histolytica* may pass in the fly's vomitus up to sixty-four minutes after ingestion and in the feces up to four hours and twenty minutes after swallowing, such cysts may be considered to have much to do with amoebiasis on a community basis, especially in the more backward rural sections.

According to this author's earlier work (1942), the genus of the fly concerned seems to play an important part in determining the length of time during which the parasite remains viable in the insect's body. Culturable cysts were recovered from the crop and rectum of *Sarcophaga* 180 minutes after ingestion, but in the gut of *Musca* the time span was 240 minutes. Again, the vomitus of *Lucilia* yielded culturable cysts after 17 minutes of internal carriage, but with *Phormia* the vomitus proved contaminative for 64 minutes, at least. In the same genus, fecal droplets were positive up to 137 minutes after initial ingestion, while in the case of *Cochliomyia* the feces yielded culturable cysts over a period of 218 minutes. Trophozoites were less viable, but similar interesting differences were found. Culturable trophozoites were obtained from the crops of both *Musca* and *Lucilia* 15 minutes after ingestion, while the period was but 5 minutes for the gut, not only for these forms but also for the genus *Phormia*. Flies of the genus *Sarcophaga* yielded culturable cysts from the gut 30 minutes after ingestion, and from the crop 40 minutes after swallowing.

Pipkin (1943) also studied the possibility that filth-feeding flies might transmit the ova of parasitic roundworms. External carriage by *M. domestica* and others was demonstrated for *Enterobius, Necator, Trichuris* (*Trichocephalus*), and *Ascaris*. The flies remained contaminated for averages ranging from 1.37 to 3.47 hours. Smaller eggs, such as those of *Trichuris,* were ingested by practically all species of filth feeders, but only the larger types, such as *Calliphora,* could ingest the ova of *Ascaris lumbricoides.*

In this connection, it is helpful to recall the findings of Graham-Smith (1930a), who states that since infective organisms may remain alive in the crop of muscoid Diptera for a number of days, the habit of frequent regurgitation ordinarily insures repeated reinfection of the inner surfaces of the labella. He notes, however, that helminth ova, which several workers have observed to be present in the feces of flies, are apparently never regurgitated in the vomitus.

SCATTERED RESEARCHES ON FLY-BORNE DISEASE

The present period has witnessed very little additional data on dysentery of bacillary origin. Worthy of mention is the report by Kuhns and Anderson

(1944) on a fly-borne epidemic in a large military organization. The work of Stewart, published the same year, on experiments carried out in Algiers has already been mentioned on an earlier page.

De Souza-Araujo (1943) reported *Musca domestica* as becoming heavily infected with acid-fast and alcohol-fast bacilli from feeding at the ulcerated lesions of a hospitalized case of leprosy in South America.

Moorehead and Weiser (1946) proved the survival of a food-poisoning strain of *Staphylococcus* in the gut and excreta of the housefly by suspending *S. aureus* 611 in a dilute solution of sucrose, which was then fed to approximately 900 laboratory-reared houseflies and reisolated at suitable intervals. The exteriors of the flies were sterilized with a mixture containing 1 per cent aerosol, 1 per cent potassium hydroxide and 5 per cent formaldehyde. *S. aureus* 611 was found scattered in the footprints and proboscis marks of all groups examined three days after ingestion of the organisms, but was not recovered from the exterior by 23 washings in a preparation of broth. Only 2 of 17 suspensions of excreta and vomitus contained the organism, but it was found to survive in the digestive tract for eight days in 18 of 23 samples tested. Among wild-caught flies, 10 out of 50 yielded *Staphylococcus* by isolation methods. These authors consider that *Musca domestica* may serve as a reservoir host for this organism under suitable conditions and thus be responsible for outbreaks of food poisoning by spreading *Staphylococcus* from contaminated food, equipment, or the soiled skin or clothing of persons engaged in handling food.

The transmission of similar organisms from fly to fly as well as from fly to food or water was noted by Ostrolenk and Welch (1942a) in connection with their studies on *Salmonella enteritidis*. This well-known agent of food poisoning survives in the fly as long as the insect lives (approximately thirty days). These authors succeeded in transferring *Salmonella* infection from flies to mice, and later from the infected mice to other flies.

A preliminary report on the probable transmission of bovine mastitis by *Musca domestica* was published by Sanders in 1940. Mention has already been made of the experiments of Ewing (1942) which were designed to test the hypothesis. Sanders' study was made on a milking herd of 65 animals in the summertime. Twenty-seven of the cows were known to have streptococcus mastitis, three had staphylococcus infection, and three had no mastitis by blood-agar-plate diagnosis. Flies that had fed on skim milk containing viable *Streptococcus agalactiae* for four days showed the organism present on their body surfaces in declining numbers for a week following. After that, cultures were negative. Preparations made from tissues of the fly, however, revealed that *S. agalactiae* survives internally for at least ten days. Since both this organism and pathogenic staphylococci were available at the external apertures of the teats in practically all the mastitic animals examined, flies in the dairy barn were probably carrying the organisms both externally and internally at all times. Ewing does not think that the housefly can be considered a very important agent for the transfer of bovine mastitis, thereby differing with Sanders, who considered *M. domestica* a natural vector wherever flies have access to infected milk, but both would agree that a certain amount of fly-borne infection exists. According to Sanders' observations, the flies most easily infected healthy cows when the latter were being "dried off" before calving. Such animals stand many hours with the udder partly full, a condition particularly inviting to infection. At any rate, houseflies are known to be persistent feeders at the openings of the teats and often visit other teats of the same or a second animal within a short span of time. Sanders records that the flies sometimes inserted the proboscis deep into the orifice to seek more milk. Also, in some lactating cows, there is a very noticeable fossa at the extremity of the teat. This depression seems to form a natural anchorage for the insect's feet.

Shooter and Waterworth (1944) published briefly on the transmissibility of haemolytic streptococcal infection by flies. Twenty-seven flies caught in wards where there were streptococcic infections were permitted to crawl over a plated culture medium. Nine gave cultures of haemolytic streptococci. While this by no means proves the fly a vector of haemolytic infection, it is strongly suggestive thereof, especially when the condition spreads without explanation from one part of a hospital to another.

MISCELLANEOUS CONSIDERATIONS RELATING TO EPIDEMIOLOGY

One aspect of the disease relations of flies remains to be touched upon. This has to do with the possibility of the fly's serving as carrier host for some other arthropod of medical importance. Larval mites have already been mentioned in Chapter X, but it remained for Leon (1920) to demonstrate that ordinary body lice can be carried by flies, only to leave the insect and attach to a warmblooded host when opportunity affords. Leon's studies had to do with the prevalence of typhus in Rumania in 1917, and it may well be that flies, when abundant, can be a tangible factor in the dissemination of this rickettsial disease. However, since lice do not live too long away from suitable temperatures, it is not likely that they can survive on the fly more than a few hours at most.

CONTAMINATION OF SUCCESSIVE
STAGES IN THE LIFE HISTORY

In studies relating to the transmission of disease by filth-feeding flies, it is always important to inquire into the question as to whether or not disease organisms taken up by the larvae can survive pupation and be present in the body of the adult fly. Glaser (1923b) pointed out that *Musca domestica* on pupating encloses many bacteria which do just this thing, as demonstrated by bacterial studies on recently emerged adults. Glaser also found bacteria in the upper regions of the air passages of pupae, but the fate of these was not determined. It was shown that *M. domestica* almost always carries far more bacteria than *Stomoxys,* a fact which might readily be inferred by comparing the feeding habits of the two species both in the larval and in the adult state.

Considerably earlier than this, Graham-Smith (1912b) performed a series of experiments with the anthrax bacillus, which is a sporeformer, using three species of flies. He found that a large proportion of the houseflies that developed from larvae infected with the spores were still infected. Nonsporeformers did not survive so well. Graham-Smith concluded that only those nonsporeformers which were adapted to conditions existing in the larval intestine could ordinarily survive through metamorphosis. Examples were *Proteus morganii* and certain non-lactose-fermenting forms.

The pioneer work of Bacot (1911a,b) with *Bacillus pyocyaneus,* which he introduced into the larval food of *M. domestica,* showed that not only could the maggots harbor the bacilli until transformation, but that the organisms persisted both in the pupae and in the adult flies.

Wollman (1921a), who used a sterile technique for rearing his maggots, found that larvae of *Calliphora vomitoria, Lucilia caesar,* and *Musca domestica* which had been infected with typhoid, dysenteric, or tubercle bacilli gave rise to pupae which were still infected. He showed that the organisms were *not* passed on to the adult, but that the fly practically always contaminated itself with bacilli adhering to the exterior of the pupa. Such flies, however, remained infective only a few days.

Considerable interest attaches to the work of Gosio (1925), who observed that maggots of *M. domestica* and other species frequently ingest *Pasteurella pestis* while feeding on the dead bodies of infected animals. Such maggots complete their development in a normal manner, though numerous plague bacilli can be found both in the ventriculus and in the feces. Only small numbers of bacilli persist in the pupae. The adult flies that emerge from these are normal for a time, but soon develop large numbers of plague bacilli, and many die in from 15 to 24 hours. Uninfected control flies lived approximately seven days. Gosio mentions that medieval literature records heavy mortality among flies during epidemics of plague. Gosio considers infection by way of the larva to be far more common than direct infection of the adult.

A recent contribution to this field is that of Ostrolenk and Welch (1942a), who planted fly eggs in mash infected with *Salmonella enteritidis*. The resulting larvae, pupae, and adults all proved to be infected.

DISEASES OF PLANTS

The role of flies in the spread of fire blight of orchard fruits deserves some comment. The work of Ark and Thomas (1936) shows that the pathogen, *Erwinia amylovora*, may live for several days in the intestinal tract of muscoid flies, specifically *Musca domestica*, *Drosophila melanogaster*, and *Lucilia sericata*. Eggs from contaminated houseflies have also been found to carry the organism. Furthermore, maggots, both of *Drosophila* and of *Musca*, when fed on contaminated food may give rise to infected pupae and infected adult flies. This suggests residence in fly pupae as a possible means of carrying the infection over winter. The more obvious method of overwintering is through holdover cankers on the trunks and branches of trees. Transmission of the bacteria by flies and other insects from the oozing cankers to the newly opened blossoms has been stressed by Thomas and Ark (1934) and by Parker (1936). The establishment of secondary infections by the passage of insects from blossom to blossom is generally accepted. The importance of insects as vectors of this very important disease of pears, apples, and many other species is adequately summarized by Leach (1940).

CHAPTER XII

Public Health Relations

One of the seven was wont to say: "That laws were like cobwebs; where the small flies were caught, and the great break through."—Bacon, Apothegm 181

WOODROW WILSON once stated that laws are effective only insofar as they reflect the moral judgment that the community has come to possess. Health legislation is no exception. The achievement and maintenance of standards in regard to public health depend largely upon two important factors: (1) education of the people and (2) the enforcement of a legal code. Time has shown that in a democracy, at least, education is basic; legislation, secondary.

The sanitary codes that govern fly nuisances and similar matters in the United States today are the outgrowth of a serious educational effort which had its beginnings prior to the turn of the century and reached its climax around the year 1910.

As early as 1898 Veeder, lamenting the general ignorance of the public in regard to fly-borne disease, wrote as follows:

Even in a private house, not at all uncleanly, I have seen typhoid dejections emptied from a commode, and the latter thoughtlessly left standing without disinfection within a few feet of a pitcher of milk just left at the door, both the commode and the pitcher attracting the flies, which swarmed about and went from the one to the other.

Dr. Veeder advocated keeping a disinfecting solution, such as blue vitriol, in chamber utensils and water closets at all times. This had the added advantage of destroying all odor and thus causing the flies to cease their visits.

In 1907 D. D. Jackson called attention to the inconsistency of spending large amounts for the control of malaria mosquitoes while the problem of intestinal diseases went largely neglected. Jackson pointed out that during a year in which there were 359 cases of malaria in Greater New York City, with 52 deaths, 650 deaths occurred from typhoid and 7,000 deaths from other intestinal diseases. Jackson's report contains the following statement: "Our entire waterfront is without decent sanitary toilets, and most of the wharves are without any at all." This document was subsequently transmitted through the Merchants' Association of New York to Governor Charles Evans Hughes.

But the problem was not confined to metropolitan areas. Washburn (1910) made some rather searching observations of health conditions on the Minnesota iron range. Exposed filth of all kinds, including pathological excreta in close proximity to human food, plus enormous numbers of flies in all cities and towns, gave ample explanation for the epidemic of typhoid fever which occurred that season, as well as for a mild form of dysentery prevalent in July and August. Neither hotels, camps, boarding houses, nor houses of miners were properly screened. It was interesting to note that Finnish and Swedish workers suffered much more frequently than Italian and Austrian laborers, in spite of the fact that, in general, the Scandinavian families were cleaner in habits and environment than the other groups. It was found that the Swedes and Finns lunched frequently during the day on cold food which was left exposed on the table most of the time and which attracted many flies; these flies entered freely through the unscreened windows and doors, and in many cases must have come directly from typhoid excreta that had been deposited in open vaults without having been sterilized. The Austrians and Italians, however, ate hot meals, and the Italians, at least, used very little milk. Both these groups escaped typhoid. Nowhere could one find a better example of the danger of trusting to mere physical cleanliness, or of the need for education concerning the significance of bacterial contamination. To quote a modern Wisconsin State Board of Health bulletin: "Eye appeal is not sanitation" (Bliesner and Brown, 1945).

While these reports made their due impression upon the medical profession, scientists, and those engaged in educational work at the higher levels, the general public still remained to be convinced that common flies were a serious menace to the health of the family or the community. To meet this situation the American Civic Association undertook a campaign in plain language calculated to guide ordinary folk who were interested in improving sanitary practices in their own homes. The following list of dont's is quoted from a timely circular released by that organization:

Don't allow flies in your house.

Don't permit them near your food, especially milk.

Don't buy foodstuffs where flies are tolerated.

Don't have feeding places where flies can load themselves with ejections from typhoid or dysenteric patients.

Don't allow your fruits and confections to be exposed to the swarms of flies.

Don't let flies crawl over the baby's mouth and swarm upon the nipple of its nursing bottle.

Gradually the American people as a whole acquired a practical and intelligent attitude toward flies and fly-borne disease. As large numbers of individual citizens adopted better sanitary practices, the health standards of their

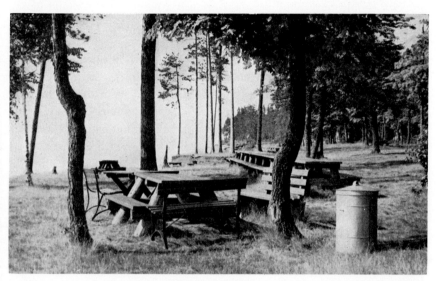

Figure 90. A high-class picnic ground in northern Michigan. Refuse cans have tight-fitting lids, and are frequently emptied by attendants. Houseflies and blowflies are at a minimum, but picnickers complain about *Stomoxys* flies, which fly in from breeding areas. (Photo by Rollin Thoren.)

respective communities became improved. There remained, of course, the inevitable minorities who, through ignorance, prejudice, or plain indifference, continued to permit the existence of fly nuisances upon their premises. This problem could only be dealt with by force of law, and the more progressive communities proceeded to enact appropriate ordinances. It must be admitted that many of the early codes were poorly drawn. Some failed to cover important phases of the subject; others were impossible of enforcement. But experience soon led to revision, and those cities and states that at first were somewhat backward in adopting sanitary codes profited greatly by the experiences of those that had pioneered in this regard.

It must be remembered that fly *abatement* rather than fly *elimination* was all that sanitarians could hope for in this period, even in the cities and towns. The suggestion of Esten and Mason (1908) is typical of the somewhat restricted viewpoint of the day. These workers, who studied the sources of bacteria in milk, found the bacterial count of individual flies to range between 550 and 6,600,000. The count increased as the season progressed, and appeared to indicate that the epidemics of intestinal disease among children fed with cow's milk were caused more often by flies than in any other way. Their principal recommendation was that all sewer openings on private or public property should have blind openings of such a nature that it would be impossible for flies to visit them.

No one will question the wisdom of this suggestion, but it obviously concerns only one phase of a many-sided problem. Unaccompanied by other recommendations, it appears to assume not only that flies by the millions were quite inevitable, but also that no marked improvement in the handling of milk and similar foods could be expected. Today, the sanitary bottling of milk and a very general adoption of pasteurization have almost entirely eliminated milk as a distributor of enteritis in areas where these practices are followed. This is especially true in states where hotels and restaurants are required by law to serve beverage milk in bottled form. Likewise, the reduction of flies to very small numbers, not only in towns but even in rural areas, was soon destined to become a practical possibility. Before ten years had passed, C. W. Howard (1917c) was advocating the "Flyless Farm," through exhibits which were shown at various state fairs and which gave to thousands of rural folk their first concept of a life free from this form of nuisance.

Two important conclusions should be obvious from the foregoing discussion: (1) that the legislative control of fly-borne diseases has many aspects and (2) that sanitary entomology is intimately involved with other important phases of public health.

PUBLIC VERSUS PRIVATE RESPONSIBILITY

Public health today implies the exercise by governmental agencies of a type of responsibility which the individual himself may not satisfactorily assume. Such responsibility falls under at least three heads: (1) the raising and appropriation of public funds to be employed for the general protection of the people; (2) the promotion of a continuing program of health education; (3) the formulation, enactment, and enforcement of appropriate laws and ordinances.

Health Protection

Under this head may be listed various services directly beneficial to the citizenry at large. These include the provision of a safe water supply, sewage and garbage disposal, quarantine enforcement, and immunizing and laboratory services. Large-scale spraying operations for insect control constitute a modern addition to the list. These services are imperative in times of national disaster, such as flood, earthquake, volcanic eruption, or enemy bombing. For example, Kearns (1942) reported that both *Musca domestica* and blowflies increased enormously as a result of breeding in rubble following the destruction of English buildings by German bombs. The breeding medium consisted chiefly of decomposing foodstuffs scattered among the bricks, stones, and other debris. By spraying freshly exposed sites with tar-oil emulsion and repeating this treatment every seven to ten days, authorities were able to achieve a fair degree of control. This type of spray repelled the egg-laying females and killed approximately 90 per cent of the eggs.

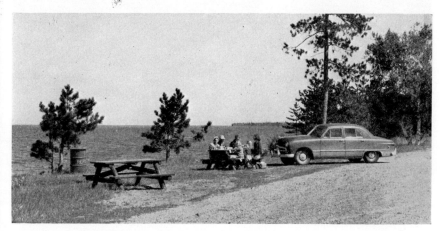

Figure 91. Desirable location for roadside table. Users will rarely stop here for defecatory purposes. Should such become necessary, exposed situation requires individual to walk a considerable distance, for privacy. (Photo by Rollin Thoren.)

The Educational Approach

This implies the education of the public by all possible means to a better understanding of good health practices, not only in regard to the personal care of the body but in regard to care of property as well. The most important phase of public health education relates obviously to communicable diseases and the part that the individual can and must play in controlling them.

Modern sanitary education usually proceeds along two general lines: (1) through the popular press, lectures, radio, motion pictures, television, exhibits, home visitation, and other channels to influence the adult population; and (2) through public and private schools, youth organizations, and the like, to make certain that the rising generation, when mature, will be prepared to assume responsibility in public health and related fields. There is also the indirect modification of adult viewpoint brought about by the transmission from children to parents of information gained during the school day.

Health Legislation

An enlightened population eventually reaches that degree of understanding which permits intelligent formulation of laws and ordinances to serve the

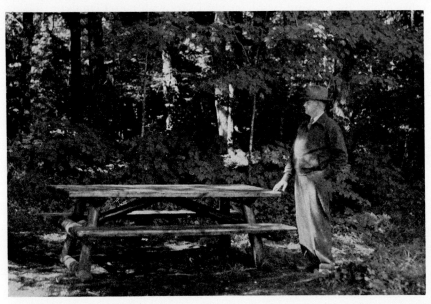

Figure 92. Abused location. Close proximity of dense vegetation invites users to defecate in near vicinity of picnic table. At the close of a holiday week, the author found a "defecatory ring" surrounding the table, within a radius of fifty feet. Fly breeding was already under way. (Photo by Rollin Thoren.)

local need. Such understanding also guarantees a degree of enforcement which only a unified majority opinion can insure. It is important that health laws be formulated in the light of the best scientific knowledge, and that provision be made for their periodic revision and improvement as new scientific information becomes available. Benefits from sanitary legislation are both direct and indirect, since enforcement not only eliminates the dangers from particular health hazards but serves likewise as a continuing educational agency, by functioning as a deterrent to potential offenders.

A good example of what may be accomplished by appropriate ordinances and strict enforcement is provided by present conditions in the Panama Canal Zone and adjacent cities. As early as 1915, in an attempt to cut the death rate among children in the city of Panama, instructions were issued for the construction, by the Panama Railroad, of a public stable of 250 stalls, to house animals previously stabled throughout the city. At the same time, steps were taken for the immediate removal of any stables on unimproved streets. The report of Siler in 1931 stated that not only the Canal Zone but likewise Colon and Panama City were quite free from flies. Siler stressed the importance of constant attention to waste disposal and the timely use of sprays. By 1935, Curry was able to report the daily removal of garbage and stable refuse from Colon, Panama City, and all towns in the Canal Zone. The beginning of the

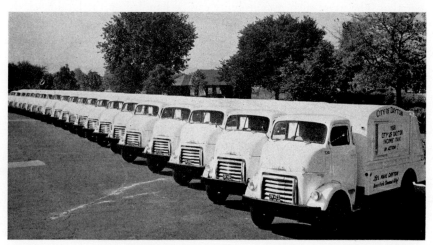

Figure 93. Planned garbage collection in a large city. An increasing number of American municipalities are investing in fleets of modern, hydraulic-hoist trucks, with sanitary bodies. (Courtesy of Gar Wood Industries, Inc.)

rainy season (May and June) and the end of that season (around December) are both times when flies tend to breed profusely and have a wide range of dispersal, so that there is migration into the sanitated areas at those times. At any other season of the year, however, the presence of a single fly in any building in the Canal Zone has become cause for comment. It should be remembered that these results were achieved almost ten years before the availability of DDT.

ECONOMY IN PUBLIC EXPENDITURE

Public responsibility on the state and federal levels is today an accepted principle, and the benefits to the population at large have surely justified the taxation involved. Cost, however, is becoming an increasingly important problem as the activity of large private foundations, which have often pioneered both in research and in education, inevitably decreases. In the United States, two reasons for this change are apparent: (1) the reduced purchasing power of the dollar, whereby the more or less fixed income of a foundation fails to cover the former scope of its work, and (2) the increased taxation of higher incomes, so that few corporations or individuals may hope either to set up new philanthropic enterprises of substantial size or to augment those already in existence.

Civilization is therefore faced with an increasing necessity for governmental responsibility in health matters, and economy in management becomes imperative. The more such responsibility can be handled on the local level, the more significant will be the return on the expenditures involved. County health organizations are exceedingly important, and should be by all means encouraged. Especially unfortunate is the situation where the county seat, for example, employs its own health officer and, being protected, ignores the health needs of the rural area round about. An example of the type of problem involved has been furnished by Stiles and Lumsden (1916), who called attention to the fact that although farmers may prevent soil pollution and fly-borne enteritis on their own farms by the use of sanitary privies, children may be exposed to these dangers at the schools and the entire family similarly exposed when they attend rural churches. The tendency toward consolidation of rural school districts, with sanitary plumbing at the consolidation center, is largely removing the first menace, but small rural churches and chapels continue to be badly neglected in many areas. Thus entire families are endangered in spite of their own high standards. In such a situation, the personal influence of the county health officer is often sufficient to bring about the necessary corrective measures, with perhaps no public cost. Similar enforcement on the state level, on the other hand, can well run into large sums spent in travel, inspection, reporting, and court procedure.

Another type of menace in rural areas may be a combination hog farm and garbage disposal, so located as to be beyond the range of nuisance laws protecting cities and towns. This type of establishment has been fairly common in various parts of the United States. For years the potential danger to health may not become apparent. When, however, activities such as road building, track laying, lumbering, or military maneuvers require the concentration of a considerable number of persons in the vicinity of such a breeding center for flies, an emergency may be said to exist.

An active local health officer will naturally be concerned in avoiding, in his area, the possible outbreak of a fly-borne epidemic originating in the unprotected camp, and will ordinarily bring pressure upon the hog farmer to utilize approved methods of fly control. If camp authorities are lax, he can also be useful in stimulating the use of flytraps, screens, sprays, flypapers, poisons, and swatters within the camp boundaries. Even large-scale measures may prove ineffective in camps, however, when the center of fly production is neglected or overlooked. Dews and Morrill report (1946) that where a dairy barn was within 500 feet of a certain installation in the Fourth Service Command, thorough treatment of the Post with DDT effected no noticeable reduction in the fly population on government property. Treatment at the source, on the other hand, proved very effective in clearing up the problem.

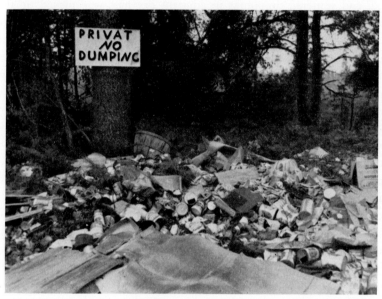

Figure 94. Private citizen's rights ignored. This attempt on the part of the landowner to protect the beauty and value of his property proved futile, in the face of careless practices. (Courtesy of Michigan Department of Health.)

FURTHER COMMENT ON RURAL PROBLEMS

Another area in which the rural health officer may function is in co-operation with the county agricultural agent. Improvement in standards of dairy-barn management comes slowly, and practical farmers are not inclined to institute new methods without logical reason. The results of investigations carried on at agricultural experiment stations must first be reduced to practical recommendations and then interpreted in a manner that the practical operator can understand, if new practices are to meet with general adoption. Popular education through well-designed publicity is well within the province of the local health officer, who, in turn, can look to the county agricultural agent to keep him properly informed.

An excellent example of the type of study that can lead to specific improvements is the report of Atkeson, Shaw, Smith, and Borgmann concerning work carried on at the Kansas Agricultural Experiment Station. This report was published in the *Journal of Dairy Science* in 1943.

The barn concerned was modern in all respects, and the establishment was producing grade-A milk. Walls were of glazed tile and the ceiling plaster was coated with enamel paint. Floors and walls were washed after each milking period, and scattered droppings in adjacent dry lots were picked up twice weekly. In spite of these high standards, *Musca domestica* remained a problem. It should be noted that the Standard Milk Ordinance Code of the United States Public Health Service, which was being observed, required screens on the milk house but not on dairy barns, since it was argued that because many flies enter the barn with the cattle, screens might act as a trap to keep them in.

Systematic counts of flies on the walls and ceilings, as well as on the arrivals themselves, in both screened and unscreened barns showed that screens very definitely improve the situation, even when the cattle are turned in and out. A great difference also was noted between clean-swept barns and bedded barns, in that while few or no flies entered with the cattle in the first case, the fly count always rose significantly after the cattle were brought into barns with bedded floors. The odor of the bedding was presumably the stimulating factor here. Even in such barns, however, the flies could be completely controlled by use of screens and sprays. Another factor proved to be residual feed in the mangers, which, mixed with saliva, is not easy to sweep out completely. The residue consequently sours and attracts flies. Scrubbing, rather than sweeping, eliminates all this, with rather dramatic results as far as the fly count is concerned. Scrubbed areas showed a count of only 16 flies per hundred square feet; swept areas, 282—a difference of almost 18 to 1.

CO-OPERATIVE ENTERPRISE

Intermediate, from an economic standpoint, between public health measures at government expense and practices carried out by the individual citizen is the possibility of co-operative effort within a restricted area, where the needs of many individuals are more or less identical and there is a common health objective. Cory and Langford (1947) have reported on such an undertaking, carried out in Maryland in 1946. One per cent DDT, as a wettable powder, was used to spray both barns and dairy cattle for a considerable number of farmers. Applied with a pressure of between 400 and 500 pounds, the DDT was effective for ten weeks on walls and for as long as six weeks on the animals. Three applications, properly spaced, gave protection against flies for the entire season. Benzene hexachloride spray, prepared from 50 per cent wettable powder, was also found very effective but was not used on or near dairy cows because of its objectionable odor.

Almost all of the farm owners and operators agreed that the protection cost less, and was more complete, than that which could have been achieved by individual effort. There would appear to be good reason to encourage cooperative fly control, especially when it can make possible the ownership of more effective machinery for dispensing the insecticides. The utilization of labor that has acquired a degree of skill in the handling of modern spray materials can also operate to insure more uniform results throughout an area or community than those usually obtained when each establishment, some experienced, some otherwise, relies upon whatever labor is available.

SPRAYING NOT A PANACEA

Community-wide use of insecticides calls for special comment. To some it may appear such an easy way out that fundamental practices tend to lose their importance in the public mind. Of interest in this connection are the controlled studies carried out by Watt and Lindsay (1948), who demonstrated that in an area where morbidity from diarrheal infection was high, both infection rate and death rate could be materially reduced by the use of insecticides. Organisms of the *Salmonella* group were not controlled as satisfactorily as were *Shigella* infections, but both types became less frequent. Relief from danger, however, was only *temporary*, as shown by the fact that fly-population curves were reversed for but a few days following each application. The seeking out and elimination of breeding places still remains, therefore, the most important procedure in the control of fly-borne diarrheal diseases. However miraculous DDT and similar compounds may seem to be in reducing the fly population of rural areas, the availability of these insecticides should not be made an excuse for neglect of the basic principles of sanitation.

It should be remembered that flies have considerable power of flight and that an individual fly laden with the virus of poliomyelitis needs only a moment of contact with food, lips, or nostrils to unburden itself of its vicious cargo. Even though a few minutes later it may settle upon a wall made lethal by residual DDT, and within thirty minutes be a dead fly, the damage to the family may already have been done, and the health and possibly the life of its members jeopardized.

Furthermore, the infallibility of DDT is not nearly as universal as was originally supposed. Its effectiveness depends upon the age and sex of the fly, the surface being treated, and the nature of the preparation employed. The work of Fay, Buckner, and Simmons (1948) will serve to illustrate certain of these points: Flies tested three days after emergence proved to be more resistant to DDT residues than any other age group, and female specimens always proved less susceptible than males. The effectiveness of DDT deposits proved to be influenced less by variations of concentration in the emulsion than by the type of surface treated. Surfaces exposed to rain retained a more satisfactory toxicity with 2.5 per cent DDT xylene emulsions than with 2.5 per cent water-wettable DDT powders.

Therefore, even if reasonably complete protection can be secured, on occasion, by the use of insecticides alone, the tremendous importance of neatness, cleanliness, and orderliness in both family and community life should always be borne in mind. It is well known that fly-borne diseases may also be transmitted in a host of other ways, associated largely with carelessness in the handling of foods and beverages, dirty floors, dirty clothing, and unsanitary personal habits. To neglect the cleaning of stables, the repair of screens, or proper covering of a cesspool on the ground that the fly problem has been solved another way is to foster habits of general neglect and carelessness in the management of the home or business enterprise. Aesthetic ideals alone should dictate a high standard of property maintenance, one of the first guarantees of a favorable health index in any community. It should be recalled that as long ago as 1912, Cox, Lewis, and Glynn showed the amount of dirt carried by flies in any particular locality, measured in terms of bacteria taken from their bodies, to be in definite relation to the habits of the people and to the condition of the streets. They emphasized the necessity for both municipal and domestic cleanliness, if the food of the inhabitants is to escape pollution.

Along the same line, Parker (1916b) showed that a fly from an unsanitary area within a city might carry from 800,000 to 500,000,000 bacteria, whereas specimens from cleaner parts of the same municipality carried only between 21,000 and 100,000. More modern work by Ostrolenk and Welch (1942b) lends additional force to these early findings. Their study of washings from the surfaces of flies showed the presence of from 2,500,000 to 29,500,000 bacteria per fly. For the colon-aerogenes group alone, the numbers ranged from 84,000 to 2,000,000. The incidence of the latter proved to depend very largely on the material on which the flies had fed. These authors state that the presence of even a very small number of flies in a food establishment constitutes a filth menace, the seriousness of which may be determined by an evaluation of surrounding conditions. A single fly' heavily laden with microorganisms may deposit large numbers of pathogens on human food in a very short interval of time.

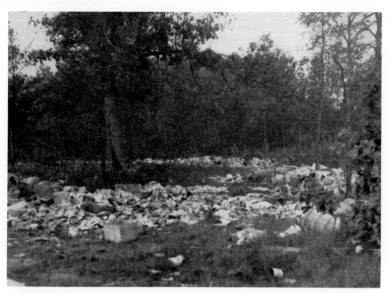

Figure 95. A bad use of an attractive spot. A potential picnic ground and recreational area has been completely spoiled for human pleasure by promiscuous dumping of unsightly and malodorous refuse. (Courtesy of Michigan Department of Health.)

SOME PROBLEMS OF CURRENT TIMES

With the general improvement of sanitary conditions in cities, especially since the reduction in the number of stables and the close supervision of those which still remain, it might be reasonable to expect an almost complete relief from the intestinal disturbances of late summer and early fall. Any active pediatrician can tesify that such is not the case. Superficial analysis might lead one to suspect that flies are not, and never have been, a major factor in the enteritis of the warmer months. Again nothing could be further from the truth. We have just stressed the fact that it requires relatively few flies, and relatively few visits from them, to contaminate food surfaces when a source of infection exists nearby.

Vacation Risks

Picture the general exodus of city populations for vacation purposes in the late summer. Not only is there the very general "week-ending" on the part of families in all walks of life, but in the United States, at least, we have the almost universal two-week vacation, during which the entire family either travels a considerable distance to a vacation spot or perhaps remains continuously on the road for an entire fortnight.

Consider now the innumerable roadside stands, especially those displaying ripe fruit ready for consumption. The hands of the fruit vendor may be the source of the original contamination, or there may be an open privy in connection with the establishment. Quite often pickers, handlers, and transporters use the roadside thicket, ditch, or open field for defecatory purposes. This is especially likely to occur if one is distressed with cramps and has little time to seek a conventional place of relief.

Once the skin of a single plum or tomato has become contaminated, either from handling or by the chance visit of a fly, that item becomes a central culture plate from which not only houseflies but fruit flies, ants, and other visitants may now proceed to inoculate the entire stock in trade.

Casual observation of the stream of purchases completes the record. Fruit appeals to the thirsty, and children especially are impatient of delay. Facilities for washing the skin of newly purchased fruit are usually unavailable in the immediate vicinity of the place of business. In fact, the provision of such facilities by the fruit dealer might even imply that his wares were dirtier than those of his competitor and therefore less desirable! Again, rare is the parent who insists on washing the fruit before the children eat it.

Millions of summer travelers cover thousands of miles each year in North America alone, seeking health, recreation, education, sport, and scenic beauty. The tendency is more and more to forsake the beaten path and the sanitated hostelries for more intriguing, more out-of-the-way places where frequently only the most primitive facilities for waste disposal may be found. Little danger lurks, to be sure, for the isolated individual or family that camps apart from other folk, but spots virtually unexplored the first season can become veritable trafficways the next, and it is in the not-quite-organized tourist and camping areas that the greatest menace to public health is found. As many as 23 typhoid carriers have been found among 1,700 apparently healthy persons, according to certain published surveys. In the light of these figures, it is disconcerting to find how very few of our summer campers have taken the trouble to secure the safeguard of a typhoid-paratyphoid inoculation before taking to the field. Under circumstances such as these, we need but a relatively small fly population to start the evil procession and convey infection from feces to food and beverage, the first chapter in the conversion of a joyous and care-free vacation period into a tour of illness, anxiety, and perhaps disaster of a tragic kind.

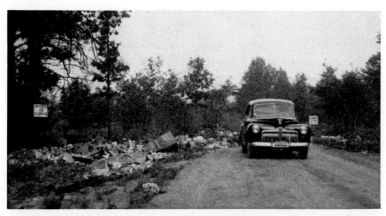

Figure 96. An unsightly and unsanitary condition along a highway, brought about by neglect of both education and enforcement. Dumping was provided for in a designated area nearby, but citizens became increasingly careless. (Courtesy of Michigan Department of Health.)

Sewage Sludge a Danger

According to a progress report prepared by Bartsch and Scott (1949) regarding pollution in the upper reaches of the Mississippi River, sludge and scum may constitute a real menace in relation to fly-borne disease. These deposits, always abundant along the banks as well as on the bottom of a sewage-contaminated stream, are frequently exposed during periods of low water and thus form a suitable medium for larval development, resulting in an increase of fly population which would not otherwise occur. Furthermore, since all such sludge deposits contain an abundance of living sewage organisms, flies have a twofold opportunity to become contaminated. The females that first seek such situations for oviposition, as well as the newly emerged flies of both sexes produced therein, are free to convey disease-producing bacteria from this source to homes, restaurants, roadside stands, and picnic grounds, where infection of food and drink may very easily ensue.

THE IMPORTANCE OF COMMON SENSE

If a reasonably thorough program of health education can be carried out in the schools, many phases of fly control will never have to be defined by ordinance. For example, the individual property owner is usually the best judge as to whether his garbage can should be housed in a container that is dog- and ratproof. If experience teaches him that there are prowlers abroad to remove the lid, upset the can, and scatter the contents, it is only sensible to conclude that better housing should be provided. A very practical container for smaller cans may be devised by sinking a section of large-diameter tile vertically in the ground. The bottom may be of cinders or gravel to facilitate drainage. This should occasionally be sterilized with Lysol or some other disinfectant. The can is lowered into the tile, where it remains until filled. The can should be

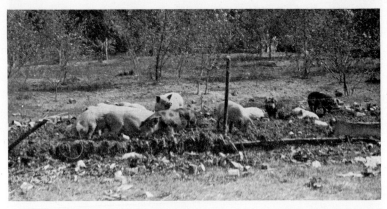

Figure 97. Disposal of garbage by feeding to hogs. This should be discouraged unless there is a feeding platform which can be given sanitary care. Many flies are generated by a situation such as this. (Courtesy of Michigan Department of Health.)

equipped with appropriate handles or bail for lifting out. A weighted or locked lid closes the top of the tile between visits.

Again, the use of paper bags to contain small units of garbage before they are consigned to the can may be of great advantage. Paine (1912) suggested this as a means of preventing maggots from remaining attached to the sides of the pails after collection. In his day it was not considered practical to insist that garbage pails be flyproof. Also, much of the garbage was flyblown before being placed in the pails. Experience will show whether such a procedure is necessary. It certainly leaves a cleaner pail after the garbage has been dumped, and in northern latitudes guards against the freezing of garbage to the sides and bottom in the wintertime.

It should be emphasized in all educational campaigns that it is the great adaptability of the housefly that makes this public health problem such a far-reaching one. Derbeneva-Ukhova and Kuzina (1938) noted that in the absence of refuse dumps, horse dung, and pig dung, *Musca domestica* used the refuse in boxes and ditches, and even the cracks in the floors of bakeries and communal kitchens, for breeding purposes. Moist earth in the vicinity of kitchen drains, or where slops of any kind have been thrown out, may itself become a breeding medium. Reasonable watchfulness on the part of the enlightened citizen can guard against seemingly harmless situations becoming sources for the production of flies.

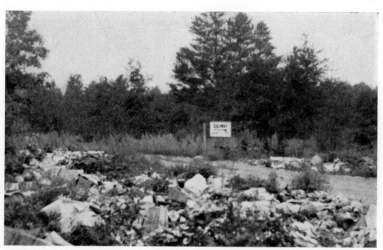

Figure 98. A situation that has got out of hand. The sign reads "Dump 1,000 feet," but users have long since taken to shortening the distance, with most undesirable results. (Courtesy of Michigan Department of Health.)

PUBLIC HEALTH ECONOMICS FROM A WORLD STANDPOINT

We should not forget that standards which have become commonplace in a country where the wealth per capita is relatively high are hardly applicable in areas where the economic ratio is reversed. This is merely another way of saying that the public health measures which a community creates for its protection will necessarily be sharply limited by the economic resources of the people.

For example, let us compare the last word in garbage disposal as carried out by an American industrial city with the approved procedure for the disposal of town wastes in India. Each is practical and up to date for the setting in which it is to be used.

The American sanitary land fill, which is fully discussed in Chapter XVIII, requires, for its maintenance, a standard wide-tread, crawler-type tractor

equipped with a bullclam bucket or shovel. A regular bulldozer and dragline
may be substituted, but in either case the investment in expensive machinery
is large. The tremendous amount of metal, glass, and paper in American refuse
makes it impractical to separate these items from organic components with
a view to using the latter for agricultural purposes. Everything is dumped
together, covered, and compressed. Miller (1948) points out that low, swampy
areas, which formerly bred mosquitoes, may thus be converted into appro-

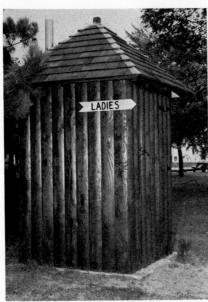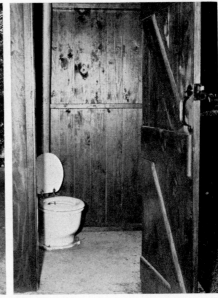

Figure 99. Modern facilities reduce fly hazard. *Left:* Ladies' toilet at state-supervised
roadside park, Muskegon County, Michigan. *Right:* Interior of the same facility, showing high standard of construction and maintenance. (Courtesy of Michigan State Highway Department.)

priate sites for parking lots, drive-in theaters, used-car displays, public parks,
and playgrounds. The emphasis on automotive interests is noteworthy, and
typically American. No special thought need be given to fly control, as the
bulk of the material is not likely to be infested before delivery, and the constant addition and compression make emergence of flies from deep layers difficult or impossible. A properly handled land fill is both rodent- and insect-free.

In India, on the other hand, the disposal of town wastes involves handling
fecal matter, as well as garbage and litter. The percentage of glass and metal is
usually not high, and the conservation of organic elements is vitally necessary
from an economic standpoint. Special machinery is rather out of the question;

on the other hand, labor is relatively abundant and inexpensive. The usual disposal is by means of a compost trench, in which 3-inch layers of dry refuse are made to alternate with 1-inch layers of excreta. The principal drawback to this otherwise satisfactory procedure lies in the fact that both eggs and larvae of various dipterous species are usually present in the excreta and refuse before these are delivered at the compost depot. The prevention of their further development in the compost trench is not easily accomplished, as some methods are out of the question because of the expense involved.

Acharya and Krishna Rao (1945a,b), in the attempt to render control both more simple and less costly, settled upon three procedures, any of which, with reasonable care, can be relied upon to be at least 95 per cent effective.

The first aims at setting up anaerobic conditions by covering the compost with a plaster composed of equal parts of cattle dung and fine earth, plus an appropriate amount of water. This is kept intact for one week, from the sixth to the thirteenth day, during which time constant supervision is provided to close up any cracks that may develop. For large-scale operations it is often difficult to secure sufficient fine earth and dung, but for disposal of small quantities, this method is very satisfactory and is quite as adaptable for treating heaps as for taking care of refuse placed in trenches. It has the disadvantage of delaying the decomposition process to some extent.

A second procedure involves placing a 2-inch layer of earth upon the compost, followed by 6 inches of dry refuse, which is burned on the sixth day. Where infestation is heavy, a second burning on the tenth day is considered necessary. This is very satisfactory in the dry season, but in wet weather a sufficient quantity of dry refuse is difficult to obtain. It is, of course, much more applicable to trenches than to heaps, and in all cases there is some destruction of humus and loss of nitrogen, due to heating and drying.

The third, and probably most satisfactory, method involves the use of a cover cloth of drill, treated with tar on both sides. If hessian cloth is used, preliminary treatment with earth-dung plaster is recommended. Such a cloth is spread over the trench, or heap, from the sixth to the thirteenth day, with the margins fixed on the ground by a layer of earth-dung plaster, above and below. Supervision with regard to cracks is necessary, as with the first method described, but as only the margins are involved, much less labor is required. As when plaster is used alone, the object is to set up conditions of an anaerobic character. Larvae, pupae, and emerging adults are thus asphyxiated. Acharya and Krishna Rao consider this the most generally useful, as well as the most economical, method of the three.

Any of these methods is superior, of course, to the so-called "Bangalore" method, consisting of the use of soil alone. While this prevents most oviposition, it obviously does not destroy eggs, larvae, or pupae which may already be present.

In regions where an abundance of green vegetation is readily available, the use of such material in composting gives excellent results. The decomposition of green vegetation generates a tremendous amount of heat and results in the complete destruction of any eggs, larvae, or pupae which may have been present in the associated rubbish, animal manure, or night soil. Pathogenic organ-

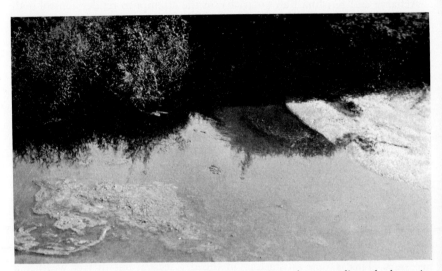

Figure 100. Fly menace, due to improper operation of sewage-disposal plant. Accumulation of sludge occurred at outlet of roadside ditch into county drain. This has since been corrected by modern sewage treatment works. (Courtesy of Michigan Department of Health.)

isms likewise disappear, and when composting is complete, the mass is entirely innocuous. Dr. J. W. Scharff (1940), formerly Chief Health Officer in Singapore, is convinced that this method has great value in suppressing fly breeding in Malaya, and holds the presence of any considerable number of flies to be indicative of careless or faulty workmanship in handling the compost.

Obviously, any planned procedure is infinitely preferable to no method at all. For example, on the eastern front in World War I, Hase (1916) reported deplorable conditions in the small villages of Poland. Solid excrement, both human and animal, was thrown on fields. Liquid refuse was poured into several gutters which joined at the lower end of the village to form a stagnant, foul-smelling pool. Hase remarks that "very little fly control was possible under these conditions."

WORLD-SPONSORED SANITATION

It has often been stated that the League of Nations failed. This was not true in the area of health research. It is of interest to recall the investigations of Lörincz, Szappanos, and Makara (1935–1936), results of which were pub-

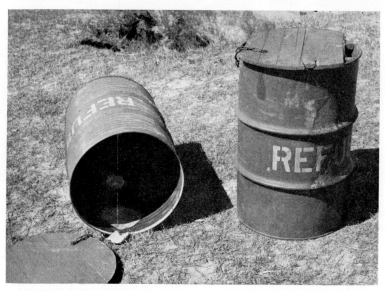

Figure 101. Supervision and upkeep are important. Lids are chained to containers, but this is no protection when cover becomes damaged or falls off. These two refuse cans were found as shown, at a roadside picnic site. Both were malodorous, and contained many flies. (Photo by Rollin Thoren.)

lished in the Quarterly Bulletin of the League's Health Organization. These studies were confined to the fly problem in Hungary. To them we owe the significant information that the further advanced the fermentation process is in the breeding medium, the longer will be the duration of the larval stage. These workers also demonstrated that traps baited with overripe or decomposing fruit attract nearly seven times as many flies as traps baited with human feces. This indicates a very pronounced tendency for houseflies to spend a great portion of their time in the fruit market and reminds us that the handling and sale of this type of food can become a significant public health problem. Interesting correlations were worked out for fly density and the incidence of typhoid. The disease followed the fly curve with a lag of approximately four weeks; August and October were the peak months for flies, and September and November, for typhoid fever. Obviously, flies are not the only cause of seasonal fluctuation.

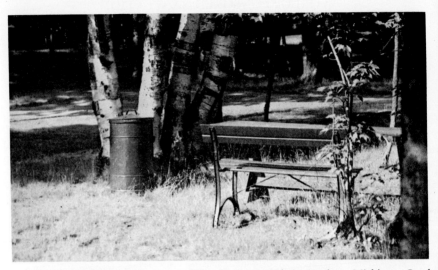

Figure 102. Inviting nook in a well-handled city park in northern Michigan. Good co-operation between visitors and park attendants keeps the area clean, sanitary, and attractive throughout the season. (Photo by Rollin Thoren.)

It is confidently expected that the United Nations, through its World Health Organization, will likewise sponsor and advance the sanitary aspects of applied science, in the interest of healthier and happier individuals. Certain phases of the program of UNESCO should also be of value in this respect.

CHAPTER XIII

Myiasis

Though he in a fertile climate dwell, plague him with flies.—Shakespeare, Othello

THE term "myiasis" is applied to the presence of the larvae of any species of fly within or upon the human or animal body. This form of parasitism may involve the skin and subcutaneous tissues, the natural apertures and adjacent cavities (such as the nasal passages and sinuses, mouth, anus, orbit of the eye, vagina), or the more internal cavities (such as the intestine, stomach, or bladder). A few, like *Hypoderma,* migrate through many types of tissue before arriving at a definite location.

Species have been grouped according to the extent to which the parasitic behavior has become confirmed:

(1) Specific myiasis. These forms are obligate parasites, and are therefore unable to complete their life cycles without appropriate hosts. The Congo floor maggot (*Auchmeromyia luteola*), the Tumbu fly (*Cordylobia anthropophaga*), the so-called human botfly (*Dermatobia hominis*), the oxwarbles (*Hypoderma*), horse botflies (*Gasterophilus*) and other botflies, and certain screwworm flies (*Chrysomya, Callitroga*) are common examples.

(2) Semispecific myiasis. This applies to infestations by species which ordinarily deposit their eggs or living maggots in decomposing plant or animal matter, but which may adopt the parasitic habit on occasion, as when ovipositing flies are attracted by the odors from sores, wounds, body discharges, or soiled clothing. The larvae of such forms may penetrate considerable distances into the cavity or lesion, but rarely or never attack healthy tissue. In this way they may actually be of benefit in removing necrotic material, and wounds infested with maggots have sometimes been observed to heal more rapidly than lesions which were maggot-free. In this connection it is important to note that the salutary effect is due less to mechanical cleansing than to the secretion of certain chemical substances which stimulate tissue proliferation. (See page 342 for discussion of therapeutic myiasis.)

Puri (1943) lists the following species as responsible for semispecific myiasis in India: *Aphiochaeta* (*Megaselia*) *scalaris* Loew, *Calliphora erythrocephala* (*Meigen*) (*vicina* R.-D.), *Calliphora vomitoria* (Linnaeus), *Chrysomya megacephala* (Fabricius), *Lucilia* (*Phaenicia*) *cuprina* (Wiedemann), *Lucilia* (*Phaenicia*) *sericata* (Meigen), *Musca domestica* Linnaeus, *Sarcophaga ruficornis* (Fabricius). Representatives of the same and related genera exhibit similar habits in other parts of the world.

Semispecific myiasis appears to depend on the adaptability of the species to a number of environmental conditions. For example, Kozhanchikov (1947) found that *Calliphora erythrocephala* (*C. vicina* R.-D.) has a very low thermal optimum, which ranges from 18° to 20°C (64.4° to 68°F). This species is thus quite unable to adjust permanently to the body temperature of mammals and birds, though it tolerates a greater range of pH than might reasonably be expected.

(3) Accidental myiasis. Here are grouped those facultative parasites which are capable of adapting themselves to the environment of the alimentary tract and other cavities with exterior connections. Eggs or larvae sometimes are deposited on human food, or upon excrement or other decomposing material which may later be introduced into the mouth, usually by way of the fingers or soiled utensils. No hard and fast line may be drawn between semispecific and accidental myiasis. Infestation of the bladder by maggots which have migrated through the tissues from the alimentary tract is surely accidental. On the other hand, urethral, vaginal, or even rectal myiasis, if due to the actual deposition of egg or first-stage larva within the orifice concerned, is scarcely to be distinguished in mode of origin from nasal, ocular, or aural. The classification will frequently depend on whether the particular species of fly has been recorded more than once from the same tissue or location. *Eristalis* (*Tubifera*), *Fannia, Aphiochaeta, Sarcophaga,* and *Musca* (*M. domestica*) are among the genera recorded as producing accidental myiasis in man.

The relation of *Musca domestica* to all these conditions is rather limited, but the phenomenon itself is of such interest, and can be so important from a medical standpoint, that a brief, general treatment of human myiasis seems quite in order in a volume of this type.

Use of the term "myasis" (note spelling) dates from 1840, when the Reverend F. W. Hope proposed a more descriptive terminology than that which had been employed by Kirby and Spence (1826) in their well-known *Introduction to Entomology*. These authors had used the term "scholechiasis" for larval infestations of all kinds. Hope, recognizing that three orders of insects are chiefly concerned, proposed that "scholechiasis" be restricted to infestations by lepidopterous larvae, that "canthariasis" be similarly employed for infestations in which Coleoptera are present, and that "myasis" be adopted for all conditions in which dipterous larvae are involved. Subsequent modification of the spelling (and pronunciation) is of rather recent origin, and represents a desirable attempt to render medical terminology more uniform. (Compare schistosomiasis, amebiasis, etc.)

Hope compiled rather extensive tables, with references to published authorities, for many countries of the world. Nine cases were positively credited to the genus *Musca,* with three more listed as "probable." Rather shrewdly, Hope suggested four methods by which human beings may become parasitized: (1) by adult insects' depositing ova on the living person; (2) by insects' depositing ova on dressed meat, through subsequent consumption of which the ova reach the stomach; (3) by persons' swallowing ova which have been deposited on too-ripe fruit, raw vegetables, and salads; (4) by swallowing ova and larvae in "impure and turbid" water.

If we add to these methods (1) the possibility of the larva seeking the host on its own initiative, as in the case of the Congo floor maggot, and (2) the utilization of a transport host, as with *Dermatobia hominis,* the summary is practically complete.

The world literature on the subject is extensive but widely scattered, and many of the references are questionable, as misidentification of species has been all too common, and misinterpretation of clinical data is frequent also. A few of the more important contributions may be mentioned:

For the United States, the paper of Dove (1937) is especially informative. Larvae of *Phormia regina* and of *Sarcophaga bullata* are discussed as occurring superficially in necrotic wounds, with *Musca domestica* more common in "filthy" injuries. Dove considers *Cochliomyia (Callitroga) americana* the most important as well as the most dangerous of American species. It is recorded from a large number of cases. Sinuses and nasal cavities are most commonly involved, though deep wounds almost anywhere on the body may be attacked.

Mazza, Jörg, and Basso (1939) give interesting data from Argentina. These include observations of *M. domestica* on carcasses in open air. Mumford (1926) records three cases of myiasis from northern England, including examples of urethral infection by larvae of *M. domestica* and *Fannia canicularis.* A useful reference in Swedish is Lampa's paper (1887), which deals primarily with intestinal forms. A number of papers in Russian, by Portchinsky (1906, 1913c, 1915, 1916), treat of human infestation with *Oestrus, Rhinoestrus, Wolhfahrtia,* and other forms.

There is extensive literature for various parts of Africa. Lewis (1933) gives important data for Kenya Colony, while Bedford (1926) has prepared a useful check list of myiasis-producing forms for South Africa. A comprehensive treatment of myiasis in Tripolitania was published by Onorato in 1922. An older but valuable paper by Roubaud (1914) gives similar information for French West Africa. For India and adjacent areas, the several papers by Patton (1920a,b,c, 1921b, 1922c,d,e,f) should be consulted.

For identification of myiasis-producing Diptera throughout the world, the contribution of James (1947) is by far the most useful. It is amply illustrated, and contains valuable keys and tables. Both adult and larval characters are treated. In discussing the various types of myiasis, James makes extensive use of the classification proposed by Bishopp and others (1926), who recognized the following categories: (1) tissue-destroying forms, (2) subdermal migratory forms, (3) larvae infesting the intestinal and urogenital tracts, (4) forms infesting the head passages, and (5) bloodsucking forms.

James expanded this to nine separate headings, thereby arriving at a classification especially useful to the clinician, who must always begin with symptoms, relating to lesions in a definite part of the body and, by subsequent investigation, locate the etiological agent concerned:

1. Traumatic (wound) myiasis.
2. Myiasis of nose, mouth, and accessory sinuses.
3. Aural myiasis.
4. Ocular myiasis.
5. Myiasis of the anal region and vagina.
6. Myiasis of the bladder and urinary tract.
7. Furuncular dermal or subdermal myiasis.
8. Creeping dermal or subdermal myiasis.
9. Enteric, i.e., gastric, gastrointestinal, or intestinal myiasis.

In Table 16, based on data compiled by James, the categories are regrouped and a tenth subdivision is added to provide for the unique bloodsucking habits of the Congo floor maggot. These tables will, it is hoped, prove of value to the pathologist or technician in guiding him toward a proper identification of the forms encountered. The last column should aid in estimating the seriousness of the infestation. Only generally accepted, authentic records are here included.

IDENTIFICATION OF LARVAE REMOVED OR RECOVERED FROM HUMAN HOSTS

First- and second-stage larvae are usually very difficult to identify. If only such early stages are recovered, the physician will do well to send his material

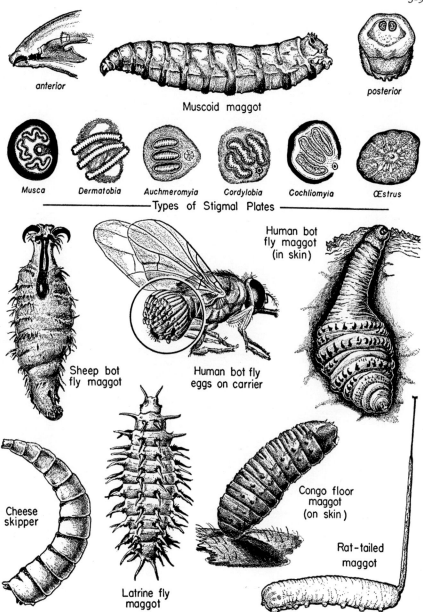

anterior

Muscoid maggot

posterior

Musca   Dermatobia   Auchmeromyia   Cordylobia   Cochliomyia   Œstrus

Types of Stigmal Plates

Sheep bot fly maggot

Human bot fly eggs on carrier

Human bot fly maggot (in skin)

Cheese skipper

Latrine fly maggot

Congo floor maggot (on skin)

Rat-tailed maggot

Figure 103. Recognition characters of larvae causing myiasis in man. (From *Manual of Tropical Medicine,* by Mackie, Hunter, and Worth [L. S. West, collaborator]; courtesy of W. B. Saunders Company.)

Table 16

A. Traumatic (developing at the site of wounds)

Genus and species	General distribution	Dipterous family to which referred	Specific semispecific or accidental
Calliphora croceipalpis	Ethiopian	Calliphoridae	Semispecific
Calliphora vicina	Temperate regions generally	Calliphoridae	Semispecific
Calliphora vomitoria	North America; Palearctic; Oriental and beyond	Calliphoridae	Semispecific
Calliroga americana	Nearctic and Neotropical	Calliphoridae	Specific
Calliroga macellaria	Nearctic and Neotropical	Calliphoridae	Semispecific
Chrysomya bezziana	Oriental; Ethiopian	Calliphoridae	Specific
Chrysomya chloropyga	Africa	Calliphoridae	Semispecific
Chrysomya marginalis	Southern Europe; India; Ethiopian	Calliphoridae	Semispecific
Chrysomya megacephala	Oriental and beyond; Australia	Calliphoridae	Semispecific
Cynomyopsis cadaverina	Nearctic and northern Europe	Calliphoridae	Semispecific
Lucilia caesar	Palearctic generally	Calliphoridae	Semispecific
Lucilia illustris	Palearctic; North America; Oriental	Calliphoridae	Semispecific
Megaselia rufipes	All continents	Phoridae	Semispecific
Megaselia scalaris	All continents	Phoridae	Semispecific
Mintho algira	Algeria; Libia; Eritrea	Larvaevoridae	Accidental
Musca domestica	Practically world-wide	Muscidae	Accidental
Phormia regina	Cooler parts of Holarctic	Calliphoridae	Semispecific
Phaenicia cuprina	Oriental; Ethiopian; Australian	Calliphoridae	Semispecific
Phaenicia sericata	Practically world-wide	Calliphoridae	Semispecific
Sarcophaga albiceps	Palearctic; Oriental and beyond; East Africa	Sarcophagidae	Semispecific
Sarcophaga barbata	All continents	Sarcophagidae	Semispecific
Sarcophaga beckeri	Southern Europe; Africa	Sarcophagidae	Semispecific
Sarcophaga bullata	Nearctic generally	Sarcophagidae	Semispecific
Sarcophaga carnaria	Europe; Central Asia	Sarcophagidae	Semispecific

Genus and species	General distribution	Dipterous family to which referred	Specific semispecific or accidental
Sarcophaga crassipalpis	Practically world-wide	Sarcophagidae	Semispecific
Sarcophaga fertoni	Europe; North Africa	Sarcophagidae	Semispecific
Sarcophaga haemorrhoidalis	Practically world-wide	Sarcophagidae	Semispecific
Sarcophaga lambens	Southern U.S.; Central and South America	Sarcophagidae	Semispecific
Sarcophaga misera (broad sense)	Practically world-wide	Sarcophagidae	Semispecific
Sarcophaga peregrina	East Asia; Oriental; Australia	Sarcophagidae	Semispecific
Sarcophaga placida	Texas; Panama	Sarcophagidae	Semispecific
Sarcophaga ruficornis	Oriental; Northeast Africa	Sarcophagidae	Semispecific
Sarcophaga striata	Warmer Palearctic	Sarcophagidae	Semispecific
Stomoxys calcitrans	Practically world-wide	Muscidae	Accidental
Synthesiomyia nudiseta	Southern U.S. and Neotropical; India; Africa; Australia	Calliphoridae	Semispecific
Titanogrypha alata	Florida; southern Texas; Cuba	Sarcophagidae	Semispecific
Wohlfahrtia magnifica	Europe; Asia; Africa	Sarcophagidae	Specific
Wohlfahrtia nuba	Northeast Africa; southwest Asia	Sarcophagidae	Semispecific

B. Lesion in the form of a creeping eruption

Gasterophilus haemorrhoidalis	Practically world-wide	Gasterophilidae	Specific
Gasterophilus intestinalis	Practically world-wide	Gasterophilidae	Specific
Hypoderma bovis	Chiefly Holarctic	Hypodermatidae	Specific
Hypoderma diana	Central and southern Europe	Hypodermatidae	Specific
Hypoderma lineatum	Holarctic; India; South Africa	Hypodermatidae	Specific

C. Lesion in the form of a cutaneous furuncle

Callitroga americana	Nearctic and Neotropical	Calliphoridae	Specific
Cordylobia anthropophaga	Ethiopian only	Calliphoridae	Specific
Cuterebra buccata	Nearctic	Cuterebridae	Specific

Table 16—Continued.

Genus and species	General distribution	Dipterous family to which referred	Specific semispecific or accidental
Dermatobia hominis	Neotropical only	Cuterebridae	Specific
Hypoderma bovis	Central and southern Europe	Hypodermatidae	Specific
Hypoderma diana	Central and southern Europe	Hypodermatidae	Specific
Hypoderma lineatum	Holarctic; India; South Africa	Hypodermatidae	Specific
Stasisia rodhaini	Ethiopian only	Calliphoridae	Specific
Wohlfahrtia opaca	Nearctic only	Sarcophagidae	Specific
Wohlfahrtia vigil	Nearctic only	Sarcophagidae	Specific

D. Lesion located in mouth, nose, or sinuses

Genus and species	General distribution	Dipterous family to which referred	Specific semispecific or accidental
Calliphora vicina	Temperate regions generally	Calliphoridae	Semispecific
Callitroga americana	Nearctic and Neotropical	Calliphoridae	Specific
Chrysomya bezziana	Oriental; Ethiopian	Calliphoridae	Specific
Chrysomya megacephala	Oriental and beyond; Australia	Calliphoridae	Semispecific
Cuterebra sp.	New World	Cuterebridae	Specific
Musca domestica	Practically world-wide	Muscidae	Accidental
Oestrus ovis	Practically world-wide	Oestridae	Specific
Phaenicia sericata	Practically world-wide	Calliphoridae	Semispecific
Piophila casei	Practically world-wide	Piophilidae	Accidental
Sarcophaga carnaria	Europe; Central Asia	Sarcophagidae	Semispecific
Sarcophaga misera	Practically world-wide	Sarcophagidae	Semispecific
Titanogrypha alata	Florida; southern Texas; Cuba	Sarcophagidae	Semispecific
Wohlfahrtia magnifica	Europe; Asia; Africa	Sarcophagidae	Specific

E. Lesion affecting the eyes, either externally or internally (ophthalmomyiasis)

Genus and species	General distribution	Dipterous family to which referred	Specific semispecific or accidental
Callitroga americana	Nearctic and Neotropical	Calliphoridae	Specific
Chrysomya bezziana	Oriental; Ethiopian	Calliphoridae	Specific

Genus and species	General distribution	Dipterous family to which referred	Specific semispecific or accidental
Gasterophilus intestinalis	Practically world-wide	Gasterophilidae	Specific
Hypoderma bovis	Holarctic chiefly	Hypodermatidae	Specific
Hypoderma diana	Central and southern Europe	Hypodermatidae	Specific
Hypoderma lineatum	Holarctic; India; South Africa	Hypodermatidae	Specific
Megaselia scalaris	All continents	Phoridae	Semispecific
Musca domestica	Practically world-wide	Muscidae	Accidental
Oestrus ovis	Practically world-wide	Oestridae	Specific
Rhinoestrus purpureus	Palearctic; India; Ethiopian	Oestridae	Specific
Sarcophaga carnaria	Europe; central Asia	Sarcophagidae	Semispecific
Wohlfahrtia magnifica	Europe; Asia; Africa	Sarcophagidae	Specific

F. Lesion affecting the auditory structures (aural myiasis)

Genus and species	General distribution	Dipterous family to which referred	Specific semispecific or accidental
Calliphora vicina	Temperate regions generally	Calliphoridae	Semispecific
Callitroga americana	Nearctic and Neotropical	Calliphoridae	Specific
Chrysomya bezziana	Oriental; Ethiopian	Calliphoridae	Specific
Fannia canicularis	All regions except Oriental	Muscidae	Accidental
Fannia incisurata	Nearctic; Neotropical; Palearctic	Muscidae	Accidental
Fannia scalaris	Temperate regions of all continents	Muscidae	Accidental
Hydrotaea meteorica	Holarctic	Muscidae	Accidental
Lucilia caesar	Palearctic generally	Calliphoridae	Semispecific
Musca domestica	Practically world-wide	Muscidae	Accidental
Oestrus ovis	Practically world-wide	Oestridae	Specific
Phaenicia sericata	Practically world-wide	Calliphoridae	Semispecific
Sarcophaga canaria	Europe; Central Asia	Sarcophagidae	Semispecific
Sarcophaga cooleyi	Warmer Palearctic	Sarcophagidae	Semispecific
Sarcophaga lambens	Southern United States; Central and South America	Sarcophagidae	Semispecific
Sarcophaga nodosa	Africa	Sarcophagidae	Semispecific

Table 16—Continued.

Genus and species	General distribution	Dipterous family to which referred	Specific semispecific or accidental
Sarcophaga placida	Texas; Panama	Sarcophagidae	Semispecific
Syrphus spp.		Syrphidae	Accidental
Wohlfahrtia magnifica	Europe; Asia; Africa	Sarcophagidae	Specific
G. Infestation occurring in anus or vagina			
Callitroga americana	Nearctic and Neotropical	Calliphoridae	Specific
Chrysomya bezziana	Oriental; Ethiopian	Calliphoridae	Specific
Sarcophaga carnaria	Europe; Central Asia	Sarcophagidae	Semispecific
Sarcophaga haemorrhoidalis	Practically world-wide	Sarcophagidae	Semispecific
Wohlfahrtia magnifica	Europe; Asia; Africa	Sarcophagidae	Specific
H. Larvae found in bladder or urinary passages			
Fannia canicularis	All regions except Oriental	Muscidae	Accidental
Fannia scalaris	Temperate regions of all continents	Muscidae	Accidental
Musca domestica	Practically world-wide	Muscidae	Accidental
Psychoda albipennis	Palearctic; Ethiopian	Psychodidae	Accidental
Teichomyza fusca	Palearctic; Neotropical	Ephydridae	Accidental
I. Larvae recovered from stomach or intestine (enteric myiasis)			
Calliphora vicina	Temperate regions generally	Calliphoridae	Semispecific
Calliphora vomitoria	North America; Palearctic; Oriental and beyond	Calliphoridae	Semispecific
Chrysomya chloropyga	Ethiopian region	Calliphoridae	Semispecific
Drosophila funebris	North and Central America; Palearctic; Africa; western Australia	Drosophilidae	Accidental
Fannia canicularis	All regions except Oriental	Muscidae	Accidental

Genus and species	General distribution	Dipterous family to which referred	Specific semispecific or accidental
Fannia incisurata	Nearctic; Neotropical; Palearctic	Muscidae	Accidental
Fannia manicata	Nearctic; Palearctic	Muscidae	Accidental
Fannia scalaris	Temperate zones of all continents	Muscidae	Accidental
Gasterophilus spp.		Gasterophilidae	Specific
Hermetia illucens	Nearctic; Neotropical; Malta; South Pacific	Stratiomyidae	Accidental
Hydrotaea meteorica	Holarctic	Muscidae	Accidental
Musca crassirostris	Palearctic; Ethiopian; Oriental	Muscidae	Accidental
Musca domestica	Practically world-wide	Muscidae	Accidental
Muscina stabulans	Practically world-wide	Muscidae	Accidental
Paregle radicum	Nearctic; Palearctic; Australia	Muscidae	Accidental
Piophila casei	Practically world-wide	Piophilidae	Accidental
Psychoda alternata	Practically world-wide	Psychodidae	Accidental
Sarcophaga bullata	Nearctic generally	Sarcophagidae	Semispecific
Sarcophaga haemorrhoidalis	Practically world-wide	Sarcophagidae	Semispecific
Sepsis sp.		Sepsidae	Accidental
Stomoxys calcitrans	Practically world-wide	Muscidae	Accidental
Sylvicola fenestralis	Nearctic; Palearctic	Silvicolidae	Accidental
Thereva nobilitata	Palearctic	Therevidae	Accidental
Tipula spp.?		Tipulidae	Accidental
Tubifera arbustorum	Holarctic; India	Syrphidae	Accidental
Tubifera dimidiata	Nearctic	Syrphidae	Accidental
Tubifera tenax	Practically world-wide	Syrphidae	Accidental

J. Larvae active bloodsuckers

Auchmeromyia luteola	Ethiopian region	Calliphoridae	Specific

to known experts in the field for study. The Bureau of Entomology and Plant Quarantine, U.S. Department of Agriculture, Washington, D.C. is glad to assist in this connection. Large maggots, however, especially those which leave the host of their own volition, are usually in the third, or last, stage of larval development, and possess well-developed characters by which normally trained technicians can make accurate identification in the majority of cases. The Key to Mature Larvae, adapted from James, is intended as a practical aid to pathologists and hospital technicians. An explanation of certain terms and structures will be found in the legend pertaining to Figure 103.

KEY TO MATURE LARVAE OF SPECIES LISTED
IN TABLE 16 *

1. (10) Head distinct, though sometimes retracted into prothorax; antennae recognizably developed and situated on a sclerotized plate; mandibles broad; no free cephalopharyngeal skeleton 2

2. (5) Head complete, never retracted into prothorax 3

3. (4) Each segment of thorax and abdomen divided into two or three annuli, some of which bear transverse, sclerotized bands on dorsal side; last segment in the form of a sclerotized air tube ...... Family PSYCHODIDAE, genus *Psychoda;* examples: *P. albipennis* Zetterstedt, and *P. alternata* Say.

4. (3) No division of thoracic and abdominal segments into annuli (though each abdominal segment may have an anterior restriction); no sclerotized air tube ...... Family SYLVICOLIDAE, genus *Sylvicola;* example: *S. fenestralis* (Scopoli).

5. (2) Head retracted into prothorax, therefore appearing incomplete; no deep incision between head and thorax 6

6. (7) Mandibles opposed, movable horizontally; body always cylindrical, with fingerlike processes around posterior spiracles ....Family TIPULIDAE, genus *Tipula* (?) (forms causing human myiasis not identified in literature beyond family).

7. (6) Mandibles adapted only for vertical movement; body of various forms, but not as in Tipulidae 8

8. (9) Body flattened in form and finely "shagreened"; abdomen with

* *Mintho algira,* family Larvaevoridae, and *Paregle radicum,* family Muscidae, are not included, for lack of reliable diagnostic characters.

spiracles in the lateral position .... Family STRATIOMYIDAE, genus *Hermetia;* example: *H. illucens* (Linnaeus).

9. (8) Body cylindrical, not "shagreened"; abdomen without lateral spiracles; last abdominal segment ending in two points, vertically disposed ...... Family THEREVIDAE, genus *Thereva;* example: *T. nobilitata* Fabricius.

10. (1) Head poorly developed, appearing as a small, unsclerotized segment; antennae absent or obscure, never situated on a sclerotized surface; mandibles replaced by mouth hooks; free, pharyngeal skeleton present 11

11. (18) Typical maggots with smooth surfaces; body tapering and narrow in front, broad and truncate behind; only the last segment with prominent tubercles or processes; posterior spiracles never borne on processes or on a respiratory tube 12

12. (15) Posterior spiracles always sunken in a rounded cavity; inner spiracular slits diverging from one another ventrally ....
.... Family SARCOPHAGIDAE: three genera, *Wohlfahrtia, Sarcophaga, Titanogrypha.* The last is represented by *T. alata* Aldrich, of which only first-stage larvae are known. The others may be separated roughly 13

13. (14) Branches of anterior spiracle few in number, never exceeding ten, and spread out fanlike; form of body more robust ......
Genus *Wohlfahrtia;* examples: *W. vigil* (Walker), *W. nuba* (Wiedemann), *W. opaca* (Coquillet), *W. magnifica* (Schiner).

14. (13) Branches of anterior spiracle more numerous in most species; tubercles above and below posterior spiracular cavity strongly developed; form of body more slender .... Genus *Sarcophaga.* At least twenty-two species are positively recorded as agents of myiasis. They are very difficult to separate even in the adult state, where the male genitalia constitute the most reliable indication of species limits.

15. (12) Posterior spiracles usually flush with the surface of the anal segment; if spiracles lie in a shallow cavity, the inner slits converge ventrally toward the median line 16

16. (17) Slits of posterior spiracles long, slender, and more or less parallel to one another .... Family CALLIPHORIDAE (in part) 56

17. (16) Slits of posterior spiracles either sinuous or short and radially

arranged .... Family MUSCIDAE
(in part) 91

18. (11) Larvae either grublike, or with tubercular or spinous processes on the segments, or with posterior spiracles on individual processes, or at the end of a respiratory tube 19

19. (42) Larvae grublike 20

20. (29) Each posterior spiracle with three well-marked slits 21

21. (28) Larvae with spines; slits of posterior spiracles not sinuous 22

22. (27) Larvae ovate in outline; spiracular slits bent at the middle; spiracular concavity slight or wanting ...... Family GASTER-OPHILIDAE, genus *Gasterophilus* 23

23. (24) Spines on anterior margins of segments arranged in a single row .... *G. nasalis* (Linnaeus).

24. (23) Spines on anterior margins of segments arranged in two rows, the anterior of which is more robust 25

25. (26) Spines large, strong, and rather blunt; at most one or two pairs of spines lacking on dorsum of segment ten; at least one to five spines present on either side of segment eleven, above the lateral line .... *G. intestinalis* (Degeer).

26. (25) Spines small, with slender points; entire dorsum of segment eleven and middle portion of the dorsum of segment ten are spineless ....
.... *G. haemorrhoidalis* (Linnaeus).

27. (22) Larvae more or less pear-shaped; spiracular slits straight and elongate; spiracles in a deep concavity ....
.... Family CUTEREBRIDAE (in part), genus *Derma-tobia;* example: *D. hominis* (Linnaeus Junior).

28. (21) Naked, wrinkled larvae with posterior spiracles widely separated; if otherwise, the spiracular slits are always sinuous ......
.... Family CALLIPHORIDAE (in part)
.... 56

29. (20) Each posterior spiracle with many small openings; slits usually indistinct 30

30. (35) Mouth hooks small and rudimentary .... Family HYPODERMATIDAE, genus *Hypoderma* 31

31. (32) Segment ten devoid of spines; posterior spiracular plate deeply excavated toward the button .... *H. bovis* (Linnaeus)

32. (31) Segment ten with spines on ventral surface; posterior spiracular

plate less conspicuously excavated toward the button 33

33. (34) Segments eight and nine with no posterior bands of spines on dorsal surface; segment ten with ventral spines on anterior portion only; posterior spiracles divergent ....

.... *H. diana* Brauer.

34. (33) Segments eight and nine with posterior bands of spines on dorsal surface; segment ten with ventral spines on posterior portion only; posterior spiracles not divergent ....

.... *H. lineatum* (Villers).

35. (30) Mouth hooks well developed, usually large 36

36. (39) Spines on body surface weak, confined to ventral surface or to anterior margin of dorsal segments ....

.... Family OESTRIDAE 37

37. (38) Posterior spiracles D-shaped, completely surrounding the button .... Genus *Oestrus;* example: *O. ovis* Linnaeus.

38. (37) Posterior spiracles crescent-shaped, never completely surrounding the button (though approaching this condition in some instances) .... Genus *Rhinoestrus;* example: *R. purpureus* (Brauer).

39. (36) Spines on body surface stronger; spines or spinous plates more or less evenly distributed .... Family CUTEREBRIDAE (in part) 40

40. (41) Thick, ovoid species, thickly beset with spines or scales; last segment short; posterior spiracles in a shallow cavity ....

.... Genus *Cuterebra* (only first-stage larva known from man).

41. (40) Elongated species, with spines in patches; last segment conspicuous; posterior spiracles flush with surface, which bears conical extension below .... Genus *Cephenemyia* (of doubtful occurrence in man).

42. (19) Larvae not grublike 43

43. (80) Body with various types of prominences on dorsal and lateral surfaces 44

44. (51) Larvae flattened, with long, filiform processes, more or less branched, borne on sides and dorsum of the segments ....

.... Family MUSCIDAE (in part), genus *Fannia* 45

45. (46) Dorsal and lateral processes similar; those in abdominal region spinulose on basal region only, never pinnate ....
.... *F. canicularis* (Linnaeus).

46. (45) Lateral processes more than twice the length of the dorsal ones; laterals pinnate nearly or quite to apex 47

47. (50) Dorsal processes reduced to mere buttons 48

48. (49) Lateral processes relatively small, the branches of adjacent processes not in contact .... *F. manicata* (Meigen).

49. (48) Lateral processes well developed, the branches of adjacent ones in contact or nearly so ....
.... *F. incisurata* (Zetterstedt).

50. (47) Dorsal processes small, but well developed and spinulose ......
.... *F. scalaris* (Fabricius).

51. (44) Larvae more or less cylindrical; with at most short, unbranched tubercles on sides and dorsum of the segments 52

52. (55) Larvae slightly flattened, usually dirty white in color and less than four mm. in length; posterior spiracles on brown, sclerotized tubercles, each with a single narrow opening ....
.... Family PHORIDAE, genus *Megaselia* 53

53. (54) Paired processes on body segments definitely hairy ....
....................................*M. rufipes* (Meigen).

54. (53) Paired, fleshy processes on body segments not hairy ....
.... *M. scalaris* (Loew).

55. (52) Larvae more nearly cylindrical; posterior spiracles in a cleft on posterior surface of anal segment; each spiracle a flat plate perforated by three slits .... Family
CALLIPHORIDAE (in part), genus *Chrysomya* (in part) 56

56. (69) New World species (limited to Nearctic) 57

57. (62) Ring of posterior spiracle incomplete and not enclosing button, which may be poorly defined 58

58. (59) Posterior margin of segment eleven with dorsal spines; posterior spiracle with a definite button ..... *Phormia regina* (Meigen).

59. (58) Posterior margin of segment eleven without dorsal spines; posterior spiracle without a definite button 60

60. (61) Tracheal trunks leading from posterior spiracles darkly pigmented ....
.... *Callitroga americana* (Cushing and Patton).

61. (60) Tracheal trunks leading from posterior spiracles not pigmented
.... *Callitroga macellaria* (Fabricius).

62. (57) Ring of posterior spiracle complete, though sometimes less distinct in the area of the button 63

63. (66) Accessory oral sclerite present 64

64. (65) Toothlike, apical portion of labial sclerite longer than greatest width of basal portion .... Genus *Calliphora;* example: *C vicina* Robineau-Desvoidy.

65. (64) Toothlike, apical portion of labial sclerite equal in length to greatest width of basal portion .... Genus *Cynomyopsis;* example: *C. cadaverina* (Robineau-Desvoidy).

66. (63) Accessory oral sclerite absent 67

67. (68) A prominent pigmented area below the posterior extremity of the ventral horn of the pharynx .... Genus *Phaenicia;* example: *P. sericata* (Meigen).

68. (67) No pigmented area below the posterior extremity of the ventral horn of the pharynx .... Genus *Lucilia;* example: *L. illustris* (Meigen).

69. (56) Old World species (limited to Ethiopian) 70

70. (75) Maggotlike larvae 71

71. (72) Ring of posterior spiracles incomplete, the button outside the sclerotized area .... Genus *Chrysomya.*

72. (71) Ring of posterior spiracles complete and enclosing the button 73

73. (74) Accessory oral sclerite present .... Genus *Calliphora.*

74. (73) Accessory oral sclerite absent .... Genus *Phaenicia.*

75. (70) Grublike larvae 76

76. (77) Cuticle with few or no spines; anterior spiracles flush with surface; posterior spiracles widely separated; slits straight and short .... Genus *Auchmeromyia;* example: *A. luteola* (Fabricus).

77. (76) Cuticle with obvious spines; anterior spiracles appearing as fingerlike processes borne on stalks; posterior spiracles approximated; slits more or less sinuous 78

78. (79) Spines of cuticle large, not in transverse rows; posterior spiracle large, with three long serpentine slits, sometimes fragmented .... Genus *Stasisia;* example: *S. rodhaini* (Gedoelst).

79. (78) Spines of cuticle small, with a tendency toward grouping in transverse rows; posterior spiracle smaller, with three short,

sinuous slits ....

Genus *Cordylobia;* example: *C. anthropophaga* Grünberg.

80. (43) Body without such processes, or at most with prolegs 81

81. (82) Posterior spiracles at the end of a long, retractile respiratory tube, which may exceed in length the body proper ....
.... Family SYRPHIDAE (in part), genus *Tubi-fera (Eristalis)*; examples: *T. arbustorum* (Linnaeus), *T. dimidiata* (Wiedemann), *T. tenax* (Linnaeus).

82. (81) Posterior spiracles at most on a short respiratory process much shorter than the body length 83

83. (84) Robust larvae, broad behind and tapering before; posterior spiracles small, closely adjacent and located at extremity of a short respiratory tube ...... Family SYRPHIDAE (in part), genus *Syrphus.*

84. (83) Body not as above; posterior spiracles on separate tubercles or at the end of a forked process 85

85. (88) Very slender larvae; posterior spiracles borne at apices of short cones 86

86. (87) Anal segment with a pair of tapered, ventrolateral processes which point slightly upward; skipping forms .... Family *Piophilidae,* genus *Piophila;* example: *P. casei* (Linnaeus).

87. (86) Ventrolateral processes of anal segment not as above; not skipping forms .... Family SEPSIDAE, genus *Sepsis.*

88. (85) Moderately stout larvae; posterior spiracles at the end of branches of a forked process 89

89. (90) No prolegs on either thoracic or abdominal segments .... Family DROSOPHILIDAE, genus *Drosophila;* example: *D. funebris* (Fabricius).

90. (89) Prolegs on last two thoracic and first six abdominal segments .... Family EPHYDRIDAE, genus *Teichomyza;* example: *T. fusca* Macquart.

91. (94) Slits of posterior spiracles straight or arcuate 92

92. (93) Slits nearly straight ....
.... Genus *Hydrotaea;* example: *H. meteorica* (Linnaeus).

93. (92) Slits distinctly arcuate ....
.... Genus *Muscina;* example: *M. stabulans* (Fallén).

94. (91) Slits of posterior spiracles strongly sinuous 95

95. (98) Slits each with two loops; posterior end of larva with setulose tubercles on ventral side 96

96. (97) Posterior face of larva almost as broad as high; setulose tubercles not particularly prominent; spiracular slits surrounding the button ...... Genus *Stomoxys;* example: *S. calcitrans* (Linnaeus).

97. (96) Posterior face of larva nowhere near as broad as high; setulose tubercles always prominent; spiracular slits not surrounding the button ....
Genus *Synthesiomyia;* example: *S. nudiseta* (Van der Wulp).

98. (95) Slits each with three loops or more; posterior end smoothly rounded ....
...........Genus *Musca* 99

99. (100) Posterior spiracles heavily sclerotized, with no peritreme (ring) .... *M. crassirostris* Stein.

100. (99) Posterior spiracles with a distinct ring or peritreme ....
.... *M. domestica* Linnaeus and *M. vicina* Macquart.

It will be noted from the Key to Mature Larvae (and from Table 16) that approximately twenty families are involved in the production of myiasis in man. Although the housefly and its immediate relatives appear only in relation to certain types of infestation, it is significant that muscoid families, in the broad sense of the term, practically dominate the picture. The very large number of Sarcophagidae, Calliphoridae, and Muscidae, for example, stand in strong contrast to the occasional representatives of the Tipulidae, Psychodidae, Sylvicolidae, Stratiomyidae, and other nonmuscoid groups.

The discussion that follows is divided into two parts. The first deals with parasitic activities of larvae of the genus *Musca;* the second, with conditions in which species of other genera are chiefly concerned.

SPECIAL RELATIONS OF THE GENUS *MUSCA* TO THE OCCURRENCE OF MYIASIS IN MAN

Musca crassirostris Stein, the adult of which possesses rasping labella and sucks blood, rarely parasitizes man in the larval state. Several cases of intestinal myiasis, however, are on record from India, probably connected, as suggested by Patton, with the religious rite of eating the five products of the cow, including a small quantity of fresh manure. An equally interesting explanation is suggested by Onorato (1922) for the occurrence of *M. crassirostris* in the alimentary tract of an indigent patient in Tripolitania. Onorato (who refers to this species as *Musca [Philaematomyia] insignis* Austen) mentions that poor folk in that country frequently search through deposits of

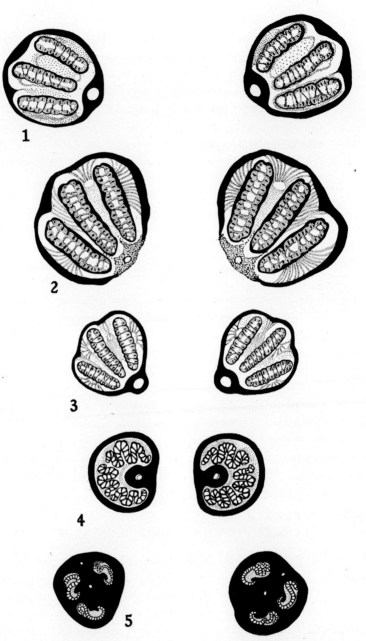

Figure 104. Posterior spiracles of third stage larvae. Myiasis-producing forms may be distinguished by the structural peculiarities of the ring, button, and slits. Distance between the two spiracles is also used. *1: Calliphora vomitoria. 2: Phormia regina. 3: Lucilia sericata. 4: Musca domestica. 5: Stomoxys calcitrans.* Drawn to scale. (Matheson, *Medical Entomology;* Comstock Publishing Co.)

horse dung for undigested grains of barley. It is easy to understand how soiled hands may have transferred eggs or larvae to the patient's food.

Musca sorbens Wiedemann, though a very common housefly in many tropical and near-tropical areas, is not known to be involved in human myiasis of any type.

Musca domestica Linnaeus, on the other hand, and its doubtfully separable variety *M. vicina* Macquart, appear rather frequently in published records, as might be expected from the nearly world-wide distribution of the species. Both intestinal and gastric infestations have been repeatedly observed, as have cases of urinary, traumatic, and cuticular myiasis. Nasal, aural, and ocular infestations are on record also. In general, a diseased condition of the tissue seems to be prerequisite for any attack not of an enteric nature, where *M. domestica* is concerned. A few modern records follow.

Frison (1925) reported on a case in Illinois in which larvae, less than half grown, were vomited by a boy recovering from pneumonia. Others were passed in the feces on the same day. The sickroom was not screened against flies, and it is probable that the eggs were deposited directly on the patient's mouth.

Kelevin and Ruibina (1940) record the recovery of eight living larvae of *Musca domestica* from the infected ear of a young boy. Flies had undoubtedly been attracted by a purulent discharge.

Urethral myiasis in Rumania due to *Musca domestica* is described by Leon (1921). The patient was a young man who had slept without pajamas because of extreme heat. He was recovering from a blennorrhea, and still had a slight discharge. Oviposition probably took place in the early morning. The body heat in the folds of the prepuce presumably stimulated hatching within a few hours. Eight larvae were discharged by the patient, along with seminal fluid, in the presence of Mr. Leon. Mumford (1926) records two cases of urethral myiasis in northern England, due to *Musca domestica* and *Fannia canicularis*.

Natvig (1932) found *Musca domestica* larvae in stools of a patient suffering intestinal symptoms. Rao (1929) reared several larvae from nasal lesions in lepers. In one of two cases the species proved to be *M. domestica*. The same author found housefly larvae associated with *Sarcophaga* in wounds. A rather interesting case is that of Rennie (1927), who found larvae of *M. domestica* in the feces of a breast-fed infant in northern Scotland. He concluded that oviposition on or near the anus was more probable than on the lips or nostrils. Yatsenko and associates discuss the case of a boy six years old who voided larvae of *M. domestica* in his urine on two occasions, a number of months

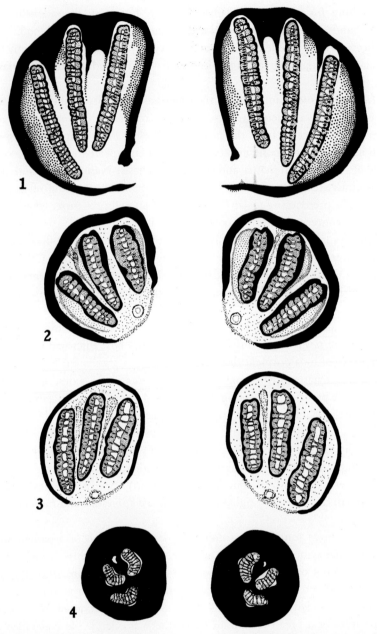

Figure 105. Posterior spiracles of third-stage larvae. These drawings are made on the same scale as those in Figure 104. *1: Sarcophaga bullata. 2: Callitroga macellaria. 3: Wohlfahrtia vigil. 4: Muscina stabulans.* (Matheson, *Medical Entomology;* Comstock Publishing Co.)

apart. Several of the larvae were seen protruding from the urethra. It was assumed that the eggs were laid on a dirty sheet in the child's bed.

Cutaneous myiasis in man due to *Musca domestica* is recorded by Patton and Cookson (1925). A rather complete account of this case has been given in Chapter VII.

An indirect relation between *M. domestica* and specific, dermal myiasis exists in the fact that houseflies, with various other species of insects, may serve as transport hosts for the eggs of *Dermatobia hominis,* well-known neotropical human botfly. The heat of the human body is apparently sufficient to cause hatching of the eggs as the housefly crawls upon the skin. The relationship is recorded by Neiva and Gomes (1917) and discussed by De Almeida (1933). Dunn (1930), in experiments performed upon himself, observed that larvae of *D. hominis* sometimes require as long as an hour and a half to burrow into the integument.

SELECTED EXAMPLES OF MYIASIS PRODUCED BY MUSCOIDEAN SPECIES NOT OF THE GENUS *MUSCA*

Anduze (1945) discusses human myiasis in Venezuela. *Dermatobia hominis* is common in that country. He also records accidental infestation by *Cuterebra,* nasal myiasis due to infestation with *Calliphora,* and gastrointestinal myiasis due to *Sarcophaga.*

Beachley and Bishop (1942) reported a case of nasal myiasis in Arlington County, Virginia, due to infestation with *Cuterebra.* A first-instar maggot was removed from the patient's nose. Another record pertaining to the same genus was published by Bequaert (1945), this time a dermal infestation of the furuncular type. The specimen, which proved to be a third-instar larva of *Cuterebra buccata,* was embedded in the skin of the chest, close to the nipple. The patient, a mature man, lived in very poor circumstances.

Pavlovsky and Stein (1924) record *Gasterophilus,* enteric parasite of horses, as a cutaneous parasite of man. A similar condition is reported by Stewart (1929) as due to the larva of *Phormia regina* Meigen.

The genus *Wohlfahrtia* is of considerable importance. *Wohlfahrtia magnifica,* which is found both in Europe and in Asia, is a serious cause of traumatic and nasal myiasis. Its biology has been thoroughly discussed by Portchinsky (1916). A number of cases of *magnifica* infection have resulted fatally. In North America, *Wohlfahrtia vigil* and, more rarely, *W. opaca* have been incriminated as causing a furuncular type of cutaneous myiasis, especially in children. A number of papers by Walker (1920, 1922, 1937) deal with *W. vigil,* which is also discussed by Kingscotte (1935) and by Silverthorne and Brown (1934). The latter authors describe three cases of myiasis in healthy infants who slept out of doors during the month of June in Montreal. Norma Ford (1932, 1936) gives a good account of the ovipositional activities of *W. vigil.* She describes how a female, under her observation, poured out a stream of white larvae on the head of a guinea pig, near the eye. In a few seconds, the actively moving maggots had disappeared among the hairs. In the case of infants, the larvae are usually deposited upon the cheek. They may migrate a considerable distance before penetrating the skin. It apparently is not necessary for the child to be in an unclean condition to be attractive to the flies.

Gerston and his associates (1933) reported on two cases of *Wohlfahrtia* infestation in North Dakota. In one, the larva was found in the base of the penis of an infant of four months. The second case involved the upper eyelid of a child eight months of age.

All members of the genus, however, do not seem to be as pathogenic as *W. vigil* or *W. magnifica.* Grantham-Hill (1933) found *Wohlfahrtia nuba* actually beneficial in the treatment of infected wounds, and considered it quite as satisfactory as *Lueilia* for maggot therapy.

Mention of cutaneous myiasis would be incomplete without reference to the tumbu fly, *Cordylobia anthropophaga* Grünberg. The female lays her five hundred or more eggs on soiled bedding, clothing, or soil fouled with human or animal discharges. The larvae hatch in about forty-eight hours and penetrate the skin of any available person or small animal. According to Cuthbertson (1942), infants and young children are more commonly affected than mature hosts. The parasites cause boillike tumors, within which all three larval stages are passed. Larval development is completed in eight or nine days, after which the larvae seek the ground for pupation. Dogs, guinea pigs, and rats are commonly infested. Rats are perhaps the normal hosts and undoubtedly serve as the principal reservoir in nature.

Patton (1935) divided the producers of specific myiasis into two groups according to whether or not the flies oviposit in close proximity to the tissues to be invaded. The African genus *Cordylobia* and the new-world genus *Dermatobia* fall into the same classification in this respect, since neither requires the presence of the host. *Dermatobia,* however, is unique in making use of a mosquito, fly, or other transport host to which the eggs are glued.

Most serious of all species from a pathogenic viewpoint is *Callitroga* (*Chrysomya*) *americana* (Cushing and Patton). This "primary screwworm" invades any wound, however trivial, and proceeds to the rapid destruction of healthy tissue. Great economic loss may result from infestation of freshly dehorned or castrated animals, or of those which have had the skin broken in some other way. Invasion of the human eye, ear, nasal passage, or sinuses is likely to result fatally if left untreated. The patient suffers excruciating pain. Frequently associated with this species is *Callitroga macellaria* (Fabricius), but this is normally a secondary invader, attracted by the odors and discharges resulting from the presence of *C. americana* or some other primary parasite. Large numbers of *C. macellaria* may, however, greatly complicate the pathology and so become a factor in bringing about the death of the host.

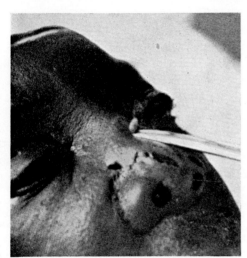

Figure 106. Patient suffering from infection with *Callitroga americana* C. & P. Over 230 larvae were removed from the nasal passages. (From *Manual of Tropical Medicine*, by Mackie, Hunter, and Worth [L. S. West, collaborator]; courtesy of W. B. Saunders Company.)

Pine tar oil has been found effective as a repellent against blowflies of animals and has also been used successfully to induce spontaneous emergence of screwworm larvae from the nasal passages in man (McGovran and Ellisor, 1936; McGovran, 1938).

The old-world screwworm fly, *Chrysomya bezziana* Villeneuve, is almost as serious a pathogen as *Callitroga americana*. Man suffers most from its attacks in India, while cattle seem more subject to infestation in Africa. Patton (1920a, 1922d) describes a total of fifty-nine cases in man and seventy-one in animals. Infestation of the nasal passages and related parts is particularly dangerous, and loss of sight or hearing is not uncommon, if the infection does not prove fatal.

An interesting case of myiasis due to *C. bezziana* is recorded by Strickland and Roy (1941), in which a larva was found within the dura mater of the spinal cord.

Ocular myiasis in man is almost always due either to *Oestrus ovis* L., common head bot of sheep, or *Rhinoestrus purpureus* Brauer, which normally develops in the nasal passages of horses. Gómez (1946) states that infestation by the former is much commoner in Spain, where only one of eighteen cases recorded since 1918 is known definitely to have been caused by *Rhinoestrus*. Gómez describes two varieties of *O. ovis,* var. *granatae,* from Granada, and var. *corsicae,* from the island of Corsica. They are distinguished by the form of the spiracles.

Oestrus ovis as a cause of human myiasis in France is recorded by Larrousse (1921) and Galliard (1934). Manine (1941) and Pédoya (1941) have published similar records from North Africa. *Rhinoestrus purpureus,* as a cause of human ocular myiasis, is discussed by Portchinsky (1915).

An example of ophthalmomyiasis caused by a species other than these is recorded by Nájera Angulo (1942). He describes the case of a ten-year-old boy who developed marked edema after being "stung" in the eye, and from whom were removed three larvae of *Wohlfahrtia magnifica* forty-eight hours later. Another record, likewise from Spain, reports approximately 140 *W. magnifica* larvae from a human eye!

Such records, however, are not common. James (1944) points out that the supposed occurrence of *Wolhfahrtia vigil* in a cyst in the human eye, as reported by Felt, is in error. Subsequent publication of a photograph makes clear that *Oestrus ovis* was the species involved.

ENTERIC MYIASIS

A case of gastrointestinal myiasis extending over a period of several years is recorded by Vartiainen (1946). At the age of forty-four, the patient, a farmer's wife, began to notice symptoms of mild abdominal distress. This continued for some six years, after which the pain became more severe, with occasional attacks of colic. During the next four years, the patient observed numerous larvae in the feces, especially during the summer months. The few that were identified proved to be of the genus *Calliphora*. It would appear that some peculiarity in personal habits must have favored the reinfection of this woman, year after year.

Intestinal myiasis has also been traced to *Lucilia*. Webster (1945) describes a patient who suffered from intermittent diarrhea for six or seven months. Third-instar larvae were eventually passed in the stools. The host proved also to be harboring *Ascaris lumbricoides*.

Probably 75 per cent of all gastrointestinal myiasis in man is caused by either *Fannia scalaris* (Fabricius) or *F. canicularis* (Linnaeus). The peculiar, flattened larvae with their characteristic dorsal and lateral processes are not easily mistaken. Hewitt (1912b,d) has summarized the biology and pathogenesis of these forms, which may also infest the urinary tract. There are many subsequent records. *Fannia scalaris* is generally known as the "latrine fly"; *F. canicularis,* as the "lesser housefly."

The whole question of gastrointestinal myiasis has been much discussed and several responsible investigators have challenged the authenticity of published records.

Komárek (1936) found that the larvae of *Calliphora vomitoria, Sarcophaga carnaria, Musca domestica,* and *Piophila casei* cannot survive long in the absence of atmospheric oxygen and that they are quickly killed by the digestive juices of cats. Causey (1938) performed similar experiments, using both cats and dogs, and observed that all larvae were either killed or immobilized in the stomach within three hours. Upon subsequent passage into the intestine, they were digested. Earlier works by Desoil (1924) showed that though ova of *Calliphora vomitoria* could resist the effects of gastric juice "in vitro" for a period equal to that required for normal digestion, other factors made survival "in vivo" doubtful or impossible. He concluded that for this species, at least, intestinal myiasis may not be produced by swallowing of the eggs.

Kenney (1945) fed living maggots of *Calliphora, Sarcophaga,* and *Musca domestica* to sixty human volunteers. All but ten suffered gastrointestinal symptoms, such as nausea, vomiting, cramps, or diarrhea. Within forty-eight hours, however, all larvae had been eliminated, either by way of the vomitus or in the stools. Only a very few larvae were still alive. This put an end to all symptoms and led Kenney to conclude that a true myiasis had not existed. Strickland and Roy (1940) failed to infect rabbits with first-stage larvae of *Musca domestica* fed in milk.

In spite of these demonstrations, there seems no doubt that genuine enteric myiasis does occur from time to time, when chemical and physical conditions within the patient's alimentary tract are such as to favor survival of the parasites. That many individuals are habitual "air swallowers" is well known. In such cases, the larvae should have little difficulty in obtaining at least a minimum supply of oxygen. Again, human beings vary greatly in the amount and concentration of hydrochloric acid produced in the stomach. Carnivores especially are usually characterized by a heavier secretion of hydrochloric acid than man, a fact which tends to make the cat (or dog) somewhat unsuitable as a test animal where borderline conditions may be involved. Riley (1939) has made a judicious analysis of the arguments on both sides, and concludes that intestinal myiasis, though of relatively rare occurrence, is an established clinical condition, a conclusion substantiated by the repeated observations of reputable physicians and entomologists.

THERAPEUTIC MYIASIS

In the period following World War I, the use of maggots in the treatment of certain traumatic conditions and infections became very popular among clinicians, particularly those groups whose duties involved the handling of chronic osteomyelitis.

Livingston and Prince (1932) point out that as early as the sixteenth century, Paré had noted the very satisfactory healing of infected wounds in which larvae of blowflies had become established. Larrey, surgeon to Napoleon, made similar observations during the Syrian campaign. World War I, with its emphasis on trench warfare, furnished many excellent examples, as a result of wounded soldiers' being stranded in no man's land for sometimes as many as seven days without hospital attention. Those whose wounds had become flyblown were almost always in better condition than the others. Fever was less common and healthy granulation tissue had taken the place of pus and other debris.

Baer, in two papers (1929, 1931), advocated the use of maggot therapy in cases of osteomyelitis and reported on various cases so treated. His interpretation of the reasons for success may be summarized as follows:

(1) The maggots clear away tissue sloughs and minute fragments of bone by digestive action.

(2) Wounds infested with maggots tend to become alkaline, and thus inhospitable to many pathogenic bacteria of acidophilic nature.

(3) Certain biochemical effects are produced which greatly stimulate the healing process.

Since the death of Baer, the third point has been more extensively investigated, and has proved to be by far the most important.

Stewart (1934) added the following observations and suggestions:

(1) Bacteria ingested with necrotic tissue are practically all killed by the acids in the mid-gut of the larva.

(2) Alkalinization is accomplished chiefly by the excretion of ammonia and calcium carbonate.

(3) The exuded calcium carbonate stimulates phagocytosis.

(4) Bacterial exotoxins are presumably rendered inert by the acids of the larva's mid-gut.

(5) The formation of granulation tissue may be due to stimulation by exuded calcium ions.

Robinson, in a series of papers (1935, 1937, 1940a,b), has thrown much added light on the nature of larval secretions. Both allantoin and urea are produced by the maggots, the urea probably resulting from a splitting off of one of the side chains of allantoin, through hydrolysis. Both these substances have marked healing properties, a principle discovered by Macalister in 1912 but apparently forgotten until the use of maggot therapy called attention to the biochemistry involved. Robinson also pointed out the tissue-stimulating qualities of ammonium bicarbonate, another product of maggot metabolism. Its occurrence is associated with the enzyme urease in the tissues of the larvae. A sterile solution of the bicarbonate in concentration of 1 or 2 per cent, applied with gauze packs, shows healing properties comparable to those of allantoin.

Earlier studies by Robinson and Norwood (1933, 1934) had particularly emphasized the destruction of pathogenic bacteria in the alimentary canal of the living larvae. Bactericidal substances are also undoubtedly given off in the natural excretions of the maggots. In this relation, Simmons (1935a,b) has demonstrated the presence in such excretions of a thermostable substance capable of destroying *Closterium welchii, Staphylococcus aureus,* and a number of hemolytic streptococci.

The selection of suitable species for use in maggot therapy requires knowledge of the feeding habits of the larvae. *Lucilia sericata,*[1] *Lucilia caesar, Phormia regina,* and *Wolhfahrtia nuba* have been preferred, as these species tend to confine their activities to necrotic tissue and thus are unlikely, of themselves, to bring about a myiasis of pathological type. Forms such as *Callitroga americana, Chrysomya bezziana,* or *Wohlfahrtia magnifica* are, of course, entirely unsuitable. The use of *Musca domestica* for this purpose seems to have been confined largely to European countries. Paramonov, in two papers (1934a,b), discusses maggot therapy in the treatment of gangrene, osteomyelitis, and similar conditions, and reports specifically on the experiments of Dr. W. M. Schkaláberd, of Kiev, with housefly larvae. Twenty to thirty larvae of *Musca domestica* were placed in wounds of three cases where gas gangrene had become established and amputation seemed the only possible procedure. After forty-eight hours, healing was proceeding so satisfactorily that any thought of amputating was abandoned. *Musca domestica* would certainly be safer than *Calliphora,* for example, as it is less likely to invade healthy tissue.

[1] Not all strains of *L. sericata* are equally benign. In China it produces a serious myiasis. It is also recorded as dangerous in Africa and in Europe. The older larvae, especially, tend to bore deeply in healthy tissue.

In recent years, the use of maggots has been rather generally abandoned in favor of direct treatment with allantoin, urea, and ammonium carbonate. Not only is this more satisfactory from the viewpoint of avoiding injury by the larvae; it also insures against introducing dangerous infection from other sources. In the early days of maggot therapy, cases of tetanus were sometimes traced to contaminated larvae. The development of special techniques for the sterile rearing of maggots for surgical use soon solved this problem, but the rather tedious task of maintaining sterile colonies still remained. Today maggot therapy may be considered of historical rather than current importance. A concise summary of the subject may be found in Steinhaus' excellent volume, *Insect Microbiology* (1946).

This chapter may appropriately be terminated with a somewhat quaint observation by B. D. Walsh (1870), who recognized the significance of larvae in human stools and ventured a bit of apt advice for those who cared to heed it:

Moral—Avoid eating decayed fruit . . . and from fruit which is only partially decayed pare away carefully the unsound parts before you introduce the sounder portions into your stomach. Every entomologist knows what a pleasing pursuit it is to breed insects through all their stages in appropriate vessels; but to breed them in one's own body is rather too much of a good thing.

CHAPTER XIV

Are Flies Beneficial?

Achilles: But I have grievous fear lest, meantime, on the gashed wounds of Menoitios' valiant son [Patroklos], flies light and breed maggots therein and defile his corpse—for the life is slain out of him—and so all his flesh shall rot.—Homer, Iliad

ACHILLES' familiarity with nature's instruments for the destruction of animal bodies reminds us that without these agencies the world might well be a very different place from what it is. Without them the continuous and rapid overturn of both organic and inorganic food materials, which seems so commonplace today, might become extremely difficult, if not impossible. Along with saprophytic bacteria, various fungi, and certain protozoans, insects and their larvae reduce prodigious amounts of plant and animal debris to simple form. This material thus becomes available again for utilization in the basic nutrition of photosynthetic plants. It is difficult to imagine a world piled high with the dead bodies of overage trees, whales, and dinosaurs, yet such indeed might be the picture, had not lesser forms of life survived to perform this significant function.

Thus we are challenged, even as we gird ourselves for the possible extermination of these enemies of humankind, by the realization that all forms of life are interdependent, that nothing is wholly good or wholly evil from the standpoint of nature's economy, and that it is only our own anthropocentric approach which determines whether a species shall be considered useful, useless, or detrimental. In all fairness to biological principle, we cannot justifiably condemn the fly as unfit to live in modern society without first hearing the argument for the defense, slender as that argument may be.

In five respects, at least, muscoid Diptera are capable of benefiting man. The first, already referred to, consists of the ability of the larvae to assist in the reduction of plant and animal remains. The second pertains to the use of larvae to stimulate the healing of infected wounds. A third benefit results from the activity of dipterous larvae as parasites within the bodies of noxious insect hosts. A fourth and obvious benefit derives from the immense numbers of flies, larvae, and pupae which feed and nourish other forms of animal life valued by man. Of lesser consequence, but not to be overlooked, is the flower-visiting habit which many adult Diptera practice, thus assisting in pollination and subsequent reproduction of green plants. In addition, there are certain less tangible benefits which, for want of a better term, may be called aesthetic and which are no less real because of their less mundane qualities. We shall consider each of the foregoing possibilities in turn.

FLIES AS SCAVENGERS

Sibthorpe (1896) voiced an opinion not uncommon in his day, namely, that flies perform a very important function as scavengers and that their activities therefore actually contribute to the abatement of cholera in a community! While the latter concept seems diametrically opposed to the truth, the first portion of the statement deserves some analysis.

The essential distinction here is between the activities of the larvae and the behavior of the adult fly. The latter, by her restless migrations, is an unpardonable offender against the laws of sanitary science. The larva, however, remaining as it does in close proximity to the place of its origin, spreads little or no infection (except as certain organisms may occasionally remain in larval tissues, survive pupation, and so be available for distribution in the excretions of the winged insect).

The rapidity with which larvae, when present in numbers, can reduce animal bodies to skeletons is striking. Conditions must, of course, be favorable. Warm summer temperatures are most ideal, for obvious reasons. First, bacterial decomposition gets under way more promptly if temperatures are rather high, thus contributing to the odors which emanate from carcasses and excite the olfactory structures of female flies ready for oviposition. Well known among the odoriferous substances produced by putrefaction is cadaverine, a nitrogenous base with the chemical name *pentamethylenediamine* and the formula $NH_2CH_2(CH_2)_3CH_2NH_2$. To human beings, its odor is most repellent! Among the organisms capable of producing cadaverine is the Finkler-Prior bacillus (*Vibrio proteus*), also *Vibrio comma*. Other substances attractive to ovipositing flies are ammonia, urea, and carbon dioxide, all more or less universally present when animal bodies decompose. The same higher temperatures which favor the production of odoriferous substances likewise favor activity on the part of the flies, which roam farther and change position more frequently on warmer days. It is also well known that the larvae, once established, feed more ravenously and complete their development more quickly at temperatures in the upper bracket of the tolerated range.

Another factor, closely related to the above, is sunshine. It is the author's personal observation that houseflies and blowflies seem to find exposed carcasses more readily on sunny days than in dull, cloudy weather, if temperature conditions remain the same. In this relation, it should be borne in mind that when a storm is brewing, the behavior of flies sometimes becomes most erratic (see Chapter IX). This diversion from normal activity may well account for the flies' seeming to overlook opportunities for oviposition when atmospheric pressures are suddenly disturbed.

A third and very important limiting factor is the intensity of the wind. With no wind at all, the attractive odors spread only by diffusion, or perhaps slightly by convection, as decomposition causes the carcass to develop a temperature higher than that of the surrounding air. In either case only flies in the immediate vicinity are quickly attracted to the scene. At the opposite extreme, a strong wind or gale is likewise deterrent to ready visitation by flies, for two reasons: From the windward side no flies are attracted at all, as the strong wind sweeps all odors in the opposite direction. On the leeward side, though the odors are carried great distances, the insects are unable to make headway against the wind, and must await its subsidence before they are able to locate the source. Ideal for the encouragement of oviposition are light, variable winds, the gentler the better, in most instances. Undiluted odors drift long distances on such air currents, yet the females have no difficulty in flying upwind to locate a suitable place to lay their eggs. Also, if there are frequent changes of direction, a much wider area will receive the stimulus than when air movement continues in the same direction throughout the day.

It is not certain whether relative humidity is a strong factor either in the dissemination of odors or in the responses of the fly to olfactory stimulation. To the human subject, at least, odors usually seem more pronounced in moisture-laden air.

The activity of the larvae in the carcass is less apparent at first, more obvious as days go by. The capacity of the second-stage larvae to devour food is many times that of the first, and the third stage is truly remarkable for its voraciousness. The catholicity of taste of housefly maggots enables them to utilize practically any portion of a carcass, regardless of the state of decomposition. Hourly arrival of new ovipositing females, plus the return of first-brood adults to oviposit in the same environment, causes the process to pyramid in the second and third weeks, until perhaps the entire carcass (or cadaver) appears to be made up of nothing but a crawling mass of eager, writhing maggots, seeking the last available residue by which life may be sustained. And so the process terminates, the final, half-starved brood either transforming at substandard size or failing to pupate altogether. Under wilderness conditions the mechanism is most adequate. Where human beings live as neighbors, however, it will not serve. Too much time is required, during which offensive odors prevail, flies transfer bacteria from the decomposing animal to human habitations, and, what is far worse, thousands of flies are produced which range afar and menace human health in a hundred other ways. Under civilized conditions, then, the beneficial effects of flies, acting as scavengers, appear to be entirely nullified by the dangers and inconveniences involved. Consignment to the glue factory for larger animals and incineration for the smaller, or deep burial for all, should be standard practice in rural areas in a modern age.

LARVAE AS AGENTS IN THE HEALING OF WOUNDS

This phase has been treated more or less fully in Chapter XIII. Apparently very little real benefit results from mechanical cleansing of the wounds by the feeding activities of the larvae. Of much greater value are the products of larval metabolism, such as allantoin, urea, and ammonium carbonate. Of course, only those species which refrain from destroying healthy tissue are beneficial in this respect, or can be used in maggot therapy.

LARVAE AS PARASITES OF NOXIOUS FORMS

There is no record that *Musca domestica* or any other member of the genus acts as a parasite of insects or other arthropods. Within the muscoid series, however, occurs the large and widespread family known as the Tachinidae, now generally considered as including the Phasiidae and Dexiidae of various writers. So conceived, the Tachinidae are probably the most beneficial single family of insects known. These species spend the larval period as rather poorly adapted parasites within the bodies of Arthropoda. In almost all cases the host is eventually killed or at least rendered incapable of reproduction. The importance of such parasites as a factor in the natural control of economic pests is enormous. True, the honeybee and silkworm also have their tachinid parasites, but such hosts are exceptional and the vast majority of these flies prey upon forms which man greatly desires to reduce or eliminate. As long ago as 1908 Williston listed 400 species parasitic on Lepidoptera, 70 on Hymenoptera, 40 on Coleoptera, 20 on Orthoptera, 5 on Hemiptera, and 5 on Diptera. Since then many additional records have been added. Earwigs and sow bugs are also listed among tachinid hosts. Lepidoptera, Hymenoptera, and Diptera are usually attacked in their immature stages, while Orthoptera, Hemiptera, and Coleoptera are commonly parasitized as adults.

The manner in which the adult fly deposits its egg (or larva) on or near the host differs with the species. Prell (1914) recognized six biological groups, based on reproductive habits. In Group 1, which includes perhaps 75 per cent of all Tachinidae, the large, whitish eggs are merely glued fast to the external surface of the host's body. The larvae hatch and bore directly through the integument. There is evidence (West, 1923) that occasionally the host manifests an immunity and that the larvae, though successful in their invasion of the host, may nevertheless fail to develop. The second group, which includes such forms as *Hyalomyia,* possess sharp, pointed ovipositors by which the female is able to insert the egg more or less deeply within the tissues of the host. In Group 3, the flies deposit tiny "microtype" eggs on foliage of the plant species which the host caterpillar uses as food. Digestive juices of the host stimulate hatching of the egg before it can be swept out of the alimentary canal with the frass. This method is obviously wasteful of eggs unless the hosts are so abundant as to strip the foliage almost completely. *Blepharipa scutellata* is a parasite of such habits.

The remaining groups differ from the first three in that all species are larviparous. In Group 4, of which *Blepharipeza* is an example, the living larva is deposited directly upon the integument of the host. The parasite penetrates the cuticle at once. Most members of the subfamily Dexiinae are believed to employ this method. Group 5 differs in that the females possess an intromittent ovipositor by which the larvae are inserted into host tissue. *Compsilura, Lydella,* and *Vibrissina* are representative genera. The last group, exemplified by *Panzeria,* deposits the living larva in the general vicinity of the host. The larva is often attached to a twig on which the caterpillar has left a silken thread and along which it will probably return. The little larvae become very excited as the host approaches, wave their heads about, and, if contact is established, attach themselves to the host insect by means of their mouth hooks. Penetration of the integument follows immediately.

Pyraustomyia penitalis is perhaps unique in depositing "eggs" near the entrance hole of its borer host (*Pyrausta*). After hatching, the first-stage maggot by its own activity seeks and invades the body of the host insect.

Regardless of mode of entry, the first-stage larva usually lies free, either in the body cavity or in the foreintestine of the host. There it absorbs both oxygen and nourishment from tissue fluids and rarely attacks the host tissue. Second and third stages, however, require a greater air supply, which they usually secure by making an opening in the host's body wall by means of their mouth hooks. The host tissue, thus irritated, responds by invaginating in such a way as to form an "integumentary funnel." The parasite lives from then on in this funnel of host tissue, with the posterior spiracles directed outward, whence comes its air supply. Sometimes the integumentary funnel extends from a tracheal trunk, rather than from the body wall. The parasite molts to the third stage *in situ*. When nearly full grown, the maggot actually becomes a predator and devours the vital organs of the host. If a number of larvae should find themselves competing for nourishment within a single host, it is usually only the largest and strongest which survives. Cannibalism is common.

Pupation may take place either in the soil or within the dried skin of the host, depending on the particular species of fly.

Most Tachinidae are able to parasitize a number of closely related host species of reasonably similar habits. They are thus able to maintain themselves by use of second- and third-choice hosts during periods in which the preferred host may be numerically scarce.

FLIES AS FOOD FOR OTHER ORGANISMS

One has only to observe a flock of chickens about a barnyard manure pile to realize that maggots go far in providing nourishment for scratching birds. In this connection, Feldman-Muhsam (1944a) has even suggested the intentional rearing of fly larvae for use as poultry food. He recommends wetting of the dung at the proper stage of development, so that the larvae will migrate from the interior and fall into a dish, or vessel, conveniently arranged. Very large numbers can be obtained by this method, which also lends itself to the feeding of insectivorous birds confined in zoological gardens, usually a vexing problem for caretakers and veterinarians. The same technique may be employed to produce pupae needed for experimental purposes.

A chemical analysis of the fly maggots shows that they contain very close to 71.4 per cent water, 18.6 per cent protein, 5 per cent fat, and 5 per cent of other substances, chiefly carbohydrates and salts. The vitamin content of active maggots is somewhat interesting. They are rich in riboflavin, which is present to the extent of 3 milligrams per 100 grams of larval tissue. Carotins make a poorer showing, totaling only 0.4 milligrams per 100 grams of larva. No true vitamin A content has yet been found.

The use of artificial manure, such as macerated leaves of dock, has been attempted at experimental stations as a lure for ovipositing flies. Pans of such material in which larvae are developing may be placed in various situations where they will be found by growing pheasants, for example, a species which requires an abundance of protein food. The provision of a constant supply of maggots, regardless of weather conditions, is not always easy, and for this reason many regard the procedure as somewhat impractical. The principle, however, is sound, and should prove of future value in various phases of game management.

The contribution which larvae and pupae make to the diet of walking and scratching birds, great as it is, is probably not to be compared with the tonnage of adult insects consumed by birds in flight. How great a percentage of this consists of muscoid forms is difficult to say, but that common flies contribute their appropriate share need not be doubted. In this connection, day-flying insectivores, such as the flycatchers (Tyrannidae), of course stand to profit more abundantly than crepuscular or nocturnal species, such as night-hawks and whippoorwills, which feed at a time when muscoid Diptera are rarely or never on the wing.

POLLINATION OF FLOWERS

Musca domestica is rarely, if ever, a flower feeder. With a proboscis so poorly adapted for probing into nectaries, it is not to be wondered at that the housefly prefers the honeypot of the human table. Malodorous flowers do, indeed, attract flies, especially females seeking a spot for oviposition, but such visitations are too rare to be significant in normal pollination, which depends fundamentally upon the insect's entering a number of flowers of the same species in fairly rapid succession.

As in the case of larval parasitism, however, other closely related groups of Muscoidea have habits which entitle them to mention as pollinating types. Tachinidae and Sarcophagidae are both of great importance here, and since a considerable number resemble the housefly very closely both as to size and coloration, it frequently happens that the casual observer considers them to be *Musca domestica* engaged in activities more worthy than their usual reputation implies. A few observations from the writer's own experience are perhaps not out of order at this time. All Tachinidae, so far as known, feed in the adult stage on pollen, nectar, or both. The length and shape of the proboscis and the structure of the labella determine the type of flower likely to be visited. In the early spring the marsh marigold, *Caltha palustris,* furnishes good picking for certain species of *Phasia*. Later, and indeed all through the summer, at least in New York State, the larger Umbelliferae, *Pastinaca sativa, Daucus carota,* and *Angelica atropurpurea* yield many specimens of *Ernestia,*

Tachina, and *Peleteria.* Indian hemp (*Apocynum*) seems to be a favorite with *Cistogaster, Archytas,* and *Trichophora.* Still later in the season, the common daisy, *Chrysanthemum leucanthemum,* is often visited by the fairly common tachnid *Phasia occidentis.*

The presence of Tachinidae on blossoms is not necessarily an indication that the fly is seeking food. Thus *Celatoria diabroticae,* a parasite of cucumber beetles, may normally be taken from melon and cucumber vines, as may *Trichopoda pennipes,* which parasitizes the common squash bug, *Anasa tristis.* The writer has taken *Exorista pyste* from the flower head of *Pastinaca,* only to find a moment later that the net contained also a larva of the parsnip web-worm, *Depressaria heracliana,* covered with tachinid eggs of the macrotype sort, while to the extruded ovipositor of the fly adhered an egg of similar type. Obviously, these parasitic flies seek flowers in order to find their hosts, as well as to find sustenance. Any conveyance of pollen incidental to reproductive activities on the part of the flies must necessarily be added to whatever benefit the plant derives from intentional visitation of its flowers for nutritional purposes.

PHILOSOPHY AND AESTHETICS

No one will deny that the aesthetic enjoyment of flowers for their own sake is as important an experience in the total development of man as is the consumption of their seeds and fruits. From such a standpoint, it is not difficult to admit soul-satisfying experiences for which the activities of insects are largely responsible. In the early pages of this volume I mentioned the sound of flies as sometimes contributory to an atmosphere of rural contentment. In more than a small way, our winged hexapods form part of the aesthetic background against which man grows to maturity and out of which come both the prose and poetry of human experience. The baying of hounds in marsh-land, the voices of crows and gulls at noontime, the rustle of the wind in foliage, the murmur of moving water, and the mystery of echoes among mountains are not complete without the chirp of the cricket, the whir of the locust, the shrill din of the cicada, and the hum of common flies.

Another contribution to beauty derives from the color and design of a number of species whose metallic surfaces throw back reflections of green, blue, and purple in the sunlight and not only arrest the attention of those sensitive to artistic stimulation but likewise intrigue the student of biophysics, who, wrestling with his problems of diffraction, refraction, and absorption, sees in such creatures a possible avenue of approach to the better understanding of what man calls light and the laws that govern its behavior. Notable for their metallic coloration are such forms as *Lucilia, Phormia,* and *Calliphora.* The same species may be said by their very life cycles to symbolize man's highest aspirations and most sacred hopes. When one contrasts the darkness, sordidness, and unremitting toil which characterize the life of the sightless maggot with the freedom, beauty, unrestricted movement, and procreative power which the adult winged creature may enjoy, one finds an almost perfect symbol for the continuing nature of the universe. We are reminded of a well-known biblical quotation:

"It is sown in corruption, it is raised in incorruption. . . . For this corruptible must put on incorruption, and this mortal must put on immortality" (I Cor. 15:42,53).

It will be noted, however, that the various economic and aesthetic benefits which have been credited to muscoid Diptera would be very little diminished if *Musca domestica* did not exist. Blowflies are at least as capable scavengers, and several genera are more suitable than *Musca* for maggot therapy. The housefly never makes a habit of parasitizing noxious forms, and its visits to flowers requiring insect pollination are exceedingly rare. Even the pleasant hum of flies in summer can be credited as properly to *Stomoxys, Muscina,* or species of Calliphoridae. Nor is the adult housefly a creature of striking beauty. In summary, then, it must be said that although the superfamily Muscoidea includes a considerable number of human benefactors, it also contains many black sheep. Among these, *Musca domestica* is certainly the blackest.

Even so, the record is not all bad. There remains the unquestionably great value of the species as an experimental animal. In this field *Musca domestica* perhaps excels all other insects, and has surely succeeded in winning for itself a place in the sun. For example, bodies of dead houseflies have been used to furnish protein food for the rearing of mosquito larvae for experimental purposes. Again, the wings of a housefly are used in an instrument at the Mount Wilson Observatory which measures the heat radiated by the stars. The next chapter will describe at some length the techniques employed by investigators and manufacturers in utilizing the fly as a test animal for the standardization of insecticides.

We are thus justified in closing our discussion on a sympathetic note. An answer has apparently been found to the query of an anonymous but oft-quoted poet, "Poor little fly! Ain't you got anyone to love you?"

CHAPTER XV

The Fly as an
Experimental Animal

The fly sat upon the axle-tree of the chariot-wheel, and said, "What a dust do I raise!"—Fables of Phaedrus, *bk. iii, fab.* 6

IN THE growth and development of modern science, a comparatively small number of plant and animal species have taken their places as particularly useful to the investigator. The best-known insect in genetic research is the tiny fruitfly, *Drosophila melanogaster*. Equally important in medical and economic entomology is *Musca domestica,* the test species by which the merits of modern contact insecticides are largely evaluated.

Entomology as a distinct science and profession came into being chiefly because of the economic importance of those insects which destroy man's food supply, threaten his health, jeopardize the well-being of his domestic animals, or prevent the survival of plant forms on which he depends for clothing, shelter, and medicine.

To combat the insect menace, manufacturers have brought into existence an unbelievably great number of insecticides and repellents, each calculated in its own way to eliminate, control, or discourage the presence of various noxious forms. The standardization of these numerous products, however, so necessary for the protection of the purchaser, has posed a difficult problem not only for civil and military authorities but likewise for the manufacturers, most of whom value the satisfaction and good will of their clientele and have no desire to sell materials under false pretenses.

Among insects, the common housefly is far out in front as the best laboratory animal for determining the relative efficiency of insecticides, attractants, and repellents. The only species which may be said to compete with *Musca domestica* for first honors is the cockroach, which, since it has chewing mouth parts, is a type especially suitable for the testing of stomach poisons. For the standardization of contact sprays, on the other hand, houseflies have come to be regarded as indispensable, and the number used for routine testing by commercial houses, government agencies, and private investigators is virtually enormous. The remarkable fecundity of the species and the ease with which it may be cultured, as well as the relatively short life cycle, which makes possible the production of vast numbers within a few weeks' time, all contribute to the appropriateness of *Musca domestica* as an experimental type.

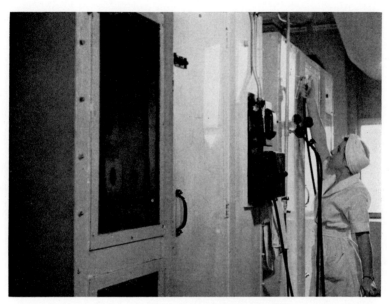

Figure 107. Interior of insecticide testing laboratory. Technician is releasing spray into Peet-Grady chamber. Foreground shows battery of rearing cages. (Courtesy of John Powell & Co., Inc.)

The first use of houseflies for such a purpose goes back many years, but the perfection of apparatus for accurate testing procedure is a rather modern achievement. Today it may be said that the housefly is, in truth, the entomologist's white mouse, the controlled culturing and rearing of which has become a procedure as highly technical as that employed for the maintenance of type cultures of bacteria or for the production of disease-free strains of rodents for use in clinical diagnosis.

For convenience, the discussion which follows is divided into two parts: (1) rearing and culturing techniques, and (2) standard testing procedures.

THE REARING OF *MUSCA DOMESTICA* FOR
EXPERIMENTAL PURPOSES

The media employed by experimental workers for the rearing of flies have been many. Horse manure, a natural medium, may be employed successfully in the laboratory if it can be made available in a fresh condition as often as desired. The best procedure is to pasteurize the manure at 160°–165°F (71.1°–73.9°C) for two hours, then allow it to cool. The manure should then be packed rather loosely in battery jars, leaving only room to fit on the covers.

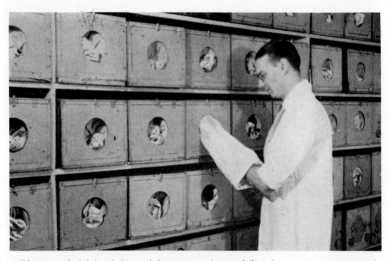

Figure 108. Maintaining a laboratory colony of flies for use in testing work. Dried-out pupae are placed in rearing chambers. Flies emerge five days later. (Courtesy of John Powell & Co., Inc.)

Jars 9 inches high and 6 inches in diameter are of convenient size. A yeast culture made up of 1 pound of yeast to 1,700 cubic centimeters of water should be in readiness. One hundred cubic centimeters of yeast culture are added to the manure in the jar. More or less than this amount may be used, depending on the amount of moisture in the manure, but it is best to have a thin layer of quite dry manure at the top as the time of pupation draws near.

A more reliable medium, in that it can be made up in the laboratory at any time, is prepared by mixing together 200 g. of alfalfa and 400 g. of coarse, soft wheat bran. The mixture is placed in a battery jar and moistened with about a liter of yeast suspension prepared by combining 10 g. of compressed yeast with 16 ml. of malt extract in the required amount of water. Thorough mixing of all ingredients is important. Experience will determine the correct degree of dryness to prevent the growth of molds.

Some workers use powdered milk as a rearing medium. Oat hulls in combination with various other ingredients are also satisfactory. Such modifications are discussed in greater detail in the pages that follow.

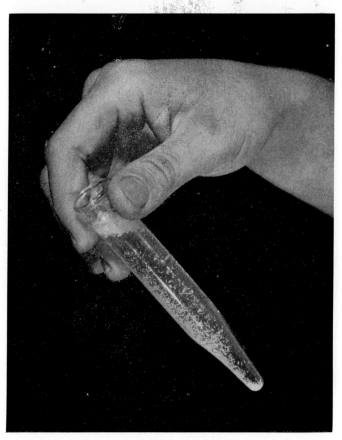

Figure 109. Fly eggs in centrifuge tube. These will next be placed in breeding jars. (Courtesy of Standard Oil Company [N.J.]; photo by Bubley.)

Transferring the Eggs

In the breeding cages, it is desirable to provide moist cotton on which the flies may oviposit. If it is desired to estimate the number of eggs being transferred to the rearing medium, they may be shaken gently in a little water. After the eggs have settled, the number present can be very closely calculated by assuming that one-tenth of a milliliter of settled eggs contains about 500. In rearing flies for testing, it is recommended that eggs be taken from at least two laboratory cultures. Under good conditions, a survival of 75 to 90 per cent may be expected; in other words, 2,000 eggs placed in a jar of properly prepared medium will yield from 1,500 to 1,800 flies.

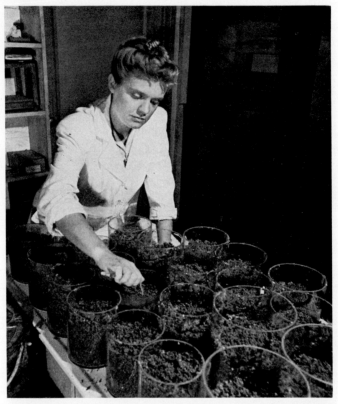

Figure 110. Placing fly eggs in breeding jars. The laboratory assistant is here pouring a suspension of housefly eggs upon a medium suitable for larval development. (Courtesy of Standard Oil Company [N.J.]; photo by Bubley.)

Handling of Larvae, Pupae, and Adults

By the eighth or ninth day, the larvae should have completed their development and will be found undergoing pupation near the surface. The pupae may be separated from the medium by lifting off the upper half inch of the latter and spreading it upon a tray. A blast of air is then directed upon the particles of media until these become dry enough to blow away and leave the pupae relatively clean. These are gently but thoroughly mixed and weighed into batches of approximately 500 each (if large-group procedure is to be used). Each batch, contained in a shallow dish, is placed in a separate cage and appropriate food is provided for the emerging flies. Milk, diluted 50 per cent with water, is very commonly used. A 40 per cent solution of formaldehyde, diluted 1 to 1,500 with the above mixture, will delay the souring of the milk and is not toxic to the flies.

The foregoing procedures have been found especially successful by H. H. Richardson (1932a) and are included by Galtsoff *et al.* (1937) in their well-known *Culture Methods for Invertebrate Animals.*

Eagleson (1943) advocates the use of a somewhat simpler medium consisting of crimped oats and water, the unhulled oats having been crushed between rollers. Eagleson places 2 kg. of the crimped oats in an unrusted, galvanized washtub and wets them down with approximately 4 liters of water. Care should be taken that there is no free water standing at the bottom. The hulls are said to prevent the formation of undesirable gummy masses. The medium should not be more than 5 to 7 cm. deep, as more than this favors acid fermentation of the lower layers. The addition of yeast is not necessary, as yeast fermentation is spontaneous from spores present in the dry oats. He does not advise stirring the medium. Daily sprinkling with water is required.

Eggs will meanwhile have been deposited on food dishes in the adult cages. These are shaken in water in a graduated cylinder of 10 cc. capacity. About 2 cc. of settled eggs are added to the freshly soaked oats. It is not necessary to wait for preliminary fermentation to set in.

The tub is covered with a canopy of muslin which serves both to conserve moisture and to prevent contamination by flies that may be free in the laboratory. If a sufficient number of larvae hatch out, there will be no danger of mold. After two days, the cover should be removed. This encourages the drying of the walls and thus prevents the escape of the more mature larvae, which tend to migrate when four to six days old.

As soon as pupation starts, the entire culture is spread on a sieve of hardware cloth, of a 6-mm. mesh. This is suspended in a frame above a funnel. The maggots, seeking an appropriate place for pupation, move downward and drop through both sieve and funnel into a shallow metal pan containing damp excelsior. The edge of the pan is made to overhang in an inward direction, to prevent the escape of the larvae. When all have fallen into the excelsior, a sheet metal cover is put in place. This provides a moist and dark environment, comparable to natural conditions.

When the time approaches for emergence of the flies, the excelsior containing the pupae is laid on a wire sieve of the type used in a mill for fanning grain. The mesh should be 2.8 × 20 mm. A second sieve, with a mesh 2.5 × 20 mm., is arranged beneath. Shaking and gentle brushing will cause dust and undersize pupae to pass through both sieves. Excelsior and oversize pupae remain on top, while normal pupae of uniform size accumulate between the screens. These are poured into small dishes of about 150 cc. capacity. Each dish, which will contain approximately 3,000 pupae, is then placed in an emergence cage.

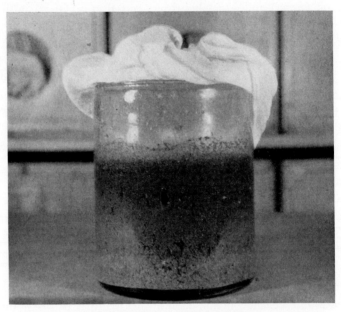

Figure 111. Method of rearing flies for experimental purposes. The medium in the jar contains housefly maggots. (Courtesy of John Powell & Co., Inc.)

Eagleson advocates an octagonal cage, horizontally disposed, with the screen projecting 1 cm. at the open end. This is for sewing on a sleeve made of sheeting. The sleeve is turned inside out, the edges are made to match, and the stitching is completed, after which the sleeve is drawn forward once more. The sleeve may be gathered by a cord or tied in a single knot. The back of the cage is of wood, in which an aperture seven cm. in diameter is closed by a gate of 26-gauge galvanized iron. This is to provide for rapid emptying of the cage. Flies will usually emerge quickly from this aperture if the cage is covered by a dark cloth. After each use the cage is scrubbed with soapsuds and the wood surfaces are given three coats of waterproof enamel paint.

To feed the adult flies Eagleson uses a formula with the following ingredients:

> Water, 500 ml.
> Shredded agar, 10 g.
> Pulp of ripe banana, 200 g.
> Sugar, 150 g.
> Skimmed milk, 1 liter
> Formalin, 0.5 ml.
> Gelatin (crude chips), 25 g.

The sugar and agar are added to the water and heated until the agar dissolves. Banana pulp and gelatin are next added and a boiling heat is maintained until the gelatin also goes into solution. The formalin and milk are stirred in cold, and the medium is then placed in a refrigerator to congeal. A final stirring just before the medium solidifies will insure even distribution of the banana pulp. If the bananas used are not sufficiently ripe, the milk may curdle. This may be prevented, however, by the addition of 2 g. of bicarbonate of soda.

The medium, as prepared above, is in the form of a soft gel which will neither drown the flies nor ensnare them. It can be stored up to three weeks in a refrigerator and at 30°C (86°F) lasts three or fours days without souring or undergoing putrefaction. Eagleson feeds it in 15-cm. chinette (glazed) paper plates which are discarded after use.

The same author advocates a temperature of 28°C (82.4°F) for the adult flies and a temperature of 33°C (91.4°F) for the larvae. The latter temperature was determined as most suitable for maintaining the crushed oat medium. As indicated in an earlier chapter, larvae thrive at temperatures up to approximately 40°C (104.0°F). A relative humidity of 25 to 30 per cent was found most desirable. Eagleson points out that sunlight or even daylight is not required, stating that he has reared dozens of generations in a basement.

Bickoff (1943) prefers a modification of Richardson's technique. Bickoff uses three-and-a-half-gallon pans, in each of which are placed one-third of a pound of alfalfa meal and two-thirds of a pound of bran. These are mixed dry, after which are added 850 cc. of water containing one ounce of yeast. The entire mixture is then stirred until uniform. Using a calibrated pipette, the technician measures out approximately 7,500 eggs, which are then placed upon the mixture in the pan. Bickoff advocates a temperature of 32°C (89.6°F) and a relative humidity of 50 per cent.

At the end of three days, the entire contents of the pan are transferred to a second pan in which the same quantity of the same mixture has been made up the day before. Pupation should be nearly complete in seven to nine days, at which time the mash will be almost dry and easily fragmented. The dried mash containing the pupae is then shaken through a sieve. Large lumps (which rarely contain pupae) are discarded. An air blast is used to separate medium from pupae, of which approximately 5,500 may be expected from each batch.

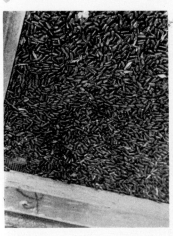 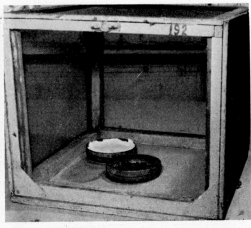

Figure 112. Left. Rearing flies for experimental purposes. This drying screen holds 25,000 puparia. (Courtesy of John Powell & Co., Inc.)

Figure 113. Right. Numbers controlled in pupal stage. Five hundred puparia are placed in an open cup in the rearing cage. The second container holds food for the emerging flies. The entire batch will be used in a single test. (Courtesy of John Powell & Co., Inc.)

Allen, Dicke, and Brooks (1943) used Richardson's medium but introduced certain technical procedures of their own. Their flies were reared at 85°F (29.4°C) and at a relative humidity ranging between 60 and 70 per cent. The larvae were separated from the medium one day before pupation by placing the mass in a funnel that was provided with a succession of three screens of 4-, 8-, and 12-mesh gauze, respectively. Exposure to light caused the larvae to work their way down through the screens into a receptacle containing dry sand. At the end of 24 hours, the pupae were separated from the sand by sifting. This utilization of only those which pupated the first day served to insure reasonable uniformity as to time of emergence of the adult flies. Shortly before this occurred, the pupae were transferred to testing cages of 14-mesh construction. Wicks of rolled cotton wool provided a continuous supply of milk and water for emerging flies. During the actual running of the tests, these wicks were replaced by corks. Immediately after, wicks supplying sugar solution were introduced, to provide for the nourishment of surviving flies.

Basden (1947) also published some interesting modifications of accepted rearing techniques: Flies not more than one day old are etherized, and 80 perfect specimens of each sex are selected by examination of the genitalia. From such a colony sufficient eggs are obtained each day to produce approximately 4,000 puparia. A new oviposition cage is set up once a week. According to Basden, flies oviposit as well in complete darkness as when illuminated for 8 out of 24 hours. Instead of transferring a definite volume of eggs to freshly mixed food, Basden prefers to allow all the eggs to hatch, then mix the contents of the oviposition jar with the food material.

Basden's rearing medium, which he finds more satisfactory than either Richardson's formula or the modification thereof usually employed in Peet-Grady testing, differs from these as shown in Table 17:

Table 17

Richardson	Peet-Grady	Basden (formula no. 6)
3.25 lb. (1,474 g.) wheat bran	3.96 lb. (1,800 g.) coarse wheat bran	4 lb. (1,814.5 g.) middlings
1.75 lb. (794 g.) alfalfa meal	1.98 lb. (900 g.) alfalfa meal	2 lb. (907.25 g.) grass meal
5,250 cc. water	4,050 cc. water	6,000 cc. tap water
25 cc. "Diamalt"	75 cc. malt extract	60 g. dry malt extract
56 g. baker's yeast	45 g. compressed yeast	45 g. dried yeast

The first puparia form three or four days after the newly hatched larvae are mixed with the culture medium, that is, five or six days after the oviposition jar is placed in the cage containing young adults. Three days later all may be considered to have pupated, and the puparia are removed from the culture medium.

Basden collects his puparia by tipping the cultures into water. All puparia more than five hours old will float, and are decanted. Any larvae present, very young pupae, and all food (if it is wet enough) sink to the bottom. The procedure is as follows:

(1) Water at 27.5°C ± 0.5° is run into a tank.

(2) The culture is tipped into this and the whole mixture is stirred gently by hand to break up the food and release the puparia.

(3) After three or four minutes, to allow for settling, the puparia are carefully skimmed off the surface by use of gauze scoops.

(4) The puparia are transferred to a second water bath, where settling and skimming are repeated.

(5) The puparia are placed on absorbent paper and dried in a current of air. When dry, they are placed in cages for emergence. On the seventeenth day the flies are ready for use.

A method asserted to be both more convenient and easier to use than those of Richardson and Eagleson has recently been described by Frings (1948).

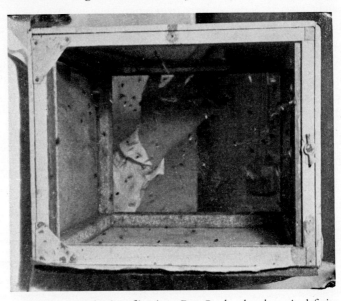

Figure 114. Releasing flies into Peet-Grady chamber. A definite number of specimens, of known age and sex ratio, are permitted to enter the Peet-Grady chamber for testing. (Courtesy of John Powell & Co., Inc.)

A small mass of fermenting dog biscuit (moistened with yeast) is kept in a covered jar as "seed." To this is added a sufficient amount of moistened biscuit for a few days' operation. When the whole mass has become fermentive, convenient portions are removed either for oviposition or for rearing. For oviposition, the material is placed in the cages in beakers or small museum jars. Frings states that "the number of eggs laid by the flies on a small amount . . . is almost unbelievable."

The rearing containers are two-quart Mason jars with two-piece lids, of which the central disc consists of 60-mesh screening. The eggs or young larvae are added to about 2 inches of medium. It has been noted that housefly larvae tolerate wider differences in moisture content than do the larvae of blowflies. Fine wood shavings or coarse sawdust may be added as the larvae grow older, to offset the accumulating moisture; the larvae accomplish the necessary mixing by their own activity.

More sawdust is added as pupation draws near, and when pupae begin to appear, the entire mass is poured into a shallow pan to permit further drying.

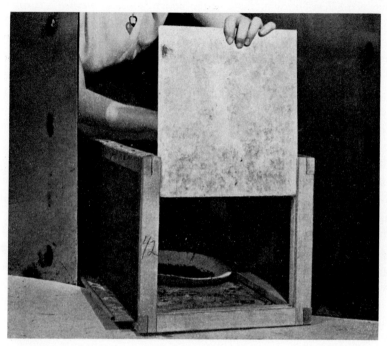

Figure 115. Pupal cases remain after release of flies. If any of the flies should fail to transform, their number can be determined by counting the unruptured puparia. This picture was made immediately after the flies had left the rearing cage and entered the Peet-Grady chamber. (Courtesy of Rohm & Haas Company, Philadelphia.)

Larval density has a bearing on normality of the adult flies, which are most satisfactory when approximately 9 g. of biscuit are allowed for each one hundred specimens. Two inches of medium in a Mason jar will thus support about 2,000 larvae. The medium is said to be remarkably free from disagreeable odor.

STANDARD TESTING PROCEDURES

As stated above, the large number of proprietary compounds claimed by manufacturers to have insecticidal value has resulted in the necessity for standard procedures by which the relative efficiency of the various products may be evaluated.

The Peet-Grady Test

In 1928, Peet and Grady published a technique which has since become known as the Peet-Grady method, and in which *Musca domestica* is employed as the test species. In the original procedure, not less than one hundred flies were used and the test chamber was kept at 85°F. The flies were liberated in the chamber at a concentration not to exceed one per cubic foot. The insecticide was then introduced by means of an atomizer through half-inch holes, the mechanism being such that both the amount of the insecticide and the pressure of the spray might be measured and controlled. After 12 cc. of insecticide had been introduced, all doors and other apertures were kept tightly closed for a period of ten minutes.

All flies found clinging to the walls or ceiling were then counted, and all dropped flies were transferred to a clean cage for observation. Those which recovered within 24 hours were then added to the wall and ceiling count, being considered to have escaped the action of the insecticide.

The chamber should be so constructed that only the biological element is subject to variation. The condition of the insects, the angle of the spray, the fineness of the spray, atmospheric conditions, the concentration of the insecticide, the carrier employed, the temperature, humidity, and the period of exposure are all kept as constant as possible during successive tests. Various modifications of procedure calculated to improve the reliability of the results have been introduced by these and other workers over a period of years.

The National Association of Insecticide and Disinfectant Manufacturers adopted the Peet-Grady method as an official procedure in 1932, and has since recognized two forms of the test for evaluating various liquid sprays in comparison with an official test insecticide [1] (O.T.I.). The small group procedure is similar to the original technique in that the insecticides are tested against lots of 100 flies, prepared while the flies are either in the pupal or the adult stage. Sex ratios are as found in nature. To compensate for biological variability, ten paired tests are run, and the results are averaged for record. In each test, the unknown insecticide is compared with an O.T.I. of previously determined potency.

---

[1] It has usually been the policy of the National Association of Insecticide and Disinfectant Manufacturers to make the Official Test Insecticide available to all firms or laboratories, whether members of the association or not.

In the large group method, 500-fly lots are employed. These are prepared in advance by placing at least 500 pupae in each cage and waiting for emergence. Sex ratios are made uniform, so that any differences in susceptibility due to sex will be eliminated. For tests to be official, the apparatus must conform to specifications.

The rearing room is maintained at a temperature ranging between 80° and 85°F, and at a relative humidity above 40 and below 70 per cent.

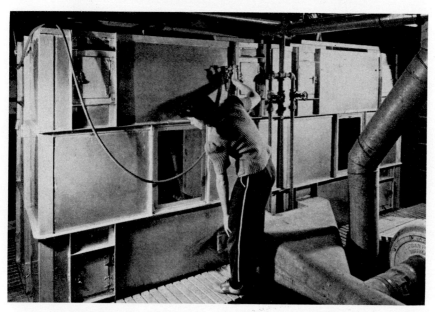

Figure 116. Peet-Grady testing chamber in use. Technician operates valve releasing insecticide into chamber in the form of a fine spray. Glass window permits direct observation of flies. (Courtesy of Rohm & Haas Company, Philadelphia.)

The testing room must be separate from the rearing room, lest traces of insecticide come in contact with the insects prior to the test. It is maintained at a temperature of 75° to 85°F; the relative humidity is unimportant, though a range between 40 and 70 per cent is considered desirable. There must be provision for an air intake, with an outside source of air of approximately the required temperature. The room should be of sufficient size to permit the operator to move freely about the test chamber that stands within.

The Peet-Grady test chamber may be made of either wood or metal. All bracing should be external, as the inside must be free from ledges, projections, crevices, or cracks. The inner surface is made smooth and of a material impervious to ordinary insecticides. The chamber itself is a 6-foot cube, a 1-inch deviation being permitted in any dimension.

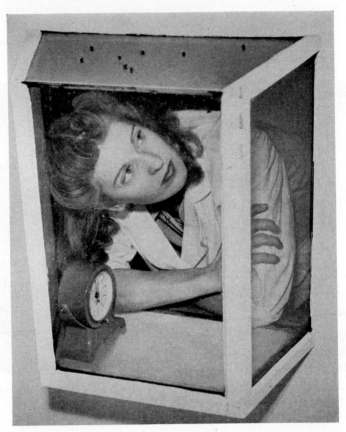

Figure 117. Observation window in Peet-Grady chamber. Entomologist is observing the effect of spray recently released into chamber. A count of flies still on the wing is made at the end of five minutes. After ten minutes the entomologist will enter the chamber and count the knocked-down flies. (Courtesy of Standard Oil Company [N.J.]; Photo by Bubley.)

The roof should contain a glass window above which is suspended an adequate source of illumination. Windows should be provided on at least one wall, preferably on two opposite walls, so as to permit adequate observation. A tight-fitting door, large enough to permit the operator to enter, is required. This should be hung so that the inner surface is flush with the inner wall of the chamber when the door is closed.

To provide for thorough ventilation after every test, there must be an air duct leading from the chamber to a point outside the building. This is equipped with an exhaust fan capable of moving not less than 1,000 cubic feet of air per minute. The air duct should be protected by a 10-mesh screen. Some chambers are equipped with a screen door in addition to the solid door, and this provides for the intake of sufficient air to replace that which is pumped out. Ordinarily, however, it is preferable to have portholes, 6 inches in diameter, located in the corners of the chamber, one in each of the eight corners, if possible. None of these should be on the same level as the exhaust aperture. Ventilation ports should be provided with tight-fitting, hinged covers that open outward. They should be covered with screen on the inside.

For introducing the insecticide, 1-inch holes are recommended. These should be not more than 18 or less than 6 inches from the ceiling. Some chambers have a single intake hole in the center of each wall; others have them within an inch of the corner on each side. For official tests, the atomizer is required to be a De Vilbiss Special No. 5004, and must be operated with air at 12.5 lbs. pressure per square inch, ±0.5 lb. Air must be free from condensed moisture, oil, or particles of dust. The atomizer is set to deliver 12 cc. of base oil in not less than 23 or more than 25 seconds. The nozzles are made to oscillate in a horizontal plane to insure even distribution of vapor. This also avoids wetting of the ceiling and walls.

For testing, the flies are confined in cages with a square base and detachable floor. At least two sides and the top are made of 16-mesh screen. Another side is fitted with either a rubber membrane or a sleeve-type opening.

Flies that have been ovipositing for two days will be of the proper age for testing, that is, four to five days old. The floor of the Peet-Grady chamber is covered with unsized, nonglazed paper of an absorbent type. Paper of 60 to 80 lbs. weight seems most satisfactory. In the large-group method all the flies in one cage are transferred to the testing chamber. All ventilating apertures are closed, and care is taken that no window is more shaded than any other. Twelve ml. of insecticide are then fed into the chamber through the spray holes at 12.5 lb. pressure, the temperature being maintained between 80° and 85°F. Ten minutes after the spraying is begun, portholes are opened and the chamber is ventilated.

A few unparalyzed flies may be found at the expiration of the ten-minute exposure. These are first counted and removed, after which the paralyzed flies are gathererd and transferred at once to clean cages of the type described. Care must be taken to avoid injuring the flies, as a certain percentage will recover from the exposure and this percentage is significant. Best results are obtained with a vacuum device which picks up the flies by gentle suction and passes them into a receptacle of sufficient size to insure against harmful crowding. Counting of the paralyzed flies may be done either at this time or after their transference to the recovery cage.

In the cage is placed a ball of cotton wrapped in gauze and saturated with a 10 per cent sugar solution. Any type of food may be used, but it must be near the floor of the cage so that enfeebled flies may reach it, and should

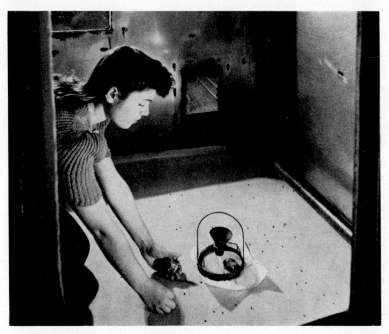

Figure 118. Counting the kill inside Peet-Grady chamber. A mechanical counter is used. (Courtesy of Rohm & Haas Company, Philadelphia.)

not be of such consistency that the flies can drown in it. After 24 hours in the rearing room, the recovery cage is examined and the final count is recorded. This is best accomplished by removing from the cage all individuals that show no sign of life on being touched. These may be counted as dead. If all paralyzed flies were counted on removal from the test chamber, no further counting is needed. If not, it will be necessary to kill the recovered flies still in the cage. This is best done by placing the latter in an oven at 170°F. These may then be counted and the data assembled. The following relationships will be apparent: (1) Number of recovered flies plus number found dead after 24 hours equals the number paralyzed. (2) Number of

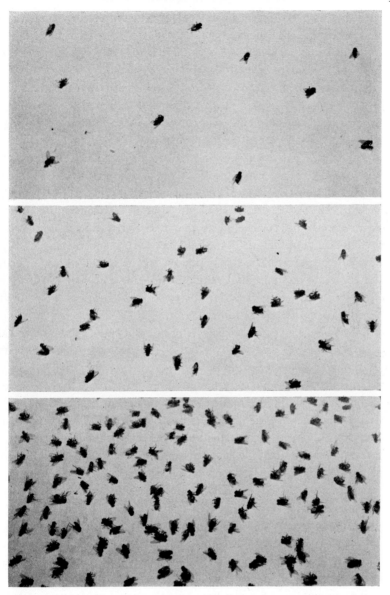

Figure 119. Progressive knockdown with continued exposure to pyrethrum. *Upper:* Knockdown one minute after treatment with a 5 per cent pyrin spray. *Center and lower:* Knockdown after three minutes and ten minutes, respectively. (Courtesy of John Powell & Co., Inc.)

paralyzed flies plus number not paralyzed after ten-minute exposure equals total number of flies used in test. (3) "Knockdown" may be expressed as the percentage of total flies which were paralyzed. (4) "Mortality" may be expressed as the percentage of total flies counted as dead.

Before the test chamber can be utilized for a second test, the walls must be thoroughly cleaned by wiping with a clean cloth saturated with an effective solvent, such as alcohol containing 10 per cent of acetone. Such cleansing is sufficient for a short series of tests, but at intervals the chamber should be cleaned thoroughly with soap and water. Any toxic residue can destroy the value of successive tests, hence the great importance of perfect cleanliness, especially when new compounds are being tested.

Each year, the National Association prepares an official test insecticide to be used in testing other compounds. It may or may not differ from that used the previous year. The O.T.I. kill must fall between 30 and 55 per cent. If the insecticide to be tested falls within 5 per cent of the mortality figure for the O.T.I. it is given a rating of "B." Should it exceed in efficiency the O.T.I. by from 6 to 15 per cent, it is rated "A" or *good.* A kill 16 per cent or higher above the O.T.I. entitles the product to a rating of "AA" or *excellent.* No unknown insecticide is given an official rating unless its knockdown percentage is equal to that of the O.T.I. A variation of (—) 2 percentage points, however, may be allowed.

Bliss (1939) is responsible for a modification of the Peet-Grady technique by which it is possible to determine exactly the extent of the difference in toxicity between the material being tested and the O.T.I. This calculation is based on determining the exact amount of the official test insecticide which will give the same mortality as a measured unit of the sample. If a quarter unit of the standard gives the same mortality as one unit of the sample, the latter is listed as 0.25, or a 25 per cent toxicity rating. All tests must necessarily be run on the same culture of flies.

Eagleson (1940) preferred the Bliss method in determining the toxicity of livestock sprays. His flies were placed in cylinders exposed in a spray tunnel. After the insects became paralyzed they were placed in recovery cages and the results were observed. He found mortality to be from 14 to 20 per cent higher among protected flies than among aerated specimens. Eagleson's spray tunnel (1941) was made to simulate conditions as they normally exist in well-aired barns. Strict reliance upon Peet-Grady tests was found inadequate for evaluating the killing power of insecticides as used under practical conditions.

After testing, Eagleson placed his flies in a recovery cabinet with a stream of air circulating through it. Since the spray-tunnel technique is more rapid than the Peet-Grady method, the mortality from other causes becomes negligible. Eagleson counted his flies without removing them from the cylinder. The method has one great advantage in that it can be used to study the ability

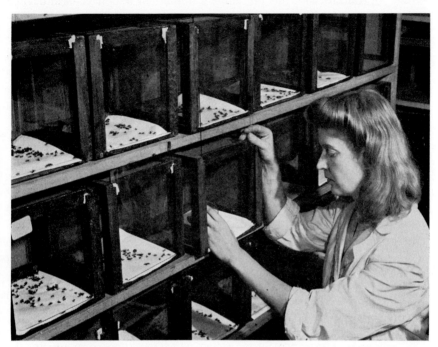

Figure 120. Recovery cages. Flies that have been knocked down by insecticide in the Peet-Grady chamber are placed here for twenty-four hours. A count is then made to determine the percentage of recoveries. (Courtesy of Standard Oil Company [N.J.]; photo by Bubley.)

of the insects to recover from mild doses of any spray. This factor, usually not well known, strongly limits the efficiency of many sprays in general use.

In most of his tests, Eagleson demonstrated that though male and female flies seemed about equally susceptible to the hypnotic dose of the material being tested, the lethal effect was more pronounced among the males. It becomes important, therefore, that the proportion of males and females be uniform for all tests in a series. Eagleson and Benke (1938) found that an equal number of males and females could usually be assured through sorting the pupae by means of two wire screens. One should have a mesh of $\frac{6}{64} \times \frac{3}{4}$ inch; the other $\frac{7}{67} \times \frac{3}{4}$ inch. Abnormally large pupae pass through neither screen; undersize pupae, through both.

Other Cylindrical Chamber Tests

The Peet-Grady chamber, of course, is of a type in which the insects are free to distribute themselves throughout a considerable space prior to exposure. In contrast with this procedure a number of tests have been devised in which the insects are confined in a smaller area. The cylindrical chamber of Tattersfield and Morris (1924) is of such a type. It insures greater uniformity of spray application and is adaptable for use with both crawling and flying insects. Water, oils, or other liquids may be employed equally well as the carrier fluids. The apparatus is essentially a glass jar with an atomizer fixed in the lid. This throws a fine spray on the insects, which are placed in a dish inside the jar. The cylinder should be mounted on a leveling platform.

The Turntable Method for Comparative Testing of Liquid Contact Insecticides

Based on the cylinder of Tattersfield and Morris, an apparatus which costs less than the Peet-Grady chamber, requires less space, and operates more quickly was brought forward by Campbell and Sullivan in 1938. As later perfected, this consists of a metal turntable, preferably of aluminum, 46 inches in diameter and mounted on a triangular frame of angle iron. Upon the turntable are mounted ten large aluminum cylinders, each 8 inches in diameter and 17 inches high. Immediately below each of those cylinders, and attached to the under side of the table, is a small cylinder or "cage holder" 4 inches deep and 6 inches in diameter. Arising from the center of the turntable is a vertical brass pipe, at the top of which is a supporting arm for the spray gun. Beneath this, the cylinders may be rotated.

Air is piped to a valve and gauge panel in front of the table, where it is split into two lines. The pressure in one line is controlled by a reducing valve and recorded on the gauge. The pressure in the other line is not controlled, its function being merely to operate the valve in the nozzle of the spray gun while the controlled pressure line atomizes the liquid to be sprayed.

From the valve, the two air lines extend beneath the table and enter the ball-bearing assembly at the center. One rises through the center of the brass standpipe. The air from the other is carried upward through the annular space between the inner and outer pipe. The two serve the double purpose of supporting the spray gun and conveying air, under pressure, to the nozzle. Bent copper tubing makes the final connections.

The turn table is composed of two layers, the upper of which has a somewhat smaller diameter than the lower. The cylinders fit into holes in the upper layer and rest on a circular lip formed by the lower element. At these points the layers are separated by a ⅛-inch slot into which a stainless steel plate may be inserted from the outside.

For the test, a 5½-inch Petri dish containing about 100 houseflies, and covered with screen, is placed in one of the ten cage holders, and the latter is closed by inserting a stainless steel slide. The cylinder next to the right is then transferred to the "loading" position and the process is repeated until all ten places have been made ready.

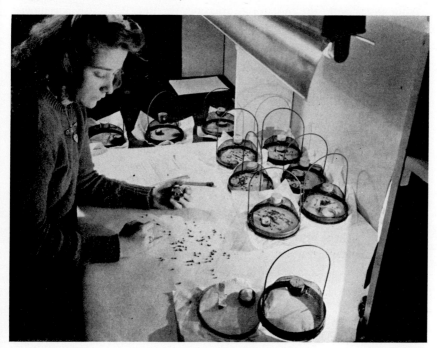

Figure 121. Counting dead flies after Peet-Grady test. Technician is using a mechanical counter to record mortality twenty-four hours after exposure to insecticide in testing chamber. (Courtesy of Rohm & Haas Company, Philadelphia.)

Liquids to be tested are measured into test tubes, 5 cc. to a tube. The contents of one tube are then poured into a thistle tube which leads to the spray gun. An automatic device exactly centers the hole in the cover of each cylinder as the latter comes into position beneath the nozzle. By opening the hand control valve on the gauge panel, the operator causes the two pressure lines to function and the entire charge is sprayed into the cylinder. The valve is then closed and the steel slide is pulled out. The cylinder settles to the level formerly occupied by the slide, and the mist settles into the cage holder without escaping to the outside.

If the second test tube contains a different insecticide, the nozzle is cleaned by spraying through it a solvent, such as acetone, a reservoir of which can be made available by fusing to the thistle tube a glass tube, with stopcock, leading from an Erlenmeyer flask. The sprayed solvent is received into a cloth with the nozzle over a space between two cylinders.

By turning the table at 30-second intervals, ten samples can be sprayed into as many cylinders in a total of 5 minutes.

After exposure to the mist for 10 minutes, the first Petri dish is removed and the paralyzed flies are transferred to a small, cubical cage. Others are removed at intervals of 30 seconds, so that all will have been exposed for the same 10-minute period. Operating on such a schedule, the investigator completes the entire procedure in a quarter of an hour.

A Less Expensive Chamber

A much cheaper device for testing contact insecticides against *Musca domestica* has been constructed by Hoskins and Caldwell (1947). This consists of a cylinder twelve inches in diameter and forty inches long, so mounted that the long axis is nearly, but not quite, horizontal. The fly cage is placed beneath a hole in the bottom, near the lower end of the chamber, opposite the point of entry for the spray. This arrangement permits the larger droplets to settle out before the spray cloud, which consists of small droplets only, makes contact with the flies. Ease of cleaning and rapidity of operation are the principal arguments in favor of its use.

Testing Residual Insecticides

Constructive criticism of the Peet-Grady method for the evaluation of household fly sprays has been advanced by Waterhouse (1947), who points out that the procedure was devised primarily for testing insecticides which behave after the manner of pyrethrins, with a quick knockdown effect. The method is not as suitable for comparing preparations which contain DDT, the action of which is considerably slower. A chemical assay of the DDT present is seen to be necessary as an adjunct to the biological test. It is therefore obvious that the comparative value of various toxicants can no longer be measured entirely by the use of mists and sprays. Residual films have become important, and our testing methods must be revised, especially since insects now frequently come into contact with layers of crystals or other particles, rather than with drops of a solution.

Busvine and Barnes (1947) have recently devised a method for testing the toxic effect of such dry insecticidal films. These authors make use of Watkins

No. 1 filter papers, 9 cm. in diameter. One cubic centimeter of acetone is sufficient to soak a single paper. Solutions of the various insecticides are prepared in eight different concentrations, so that one cc. of liquid will give a deposit of 10, 5, 3, 1, 0.1, 0.01, 0.001, or 0.0001 mgm. per square centimeter on the filter paper. In applying the solution, the paper is balanced on pin points and the liquid is added spirally from a 1 cc. hypodermic syringe. First-stage drying is accomplished by fanning. The papers are then allowed to dry several hours further before use.

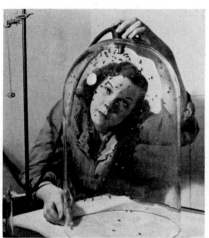 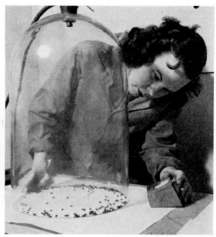

Figure 122. Left. Small-chamber testing. Entomologist is spraying insecticide into a bell jar containing healthy, laboratory-reared flies. (Courtesy of Standard Oil Company [N.J.]; photo by Parks.)

Figure 123. Right. Timing the action of an insecticide. The entomologist uses a stop watch to determine the effectiveness of the spray. (Courtesy of Standard Oil Company [N.J.]; photo by Parks.)

The method of exposure varies with the type of insect being studied. Flies are confined between two Petri dishes, each lined with a filter paper. With Gammexane, which tends to give off toxic vapor, the papers are placed at least 2 cm. apart and ventilation is provided by enclosing the system in a ring of mosquito bar.

The percentage kill of different insects is calculated on the assumption that the number of particles picked up by the insect is directly proportionate to the number per unit area. It is further assumed that the toxic effect is related to the logarithm of the number of particles on the insect. For *Musca domestica,* exposed two hours at 30°C, the results shown in Table 18 were obtained.

Table 18

Insecticide	Deposits: mg. per sq. cm.							
	10	5	3	1	.1	.01	.001	.0001
(1) DDT	—	—	—	100	100	97	41	—
(2) Gammexane	—	—	—	—	—	100	100	100
(3) Pyrethrum	—	—	—	100	55	32	—	—
(4) Rotenone	100	—	67	25	—	—	—	—

The DDT used was pure para-pará DDT, with a melting point of 108°C (226.4°F). The designation *gammexane* refers to a pure preparation of the *gamma* isomer of benzene hexachloride, melting point 112°C (223.6°F). The pyrethrum employed for these experiments tested 20 per cent pyrethrin content. A crystalline form of rotenone was used.

From these data, it is calculated that a kill of 50 per cent might ordinarily be expected from a deposit of .001 mg. per sq. cm. of DDT, a .00001 mg. of gammexane, .08 mg. of pyrethrins, or 2 mg. of rotenone. In an oil spray, the number of milligrams of toxicant per kilogram of body weight necessary to produce a kill of 50 per cent is approximately 6–9 mg. of DDT, 2–3 mg. of gammexane, 31–38 mg. of pyrethrins. Rotenone is not ordinarily tested in this manner. It will be seen that the relative toxicity of the films of undiluted insecticides is considerably different from that of the same insecticides in oily solution.

As for the residual effect, it has been found that the very sparse films of gammexane soon lose their toxicity, apparently by evaporation. Pyrethrum films are somewhat more enduring, while DDT persists the longest. Data of this sort are obtained by storing the saturated discs of filter paper and testing at definite intervals of time.

Special Tests and Investigational Techniques

For testing the reaction of flies to stimuli of an olfactory character, Eagleson (1939) has devised a relatively simple apparatus, consisting of a U tube of adjustable length, with wire screen partitions closing the free ends of the two arms. The flies are imprisoned in the tube and one arm is then perfused with the odor of the repellent or attractive material to be tested. At suitable intervals, the observer counts the number of flies resting on each of the screen septa. The degree of attraction or repulsion is calculated according to the formula $R = \dfrac{100\,(E - c)}{c}$, in which $E =$ experimental ratio of populations after introduction of the odor and $c =$ the control ratio of populations before the test. R indicates "reactance," which may be represented by a point on a scale ranging from $+100$ to -100, where 0 is the dividing line between attraction and repulsion.

This apparatus is not different in principle from that of Ingle (1943). After using blue light to attract the flies to a certain general location, Ingle observed the numbers which alighted on untreated screens as compared with the count on a screen treated with some specific repellent, attractant, or other odoriferous substance.

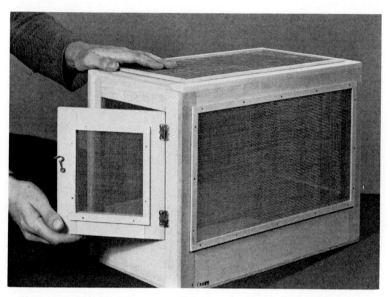

Figure 124. Insect rearing cage. This type is suitable for general use, including the rearing of flies. The mesh of the screen should be sufficiently fine to prevent smaller specimens from making their escape. (Courtesy of Ward's Natural Science Establishment.)

For transferring flies from a cage trap to a glass container, Harris and Down (1946) describe a simple device consisting of a box into which the cage is placed after a few hours' trapping. The cage should have a hole in the top, fitted with a removable stopper. The latter is removed and a cover is placed over the box. There is a hole in this cover over which a glass container is inverted. The cover is then shifted so that the aperture is directly above the hole in the trap. Positive phototropism causes the insects to fly upward.

The temperatures and relative humidities employed by experimental workers for the maintenance of fly colonies vary considerably. Tischler (1931b) was successful at 85°–90°F (29.4°–32.2°C). Thomssen and Doner (1938) prefer 80°F (26.7°C), maintaining this level by means of a thermostat. Like most workers they make no attempt at precise control of humidity, as the moisture given off by the rearing mechanism is usually adequate in this regard. In breeding flies throughout the year for insecticide tests, Grady (1928) made use of a constant temperature of 86°F (30.0°C). By employing a trough of wetted sawdust under a steam coil he was able to provide a relative humidity

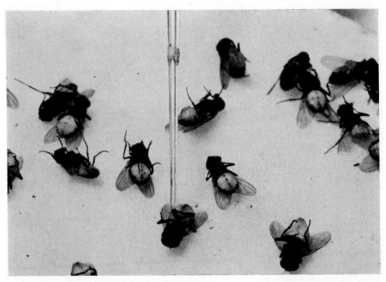

Figure 125. Drop-testing a potential new insecticide. The flies are immobilized by chilling, then placed on a cold slab. A drop of the material is placed on each one, after which the flies are placed in a recovery cage. At the end of twenty-four hours, a record is made of the percentage killed. (Courtesy of Standard Oil Company [N.J.]; photo by Bubley.)

of 40 per cent. Derbeneva-Ukhova (1935a) kept his virgin females for ovarian studies at 26°C (78.8°F), with a relative humidity of 40 to 45 per cent. Cox (1944) reared his larvae at 80°–85°F (26.7°–29.4°C). Reference to Chapter VIII will explain why such latitudes are allowable.

If the experimenter should desire to maintain control of the relative humidity in a small chamber, the method of Buxton and Mellanby (1934) is recommended. A stock solution of sulphuric acid is prepared by combining equal volumes (not weights) of concentrated acid (A.R.) and distilled water. If the original acid had a specific gravity of 1.841, that of the stock solution will be 1.550 after it has cooled (100 cc. acid + 100 cc. H_2O = 183.5 cc. of stock).

Table 19 shows the relative humidity produced in the atmosphere by various mixtures of water and stock solution. It will be noted that the specific gravity declines proportionately as the concentration of acid is reduced.

Table 19

RH%	Stock H_2SO_4, cc.	Water, cc.	Specific gravity
20	709	114	1.486
30	686	226	1.41
40	539	306	1.38
50	514	396	1.33
60	374	420	1.295
70	348	510.3	1.25
80	294	640	1.19
90	161	712	1.125

Buxton and Mellanby state that in the tropics better results are obtained by using graduated solutions of potassium hydroxide.

It is sometimes desirable to measure quantitatively the spray material accumulated by an insect as it flies through an insecticidal mist. David (1946) has devised a colorimetric method for determining this. A measured quantity of the red dye Sudan III is first dissolved in benzene, which is then added to an equal volume of odorless kerosene containing the insecticide. After exposure the insects are extracted in odorless kerosene, and the extracts are compared with a standard dilution of the dye.

David was thus able to determine the *surface median lethal dosage* for pyrethrins, for DDT, and for benzene hexachloride. For male houseflies the maximum median lethal dose was 6 mg. of DDT per kg. of body weight, 2 mg. of benzene hexachloride (666), and 31 mg. of pyrethrins. Females were more resistant, requiring 9, 3, and 38 mg., respectively.

CHAPTER XVI

Field, Museum,
and Laboratory Techniques

I saw a flie within a beade
Of amber cleanly buried.
—*Robert Herrick, "The Amber Bead"*

IN ALL biological studies it becomes desirable, from time to time, to pre-serve representative specimens, either for future observation or as proof and record of experiments performed.

The techniques best suited for the collection and preservation of filth-feeding Diptera do not differ essentially from those employed by the general entomologist. These techniques, however, are not always included in the training of teachers, laboratory technicians, or medical personnel who, through an interest in public health and sanitary education, may be called upon to conduct surveys, give instruction, or assemble collections of medically important forms. For this reason, it appears desirable to include in the present work a chapter summarizing both field and laboratory techniques, and pointing out those modifications of procedure which are of particular value in the study of muscoid flies.

COLLECTION OF ADULT FORMS

The traditional insect net, so useful in capturing Lepidoptera, Coleoptera, and other insects in the field, has but limited use in the capture of filth-feeding flies. It is, nevertheless, an essential part of one's equipment. The fabric should be relatively transparent and of not too fine a mesh. Both features contribute to the ease with which the specimen may be seen after capture and transferred to a suitable container or killing jar. Color, also, is important here. Since the body of the fly is relatively dark, the specimen is much easier to locate against a white background than against a black or khaki-colored fabric. There are times, however, when this advantage may well be sacrificed for safety, as in survey work during military campaigns, where white might attract enemy attention and lead to disclosure of the disposition of troops.

The shape of the net is of some importance. A conical design is preferable to a U-shaped pattern, as it favors the transfer of the insect from net to bottle. This is because flies are positively phototropic, and, therefore, tend to fly upward when confined. Except when cold or other factors make them sluggish, houseflies, blowflies, and similar types will rarely escape if the point of the

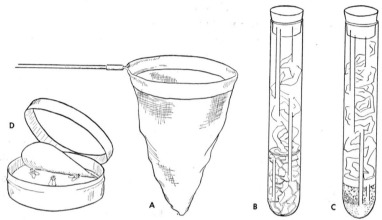

Figure 126. Collecting tools. *A:* Net, preferably of white material. *B:* Chloroform tube. Scraps of rubber, soaked in chloroform, release vapor gradually. *C:* Cyanide tube. Potassium cyanide, covered with sawdust, reacts slowly with air to produce cyanide gas. Both tubes contain crinkled lens paper to keep specimens from matting. *D:* Pillbox, for carrying specimens in the field. Discs of soft tissue protect successive layers.

net is held uppermost and the insect is permitted to follow its natural instincts. In the attempt to escape by flying upward, the flies soon find themselves trapped in the tip of the net, where they betray their presence either by a loud buzzing or by crawling about in the limited space which the extremity provides. The collector may then introduce his tube or bottle through the mouth of the net, with his free hand, and thus encompass the insect from below. In its first reaction to fumes from the killing agent, the insect usually makes a short flight downward, at which time the collector may close the mouth of the tube by thumb or finger and withdraw it from the net. As soon as the fly becomes sufficiently affected to make escape unlikely, a cork or stopper is substituted for the thumb or finger, and the specimen is secured. Large flies may often be held stationary in the net by light pressure of thumb and finger from the outside while the tube is introduced below. For small specimens likely to be damaged by such handling, this is impractical.

THE KILLING TUBE

A 6-inch test tube, of heavy glass, approximately 1 inch in diameter makes the handiest and most practical type of killing tube for use in the field. It fits conveniently into any large pocket, can be readily grasped with the fingers of one hand, and is easily stoppered by a man's thumb. The poison of choice for insect killing tubes is potassium cyanide (KCN), which is available from supply houses in the form of a white powder. It is one of the more dangerous poisons and bears the skull and crossbones label. Care should be exercised in handling potassium cyanide and, of course, one should avoid breathing the fumes. If cyanide poisoning is suspected, a physician should be summoned at once. Meantime, antidotes may be administered. The inhalation of ammonia is recommended, as well as the administration of a teaspoonful of hydrogen peroxide by mouth. If available, 20 grains of potassium carbonate in one ounce of water, followed by a solution of 10 grains of ferrous sulphate and 60 minims of tincture of iron chloride in one ounce of water, is usually effective. Curran (1934) points out that one of the most efficient antidotes for cyanide poisoning is the intravenous injection of methylene blue. Dosage will depend upon the age and weight of the patient, and on the judgment of the physician. Ordinary precautions consist of keeping all containers tightly closed when not actually transferring the salt, holding the breath when directly over the material, and seeing that the room is well ventilated. Any spoons or other apparatus used in handling cyanide should be kept for that purpose only and should never be allowed near food.

To prepare the killing tube, place approximately ½ inch of the potassium cyanide in the bottom and cover with a like amount of sawdust, not too coarse. The sawdust should be tamped slightly, then sealed in place by one of two methods. A neat and permanent arrangement results from pouring a small quantity of freshly mixed plaster of Paris upon the sawdust. This hardens almost immediately and prevents both the sawdust and the cyanide from working up into the tube and inflicting mechanical damage upon the specimens. An alternative procedure is to prepare two or three discs of blotting paper of such a diameter as to fit snugly within the tube. When these have been pushed down tightly with a stirring rod or similar tool, the tube is ready for use. The potassium cyanide reacts slowly with the moisture in the air to form cyanide gas (HCN). Such a generator will serve a full year, and sometimes longer, depending on the rate of the reaction. If captured flies do not succumb within a few minutes, it is an indication that the supply of moisture is insufficient. A drop or two of water upon the plaster or blotting paper will correct this, though such a procedure is usually unnecessary. When the tube loses its killing power, it may either be cleaned out and recharged or thrown away. Those sealed with plaster are usually discarded because of the difficulty of removing the seal.

For short-time service, many collectors prefer a chloroform tube. This is easy to prepare and is safe to have about where there are pets, children, native helpers, or irresponsible workmen. Old rubber tubing or heavy sheet rubber is cut into bits not more than a ½ inch in greatest dimension. These are placed in the bottom of an empty tube, to the height of about 2 inches, and sufficient chloroform is added to cover them. The tube is corked and the rubber is allowed to soak up the chloroform. Any liquid not absorbed by the rubber within twenty minutes should be poured off, after which a disc of cork or cardboard should be snugly fitted to hold the rubber in place. Such a disc will retain its position more satisfactorily if a layer of cotton is first employed to give an even surface. The rubber will give off chloroform vapor slowly over a period of weeks or even months.

Whichever type of killing tube is employed, it is a good plan to place in the tube a few strips of wrinkled lens paper or toilet tissue. These will serve, first, to entangle the newly captured insect and thus reduce the likelihood of its escape while the cork is being inserted. Its second, and more important, function is to prevent specimens from matting together in the bottom of the tube. Antennae, legs, and bristles may become detached and wings may be spoiled for study if such a precaution is not taken. Even so, no very great number of specimens should be allowed to accumulate in a killing tube, especially if they are to be studied with a view to identification of species.

The collector should carry with him in the field a number of small pillboxes, salve boxes, or similar containers to which the specimens may be transferred. Each of these should be made ready before setting out, by placing therein shredded tissue paper or tissue discs for the reception of the specimens. The use of discs has one advantage in that specimens from a given collecting station or locality may be arranged between two adjacent sheets while those taken at another point occupy the next tier, and so on. In no case should the number in one tier be so great as to result in matting together.

For taking more than a few specimens from any particular location, the trap should be substituted for the net. Flytraps, described and discussed in Chapter XVII, are exceedingly useful in obtaining a generous sample of prevailing forms and in indicating the relative abundance of the species concerned. Type of trap, choice of bait, location, and method of mounting will vary with climatic conditions and with the habits of the species desired. When specimens are to be saved for laboratory study, more frequent tending of the trap is necessary than when the object is merely the destruction of the flies. In the latter case, the pouring of boiling water upon the trap is a common practice, but when museum specimens are sought, killing with pyrethrum spray is probably the best procedure. The flies are then spread upon a white cloth, paper, or tray, and the undamaged individuals are selected for transportation to the laboratory.

Subsequent treatment will depend upon the purpose to be served. For immediate dissection, no preservation is required. For subsequent dissection or histological study, preservation in a suitable liquid medium is essential. Traditional preservatives are (1) 70 per cent alcohol and (2) dilute solutions of formaldehyde (2 to 10 per cent). Mixtures of the two are sometimes used, as alcohol alone tends to harden the tissues to an undesirable degree. Formaldehyde also accomplishes better fixation of cells and tissues for microscopic study than does alcohol. A small amount of glycerine may be added to the preservative for further insurance against excessive hardening.

PINNED SPECIMENS

The majority of adult specimens will, of course, be pinned and preserved as dry mounts in museum cases. Houseflies and related forms are of convenient size for direct pinning without the use of points, minuten, or other special supports. A number 2 or, for large Calliphoridae, a number 3 pin is most satisfactory. Finer pins tend to bend when transferring specimens. Coarser ones mutilate the specimens and may obscure important taxonomic characters. Pinning within a few hours after collection is most desirable, as the specimen is still flexible and there is little danger of losing legs or antennae through necessary manipulation. The author has found it convenient to spread newly collected specimens on a white paper background. Many will fall naturally with the lateral surface uppermost. Those which fall on their backs may be turned by means of forceps or dissecting needles. The point of the pin is then brought to the dorsal surface of the thorax, while the specimen is prevented from sliding away by gentle blocking with forceps or finger tip. The pin should be inserted just posterior to the transverse suture and preferably a little to the right (some prefer left) of the median dorsal line. The avoidance of the absolute center is to leave unobscured any bristle, pigment spot, or other character which may be located in that area. Destruction of similar characters on one side is not so serious, as their counterparts on the opposite side are left entire.

When the pin has penetrated the cuticula, the specimen may be lifted and the process completed by thrusting the pin through the thorax while the insect is loosely cradled between the thumb and finger of the opposite hand.

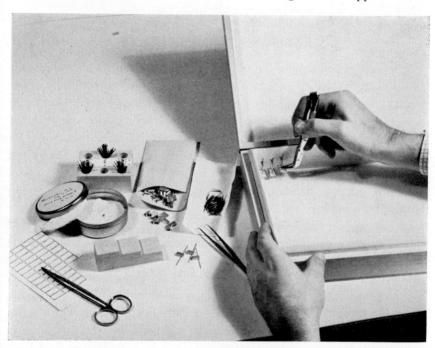

Figure 127. Standard laboratory equipment. *Left to right:* Labels; scissors; pin block; storage tin; step block; cork supports for minuten; corks on No. 2 pins; package of minuten; forceps; Schmitt box; use of pinning forceps. (Courtesy of Ward's Natural Science Establishment.)

Care should be taken that the pin runs vertically through the thorax, at right angles to the long axis of the body. This makes an attractive mount, symmetrically disposed. The pin should be pushed through until approximately eight millimeters remain between the pin head and the dorsum of the insect. Attention to this insures pleasing uniformity throughout the collection. With the insect at this level, ample room exists for the attachment of necessary labels below the body of the fly. Before the specimen hardens, attention should be given to the position of the wings, legs, antennae, and proboscis. These may be manipulated by use of pins or dissecting needles and should be so arranged as to produce a pleasing, symmetrical effect and at the same time display important taxonomic characters. Pollen, dust, and other extraneous matter may be removed at the same time, preferably by means of a camel's-hair brush. These procedures are best carried out under low power of the binocular microscope, with the pinned specimen supported by an L cork or similar device. Specimens thus prepared may be arranged on a "tack" board of cork, balsa, or celotex, to await further attention.

LABELING THE SPECIMENS

Labels are exceedingly important. It is a frequent comment about museums and laboratories that specimens which bear no labels are scientifically worthless. Locality and date of collection should be shown on a small label below the specimen. The greater dimension should parallel the long axis of the insect. This is to conserve space in the museum box. All labels throughout the collection should be so arranged as to be read from the same side. The writer prefers the left. Labels may be written by hand with India ink and a crow quill pen, but it is difficult to achieve legibility unless the label is unduly large. The labor involved is also enormous where large numbers of specimens are concerned. Printed labels are, therefore, always preferable and should be procured whenever extensive collections are intended. Some printing establishments have type sufficiently small to make direct printing a practical procedure. The author has found it more satisfactory, however, to make a master copy, using a typewriter equipped with a new black ribbon. The sheet may consist of a number of columns, each of which deals with a different locality. Only when an expedition has completed its work and no more collecting is contemplated is it practical to include dates. In preparing labels for future use, a space should be left for insertion of the date in ink.

The master sheet, prepared as described above, may then be photographed and a zinc cut prepared on a reduced scale. The amount of reduction will vary with the need, but the finished label, when closely trimmed, should ordinarily not exceed ⅝ inch in length or ¼ inch in width. Long names, or statements identifying unusual localities, will sometimes require more space. A heavy grade of bond paper is usually adequate for printing. Thinner material curls and discolors in a short time, while a heavier card is difficult to penetrate with the pin. In using a sheet of labels, the technician usually fills in all dates, then cuts the labels with scissors or a trimming board. There are many practices in abbreviating dates. The writer prefers the use of Roman characters for the month, regardless of position. Either 12-X-'49 or X-12-'49 can be used to represent the twelfth of October, 1949, whereas 12–10–49 might be interpreted as either October twelfth or December tenth.

Below the locality label may be arranged others giving additional data. Collector's labels are not often used, but when employed may be placed as shown in Figure 128. The use of the lot label has come into very general practice in many institutions and provides a clue to information available in folders, files, or notes. For example, if one encounters a specimen bearing the label $\boxed{\begin{array}{c}\text{Lot 3}\\\text{Sub 4}\end{array}}$, by turning to the appropriate lot book or file, he may discover

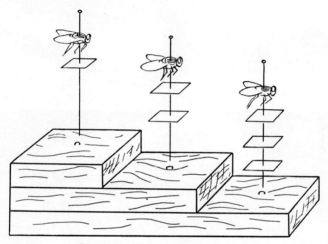

Figure 128. Step block. Labels may be fixed at definite levels by use of holes drilled in the three steps.

that Lot 3 includes all insects collected in the vicinity of Calcutta, India, in connection with the experimental trapping of filth-feeding flies, by a certain investigator between the dates of July fifteenth and August first. The designation Sub 4 will perhaps refer to flies of the genus *Musca,* the identification of which has been vouched for by a certain well-known authority on the group. More than one lot label may be attached to a specimen, if occasion warrants. The height of the labels may be regulated by use of a step block (Fig. 128). All labels in the collection can thus be made uniform for height.

PRESERVATION AND STORAGE

Since chitin undergoes no degeneration under ordinary atmospheric conditions, pinned specimens will remain intact for many years if carefully handled and protected from shocks or sudden jars. They do, however, become more and more brittle, and if exposed to light may eventually lose their distinctive coloration. In spite of great care, feet or antennae of dried specimens will occasionally be broken off. It is entirely feasible to restore such parts

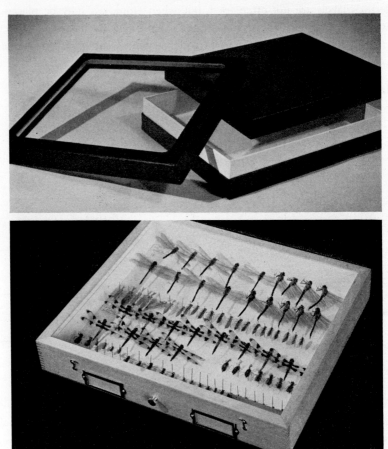

Figure 129. Types of insect boxes. *Upper:* Student-type box, of cardboard. Cover may be solid, or of glass, as shown. This type of box is not pestproof. *Lower:* Cornell-type drawer, with removable glass lid, so fitted that box is practically pestproof. (Courtesy of Ward's Natural Science Establishment.)

to their proper position, using either white shellac or the insect paste sold by biological supply houses. The technician should be absolutely sure, however, that the structure belongs to the specimen in question, as great confusion has arisen when parts of two species have been accidentally associated by well-intentioned but ignorant or thoughtless persons. Classification of such technical monstrosities is, of course, impossible.

Protection against pests of various sorts often constitutes a serious problem. Specimens left uncovered are sometimes completely destroyed by ants or mice in a single night. Even well-housed collections suffer from the attacks of clothes moths, larder beetles, and buffalo bugs, and constant vigilance must be exercised if a collection is to be kept intact. The type of box employed to contain the pinned specimens should be one as nearly pestproof as can be provided with the funds available. All-cardboard boxes should be used only temporarily, as they are in no sense pestproof. They are sometimes useful in

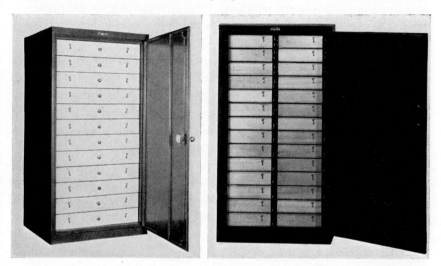

Figure 130. Museum cabinets for housing pinned specimens. *Left:* Unit for housing full-width Cornell-type drawers, with glass tops. *Right:* Two-column unit for housing conventional Schmitt boxes, with wooden lids. Carefully fitted doors render these cabinets as nearly pestproof as possible. (Courtesy of Ward's Natural Science Establishment.)

the field, however, as they are light in weight and are inexpensive. Wooden-frame boxes with cardboard top and bottom are considerably better, but only the all-wood types can be relied upon to protect the specimens over an extended period of time. Most generally used is the *Schmitt*-type insect box, with an inside collar about which the top fits closely when the box is closed. The collar may be slightly rounded to insure against an abrupt inrush of air when the box is opened. Fragile specimens are sometimes damaged by the suction.

Regardless of the type of box employed, the bottom must be lined with some substance suitable for the reception of the pins. Sheet cork is very desirable but is difficult to obtain. Composition cork is a desirable substitute, provided the cement which holds the particles together is not of such a nature as to corrode the pins (Klots, 1932). Celotex, peat, and soft grades of balsa wood have also been used. Manufacturers usually give the interior an attractive appearance by gluing white glazed paper upon bottom, sides, and lid.

Museums and institutions commonly employ a cabinet-drawer type of box with a removable glass lid. These are slid upon racks which may, if desired, be contained in cabinets with tight-fitting doors. The bottoms of the drawers can be of material suitable for holding pins, or the specimens may be pinned into small cardboard boxes which are then arranged within the drawer in rows. The exposed side of the drawer should bear a label indicating the contents.

For teaching and demonstration purposes the Riker mount will sometimes be found practical. Such a mount consists of a shallow cardboard box filled with cotton, on which the specimen is placed. A series of specimens of a single species may be placed side by side, some in dorsal view, some in the lateral position, some with the ventral structures exposed. The lid, which is of glass, is then placed in position and the margin is sealed, passe-partout fashion, with gummed tape. No pins are used in preparing the specimens.

When it is anticipated that the specimens will be carefully scrutinized with a view to determining genus and species, it is a good practice to expose the male genitalia so that these structures may be taken into account by the taxonomist. A simple technique has been described by Aldrich (1916), who was especially interested in the Sarcophagidae. It is, however, applicable to any muscoidean type. The fresh specimen is held between the thumb and finger and examined under the low power of a binocular dissecting microscope. With a dissecting needle, the extreme tip of which has been bent at right angles, the forceps of the genitalia are drawn backward as far as they will go without tearing the tissues. This operation should be repeated a few times to stretch the muscles and ligaments so that retraction no longer tends to occur. The pinned fly is then arranged upon an L cork in such a fashion that its side is in contact with one surface. A second pin is used to hold the genitalia in the extended position, and the specimen is allowed to dry for two or three days.

Old pinned specimens which have been in a collection for some time can be prepared for study of the genitalia by placing in a relaxing jar for twenty-four hours or longer, after which the parts may be withdrawn as described above. The preparation of relaxing chambers is discussed on page 394.

Repellents, to discourage insect pests, should be placed in all boxes containing specimens. Naphtha (or camphor) may be placed in a small cardboard box with a cover of fine mesh wire. The box is then securely pinned in one corner. Through the wire pass the fumes but not the crystals or powder, which might damage the specimens. If the repellent is replaced as soon as it is exhausted, usually no infestation will occur. Once pests have become established, however, repellents are not sufficient. A small amount of dark sawdust beneath a pinned specimen is usually indicative of pest activity. It will then be necessary to fumigate. Carbon disulphide, carbon tetrachloride, and paradichlorobenzene have all been used extensively for this purpose. Carbon

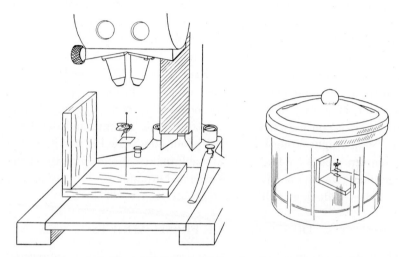

Figure 131. Left. Use of "L" block. Made of cork or balsa wood, this type of support permits the specimen to be arranged in any desired position for examination under the binocular microscope.

Figure 132. Right. Relaxing jar. Moist sand creates sufficient humidity to render specimens pliable in about twenty-four hours.

disulphide is probably the least desirable, being inflammable, rather malodorous, and somewhat poisonous to man. It may also corrode certain types of pins and has been known to stain both box and specimens. Carbon tetrachloride, though also a liquid, lacks most of these undesirable features. A teaspoonful may be poured upon the bottom of the box and left to evaporate. Paradichlorobenzene is probably most convenient to use in that it is available as small white crystals which may be placed in an open container in one corner of the box. Whatever type of fumigant is used, the box cover should then be tightly closed to permit the insecticide to do its work. Any evidence of infestation should be removed, so that on subsequent inspection the debris will not be interpreted as indicative of a fresh invasion.

RELAXING DRIED SPECIMENS

When specimens reach the laboratory in a dried condition it is futile to attempt to pin them, as loss of legs and other parts is sure to occur. They should be placed in a relaxing chamber for perhaps twenty-four hours to make the parts once more flexible. A small chamber for relaxing a very few specimens may be contrived by placing a lump of moist cotton inside a Petri dish. The specimens will be easier to see and, therefore, easier to handle if a disc of filter paper is first placed in the bottom. A more permanent type of relaxing chamber adapted for handling a considerable number of specimens may be made by placing at least an inch of sand in the bottom of a stone crock, battery jar, or large culture dish. Sufficient water is then added to render the sand distinctly moist throughout, and a few drops of phenol are sprinkled about to prevent the growth of molds. Two or three layers of paper toweling may then be placed on the sand. The insects are laid on this, and the vessel is closed with a tight-fitting lid. A twenty-four-hour period is usually sufficient for complete relaxation. It is rarely advisable to leave specimens in the chamber longer than two days in any case, as extended exposure to the moist air causes a secondary stiffening of the parts.

DISSECTION OF FRESH ADULTS

For various reasons, one may wish to dissect the adult fly. A demonstration of the alimentary canal, including the crop, has great teaching value for students of medical entomology. The age and breeding condition of captured females may be interpreted from the condition of the reproductive organs. It is sometimes desirable to isolate a definite portion of the food canal with a view to making a bacterial culture from the contents. For such work, the binocular dissection microscope is indispensable. The writer prefers to use two dissecting needles, one of which has a spear-shaped head. Such a needle may be used as a miniature scalpel to cut through tissue while adjacent structures are held fast by a needle of the ordinary type. Some investigators prefer to have each needle ground to resemble one blade of a pair of scissors. By approximating the two flat surfaces, a shearing action is achieved. Only needles of high-grade surgical steel will retain a cutting edge sufficiently keen for this purpose.

Excellent miniature dissecting needles may be contrived by utilizing either the snipped-off tips of number oo insect pins or standard "minuten nadeln," ground to a point. By use of pinning forceps, either can be pressed into the end of a throat-swab applicator, which thereafter serves as a handle. Undesirable movement in the manipulation of such light equipment, due to tremors of the fingers, may be overcome by placing a lump of plastic clay on either side of the object to be dissected. By allowing the side of the applicator to rest on this, a stable fulcrum is provided and tremors are largely eliminated. The point of contact should be considerably closer to the needle than to the hand of the operator, so that rather free manipulation of the base results in but limited movement at the tip.

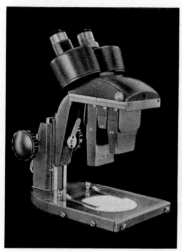 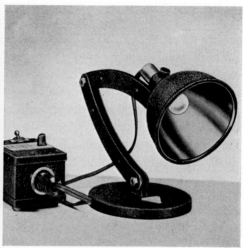

Figure 133. Widefield binocular microscope. A good binocular is indispensable for taxonomic work. It is also invaluable in dissection. (Courtesy of Bausch and Lomb Optical Co.)

Figure 134. An effective illuminator. Adequate illumination for the microscopic study of opaque specimens is of great importance. Adjustable support insures control of direction. This model is connected with a rheostat. (Courtesy of Bausch and Lomb Optical Co.)

Dissection may be carried out on the microscope stage, on a plain glass slide, in the well of a hollow-ground slide, or in a watch glass. The hollow-ground slide is probably to be preferred. A very good plan is first to pour a small quantity of melted paraffin into the bottom of the depression. Just before the paraffin solidifies, the specimen is gently pressed against it by means of forceps. The insect is thus retained in the desired position, releasing both hands of the technician for actual dissection.

IMMATURE STAGES

The collection of eggs, larvae, or pupae, either for demonstration purposes or for subsequent study, involves a somewhat different procedure. If no histological work is contemplated, these stages may be merely dropped into 70 per cent alcohol. This both kills and preserves the specimen, which may be kept in the same medium indefinitely.

Specimens preserved in alcohol are usually stored in homeopathic vials of two-, four-, or six-dram capacity. These may be fitted with screw tops, but ordinary corks are usually quite satisfactory and are less expensive. With an "active" collection, inspection is usually frequent enough to provide for replacement of evaporated alcohol before the specimens become dry, but if a collection is to be stored without attention for a considerable time, the corks should be sealed in place with paraffin. Valuable material may thereby be protected against desiccation. Delicate specimens, once dried out, are usually valueless, but if not too wrinkled, they may sometimes be restored by soaking in water for a number of hours. After they have regained their normal appearance, the specimens are again transferred to alcohol.

The classification of material preserved in alcohol is best accomplished by pouring the contents of the vial into a watch glass. If preferred, a single specimen may be placed, with forceps, upon a hollow-ground slide. A binocular dissection microscope should be used. To avoid glare, partial drying of larvae and puparia may be permitted, but such specimens should not be left exposed to air too long, lest wrinkling occur.

STORAGE AND ARRANGEMENT OF SPECIMENS PRESERVED IN ALCOHOL

If the collection is a small one, the vials may be stored in small boxes or trays, the unoccupied portion being blocked in some way to prevent the bottles from falling over. The upright position of the vial is important, as otherwise the preservative may leak out or the specimens may become discolored by disintegration of the cork.

A collection of substantial size is best housed by providing a cupboard in which removable vertical frames of strong wire netting are fitted into slots above and below. The slots are usually made ¼ inch wide and ¼ inch deep. The frames consist of squares of wire netting of approximately ¼-inch mesh, with the edges bound by a strip of sheet metal folded lengthwise to cover the raw edge. Each vial is suspended by a hook of copper wire, previously wrapped around the neck of the vial itself. A large number of vials may be very quickly fitted with these hooks. A spool of flexible wire and a pair of cutter pliers are all that are needed. If the vertical frames are placed 1¾ inches apart, there will be ample room for the specimens. Vials may be arranged in any convenient order. For example, all representatives of a given family may be attached to one frame with the genera in separate rows. Group labels may be written or typed on strips of paper or light cardboard and woven into the meshes of the frame. The system lends itself to unlimited expansion and to ready interpolation of new material.

Labels stating locality and date of collection, name of collector, and other pertinent information should be written in pencil on small strips of paper and

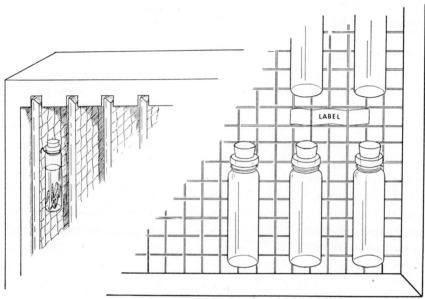

LABEL

Figure 135. Left. Housing of alcoholic specimens. Vials are hooked, by wire, upon vertical wire-cloth frames, which slide into grooves of wooden cupboard. *Right.* Face view of frame, on larger scale, with label woven into mesh of screen.

placed in the vial, with the specimen, at the moment of collection. There will then be no danger of confusing the data when the specimens are taken to the laboratory. Pencil is preferred for two reasons: (1) it is always available under field conditions; (2) it will not run or fade out in alcohol, no matter how long the specimens are kept. Subsequent study will usually require duplication of the data, as specimens are divided into smaller lots. Genus and species labels must also be added when identification has been confirmed. India ink may be used for this purpose if it is allowed to become thoroughly dry before immersion in the alcohol. Gummed labels stuck to the outside of the vial are not very satisfactory. In the course of time they usually loosen and fall off, leaving the specimen without identification. They also obscure the contents of the vial, so that casual examination becomes difficult or impossible without removing the specimens.

WHOLE MOUNTS OF IMMATURE STAGES

Eggs and very small larvae, which require higher magnification for satisfactory study, should be mounted on slides. In anticipation of this, it is best to kill the specimens by dropping them into hot water, followed by a few hours in 50 per cent alcohol. Transference to 70 per cent alcohol, then 80 to 85 per cent, is recommended procedure. The gradual increase in concentration of preservative reduces the likelihood of shrinkage and distortion. When ready to proceed with mounting, the technician transfers the specimens to 95 per cent alcohol. This usually accomplishes sufficient dehydration to permit mounting without treatment with absolute alcohol, but if absolute is available, its use will insure best results. One or more changes of 95 per cent alcohol may be employed. The usual procedure is to transfer the specimen from 95 per cent (or absolute) alcohol to xylene for clearing. The cleared specimen is then mounted in balsam, between a slide and cover glass. Direct mounting in Euparal from higher alcohols is also a common practice. The preparations become more clear with age.

Third-stage larvae, being thick-bodied, do not usually make neat balsam mounts. The preparation is often too opaque to permit observation of details, and the cover glass rides so high that there is not sufficient working distance for the high-power objective. If mounts are desired, however, these difficulties may be overcome by first soaking the specimen for a time in 10 per cent caustic potash to reduce opacity, then slitting along the side to permit squeezing out of the dissolved internal tissue. The larva should then be gently but thoroughly washed to remove residual alkali. Dehydration by immersion in alcohols of increasing concentration is followed by clearing and mounting in the usual manner. The cover glass should be supported by three or four fragments of glass, peripherally arranged. This will prevent distortion of the specimen as the balsam dries.

To insure a direct view of the posterior spiracles, which are much used in classification, it is a good plan to slice off the posterior area with a razor blade or very sharp scalpel while the specimen is still fresh. This unit is mounted near the body portion, which is disposed either for lateral or dorsoventral observation. Some workers prefer to discard the middle portion of the larva, retaining only the posterior spiracles and the anterior segments. Practically all items of taxonomic interest, including the mouth hooks, pharyngeal apparatus, and anterior spiracles, are thus preserved, while a bulky mount is avoided.

The caustic potash technique described above is well adapted for the occasional mounting of adult structures, such as antennae, feet, or male genitalia. If soaking in 10 per cent potassium hydroxide does not reduce the opacity of the chitin, gentle boiling will bring about the desired effect. Some workers recommend immersion in 50 per cent nitric acid to reduce the opacity of chitin. Frequent inspection is required to prevent the solution of the chitin from proceeding to an undesirable extreme.

DRY MOUNTS OF WINGS

The mounting of wings deserves special comment. Since the index of refraction of the veins of insect wings is very nearly the same as that of balsam (and of glass), the mounting of wings in Euparal or balsam is not usually recommended. The more delicate and more transparent veins become almost

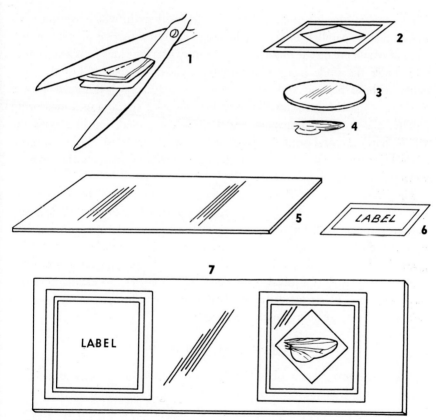

Figure 136. Making dry mounts of wings. *1:* Cutting diamond-shaped area from gummed label. *2:* Cut label, unfolded. *3:* Cover glass. *4:* Wing to be mounted. *5:* Glass slide. *6:* Identification label. *7:* Mount, complete.

invisible. The writer prefers a dry mount, as shown in Figure 136. The cover glass is held in place by a slide label, the center of which has been cut out with scissors. In such a mount, the veins stand out sharply. In most species, the veins have sufficient natural transparency to permit illumination from below.

Housefly pupae are too bulky to be mounted entire. In certain families of flies, however, where species run smaller, the pupae have been studied in this way. Thus De Meijere (1925) prepared both larvae and pupae of Agromyzidae by killing in hot water or alcohol and clearing in strong carbolic acid. He mounted them in Venetian turpentine, either from alcohol or carbolic acid. Pupae that had become too dark were bleached in Diaphanol for several hours before being transferred to the slide for mounting.

TRANSPARENT PLASTIC MOUNTS

The preservation of prehistoric insects in fossil resin, which we now call amber, may be paralleled today by the use of clear, transparent plastics, several types of which are on the market for laboratory use. Best known is a substance sold under the trade name of Castolite, a clear, transparent liquid which pours without heating and sets at low temperatures when mixed with a hardener. Supply houses usually offer for sale a kit containing a measuring pipette, glass mold, sandpapers, and buffing compound, together with the plastic, hardener, and printed directions for use. When finished, the casting is as clear as pure glass and the fly or other specimen embedded within may be viewed from any angle.

The smoother the mold, the less buffing and sanding will be necessary to give the cast a satisfactory surface. Care should be taken to see that dirt, dust particles, and water have no contact with the equipment, as any contamination of the plastic is likely to show up as a flaw in the finished work. Plexiglass, Bioplastic, and Lucite (ethyl or methyl methacrylate) are other commercial plastics of equivalent properties. Kampmeier and Haviland (1948) have been particularly successful in adapting plastic techniques to the preservation and display of bulky anatomical specimens.

HISTOLOGICAL TECHNIQUES

When the investigator plans a microscopic study of tissues and cells, ordinary methods of preservation are rarely adequate. A fixing agent must be used. The purpose of fixation is to preserve all the elements of tissue structure as nearly as possible as in the living animal. This is accomplished by either rendering the chemical constituents insoluble or substituting for them in such a way that the structural relations are preserved with the least possible degree of distortion. No fixing agent is equally satisfactory for all types of cells or for all portions of a single cell. The choice of fixative will, therefore, depend in part on the results desired. Besides alcohol and formaldehyde, which have but limited value when used alone, Kingsbury and Johannsen (1935) list the following general fixatives as most satisfactory: osmic acid, platinic chloride, picric acid, acetic acid, chromic acid, mercuric chloride, potassium dichromate, copper dichromate, and nitric acid.

Practially all fixing solutions used in histological laboratories are mixtures of two or more of these chemicals, the particular combination being known usually by the name of the worker who first employed the formula. We thus have Zenker's *dichromate, sublimate-acetic* preparation, Bensley's *osmo-acetic-dichromate*, Orth's *formol-dichromate*, von Rath's *picro-aceto-sublimate*, Fleming's *chromo-aceto-osmic* fixative, and a number of others. In such preparations, the different substances supplement each other and tend to counteract one another's defects. For any particular species or tissue, a certain amount of experimentation is usually necessary.

Entomological specimens, being small, are usually put into the fixative entire. They may be dropped alive into the preparation, which thus both kills and fixes, or the technician may prefer first to kill in hot water, then transfer to the chosen fixative.

Using four-day-old larvae of *Musca domestica*, Kramer (1948) succeeded in perfecting a technique for obtaining satisfactory differentiation of insect muscle *in toto*. The steps are as follows:

1. Drop living larvae into Bouin's fluid [1] at 30°C and allow them to remain for 8 to 10 hours. The Bouin's solution should be prepared with formalin which has been neutralized with magnesium sulphate. The larvae live from 2 to 4 hours, which favors penetration of body tissues by the fixing agent.

2. Transfer specimens to 50 per cent ethyl alcohol for ten minutes.

3. Transfer to 70 per cent ethyl alcohol for 1 hour.

4. Place in 95 per cent ethyl alcohol for ten minutes.

5. Transfer to 0.5 per cent eosin solution in 95 per cent alcohol and allow to remain for 6 to 8 hours.

6. Return to 95 per cent alcohol and mix in 4 to 6 drops of oil of wintergreen every hour for 4 to 5 days. Shriveling will result if the oil is added too rapidly. The dish should be kept covered to avoid evaporation.

7. Allow alcohol to evaporate and transfer larvae to oil of wintergreen.

[1] Picro-aceto-formol, consisting of picric acid, saturated aqueous solution, 75 cc.; formalin, 25 cc.; glacial acetic acid, 4 cc.

Under artificial illumination the larvae appear yellow-green in color. The muscles and their attachments are easily observed through the transparent cuticle. They are also easily differentiated from the fat bodies and other internal structures, a difficult matter under previous techniques.

In the technique described above, it will be noted that the three important steps, dehydration, clearing, and mounting, are carried out in the order named, as with specimens where no differentiation of internal tissue is attempted. The additional procedure, however, staining in eosin, is of particular significance. The point at which staining is carried out will depend upon the nature of the solvent in which the stain is carried. In this case, since the carrier is 95 per cent alcohol, the larvae are first passed through increasing concentrations of alcohol until that level is obtained. No shriveling, swelling, or other distortion occurs, therefore, while the stain is being applied, and a uniform penetration is assured. If the stain had been in aqueous solution, it would have been necessary to transfer from fixative to one or more changes of water to secure equivalent results. After being stained in aqueous solution, the specimen must then be passed through 50, 70, and 95 per cent alcohol to remove the water. In passing a specimen from one reagent to another, it is wise to press the tip of the forceps (and the specimen) against a bit of folded gauze before immersion in a succeeding fluid. The contact dries the specimen and thus guards the new reagent against significant contamination by the first.

PREPARATION OF SPECIMENS FOR SECTIONING [2]

Only rarely are histological relationships observable in whole-mount preparations. For discriminating studies, the use of the microtome is essential. For insect specimens, freehand sectioning without embedding is usually impractical; even if attempted, it amounts to little more than a modified gross dissection. On the other hand, if one takes the time and trouble to embed the specimen (or a part of it) properly, he may as well employ machine sectioning, as thinner and more uniform sections will thereby be secured than can possibly be produced by hand.

As with vertebrate tissue, four methods of embedding are available: (1)

[2] The pages that follow are not intended as a substitute for standard works on histological technique. The object is rather to call attention to procedures which experience has shown most useful in studying the tissues of insects, and particularly the muscoid Diptera. For additional details, for alternate techniques, and for many precautionary and corrective procedures, the user should consult the well-known volumes by Gage, Guyer, Lee, Mayer, Wright, McClung, Conn, Kingsbury and Johannsen, and various others.

the celloidin method, (2) the paraffin method, (3) the celloidin-paraffin method, and (4) the freezing method. All are similar in that the tissue spaces are completely filled by a substance which imparts uniform consistency and a certain amount of support. In frozen sections, ice substitutes for the paraffin or collodion.

The Celloidin Method

The embedding material is collodion, a solution of pyroxylin (nitrocellulose) in ether and alcohol. Tissues, however preserved, must first be dehydrated by immersion in alcohols of increasing concentration. Several changes of 95 per cent are desirable, and the last change should be to absolute alcohol, if it is obtainable. Several days in alcohols of higher concentration will do no harm, and ensure a more complete dehydration. The specimen is then transferred to a solution consisting of equal parts of pure ether and absolute alcohol, where it is allowed to remain from 12 to 24 hours. At the end of this time, the ether-alcohol is poured off and replaced with a 2 per cent solution of celloidin in the same solvent. A day or more is usually allowed for penetration, after which the thin solution is poured off and a 5 or 6 per cent solution of celloidin in ether-alcohol is used to replace it. The specimens should be allowed to remain in this medium for several days. Evaporation will usually increase the concentration to perhaps 12 per cent. A further change to 12 per cent celloidin is desirable in any case.

The most satisfactory method of embedding is by use of a small paper box.[3] A good quality of writing paper is first rubbed with vaseline, after which the excess is removed with lens paper or a bit of cloth. The paper is next folded to form the box, the greased surface being on the inside. This is to prevent the celloidin from adhering to the paper. The specimen is then placed in the box, its position adjusted with a view to future sectioning, and the 12 per cent celloidin added drop by drop, until the specimen is deeply covered and the box is practically filled. The celloidin may be rendered solid by placing the mass under a bell jar and permitting evaporation to take place. Initial hardening is usually achieved by pouring a little chloroform into the jar. After a brief exposure to the vapor, the celloidin is transferred to a container of chloroform for a period lasting from 6 to 24 hours. This removes all ether-alcohol and completes the hardening process.

Depending on the purpose to be served, the block is stored either in 67 to 82 per cent alcohol or in "clarifier," composed of three parts of xylene to

[3] See figure 137 for detail of this procedure.

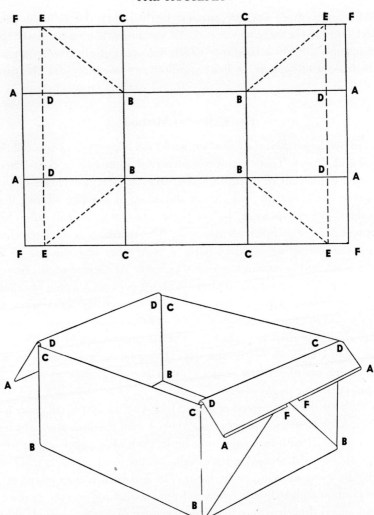

Figure 137. Preparing paper trays for paraffin blocks. *Upper:* Method of folding. *Lower:* Finished tray. (Adapted from Kingsbury and Johannsen, *Histological Technique;* courtesy of John Wiley & Sons, Inc.)

one of castor oil. The purpose of the clarifier is to render the preparation quite transparent, thus facilitating better orientation of the tissue for sectioning. In either case, when one is ready to cut the sections, the paper box is removed, the blocks are trimmed to resemble a four-sided, truncate pyramid, and the base is attached to the holding mechanism of the microtome. This is best accomplished by drying the base of the pyramid with a cloth, after which a small quantity of 6 per cent celloidin is poured upon the surface of the holder, which may be of either wood or metal. Firm pressure of the celloidin block against the holder will result, in a few minutes, in a rigid mount. The holder may now be clamped in place and sectioning may be started.

With a first-class knife and under favorable conditions, sections can be cut as thin as 6 microns. With celloidin, however, most technicians do not undertake sections less than 10 microns in thickness. The celloidin block should be so oriented that the greater mass is opposite the side which first contacts the cutting edge. For celloidin sectioning, the knife is set at an angle of approximately 18 degrees, so that a drawing stroke can be achieved. The knife should next be flooded with either alcohol or clarifier, whichever was used earlier. The tissue block is flooded in a similar manner. A slow, steady motion of the knife is most effective.

The above procedure is known as "wet sectioning." A dry method of sectioning celloidin blocks is sometimes followed by substituting thin cedar oil for castor-xylene as a clarifier. Immersion in a mixture of chloroform and cedar oil is followed by final clarification in oil alone. The cedar oil does not dissolve the celloidin, and the blocks, when cleared, may be stored dry in stoppered bottles.

The Paraffin Method

The tissue must first be thoroughly dehydrated by immersion in strong alcohol. If, after fixing, it has been stored in 80 to 95 per cent alcohol, a change or two of 95 per cent is sometimes sufficient, but final dehydration by use of absolute alcohol is always preferable. Several days should be allowed for passage through the alcohols.

Dehydration is followed by immersion in a clearing agent for from 2 to 24 hours. In common use are xylene, carbol-xylene, benzene, toluene, cedar oil, and chloroform. A complete list would include many others. Whatever clearing agent is used, it must be miscible with alcohol and must also be capable of dissolving paraffin, with which the tissue must next be infiltrated. The steps will differ according to the clearing agent used. For xylene, it is best to transfer the specimen first from absolute alcohol to a mixture composed of equal parts of xylene and absolute alcohol. The tissue is then placed in pure xylene, where it should remain until clear. The first step in infiltration consists of transfer to a mixture of equal parts of xylene and paraffin. The melting point of the paraffin should be around 38°C. A temperature in this vicinity should be maintained for perhaps a two-day period, during which time the xylene will slowly evaporate. This step is followed by a change to pure liquid paraffin, melting point 54°C. There are many types of paraffin ovens on the market which maintain a suitable temperature. One change to fresh paraffin is usually desirable. In the case of very small objects, infiltration is usually complete within an hour, but a longer period does no harm. If one is working with an entire insect, such as an adult fly, the body wall should be slit or perforated to ensure more thorough penetration.

For embedding, one should use a fresh lot of paraffin, the hardness of which

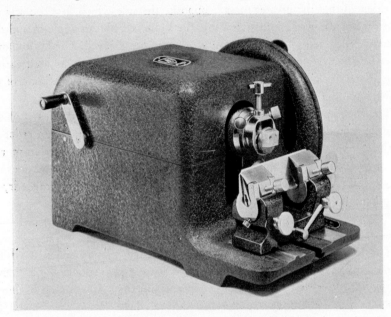

Figure 138. Rotary microtome, with blade in place. Trimmed paraffin block is attached to metal holder for sectioning. (Courtesy of American Optical Company.)

will depend upon the probable temperature of the room in which the sections will be cut. In summer, paraffin with a melting point as high as 60°C (140°F) may be required. It is desirable that the last change during the infiltration process be to paraffin of the same melting point as that selected for embedding. As when celloidin is used, the small paper box makes the most practical receptacle. Glass containers such as watch glasses may also be used by smearing the interior with a film of glycerine. Some workers prefer two L-shaped units of metal which may be so arranged on a metal plate as to form a mold of any desired size. In either case, one should use as small a container as will suffice to embed the specimen properly. This will ensure rapid cooling and thus reduce the likelihood of crystallization. When poured, the paraffin should be several degrees above its melting point, but not so hot as to alter the condition of the tissue. Prompt cooling of the block is essential in order to ensure a homogeneous condition. This is best accomplished by floating the paper box on cold water until a substantial film forms on the surface of the paraffin. The block is then immersed. Under tropical conditions, where perhaps neither ice nor cold water may be available, floating on ether-alcohol in

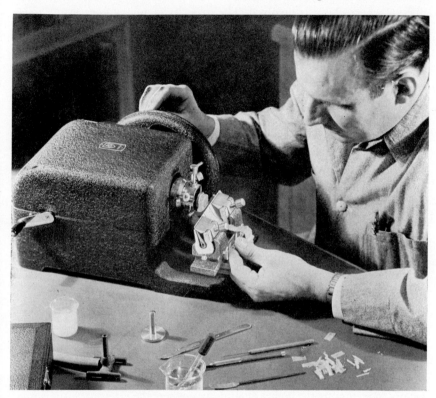

Figure 139. Microtome in operation. Paraffin sections are being removed as a continuous ribbon. (Courtesy of American Optical Company.)

a shallow dish will be found practical. Dropping 95 per cent alcohol on the newly formed film is also helpful.

After cooling, the block can be stored indefinitely. In anticipation of sectioning, it should be roughly trimmed so that opposite sides are more or less parallel. If the specimen is large, the holder may be heated and the block melted on. With insect specimens, however, the block is almost always small, and a more careful procedure should be followed. The crudely trimmed block is first fused to the holder by use of a heated needle. When cool again, the block is trimmed closely and carefully so that the upper and lower faces are absolutely parallel with one another. Mechanical trimmers are a great help in accomplishing this. The holder is then clamped in the microtome, with the upper and lower edges of the block parallel to the cutting edge of the knife, which is set horizontally. Most microtomes permit the use of either a standard heavy knife or a safety razor blade, held in a special clamp. The former is far superior where chitin is involved. The majority of microtomes in use today are of the rotary type.

For paraffin sectioning the knife should be dry and very sharp. It is usually possible to obtain thinner sections by this method than by the use of celloidin. A rapid stroke is used; if temperature conditions are suitable, successive sections will adhere in the form of a continuous ribbon. Although a slight amount of distortion is usually unavoidable, the paraffin method is generally considered superior to the celloidin method for smaller specimens. If the sections roll, it is an indication that the paraffin is too hard or that the room temperature is too low. This may often be corrected by placing an electric light at an appropriate distance from the microtome. If the sections crush together, the room is probably too warm. Sections may be transferred directly to a clean slide or, more commonly, laid on trays to await separation and mounting. Various small tools will be found useful in handling the ribbons, such as needles, scalpel handles, camel's-hair brush, or a small spatula. One should be careful in expelling the breath or in exposing the sections to drafts from doors, windows, ventilators, or electric fans, as they can be very easily scattered and perhaps rendered useless. If serial mounting is desired, it is of the utmost importance that the original relation be preserved.

Paraffin-Celloidin Method

The combined use of paraffin and celloidin will be found especially satisfactory in sectioning the bodies of adult flies, where the external chitin is much harder and more brittle than the softer tissues immediately beneath. It is also used in connection with embryological studies for sectioning ova, where the external chorion is so much more rigid than the yolky material within.

Tissue should first be infiltrated with thin celloidin (2 per cent) in ether alcohol. This is followed by 5 per cent and finally by 8 per cent. A period of 24 hours in each concentration is essential. The celloidin, with the specimen, is then poured into a watch glass and the latter is placed in chloroform vapor beneath a bell jar to hasten evaporation of the solvent. At the end of an hour and a half, the celloidin is usually firm enough to permit trimming into a small cube, which should be scarcely larger than the specimen itself. A number of such cubes are next placed in a watch glass containing chips of 40°C paraffin plus an equal volume of chloroform. After 24 hours at 40°C, the celloidin blocks are transferred to 50°C paraffin, which is changed once or twice during the next hour. Final transfer to paper boxes or glass molds greased with glycerin is followed by covering with fresh paraffin. A few minutes in the oven, then quick cooling, completes the process. The paraffin block may be trimmed to any convenient size, but the celloidin should not be exposed, as ribboning of the sections would thereby be prevented.

Tissuemat

A special embedding compound sold by supply houses under the trade name of "tissuemat" has become popular with many workers. Chemically similar to paraffin, it is superior in certain physical characteristics. It is usually supplied as flakes or small cubes, facilitating rapid melting. There is little or no shrinkage of tissue during the embedding process, and distortion due to sectioning is rare. With proper handling, crumbling and cracking do not occur, and very thin sections may be obtained. It is especially useful where ribbon sections are desired. Tissuemat may be obtained with various melting points, ranging from 50°C (122°F) to 62°C (143°F).

Use of Dioxane

Elimination of a number of steps necessary in conventional histological technique may be accomplished by the use of diethyl dioxide (dioxane), which serves both as a clearing agent and as a general solvent. Kitzmiller (1949) reported dioxane especially useful in insect microtechnique. He points out that dioxane is miscible not only with certain fixatives but also with water and with tissuemat. Kitzmiller worked chiefly with aphids, but the technique is adaptable for other forms. He recommends immersion in Bouin's fixative for at least an hour. Storage in Bouin's for several days will do no harm. Specimens are next transferred to dioxane for one hour, then changed to fresh dioxane for overnight. Infiltration with tissuemat for two to several hours is followed by embedding in tissuemat with a melting point of 56°–58°C (132.8°–136.4°F). Kitzmiller added calcium oxide to the stock bottle of dioxane to reduce the water content. He also ensured dehydration of the tissues while in dioxane by making use of a desiccator in which calcium oxide was contained.

The only disadvantage in the use of dioxane lies in the fact that it is rather toxic to man. However, if the room is kept well ventilated, and if all operations are carried out under a closed hood, there should be no difficulty on this score. The greatest argument for its use is that dehydration is accomplished without hardening of the exoskeleton, a disadvantage where alcohols and xylene are employed.

Kitzmiller cautions against allowing the tissuemat to rise above 59°C (138.2°F) during the embedding process, as this destroys the tissue. He prefers plaster of Paris molds for embedding, as recommended by Solberg (1939). These are made with sloping sides, an arrangement which results in automatic ejection of the cast when the tissuemat, cooled by immersion in ice water, undergoes shrinkage.

Freezing Method

This method is most used in pathological laboratories for quick clinical diagnosis. But it is also of value in the study of insects, especially when certain conditions arise: (1) when the tissue is too hard to be cut satisfactorily by use of either celloidin or paraffin; (2) when it is desired to examine tissues for the presence of fats, which are normally dissolved out by solutions used in connection with the other methods.

Three procedures are available. The simplest is the freezing and cutting of the fresh specimen which has never been placed in preservative. The second involves tissues which have been fixed. (Such tissues must be thoroughly soaked in water before being frozen.) The third, which requires time but ensures better preparations in the end, requires saturating the tissue with some substance which does not crystallize when frozen, as does ice, but simply hardens into a homogeneous mass. One way of producing such a congelation is by use of aniseed oil. The tissue must first have most of the water removed by passage through the alcohols, but complete dehydration is not essential. Transfer from 90 per cent alcohol to aniseed oil is entirely feasible. After 24 hours in aniseed oil, the tissue is ready to freeze and cut. This procedure is often followed with tissue that has previously been stained *in toto*.

Another substance sometimes used to achieve the same end is gum arabic, which is miscible with water. Tissues that have been kept in alcohol should be soaked in water for perhaps a day, then removed to a thick aqueous solution of the gum. After 24 hours the mass may be frozen and cut.

The usual procedure is to place upon the carrier of the microtome a drop of gum arabic or aniseed oil. This is then sprayed with either carbon dioxide or ether to initiate freezing. With the first evidence of hardening, the tissue, together with an abundance of solution, is placed upon the drop and freezing is completed by use of the spray, beneath an inverted cup. A wedge-shaped knife is used. As with the paraffin method, rapid strokes assure the best results.

If gum arabic was used, the sections are transferred to water. The gum washes away and the sections are then ready to be stained. If aniseed oil was the freezing medium, it may be removed by transferring the section to 95 per cent alcohol. Sections already stained *in toto* need only be transferred to pure aniseed oil or some other clearing agent preparatory to mounting.

Transferring Sections

Celloidin sections, if thick, are best transferred by forceps or a brush. If very thin, it is best to use tissue paper. The sections, which will be clinging to the knife, are flooded with clarifier, the knife is partially dried by means of a pipette, and the paper is pressed gently against the sections. When the paper is lifted, the sections will come with it. Firm pressure through the paper then fastens the sections to the slide, after which the paper is removed with a rolling motion. It is a good plan to repeat the process two or three times with fresh paper. This removes all excess clarifier. The tissue is next made wet with ether-alcohol, applied by means of a pipette. This softens the celloidin temporarily, with the result that, when the solvent has evaporated, the section is usually well sealed to the slide. Since celloidin sections must not be allowed to dry out, the slides should be stored in 95 per cent alcohol to await staining and mounting.

Paraffin sections are always somewhat wrinkled when first cut. A good procedure is to place the slide on a warming table and flood it with distilled water. The sections are then floated on the water, which, as it becomes warmer, causes the paraffin to spread. When expansion is complete the slide is lifted and the water is poured off. If one end of the paraffin ribbon is held in place by the tip of a dissecting needle, the sections will settle upon the slide in the desired position. Drainage may also be effected by means of a pipette. A little further warming will drive off the remaining water, though evaporation for a few hours at room temperature is usually preferred. Sections of insect tissue are ordinarily so small that they adhere quite satisfactorily to the slide during the staining process. If one anticipates trouble, however, the use of Mayer's albumen fixative is recommended. This is prepared by combining 1 g. of sodium salicylate with 50 cc. of glycerin and 50 cc. of egg white. A small drop placed upon the slide and thinly spread with a clean finger tip is sufficient. The slide is then flooded with distilled water, as described above. Albumen fixative may be used to fasten celloidin sections also, though celloidin usually adheres very well without it.

Frozen sections are usually first floated into water, then transferred to the slide with a camel's-hair brush. The water is drained off and the sections are

pressed smooth by means of absorbent paper. To fasten the sections to the
slide, a few drops of absolute or 95 per cent alcohol are sprinkled on, to be
followed immediately by a 0.5 per cent solution of celloidin. After evaporation
of the solvent, the section will adhere firmly to the slide.

STAINING TECHNIQUES

Reference has been made to staining *in toto,* but section staining is more
generally used, as it may be relied upon to produce a higher degree of differentiation. The first step is usually the removal of the embedding medium.
Paraffin may be removed by immersing in xylene for a few seconds. Celloidin
yields to ether-alcohol, absolute alcohol, oil of cloves, or acetone. The removal
of celloidin may be postponed until after staining and dehydration, if the
technician so desires. The steps that follow are those normally followed for
paraffin sections:

From xylene the slide is transferred to 95 per cent alcohol. If an alcoholic
stain is to be used, staining follows at this point. Dehydration by use of high-
percentage alcohols is then followed by clearing and mounting in balsam. If
an aqueous stain is intended, the slides are removed from 95 per cent alcohol,
passed through alcohols of decreasing concentration, and placed in water.
A common practice is to follow with a nuclear stain such as aqueous haematoxylin, then wash in water, counterstain with aqueous eosin or picro-fuchsin,
and wash again. Dehydration preparatory to clearing is accomplished by
passing through alcohols to 95 per cent or absolute. Should the counterstain
be of alcoholic nature, the same procedure will hold.

A large number of stains are available for histological work. Besides those
mentioned, methylene blue is often used by entomologists, particularly in the
study of the nervous system. Borax carmine is entirely suitable for staining
in toto, as is Mayer's HCl Carmine. Mallory's Phospho-tungstic Haematoxylin is useful in the study of muscle and connective tissue. Alkaline methylene blue gives best results after fixing agents that contain mercuric chloride,
such as Zenker's solution. Methyl green is sometimes used to stain the nuclei
of fresh tissue. Congo red makes a good counterstain after haematoxylin. Picric
acid is another which at the same time acts as a differentiating agent. If one
has special needs, he should consult the standard technical literature.

The purposes of staining are two: to give the tissues a color contrast with
their surroundings, and to differentiate particular structures, substances, or
cells. The second is the more important. Commonly used stains may be or-

ganic or inorganic; at the same time, they may be acid, basic, or neutral. Some are especially adapted to show nuclear structures; others are known as plasma stains. Some are used only for very special purposes. Occasionally, impregnation techniques are employed in which structural differentiation is accomplished by the precipitation of substances such as silver nitrate or chloride of gold.

Staining *in toto* is normally done after the fixer has been washed out and before the tissue is embedded. A nuclear stain is usually employed. Carmine, cochineal, and haematoxylin are equally serviceable. After sectioning, a counterstain may be applied. Following carmine, Lyons blue is commonly employed. In a great many cases, however, it will be found convenient to leave all staining until sections have been made—in other words, to use section staining entirely.

For double staining, the most popular combination is probably haematoxylin and eosin. But no matter which stains are selected, it is well to remember that staining is either *progressive* or *regressive*. In progressive staining, the process is closely watched and the staining is halted when the intensity of the stain reaches a desired point. With the regressive method, the tissue is deliberately overstained, after which the excess color is removed by action of a differentiator, such as alcohol, acetone, or oil of cloves.

Some stains require a mordant to make them take. This is a chemical substance that has a chemical affinity both for the tissue and for the stain. The principle is often incorporated in the fixing agent or sometimes in the stain itself, as, for example, in aluminum haematoxylin.

The time of staining may be determined experimentally for a particular lot of stain and for sections of uniform thickness and fixation, after which a number of sections may be put through according to a predetermined schedule. It is always better, however, to watch the staining (or differentiating) beneath the microscope and terminate the process when the desired condition has been reached. Dilute solutions, acting over a considerable period of time, give more uniform results than concentrated ones, acting for only a brief period. The method of applying stains (and differentiators) will vary with the circumstances. Immersion of the slides, either horizontally or vertically in suitable staining jars, permits staining of a large number at the same time. On the other hand, flooding the individual slide with stain by means of a pipette, over a staining tray, has two advantages: microscopic observations may be carried out without disturbing the position of the slide, and there is less likelihood of losing paraffin sections.

MOUNTING TECHNIQUES

Reference has been made to mounting in balsam as the usual and common method of preparing permanent mounts. Assuming that the specimen has finished clearing, one should first drain off the clearing agent, then permit the section to remain in air until the surface shows a slight tendency to dullness. A small drop of neutral Canada balsam is then placed upon the section, and the cover glass is dropped into place. If desired, the balsam may be placed upon the cover glass, which is then inverted. Xylene, toluene, and benzene are among the several substances used as balsam solvents. Damar balsam may be used as a mounting medium, but it sometimes becomes cloudy with the passage of time. Euparal, which is a mixture of certain gums and oils, may be used to mount specimens directly from 95 per cent alcohol without the employment of a clearing agent.

Drying of the balsam mounts may be hastened by exposure to a moderate amount of heat. After thorough drying, the surplus balsam may be scraped away and the margin of the cover glass wiped gently with gauze dipped in xylene. Subsequent sealing of the margin with Brunswick black, gold sizing, or similar material gives a neater appearance and guards against the preparation's turning yellow with age.

With objects of unusual thickness, a ring of glass or hard rubber may be employed to support the cover glass. If these are not available, a ring of shellac cement may be built up by spinning the slide on a turntable, using a camel's-hair brush. Two coats of shellac, applied by brush and turntable, are usually sufficient.

Balsam may also be used to prepare a shallow cell. Besides balsam, damar, and euparal, various glycerin preparations have been employed for mounting purposes. Pure glycerin, glycerin and acetic acid, and glycerin with carmine, Congo red, or some other stain are used in this way. All glycerin jelly mounts should be sealed. After drying for 12 to 24 hours, superfluous jelly is scraped away and the mount is cleaned up by wiping with a cloth moistened with water.

To illustrate different methods of feeding in flies, Graham-Smith (1930a) fixed the proboscides in various attitudes, in absolute alcohol. They were then treated with alcoholic sodium hydrate solution, and were later cleared and mounted in appropriate cells, without pressure.

If glass, rubber, or metal rings are used in preparing dry mounts, they must be cemented to both cover glass and slide.

Another popular mounting medium is "clarite," a water-white, chemically homogeneous synthetic resin developed by Groat (1939). It is a cycloparaffin or naphthene polymer with a melting point of 145°–155°C (293°–311°F). Clarite is particularly advantageous when the slides are to be used in a micro-projector in which the source of illumination is a carbon arc. Because of high temperatures generated by the arc, media of lower melting point are apt to fuse and run. Clarite has the reputation of remaining neutral in reaction, no matter how long the preparations are kept. Neither does it become dis-colored. For general use a solution consisting of 60 per cent clarite and 40 per cent toluene is recommended.

LABELING SLIDES

Labels are perhaps more important for microscopic slides than for other types of museum specimens. This is because there must be a record not only of the source of the tissue but also of the treatment it has received in the course of its preparation. Two methods are generally employed for marking slides: (1) the use of shellac or similar material; (2) the use of gummed paper squares.

The first involves coating one or both ends of the upper surface of the slide with thin Canada balsam or a mixture of varnish and xylene. When dry, this makes an excellent surface on which to enter data with India ink. A second coat of balsam or shellac protects against defacement.

Less time-consuming, and quite as satisfactory, are gummed labels pur-chased from supply houses; these are approximately one inch square, with or without ruled lines. If the slide is thoroughly clean, there is little danger of their curling or dropping off. Data should be entered with India ink, and should include a number that refers to notes or files in which full information concerning the specimen may be found. It is customary to give on the label the thickness of the cover glass and of the section, in microns. The name of the species, the organ involved, and the direction of the cut are likewise im-portant. The fixing agent and the stains employed are usually indicated in abbreviated form, followed by the date of mounting. A second label, at the opposite end of the slide, may be used to give a more detailed account of the technique followed and the particular purpose or objective sought in making the preparation.

Mounts of more than ordinary value may be permanently identified by scratching a serial number into the glass by means of a diamond-point tool.

SPECIAL PROBLEMS CONCERNING CHITIN

Flies, like other arthropods, have, of course, an exoskeleton of chitin, the presence of which often causes great difficulty in sectioning. The knife may quickly become dull, and subsequent sections may be ruined or badly mutilated. The best procedure is probably to utilize chiefly flies which have just emerged from the pupal state. Histological findings should, however, be checked against corresponding sections from more mature specimens, as certain structures (e.g., the ptilinum) undergo considerable modification after emergence. Larvae, of course, are most easily studied just after molting.

If one does not desire to study the cellular structure of the hypodermis, a practical procedure is to embed the complete insect in the usual manner, then trim away the paraffin very carefully until the chitinous layer has been removed. The residue is then re-embedded and sectioned in the usual way.

Reference has already been made to the paraffin-celloidin method as particularly useful where chitinous structures are involved.

Special techniques for softening the chitin prior to sectioning have been tried, with varying success. Soaking the specimen for a number of days in a mixture of alcohol and fluid soap is recommended. Similarly, immersion for 24 hours in a solution of hypochlorite of potash or hypochlorite of soda (20 per cent) tends to soften the chitin by partially dissolving it. The use of a suitable fixing agent is also important. Henning's, Frenzel's, and Gilson's fixatives are especially suitable, as they contain nitric acid. The special reagent known as Diaphanol is often useful in softening and bleaching chitinous structures. Tissues are placed in Diaphanol from 63 per cent alcohol, and left for two or three days. This is followed by the usual dehydration preparatory to embedding.

For a study of the chitin itself, the Diaphanol may be followed by prolonged immersion in water, following by staining with chlor-zinc-iodine. The chitin becomes violet. An excellent fixative for chitin is made up as follows:

80 per cent alcohol	66 cc.
glycerin	33 cc.
25 per cent HCl	2 cc.

Sections of chitin stain well with haematoxylin and picric acid. Iodine, carmine, and eosin are best for total staining. Ziehl's carbol-fuchsin is a good chitin stain, as is also Mallory's anilin-blue. Specimens previously treated with caustic potash may be stained with a solution of pyrogallic acid in alcohol or glycerin.

DEPIGMENTATION

Closely related to the handling of chitin is the removal of pigment from the compound eyes. Either Diaphanol or Grenacher's solution may be used for this purpose. The latter is composed of 70 per cent alcohol, 50 parts; glycerin, 50 parts; and nitric acid, 2 or 3 parts. The eyes are left in the solution for up to 12 hours, at 35°C (95°F).

BACTERIOLOGICAL TECHNIQUES

From the public health standpoint, a survey of the bacterial flora of the fly's body is sometimes indicated. Specimens taken for bacteriological study must be given special consideration, and, of course, should not be exposed to the ordinary killing and fixing agents, which are usually quite as toxic to the bacteria as to the fly itself.

Capture by ordinary trap or net is not too desirable, as there is always the possibility that the bacteria subsequently isolated from the fly were picked up after capture, rather than from natural sources. Both nets and traps may, of course, be sterilized prior to each collection, thus insuring against such secondary contamination of the specimens, but the sterilization of such bulky equipment is not always practical.

A very good source of specimens for bacteriological analysis is, naturally, the privy pit or manure pile. Larvae of all ages, as well as pupae, may be transferred by means of sterile forceps to screw-cap vials containing an appropriate solution. Adult flies may be taken as they emerge, and may be handled in the same fashion. Bacteriologists recommend sterile glycerol saline solution for this purpose. The formula is as follows:

Glycerine	30 ml.
Sodium chloride	42 g.
Distilled water	100 ml.

One ml. of glycerol saline is placed in each of a number of 10-ml. vials. The vials and their contents are then sterilized in an autoclave for fifteen minutes at fifteen pounds' pressure (121°C, or 249.8°F). This makes a suitable medium for transportation of specimens to the laboratory. Examination for bacterial content should not be delayed beyond twenty-four hours.

The technique to be followed from this point will depend both upon the purpose to be served and on the organisms thought to be present. For mere proof that the insect is carrying typhoid-dysentery organisms, for instance, the entire specimen may be macerated and inoculated into an enriched broth suitable for the propagation of such bacteria. If a more analytical study is to be made, careful dissection with sterile instruments will serve to dissociate the proboscis, crop, lower intestine, and other parts. Smears or hanging drop preparations are then made from specific areas for microscopic examination. If desired, cultures may be established by transfer of bacteria from the same organs or tissues.

Faichnie (1909) performed some interesting experiments to demonstrate that flies which were bred in enteric excreta might be infective in the adult state. A day-old fly that had been kept in sterile surroundings since emergence was chloroformed, transfixed with a hot needle, and singed in a flame. The specimen was then placed in sterile saline and later macerated in the same solution. A drop of the suspension was used to inoculate McConkey broth, which immediately developed a growth of *B. typhosus*. Control plates, inoculated by saline solution in which the flies had been shaken but had not yet been macerated, remained sterile. Various modifications of the experiment gave confirmatory results. Faichnie's interpretation was that the pathogen, which must have been acquired in the larval state, had survived pupation and so was present, from the beginning, in the internal organs of the adult fly. Bacot (1911a,b) improved on Faichnie's technique by sterilizing the pupae externally, thus eliminating the criticism that the flies might have reinfected themselves at the moment of emergence or just after.

A technique for sampling the flora of the pupa's interior was devised by Ledingham (1911). One extremity of the puparium, held lightly between the thumb and forefinger of the left hand, is seared and flattened by use of a small, hot iron. The treated surface is then pierced by a fine capillary pipette, which is used both to stir up the internal tissue and to draw off an appropriate amount of material that is then squirted on to culture plates.

Graham-Smith (1910) used an interesting technique in demonstrating that flies might, under certain circumstances, carry diphtheria bacilli. Adult flies were allowed to feed for thirty minutes on an emulsion of the pathogen in human saliva, and were then transferred to a clean cage. At various intervals, up to seventy-two hours, flies were killed and separate cultures were made from legs, wings, head, crop, intestinal contents, vomitus, and feces. Others were fed for one hour on a broth emulsion of the organism and examined in a similar manner. There was, of course, longer survival in the crop and intestine than on the exterior surfaces.

If suitable laboratory animals are available, infective material from crop, intestine, and other parts can be used for the experimental inoculation of such hosts, as well as for the establishment of plate or test-tube cultures.

To induce flies to feed on the lesions of yaws, Castellani (1907) removed the wings, then held the insects in place by means of a strip of gauze, the edges of which were fastened to the skin by collodion. The same device can be used to cause contaminated flies to transmit infection to artificial lesions in experimental animals. Modern workers may wish to substitute scotch tape for collodion in the above technique.

It is assumed that inoculation techniques, the use of various diagnostic media, and the employment of common bacteriological stains are known to the general laboratory worker. Those desiring information should consult the many excellent manuals now available for the use of the civilian or military technician.

SPECIAL TECHNIQUES RELATING TO SURVEY WORK

In connection with most fly-control programs, field surveys become necessary in order to test the efficacy of the control measures being used. These may take the form of village studies, with a view to evaluating results in terms of cost on a limited scale. Again, investigations of fly populations in a few selected restaurants, dairies, or abattoirs may be used to determine the feasibility of all-out fly control for an entire municipality.

But to count all the flies in an experimental area is manifestly impossible. Methods must therefore be devised by which reasonably accurate indexes of total fly populations may be secured. Random sampling is especially unsatisfactory, as flies are markedly gregarious and tend to congregate in a few attractive spots, where they are often found in very large numbers. The determination of these strategic points is therefore the first step in any sampling process.

When this has been done, sample counts are made in the areas of concentration, using one or more of a number of available methods. For example, a measured area, such as twenty-five square feet of wall or floor, may be selected for observation. At predetermined intervals an observer counts and records the number of flies found resting in the selected area. Uncontrollable variations in sunlight, and in direction and strength of air currents, tend to make the counts fluctuate greatly, but the method has its advantages in that no apparatus is required.

A very common procedure is to make use of baited traps. The flies actually taken can be counted very accurately, but the method is not ideal, inasmuch as other attractive substances in the vicinity of the trap may greatly influence the size of the catch. Also, the extent and outline of the area within which a particular bait may be attractive is greatly influenced by atmospheric conditions. Most important of all, it is very difficult to devise baits which will remain uniformly attractive during the period of the survey.

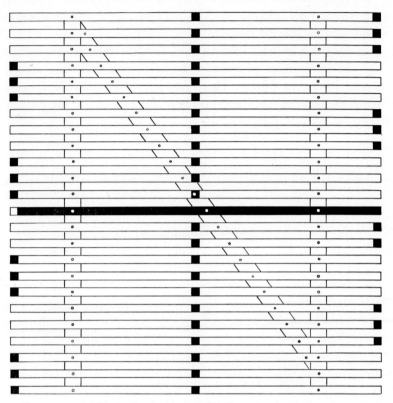

Figure 140. Scudder's fly-counting grill. Slats three-quarters of an inch broad and three feet long are arranged to form a grill one yard square. Counting is facilitated by division into quadrants and by blackening of slat tips in alternate groups of three. The small grill, eighteen inches square, is similar except that the strips are one-quarter of an inch broad and are spaced one-quarter of an inch apart. (Diagram patterned after photograph in Reprint No. 2785, *Public Health Reports.*)

A simple and reasonably satisfactory device is a strip or spiral of sticky flypaper. This method has been used effectively in Sardinia, where the strips are exposed in selected situations both before and after spraying operations. The number of flies captured over a definite period of time in an area about to be treated is compared with the number captured by a similar strip suspended in the same location after spraying has taken place. Catches on subsequent days may be used to show how long treatment remains effective and how rapidly fly populations are restored as the effect of the application wears off.

Sweeping the air with an ordinary insect net in the vicinity of favorite resting places is another possibility. It is probably the least reliable method of all,

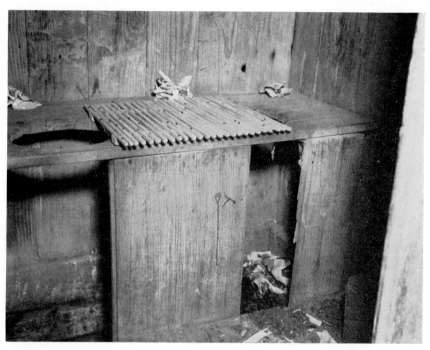

Figure 141. An obvious menace to health. Flies have unrestricted access to human fecal matter and to whatever disease organisms it may contain. Heavy fly population is indicated by number visible on the eighteen-inch counting grill. (Photo supplied by the United States Public Health Service of the Federal Security Agency.)

as so much depends upon uniform skill and timing on the part of the collector.

More satisfactory than any of these methods is the use of a standard resting surface in the form of a "fly grid" or "grill." As developed by Scudder (1947), this device makes use of the well-known fact that flies tend to utilize edges as resting places. Two types were devised. For outdoor sampling, a grill one square yard in area is used. For indoor counts, as in restaurants and soda fountains, a less conspicuous unit eighteen inches square has been found adequate. Both are constructed by tacking wood strips, a quarter of an inch thick,

THE HOUSEFLY

to a rigid, three-piece frame. To make counting easier, the larger grill is marked off into quadrants, as shown in figure 140.

The investigator first determines, by inspection, the points of greatest fly concentration or annoyance. The grill is then lowered gently into the center of this area. Flies still resting at the margin of the area are disturbed by just enough motion to put them to flight, after which all are allowed to come to rest. In approximately thirty seconds, distribution will be stabilized, and the investigator can proceed to make a rapid count of the flies resting on the grill. Scudder remarks that since houseflies are very persistent in returning to a location, only moderate caution need be exercised in handling them, but that blowflies are much more active and must be approached with greater care. For the same reason, less time can be allowed for counting than with houseflies.

The fly grill has been used extensively in connection with fly population studies in Egypt in recent years.

CHAPTER XVII

Emergency Control

Do what we can, summer will have its flies.—Emerson, "Prudence"

EMERGENCY control includes any and all procedures that may be brought to bear on situations where the fly population is already somewhat out of hand.

Emergencies may arise, for example, in connection with the movement of troops into regions or areas where the native population has no program, individual or collective, for the proper disposal of human and animal waste. Such conditions prevailed along the supply route between the Persian Gulf and the Soviet Union during World War II, and required strenuous measures in order to avoid unrestrained transmission of intestinal disorders. Similar conditions tend to exist temporarily in almost any military cantonment in the summertime whenever barnyards, pigsties, or garbage dumps exist within flight range of the reservation but, being located on private property, are with difficulty brought under the control of camp authorities.

Municipalities and recreational centers often face similar problems near the end of the summer season, when it is far too late in the year to forestall the breeding of flies and the only action that can be taken is to reduce, in some way, the great number already in existence. Meanwhile, the civilian (or military) population must be given every possible protection against the fly nuisance. Possibilities in this direction are recalled by a note published in 1918 concerning American army camps during World War I. At the time of publication some 22,700,000 square feet of screening had been used and 6,000 fly traps had been placed in operation.

MEASURES AGAINST THE ADULT FLY

The adult fly may be attacked or avoided in a number of ways. Of proven value are screens, flytraps, electrocuting devices, sprays, flypapers, poisons, and the humble but always practical fly swatter. Usually a combination of two

or more procedures is desirable, and not infrequently it becomes necessary
to attack the problem from every conceivable angle before any significant
relief can be achieved.

Screening

Screening, as a general protection against mosquitoes, flies, and other pests,
is so generally practiced in temperate zones by both urban and rural populations that we often fail to realize how generally lacking is such protection
in many regions of the world. The lack is often greatest where insect-borne

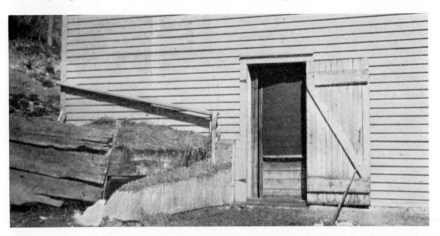

Figure 142. Combination of thrift and carelessness. The manure is stored in an open
box, but the doors and windows of the barn are screened. Prevention of breeding should
be basic in any program for fly control. (Courtesy of Michigan Department of Health.)

diseases constitute the greatest menace to human health. In general, economic
reasons lie behind the fact that this simple expedient is so infrequently employed in the very situations where it would obviously be of greatest benefit.

Houses with floors or walls of bamboo poles or similar material can never
be rendered flyproof under any circumstances. Even where dwellings of clay,
sod, or thatch are so constructed as to make screening possible, the expense is
usually quite prohibitive. Puri (1943) states that in India the vast majority
of the people cannot afford to screen their houses properly; he confines his
recommendations to the screening of hospitals, of rooms occupied by persons
with communicable diseases, and of cots and cribs used by infants, who, by
their very helplessness, are particularly vulnerable to fly-borne infections.
Muslin or mosquito netting is obviously the most suitable material for indoor
use.

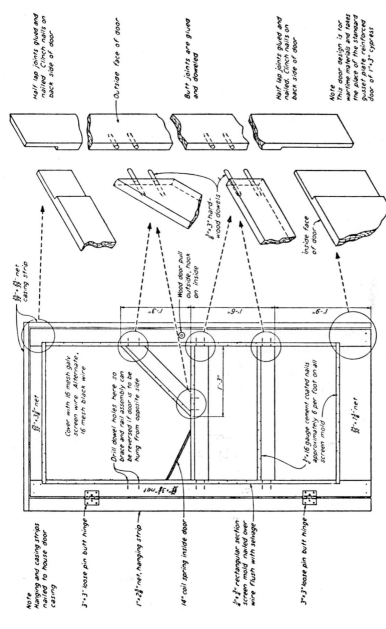

Figure 143. Practical plan for constructing screen door. All screen doors should be made to open outward. Provision for automatic closing is likewise essential. (From Kruse, C. W., and Gartrell, F. E., *J. Nat. Mal. Soc.* 4:140, 1945; used by permission of W. B. Saunders Company.)

Even among the well to do, the maintenance of screens in the tropics is a matter involving endless watchfulness and great expense. Lacquered or painted screens are wholly impractical, as they scarcely last one season. Galvanized iron is but little to be preferred, as exposure to rain soon causes rusting, which puts it also in the class of temporary materials. Copper, on the other hand, if it does not contain over 0.5 per cent of iron, is excellent, while monel metal, which consists of nickel (67 per cent), copper (28 per cent), and other metals (5 per cent), has been found particularly durable near the sea. It is, however, one of the most expensive of screening materials. Bronze, composed of nine parts of copper to one of tin, makes a very durable wire, especially if the mixture is phosphorized. Aluminum screening is also available.

In the absence of such materials, fabric or plastic screens are probably to be preferred over inferior metals. Plastic screening is surprisingly strong and durable, and does not rust or corrode. It will burn, however, when fire is held directly against it; hence, watchfulness is necessary when cigarettes or cigars are being used.

The type of support used to stretch the screening will depend chiefly on the latitude. Removable frames are a necessity in northern regions, where flies are of only seasonal concern and where exposure of the screen to the elements during the winter season tends to cause its rapid disintegration. Furthermore, in cold countries it is often the custom to conserve heat by the use of storm windows, the frames of which may be held in place by the same turn buttons or other devices which are employed to hold the screen frames in the summertime.

In warmer regions, however, where the winter season is relatively short and is perhaps more characterized by rainfall than by snow and ice, insects, including flies, will be in evidence for a much greater portion of the year, and more or less continuous screening is to be preferred. Under such circumstances, it may be feasible to fasten the netting directly upon the window frame by tacks or small nails, thus avoiding the expense of material for frames and the expenditure of time in constructing them. If muslin or cloth netting is used, the margins may be secured with lath or similar material.

There can never be any substitute, on the other hand, for the screen door. Four features are essential for the proper functioning of a screen door, and should always be insisted upon: (1) The door must fit its frame and should rest against jamb strips in such a fashion that no fly can find its way through the crack when the door is closed. (2) The door should open outward, so that any flies resting on the outside of the screen will not be carried into the house when the door is swung. (3) Spring hinges or some equivalent device should be employed to ensure automatic closing. (4) Lower panels should be protected by wood bars, wire cloth, or other reinforcement, to guard against puncturing of the screen.

Special screening is usually desirable for foods that are likely to attract flies. Hung meats, particularly, should be protected, and fresh fruits, which are usually eaten raw, ought to have protection also. The sale of fruits on the open street in fly time is one of the major causes of intestinal disturbances in many parts of the world.

The mesh of the screening is of course important. A mesh of 14 wires to the inch will exclude houseflies, blowflies, and similar species, but it is better to use about an 18-mesh screening in order to exclude smaller insects at the same time. Size of wire will modify the actual size of the aperture, and this should be taken into account. In the United States Army, the maximum aperture recommended for general use is 0.0475 inch. In the Canal Zone, hard-drawn copper wire, 99.8 per cent pure, 0.015 inches diameter, is standard. A wire this heavy gives the desired aperture with only a 16 mesh, that is, with sixteen holes along a linear inch. For comparison, a regular grade, 0.010 inches in diameter, leaves apertures of 0.0456 inches with an 18 mesh.

Attempts to reduce the apertures to the point where *Phlebotomus* and *Culicoides* will be excluded have been found impractical, as ventilation is thereby cut off and the house or room becomes so uncomfortable that few persons will tolerate it.

Plans for constructing practical and inexpensive screen doors are usually obtainable from city and state health departments. Figure 143 illustrates a type of door which has been found useful in malaria control work throughout the world.

Flytraps

It should be pointed out that flytraps alone can never afford more than partial relief from the fly nuisance; as a supplementary measure, however, their usefulness should not be overlooked.

Many types of traps are on the market, but those of conical design have been found most satisfactory for catching medium-sized muscoids of the housefly or blowfly type. While an all-metal trap is undoubtedly to be preferred, a very satisfactory device may be constructed of wooden hoops, wire screening, and wood lath. Indeed, under emergency conditions, these may be the only materials available. The accompanying diagram (Fig. 144) illustrates the basic principle of the conical trap. The aperture at the apex of the cone is usually made approximately one inch in diameter. All-metal, cylindrical traps in which the cones are removable have proved very satisfactory for military use. Cones are easily telescoped, for shipment, and by giving the outside cylinder a slightly greater diameter at the base than at the top, it is possible to telescope these units also. A large number of traps may thus be stored or transported in relatively little space.

When properly baited and placed in strategic locations, the conical-type flytrap will capture enormous numbers of houseflies and blowflies. Traps set near the doors of kitchens and mess halls usually catch a great many, especially if the location is protected from the wind. Except in very hot weather, the sunny side of a building is preferable to the shady side. For houseflies many types of bait

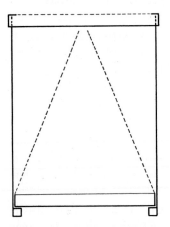

Figure 144. Scheme of conventional flytrap. Flies enter from below. Screen in cover admits sunlight. Flies, seeking light, pass upward through hole at top of screen cone and are held captive. Outer wall is usually of screening, also. Traps operating on this principle may be either rectangular or cylindrical in design.

may be used. Milk and fruit waste will answer very well. A mixture of water (three parts) and blackstrap molasses (one part) is also recommended. Bait pans should be kept well filled and should be washed at least every second week. When the captured flies form a pile one-fourth the height of the cone, the catch should be removed, as additional flies do not readily enter the trap under such conditions. Any flies that may still be living can be killed by a pyrethrum spray or by immersing the trap in hot water.

For the capture of blowflies the trap should be blocked up to give a clearance of two inches beneath the cone. Meat scraps of all kinds make good bait. Liver is especially effective, and "gut slime," a by-product of packing houses, is probably the best.

Blair (1945) reports great success in western Egypt with a type of flytrap in which the bait is in relative darkness. Flies that have fed are attracted by the light above into a trapping chamber with a cone-shaped entrance. A fairly bulky bait is recommended, with a liberal portion of meat or fish. Where odors are objectionable, fruit may be substituted. The margin of the bait tin is turned inward to prevent the escape of any larvae that may develop in the bait. Bait is replaced weekly, and the old bait and trapped flies are burned. Up to 80,000 flies were taken in two days, the record for one hour being in

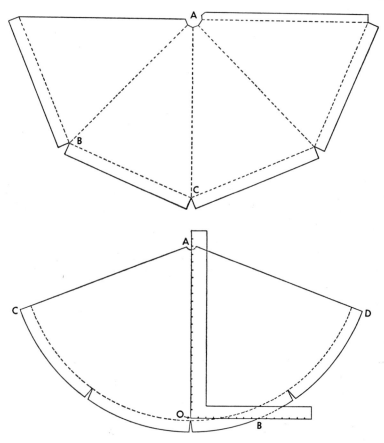

Figure 145. Interior units for conventional flytraps. *Upper:* Pattern for cutting screen when design of trap is rectangular. If line *B–C* is nine inches long, the distance from *A* to *B* or *C* should be approximately twelve inches. Folding of the screen along dotted lines produces a four-sided pyramid. (Freely adapted from Nájera, 1947.) *Lower:* Pattern for cutting screen when design of trap is cylindrical. A carpenter's square is laid upon screen so that *O–A* measures twenty-two inches; *O–B*, nine. Radius *A–B* is then used to determine *A–C* and *A–D*. Circumferential distance between *C* and *D* is fifty-seven and one-half inches. Cone is formed by causing *A–C* to overlap *A–D*. (Freely adapted from U.S. Department of Agriculture, *Farmers' Bulletin 734.*)

the vicinity of 4,500. The effective attraction radius was approximately 300 yards. Such an apparatus is of course effective only in the open and in good light.

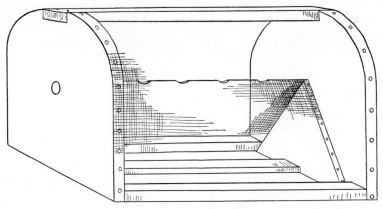

Figure 146. Small flytrap, easily made. Should be set on blocks, above appropriate bait. Flies enter from below, then make their way through holes in ridge of tent-shaped screen, into dome-shaped trap-chamber above. Withdrawal of end pins permits quick removal of interior unit.

Electrocutors

These devices are so designed that they will kill all insects that strike them. They have been found especially effective against houseflies. A screen or grid which may be hung on windows or screen doors is the commonest type used. Others are combined with trapping devices for use outdoors. A transformer is employed to convert ordinary house current into one with low amperage and high voltage. A current of 3,500 to 4,000 volts is most desirable. Ordinarily, no insect can survive even a momentary contact.

Fans

Electric fans, mounted over doorways leading to mess halls, kitchens, and places where food is stored, can be very helpful in keeping out flies. When the door is opened, flies, if present, will naturally attempt to move toward the source of the attractive odors, but because of the fan they encounter a strong air current that prevents their ingress.

Sprays

Sprays can be applied by hand sprayers, hand pumps, or power devices. The primary purpose is to bring the insecticide into direct contract with the fly, thereby causing its death. For many years, pyrethrum has been the favorite insecticide for this purpose. It knocks down the insects quickly, which not only gives satisfaction to the operator but likewise prevents the fly from continuing to spread infection after exposure to a fatal dose.

The raw product consists of the dried flowers or buds of any one of three particular species of *Chrysanthemum*. These have been intensively cultivated in Kenya Colony, where flowers have been produced with a pyrethrin content of approximately 1.3 per cent. The term "pyrethrin" is applied to any or all

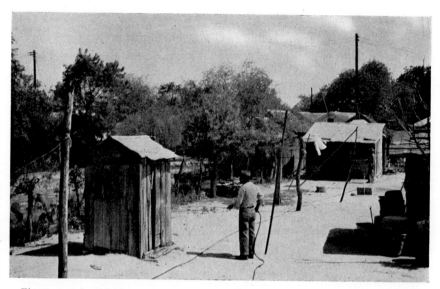

Figure 147. Insecticides not a substitute for sanitation. Power spraying of premises may reduce fly populations temporarily, but the insanitary privy remains a menace to family and community health. (Photo supplied by the United States Public Health Service of the Federal Security Agency.)

of the compounds within the dried material which are toxic to insects. These fall into two categories, referred to in the literature as pyrethrins I and II. Insect powders are prepared by grinding up the flowers. If a less potent preparation is desired, the powder may be diluted by mixing it with an inert carrier.

For spraying, the pyrethrins are extracted from the flowers by use of various solvents. For application to plants, acetone and alcohol are the preferred solvents, while mineral oil is the solvent selected when the spray is to be used against insects affecting man or animals. A concentrate containing 2 g. of pyrethrins per 100 cc. of solvent is the stock solution from which most spray solutions are prepared. Dilution with twenty times the volume of light petroleum oil or kerosene thus yields a spray containing from 0.10 to 0.12 g. of pyrethins per 100 cc. This concentration has been recommended for use against houseflies and stable flies as well as mosquitoes, eye gnats, and other forms. Practical experience shows, however, that houseflies are much more resistant to pyrethrum than are mosquitoes. The flies are knocked down readily enough, but a large percentage frequently revive, as is the case with cockroaches. Most authorities feel, therefore, that pyrethrum can be relied on for control of flies only when combined with a synergist, such as piperonyl butoxide.

If the spray is to be employed in dwellings, a perfume is sometimes added to suppress the odor. Inhalation of pyrethrum is neither dangerous nor annoying to man, except in the case of certain individuals who may be allergic to it.

The selection of the proper oil, or combination of oils, to carry the pyrethrins will depend upon the purpose for which the spray is used. In dwellings it should be of a nature to leave no stain upon furniture, walls, or clothing. In spraying animals, the oil should be noninjurious, whether left upon the skin or licked and swallowed by the same or another animal. For show animals, it must neither stain the coat nor cause undue drying or bleaching of the hair. In the case of milch cows, the solvent must not be of a nature to taint the milk.

Another function of fly spray, when applied to animals, is to repel the insects and thus save the animals considerable annoyance and irritation. A preparation which evaporates more slowly and which is more aromatic than ordinary sprays is better suited to this end. Livestock sprays are therefore usually made up with less volatile oils than household sprays, and frequently contain cloves, safrol, pine oil, or camphor.

A third purpose of spraying walls, floors, and ceilings is to render them toxic to flies for an extended period of time. For this, pyrethrum preparations are not adequate, and DDT is the most useful insecticide. This remarkable substance is treated at length in Chapter XIX and will, therefore, not be discussed further in this place, except to point out that a deposit of 200 milligrams of DDT per square foot will usually destroy flies for a month or more. According to Taggart (1946) the same concentration, in test boxes, resulted in a 100 per cent kill after 261 days!

Besides pyrethrum, extracts of derris and organic thiocyanates are used by many manufacturers in the preparation of fly sprays. Derris, and the rather similar cubé, are produced as powders by grinding the roots of certain tropical plants. The active chemical principle is rotenone. The thiocyanates are discussed at some length in Chapter XIX, which treats of the more recently developed insecticides.

Regardless of content, all of the great many commercial fly sprays sold in the United States must meet requirements specified by the National Bureau of Standards, Department of Commerce, Washington, D.C. Each product is rated against an official test insecticide (O.T.I.), agreed upon by the National Association of Insecticide and Disinfectant Manufacturers, Inc. The Peet-Grady method of testing (see Chapter XV) is employed in making the determination. If the number of flies killed by the spray in twenty-four hours falls within 5 per cent of the number that succumb to the official test insecticide, the product is given a rating of "B" and is considered satisfactory for use. A rating of "A" indicates that the kill ranges from 5 to 15 per cent higher than with the O.T.I. If the kill exceeds this, a rating of "AA" is given.

Besides possessing the desirable features already discussed, a standard household spray should not corrode metals, nor should it have a flash point below 125°F (51.7°C) when tested by the Tagliabue closed-cup method. It should not be sufficiently penetrating to contaminate closed packages of ordinary foods.

The general spraying of extended territory by airplanes is thoroughly practicable, as demonstrated by military and other experience. The interval between each application will depend upon frequency of rainfall and other factors which tend to nullify the effects of the application. This must be determined by experience. Griffiths (1946) reports that when the city of Manila was sprayed from airplanes with DDT in Diesel oil at a rate of 8 ounces of DDT per acre, Diptera of the genus *Musca* practically disappeared for a short time following each application. In this work, treatments were given at intervals of 3 to 4 weeks, which proved not sufficiently frequent for the securing of a cumulative effect. Ground sprays ten days apart during June and July had a carry-over effect, as shown by the fact that the fly population increased more slowly after each application.

Fly Poisons

Poison baits are effective in reducing the number of flies, and should not be overlooked in any all-out effort to meet an emergency condition. Old-fashioned, but probably superior to others, is formaldehyde, usually available as formalin, a 40 per cent solution of the gas in water. Three teaspoonfuls of commercial formalin are mixed with one pint of water or milk, and a little brown sugar is added to make the solution more attractive. An ordinary drinking glass is then partially filled with the mixture. The usual procedure is to line a saucer or small plate with blotting paper and place it over the glass, bottom up. The apparatus is then inverted and the glass is elevated slightly on one side by insertion of a matchstick or similar object.

A solution of sodium salicylate, plus brown sugar, has also been recommended for this purpose. Arsenic preparations, while very effective, are not usually desirable about kitchens or dwellings because of the danger to human life.

Flypapers

These are useful as supplementary control devices, particularly about kitchens and mess halls where complete exclusion of flies is difficult to achieve. Flypapers are usually available in two forms, as ribbons and in the form of flat sheets. The ribbon type pulls out spirally from a short cylinder of cardboard and may be suspended from the ceiling in any convenient manner. The lower extremity should, of course, be higher than head level. A disc or circular shelf at the bottom serves to collect any sticky material which may run downward due to high temperature of the room.

Sheets are far more effective than ribbons, though they are somewhat unsightly, especially after a large number of flies have been captured. A good procedure is to tack the flypaper to a vertical board that may be suspended in some inconspicuous place where flies are prone to congregate. A ledge should be fastened along the lower edge to prevent dripping upon furniture or the floor.

Various sticky mixtures have been used to coat flypaper. An old recipe recommended two pounds of rosin and one pint of castor oil, to be heated together until the mixture resembled molasses. This was then smeared on the paper, while hot, by means of an ordinary paintbrush.

ATTACKING THE IMMATURE FORMS

Attention should also be given to fly-breeding areas insofar as these may be under the control of the municipality, resort operator, or military authority concerned.

The selection of materials for the control of larvae will depend in part on the availability of a local supply. In Russia, chlorinated aliphatic hydrocarbons are abundant. Klechetova (1946) has conducted a series of experiments with several compounds. Third-stage larvae of *M. domestica* were confined in a concentration of 30 maggots to 100 grams of rearing medium. Each batch of 30 was then exposed to a controlled dosage of poison, of which the amounts ranged from 0.25 to 2 g. (or cc.). The most effective compounds were tetra- and pentachlorethane, both of which caused complete mortality within 48 hours at all dosages. Toxicity, however, though important, is not the sole factor in determining the superiority of a larvicide. Hexachlorethane, for ex- ample, which gave a mortality of only 91 per cent at the highest dose, is very desirable both because of its low toxicity for mammals and because it is avail- able as a powder and therefore easy to transport. Its relative insolubility in water accounts for its tardy larvicidal action. If thoroughly mixed with the medium, it is highly effective. Hexachlorethane has an additional advantage in that its odor repels adult flies and thus discourages further oviposition in the medium treated. As a repelleent, it was found to be about five times as effective as chloride of lime. Large-scale use of hexachlorethane in Moscow during 1945 gave good control throughout five of seven zones treated.

Chloride of lime is an old favorite with sanitarians for deodorizing latrines, privies, and the like, but its effectiveness as a larvicide is questionable. Dolin- skaya and associates (1946) reported on its generous use in Moscow, where complete mortality of all larvae required the application of not less than 30 ounces per square yard of surface twice a week. It was furthermore necessary to apply the lime in such a manner as to form an unbroken film. This demands a degree of responsibility not often possessed by the type of labor usually avail- able for such work; it also requires additional time. On the other hand, there is something to be said for chloride of lime as a repellent against adult flies. A substantial reduction in the number of larvae was noted where applications at the rate of only 20 ounces per square yard of surface served obviously to discourage oviposition.

Travis and Bohart (1946) give an interesting account of field tests made in Okinawa relative to the use of DDT in Diesel oil or kerosene to control larvae in latrines. One quart of 4 to 5 per cent solution per seat hole once a week was effective against *Chrysomyia megacephala* in pits built according to military specifications. Trials were also made with 5 per cent DDT in emulsified xylene, which kills more quickly, but in tight pits this proved dangerous, as a lighted match caused the xylene vapor to explode. There was some criticism of the DDT, since it did not always kill mature larvae quickly enough to prevent migration from the pit. Other materials used were Penite (a 54 per cent preparation of sodium arsenite) and paradichlorbenzene. The first was very effective in dilution of 1:40, and is particularly convenient to use, as it is not bulky to transport and any kind of water serves for mixing. It is, however, highly toxic to man. Paradichlorbenzene, like DDT, requires considerable shipping space. It is really effective only when the pits are deep, dry, and unventilated, but has one advantage in that it prevents additional flies from entering.

Olson and Dahms (1945) point out that sewage plants operating under optimum conditions ordinarily have no problem concerning the breeding of *Musca domestica* in sewage sludge. Emergencies arise from time to time, however, when it becomes necessary to withdraw the sludge before it has undergone complete digestion. This "green sludge," as it is called, dehydrates much less readily than digested sludge and thus remains an excellent medium for housefly breeding. Operators would do well, therefore, to have available a suitable means of treating the exposed sludge, when such conditions arise. Olson and Dahms made comparative tests of rotenone, DDT emulsion, DDT dust, kerosene, and other substances as available in standard preparations. Neither the rotenone nor the DDT emulsion proved to have significant larvicidal value. Both borax and kerosene, however, gave 100 per cent kill. The DDT dust, though only moderately effective as a larvicide, was effective, nevertheless, in that most of the pupae formed failed to produce flies, and the few adults which did emerge died within less than two hours.

The use of various chemical substances for control of larvae under emergency conditions was investigated by McDuffie, Lindquist, and Madden (1946). O-dichlorobenzene was applied in simulated pit latrines at the rate of 15 to 25 g. per square foot, resulting in good control of housefly larvae. Similar results were obtained by the use of 10 to 20 g. per square foot of p-dichlorobenzene. Both were effective in destroying the eggs. A 5 per cent solution of DDT was also tried, but few if any maggots were killed by it. Emerging adult flies, however, were quickly killed by contact with the residue. Maggots in carcasses were controlled fairly well by a number of substances, including thanite, benzene hexachloride, acetylene tetrachloride, and o-dichlorobenzene.

Sometimes the mere covering of the fly-breeding medium by a sufficient depth of packed soil is effective in cutting down the fly population. However, in most situations, as pointed out by Mellor (1919), it is useless to bury *larvae-infested* material under as little as four feet of clay, loam, or sand, whether loose or rammed down, as most of the flies will emerge regardless. This is because approximately 90 per cent of the larvae climb to within one foot of the surface in order to pupate.

MISCELLANEOUS PROCEDURES

Sodium hydroxide (caustic soda, NaOH) is sometimes employed to wash garbage cans and pails in connection with fly control and the maintenance of general sanitary standards. Obtainable as flakes, lumps, or rods, it is readily soluble in water, glycerine, or alcohol. Being caustic, it should be kept in tightly closed containers and should never be allowed to make contact with the bare hands.

Washing soda, also known as sodium carbonate (sal soda, $Na_2CO_3 + 10H_2O$), is quite safe to handle, and therefore useful in many situations. It is a white, crystalline powder, very soluble in water. A common use is to free garbage of fats and grease, and thus reduce its attractiveness to flies.

A dangerous but sometimes useful material is sodium arsenite ($NaAsO_2$), a white powder very soluble in water. It has been used as a spray to arrest fly breeding in compost piles, animal carcasses, and human cadavers. It is extremely poisonous, however, and must not be used near wells or springs. Livestock and children must be kept from ground that has been treated, and handlers should wear rubber gloves, as sodium arsenite is extremely caustic.

Borax, also called sodium borate ($Na_2B_4O_7 + 10H_2O$), another old favorite with sanitarians, is reasonably effective in killing both housefly and stable-fly larvae in feces, animal manure, garbage, and sludge beds. It may be applied as a powder or in water solution, by sprinkling. Manure heavily treated with borax is sometimes toxic to crops when spread on fields.

Tarpaulins, especially if rubberized, may be used to cover ricks of manure and thus prevent flies from breeding therein. This also protects the manure from disturbance by birds and other animals and tends to conserve the fertilizer value. Seams and hems should be of ample width and should be double- or triple-stitched. Eyelets should be of brass or some other noncorrosive substance. Triangular corner patches, double-stitched, greatly enhance the durability of tarpaulins.

The use of aerosols to free an area from insects for a brief period of time has been employed chiefly in connection with mosquito control, but the procedure can also be made use of in controlling flies. Brescia, La Mer, and associates (1946) have shown that fifteen gallons of DDT emulsion liberated over a front of 1,000 feet are required to control flies for a distance of 1,000 feet downwind. This means that houseflies are from four to six times as resistant to such treatment as are common species of mosquitoes. The emulsion used in these tests consisted of 50 per cent water and 50 per cent oil, by volume. The DDT content was equal to 10 per cent of the oil, by weight.

CHAPTER XVIII

Planned Control

Kill a fly in July,
  You've just killed one fly.
Kill a fly in June,
  They'll be scarce soon.
Kill a fly in May,
  You've kept thousands away.
                    —*Old English rhyme*

FLY CONTROL is a responsibility in which an ounce of prevention is worth several tons of cure. Hewitt (1914a) estimated that if the progeny of a single pair of flies all lived and could be collected at the end of the summer and pressed together, they would occupy approximately 250,000 cubic feet. Of course, no such unrestricted multiplication occurs, yet the great fecundity of the species is such that any and all measures which may prevent reproduction on the part of the original few are infinitely worth while and should never be overlooked.

Long-range planning thus resolves itself into nothing more or less than the elimination of those conditions which permit the insects to breed and multiply.

In earlier chapters, we have listed the wide variety of media, both natural and man-made, which *Musca domestica* is able to utilize for larval development. The great majority, however, of the numerous flies which characterize late summer and early fall in so many parts of the world owe their existence largely to the availability of three classes of material: (1) human feces, (2) animal manures, and (3) improperly disposed garbage. Under rural conditions the first two are of paramount importance. In cities, the third is usually of greatest concern. In military establishments, all three aspects may be involved, depending on the need for animals (camels, horses, mules), the previous civilian habits of the men, and the intended permanence of the installation. Thus slit trenches may provide adequate disposal of feces for an overnight bivouac or maneuvers of a few days' duration, but are quite unsatisfactory where large bodies of troops are to be concentrated for a considerable period of time.

GARBAGE DISPOSAL

Since the problem of garbage disposal is of concern in almost every situation, it will be considered first. Municipalities, resort operators, camp directors, and military commanders must all make provision for the disposal of food wastes

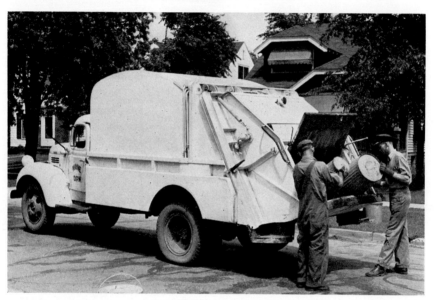

Figure 148. Modern sanitary garbage collection. Low-level loading reduces fatigue for the men and eliminates risk of injuries. Loading is faster, also. (Courtesy of Gar Wood Industries, Inc.)

and should consider only such methods as will not encourage the multiplication of flies. Farmers, who usually effect disposal by immediate feeding to cattle, poultry, or swine, nevertheless have seasonal problems, as when cellars are cleaned out and partially spoiled vegetables or fruit are thrown out and perhaps left to decompose. Garbage disposal therefore affects everyone to a greater or lesser degree.

Transportation

Hauling garbage through streets of cities and towns presents a problem certainly important in an aesthetic way, and usually important otherwise. Many larger cities still use the open truck, which starts its trip loaded with clean, empty refuse cans. At each residence the clean can is exchanged for one containing the garbage and refuse accumulated by the householder since the last collection. A tarpaulin may be utilized to cover the laden cans as these accumulate in the truck. Such a covering serves three purposes: (1) to keep the covers from jarring off the cans as the truck picks up speed; (2) to reduce the amount of odor emanating from the load as the truck works slowly along the

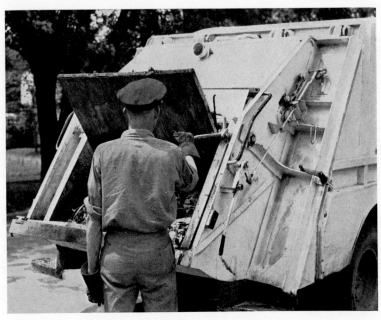

Figure 149. A truly sanitary truck for garbage collection. When the hopper is filled the door is closed, sealing both hopper and body. Nothing spills or blows away in transit. (Courtesy of Gar Wood Industries, Inc.)

street; (3) to make the appearance of the load less objectionable to passers-by.

Workmen are prone to conserve space and cans by overfilling the latter, and even dispensing with covers so that a surface layer of garbage may be distributed over the open tops. This, of course, should be discouraged, as it almost always results in the distribution of a certain amount of refuse along the highway. Such practices are most common when the work is contracted to some individual or company, to whom the cost of an extra trip may mean the difference between profit and loss. In general, it may be said that where employees of the city or village do the actual handling, there is better opportunity for health officers to supervise the work and prevent undesirable practices.

An excellent device is the bin-type collecting truck, shown in Figure 149. The bin operates by a hydraulic hoist, so that no excessive amount of strength is required on the part of the laborers.

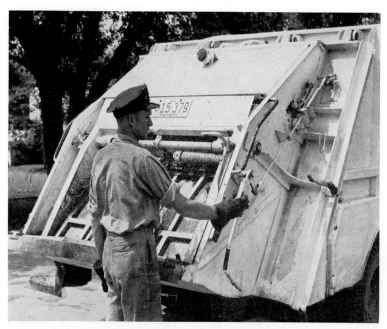

Figure 150. Great capacity means fewer trips. Operator is about to activate a hydraulic ram, which compresses garbage and rubbish into a small space, at the same time squeezing out the liquids. Drier garbage means quicker burning at dump or incinerator. (Courtesy of Gar Wood Industries, Inc.)

Disposal after Collection

The more common methods of garbage disposal are six: (1) the open dump; (2) feeding to hogs; (3) incineration; (4) grinding, followed by release into a sewerage system; (5) reduction; (6) the sanitary fill.

The city garbage dump. Of traditional usage is the sprawling dump, somewhere beyond the corporate limits of the town. It is usually the practice to keep a slow fire burning, watched over by one or more attendants, to consume the more combustible materials. Rubbish from grocery stores and other mercantile establishments contains considerable amounts of this type of refuse, and its burning accomplishes the incineration of a certain amount of moist garbage which would otherwise be left to decompose.

The great bulk of food residue, however, remains to be picked over by stray dogs, cats, hosts of rats, and, in certain areas, wild bears, not to mention human scavengers, some of whom in certain devastated countries had little other source of nourishment during the war years and early reconstruction period.

There is no question but that the open dump is economical, and this is perhaps the chief argument for its continuance, considering the modern disposal methods now available. One factor which must always be considered when a community converts from open dump to modern incineration or other methods is the large, residual rat population which the open dump always supports. To a limited extent it may be said that the rats constitute a part of the disposal mechanism, and that, with an attractive field of garbage

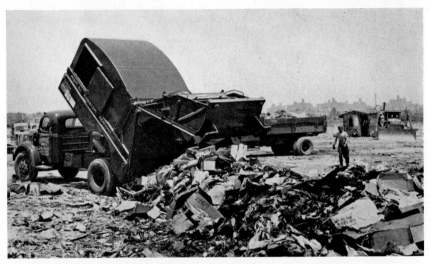

Figure 151. Easy dumping by hydraulic mechanism. A bulldozer waits, at right, to push refuse into a sanitary fill. (Courtesy of Gar Wood Industries, Inc.)

to make use of, few if any rats remain in the vicinity of private homes. With the garbage eliminated, all this is changed. The rats then scatter widely and hotels, business houses, and private households become asylums for the disinherited.

Proper anticipation of this hazard will enable the health officer to forestall most of the difficulty by putting control measures into effect before the old habitat becomes unattractive to the rodents. Potassium cyanide dust, introduced with a blow gun into the rats' burrows, has been recommended as effective. Care must be taken to plug all exists of the burrow except the one into which the poison is introduced. At the end of the treatment this also should be blocked. The cyanide salt reacts with the moisture of the air in the burrow to produce hydrogen cyanide. The rats are thus asphyxiated.

Hog feeding. The one undeniable advantage of this method of disposal lies in the fact that it utilizes the food value of the garbage. The pigs are eventually sold and a tangible profit is realized. Ashes and rubbish still remain, however, and must be provided for in other ways.

Two methods of feeding garbage have been used (Tully, 1945): Platform

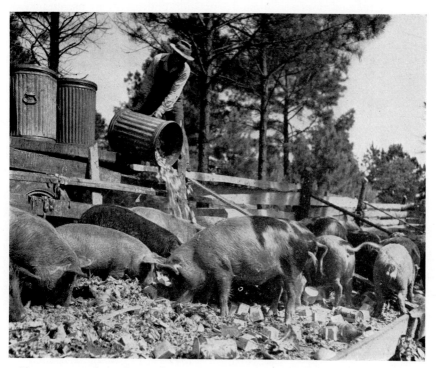

Figure 152. Garbage disposal by platform feeding to hogs. This method is much to be preferred over ground feeding, as a larger percentage of the garbage is consumed. If the platform is washed daily, no serious fly menace need ensue. (Photo supplied by the United States Public Health Service of the Federal Security Agency.)

feeding is probably preferable from a sanitary point of view; also, a larger percentage of the edible garbage is usually consumed. At the close of each day's operations, the platform should be washed down, preferably with water under pressure, and the unconsumed garbage should be collected and buried. If conscientiously followed out, this program eliminates practically all nuisance in the form of odor, and the premises present a reasonably attractive appearance at all times. Liquid waste resulting from the washing should be given tank treatment, after which soil absorption can be relied on to do the rest.

Ground feeding is more messy, results in unavoidable odors, and is far more encouraging to the production of flies. A given spot should never be used on successive days, and good management requires that not only the unused garbage but also the day's deposit of hog manure should be collected each day and buried.

Either method results in some fly breeding and inevitably encourages the rat population as well. However, if a sufficiently isolated location can be pro-

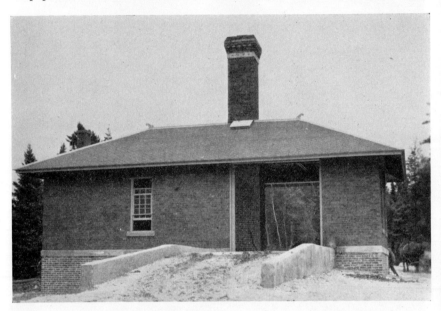

Figure 153. One type of garbage incinerator, used in a resort area. View shows inclined roadway to charging floor. (Courtesy of Michigan Department of Health.)

vided, away from all human habitation, hog feeding may prove a very economical procedure. Since the economy depends very largely upon satisfactory marketing of the pork produced, it is but sound practice to have all animals immunized against hog cholera. Another hazard attendant upon the feeding of raw garbage is the possibility of infesting the hogs with *Trichinella*. Rats also are potential reservoirs of trichinosis, and hogs which may have escaped original infection may easily acquire it by devouring a dead or dying rat. Many public health authorities hold that garbage should in no case be fed to swine until it has been cooked at a temperature sufficiently high to destroy the parasites.

Incinerators. Many municipalities have adopted incineration as a satisfactory and sanitary method of dealing with food wastes. A great many incinerator plants fail to give complete satisfaction, either because of poor design, bad construction, or careless operation. The principal features to be borne in mind in constructing the incinerator are: (1) a combustion chamber large enough to more than take care of peak loads, (2) some provision for the arresting of dust, (3) an arrangement for providing preheated air with sufficient draft to maintain necessary high temperatures, and (4) a smoke stack of sufficient height to carry off and disperse all products of combustion.

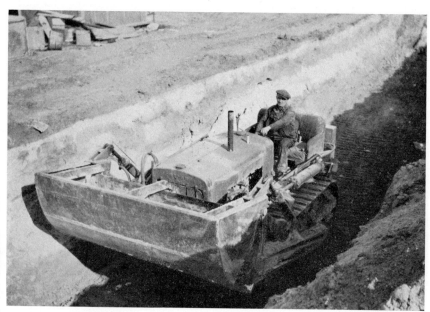

Figure 154. First step in providing for a sanitary fill. The trench may be cut with a bulldozer, power shovel, or dragline. (Courtesy Division of Health Education, Wisconsin State Board of Health.)

Skill in operation is of great importance, and the task can scarcely be left to persons of inferior intelligence or irresponsible attitude. The temperature of the combustion chamber should not be allowed to fall below 1,250°F. An average of 1,400°F is considered necessary for complete combustion. A high standard of cleanliness within and around the plant must be insisted upon. This applies also to vehicles used in hauling.

Grinding and disposal by sewer. This method may be regarded as still in the experimental stage. Obviously, only communities with adequate sewer capacity are in a position to attempt it. Some of the same disadvantages are encountered as with the use of hogs, in that metal items, such as cans, as well as other forms of rubbish not well adapted to maceration, must be collected separately or otherwise eliminated before grinding can take place. Neverthe-less, the method has attracted considerable interest in recent years, and the result of present trials should prove or disprove its practicality.

Reduction. The object of this process is the recovery from the garbage of certain valuable ingredients such as grease, glycerine, or alcohol. This is ac-complished by cooking, after which the residue is pressed dry and sold for fertilizer under the name of "tankage." Because reduction plants are expensive to build and to operate, this method of disposal is not recommended for cities

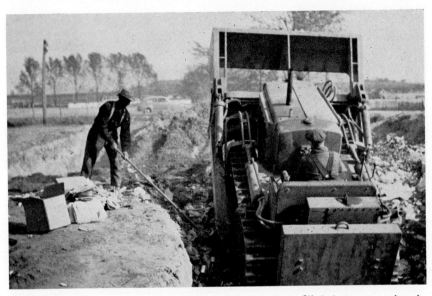

Figure 155. Compaction of garbage and refuse in sanitary fill. It is necessary that the material be thoroughly compacted before coverage. Garbage and refuse are collected and disposed of without separation, which effects a saving in both time and equipment. (Courtesy Division of Health Education, Wisconsin State Board of Health.)

of less than 100,000 population. At least two nuisances are created by the plant itself. The first relates to the offensive and penetrating odors from the cooking. The second has to do with the liquid waste or "stick liquor" that is pressed out of the tankage. This has such a high organic content that its discharge into streams constitutes a serious menace to fish. Since the income derived from the sale of grease and tankage is highly variable, few municipalities seem inclined to undertake the financial risks which this method of disposal in-volves.

The sanitary fill. The sanitary fill seems to be gaining in popularity in many American communities, both large and small. The steps involved are as follows:

1. Selection of a disposal site sufficiently isolated from residential areas to avoid adverse effect on property values. It may, however, be much closer to town than an open dump, hog farm, or incinerator, as neither odors nor fly breeding will be of significant importance.

2. Provision of proper equipment for excavation work, such as drag lines, power shovels, or bulldozers.

3. Cutting of a trench, as shown in Figure 154, by means of equipment listed above.

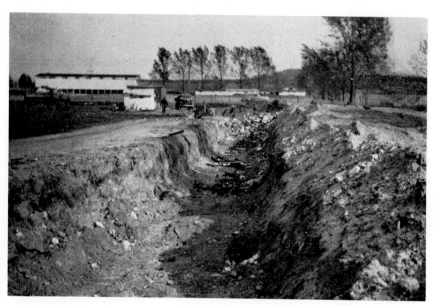

Figure 156. A sanitary fill in operation. Foreground shows excavated trench. Background illustrates completed fill and working face of garbage and refuse. (Courtesy Division of Health Education, Wisconsin State Board of Health.)

4. Dumping of mixed garbage, ashes, and rubbish into the excavation. Great economy is effected here, as separate collections of special types of refuse involve special equipment and much additional labor.

5. Thorough compaction of the refuse. This is usually accomplished by driving a roller or caterpillar type of vehicle over the pile at slow speed.

6. Prompt covering with from one to two feet of earth. Earth removed in connection with the original excavation should be piled nearby in anticipation of this need.

Each day's deposit should be covered and made a closed unit before the next day's collections arrive. Coverage of 24 inches is much to be preferred over 12, as the lesser amount cannot be relied on to give complete protection against flies, odors, rats, or the possibility of fires.

Engineers recommend that the compacted garbage should not exceed eight feet in depth; in fact, six is probably to be preferred. Care should be exercised to maintain adequate covering on the working slope as well as on the finished surface.

The success of this method will depend chiefly upon prompt handling of collections. Equipment should be planned to take care of peak loads and to keep operations normal regardless of breakdowns. In latitudes where frozen ground makes excavation difficult or impossible in the wintertime, ditches and material for covering can be made ready in the fall and the program continued through the colder season with a minimum of labor and machinery.

DISPOSAL OF ANIMAL MANURE

The greatest source of flies in the past has been the neglected piles of animal manure on farms and in the vicinity of stables. Military units have less of this type of problem than formerly, though some cavalry and artillery animals are still used, and pack animals, in the case of mountain troops, at least, are a practical necessity. A certain number of horses for sport and recreation, as well as for ceremonial purposes, will doubtless be maintained about military posts for many years to come, and whatever sanitary problem their presence creates must be given proper attention. The greatest menaces to the health of a cantonment are those situations in which native populations, not wholly under the control of the military, are maintaining animals nearby.

Care of Animal Quarters

It need scarcely be pointed out that frequent and thorough cleaning of stalls, alleyways, and feedboxes is essential in the prevention of fly breeding. Relatively small amounts of material in the corners of mangers and feedboxes can produce many flies. The best stable floors are of concrete, but even these are no guarantee against fly breeding when manure is allowed to accumulate. If plank floors are used, a little borax should be sprinkled along the cracks every two weeks. Plank floors laid above concrete are sometimes advocated for the comfort of the animals, especially if the latter must stand long hours in the stalls. Under more primitive conditions, where earth floors are necessary, the surface should be packed hard. When this becomes soaked with manure and tends to loosen, it should be removed and replaced.

Spreading on Fields

The best and most effective disposal of animal manure consists of daily spreading on agricultural land. By this means the manure is permitted to dry out quickly, in which condition it cannot support larval development. The use of modern spreaders contributes to this end by ensuring complete fragmentation. Besides preventing the accumulation of a large amount of manure in the vicinity of the barns, this method also assures maximum benefit to the soil, since all stages of decomposition take place in direct relation to the land on which the crop is to be planted. A better understanding of good agricultural practices has resulted, in recent years, in many more American farmers' following this procedure. Efficiency in removal is often achieved by standing the spreader close to the animals, indoors, so that cleaning of the stables or stanchion drops is combined with loading. Larger establishments will require a manure car supported by a track which leads out of doors, either to a definite receiving point or to a boom by means of which a number of locations can be used. In more northern latitudes direct dumping into the spreader is best carried out beneath a shed. This not only avoids filling of the spreader box with snow but also makes it less likely that the manure will freeze to the point where its solid state interferes with the action of the blades and gears. Exposure of such a valuable piece of equipment at any time of the year is certainly undesirable. In regions with a heavy snowfall, regular spreading on the fields in winter is out of the question, but of course no flies will breed so long as freezing temperatures prevail. The important point to check for here is whether manure allowed to accumulate near the animals, in closed barns, is not actually producing flies, even in the winter.

Storage in Pits or Bins

When, for one reason or another, daily disposal is not feasible, provision for storage becomes essential. If the location is somewhat permanent and the situation therefore warrants the expenditure, a box or pit of concrete construction is probably the most desirable equipment. Doors, which may be of wood or metal, close the pit from above, and if they are properly fitted, the device will be practically fly-tight. Under practical conditions this ideal may be difficult to maintain, and some prefer to arrange a flytrap at the top to receive the few emerging flies, production of which was formerly considered inevitable. Modern procedure usually dispenses with this, however, as a small additional expenditure can render the pit actually flyproof. The best-designed bins communicate both with the barn and with the outside, for ease in handling the manure. Wooden bins can be substituted for concrete if the planks are treated with creosote or coal tar.

Platforms as Maggot Traps

The use of manure platforms for temporary storage has proved to be fairly satisfactory so far as the fly problem is concerned. The best type of platform, which is of concrete, slopes downward slightly at one corner. On all four sides is a level, concrete trough in which liquid manure as well as rain water may accumulate. It is essential that some liquid be in the trough at all times. Care should be taken in stacking the manure to ensure that none overhangs the outside of the trough. The stack will of course attract flies, from whose eggs larvae will emerge. It is normal, however, for third-stage larvae which are approaching the time for pupation to forsake the high temperature of the heap and seek nearby soil for transformation. Their attempt to do this results merely in their accumulation in the trough, where they either drown or die while attempting pupation in an unsuitable environment. Cragg (1920) advocates frequent changing of water in the trough, to prevent mosquito breeding.

Various equivalents of this procedure have been advocated by different workers. Climate, geographical location, and economic factors affect local practices. A number of procedures will be briefly reviewed.

Baber (1918, 1925) utilized a metal overhang around the margin of a trench to prevent escape of larvae. This was six inches wide, and bent down one and a half inches. Besides the trench, a sump was provided for the collection of fluids. It was Baber's practice to return to the manure all liquids in both sump and trench, to assist in fermentation.

Copeman (1916) found close packing of manure directly upon the ground quite effective, providing the soil was treated with mineral wood-preserving oil at the rate of one gallon per hundred square feet.

Haydon (1922) used enclosures of wire mesh on brick or cement platforms to contain the manure. A channel sunk in the platform around the enclosure trapped the migrating larvae. Sergent and Sergent (1934) combined the wire enclosure with Baber's sheet-iron gutter lip, for composting under rural conditions. They advocated two platforms, so that the full one might be left undisturbed for a time. Many of the larvae in the gutter were consumed by birds.

Hutchison's early maggot trap (1914, 1915) consisted of a wooden platform, ten by twenty feet, made of boards one foot apart and supported by legs one foot high. This stood on a concrete base twelve by twenty-two feet, with a rim of concrete four inches high all around. Three and a half to four feet of manure were piled on the platform and one-half inch of water was maintained in the basin. The manure was sprinkled daily. Hutchison reported that 98 per cent of all larvae were destroyed.

A similar principle was utilized by Gorodetzskii and Sukhova (1936b), who advocated storage in covered boxes standing on four-inch legs. The bottoms of the boxes were of wire netting. Instead of utilizing water to entrap migrating larvae, these workers treated the earth beneath with "still residues" at the rate of 3.2 pints per square yard. Ten days later, enormous numbers of larvae were found dead upon the ground.

Ramakrishna (1935) describes four types of maggot traps suitable for use in India. All are based on the principle that the mature maggots migrate from the moist medium to seek a drier situation for pupation. He states that the manure should be kept moist and be renewed every four to five days.

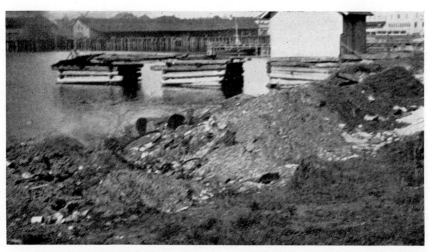

Figure 157. Poor disposal practice. Both horse manure and rubbish are here being used to fill low ground along a beach near the center of town. Use of rubbish as a fill is not objectionable if daily covering and packing are provided for, and if it does not make the location offensive. (Courtesy of Michigan Department of Health.)

The Biothermic Principle

Stacking the manure in connection with the operation of maggot traps also causes the production of a great amount of heat within the pile, due to fermentive action. This itself is destructive to most larvae.

Fay (1939) made a rather careful study of maggot control at the University of Illinois and reported that whereas larvae will develop between $110°-116°F$ $(43.3°-46.6°C)$ if the medium is sufficiently moist, $120°F$ $(48.9°C)$ is always lethal to them. For this reason the maggots usually survive only in the outer four inches. He advocates piles nine feet tall, in ricks, as having less horizontal surface. Two methods of treating the top five inches are recommended. The first makes use of sixty-pound roofing paper, overlapped three inches and held in place by bricks. By this means the temperature can be raised to a point some $40°F$ higher than that of the surrounding air. The alternative procedure employs a paper-covered burlap sheet impregnated with creosote, with the edges staked down. This is left in place for five days after the completion of the pile. By this means 90 per cent of the larvae can be destroyed. It is still necessary to provide a ditch around the bottom to trap the surviving maggots as they attempt to migrate for pupation.

Roubaud (1936) points out certain difficulties in achieving control by the biothermic method in rural France. Steam given off by horse dung quickly

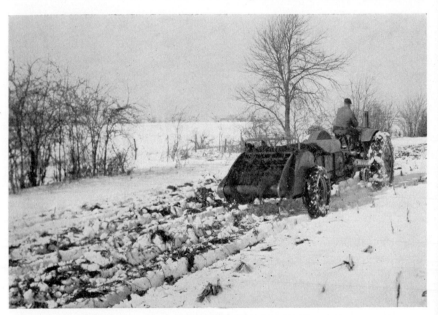

Figure 158. Prevention is better than cure. Winter hauling of manure, where climatic conditions permit, is most desirable, from the standpoint of both fly control and soil fertility. (Courtesy of Deere and Company, Moline, Ill.)

rots tarpaulins or equivalent covers. Furthermore, if any such steam passes through, flies will be attracted to oviposit on the cover itself. Another factor, really an economic one, is that covering the heap deprives barnyard fowl of the surface maggots, from the peasants' standpoint an important item in the food supply of the birds. Roubaud advocates placing fresh manure in a hollow, scooped out at the top of a fermenting pile. Most of the fly eggs will thus be destroyed by heat. Best results are achieved if this is carried out in a pit with vertical walls. Only the surface layers will then contain larvae, and these can be reached by fowls. Under such favorable circumstances a single hen may discover and consume as many as 1,000 maggots a day.

Parisot and Fernier (1934) prefer closed receptacles, in which the manure may be watered without contamination of soil. They state that the temperatures generated range from 30°–40°C (54°–72°F) higher than in ordinary stacks or heaps. These workers were particularly concerned with conditions in Lorraine, where contamination of wells from barnyard manure is an important problem.

Schuckmann (1923) considered that the heat method of handling manure satisfied all requirements, especially since it is so much more economical than treatment by chemicals.

Cory (1918) reported 95.8 per cent destruction of all maggots over a three-year period by merely packing the manure closely and watering the heap. All leached materials were returned to the manure to conserve its agricultural value.

For handling manure in town, the Sergents (1934) designed twin chambers of concrete, on pillars, so that a cart might be run beneath. Each chamber had a capacity of eighteen cubic yards, and was filled through a trap door in the top. After filling, the chamber was left undisturbed for eight days to permit fermentation. The manure was then dumped into the cart. Liquid manure was drained away by a pipe, to an enclosed pit.

Allnutt (1926) describes the Bermuda method, in which horse manure is stored in enclosures built of limestone. Each bin contains the manure from one horse and becomes filled in about ten days. Fermentation is then allowed to continue ten days more, during which time water is added daily if no rain occurs. The heat of fermentation kills most larvae, while those which do come through fall into a gutter containing water treated with cresol. An overhanging edge discourages escape from the trough. While the bin is filling, it is necessary to transfer the outside portion into the center every two days. The filled bin can be made less attractive to flies if covered with oiled earth or with straw or litter which is burned to form an ash. Such elaborate care assumes the availability of plenty of labor at low cost.

Chemical Treatment of Manure

Several chemical substances have proved valuable for the control of fly breeding in manure. It is sometimes advantageous to employ chemical treatment as a supplementary measure along with fermentation and maggot trapping.

Hellebore. This is a plant material which has the advantage of not affecting the microorganisms which accomplish fermentation and render the manure valuable from an agricultural standpoint. One-half pound of hellebore powder should be stirred into ten gallons of water. The mixture is then stored for twenty-four hours. Livestock must not be permitted access to the preparation, as it is somewhat poisonous. This amount will treat from eight to ten bushels of manure. Application is usually by means of a sprinkling can.

Borax. Borax is an old favorite for the treatment of manure but, when used in excess, may injure crops on certain types of soil. Eighteen ounces of borax to thirty gallons of water makes a satisfactory preparation. After storage for

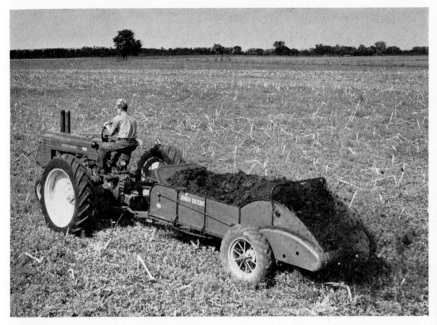

Figure 159. Hauling out manure that has been stored. If storage conditions are flyproof, there can be no criticism of such a procedure from a sanitary standpoint. The soil is most benefited, however, when fresh manure is spread immediately. (Courtesy of Deere and Company, Moline, Ill.)

twenty-four hours, it is ready for use. Two and a half gallons will treat the manure produced by one horse in a day. The rate of application is approximately eleven ounces of borax to eight bushels of manure. Manure so treated may be spread on fields up to fifteen tons per acre without danger of injury to crops. All risk may be eliminated if the manure is piled compactly, so that only the surface layer need be treated. Borax may also be used for treating the soil about garbage pits, pigpens, and chicken yards.

Sodium arsenite. This is effective against both the larvae and the adult flies. It is a dangerous poison, and also stops fermentation. Its use is therefore indicated only when the question of fly control is paramount to other considerations. Four pounds of arsenite of soda are first dissolved in fifty gallons of water. Two quarts of molasses are then added to make the poison attractive.

A 0.1 per cent solution of commercial sodium arsenite, equivalent to a concentration of two pounds per ton of manure, is reported by Howell (1942) as proving harmless to crops. Boyd (1922a) has suggested the substitution of ammonium fluoride for sodium arsenite in treating stored manures.

Sodium fluosilicate has also been advocated as a larvicide. Marcovitch and Anthony (1931) found it more effective than borax, and recommended daily spraying of the manure with a saturated solution. They found 300 pounds per acre not detrimental to plant growth.

Sodium cyanide. This chemical is not practical because of difficulty of application and great danger from cyanide gas. All immature stages of flies can be destroyed by its use, as shown by the experiments of Teichmann (1918), who found 0.1 per cent lethal for eggs, 0.25 per cent for larvae and pupae.

Chemicals with fertilizer value. A combination of calcium cyanamid and superphosphate (acid phosphate) has been found to give almost complete control of fly breeding. These are scattered dry over the manure pile at the rate of one-half pound (of each) to a bushel of manure. Water is then applied. These substances add nitrogen and phosphorus to manure, thus enhancing its value as an augmenter of soil fertility. Surface (1915) was an early advocate of the use of phosphate rock. Grandori (1938) contributed important studies on calcium cyanamid.

Crude oil. Crankcase oil or crude petroleum can be used to destroy all stages of flies in stored manure, but these render the latter almost worthless as fertilizer.

Chemical substances used to treat manure may be evaluated from three standpoints: (1) their larvicidal power (desirable), (2) their bactericidal power (undesirable), and (3) their chemical effect on the manure (which may be good or bad, as proved by subsequent effect upon crops). Cook, Hutchison, and Scales (1914) tried out many substances, and of the items then available, borax, with a larvicidal power of 99 per cent, seemed most satisfactory.

Use of Live Steam

Under certain circumstances, cooking the manure with live steam is highly satisfactory. There must, of course, be a source of steam, under moderate pressure. Boxcars that have been used for shipment of livestock may be treated in this manner, and flies in all stages of development will be destroyed. Fermentation is arrested, but will continue as soon as microorganisms once more gain access to the material. Such manure may be safely spread on lawns without danger of fly production and without reduction of its fertilizer value.

Special and Emergency Disposal

In Gallipoli (Atkinson, 1916) it was the practice to burn the manure in field incinerators. In wet weather the manure was buried at sufficient depth to prevent fly breeding. Such procedures permit no use of the excreta for agricultural purposes, and can be justified only as a military expediency. Carr

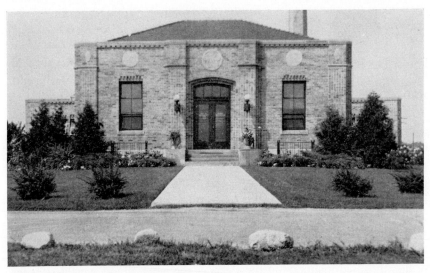

Figure 160. A modern sewage disposal plant. This view of the sewage treatment plant at Traverse City, Michigan, shows how utility may be combined with attractive landscape design. (Courtesy of Michigan Department of Health.)

(1927) also advocated incineration of manure not required for agricultural purposes, as did Davidson (1918) and McDonnell and Eastwood (1917). Marett (1915b) developed in Rouen a routine procedure wherein a narrow-gauge railway was used to carry manure to a large depression where it was dumped and covered with earth. The latter was then planted with grass and other seeds. He also employed incineration.

Brazil (1926) obtained fair results by merely mixing dry earth with animal manure, in the proportion of 1 to 2. This prevented movements of the larvae necessary to feeding. Only animal manures could be handled in this way, however, as it was impossible to obtain a homogeneous mixture with human feces.

In Denmark pig manure is much preferred over horse or cow dung as a breeding medium by flies. Thomsen (1934, 1935a, 1936, 1938) recommends a layer of cow dung over pig dung, as a deterrent. Seaweed or peat moss may be used if cow dung is not available. He also advocates a tarpaulin made of old nitrate bags, to insure biothermic control.

Brain (1918) made large-scale disposal of manure from military units in East Africa by preparing huge pits in sand dunes, 20 by 70 feet across and 10 feet deep (where clay was encountered). One foot of manure was covered

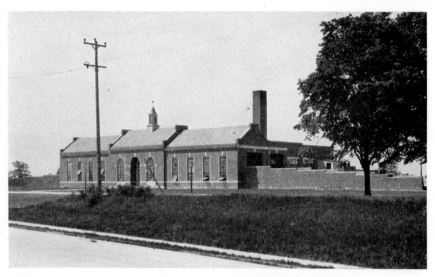

Figure 161. Sewage disposal plant at Dearborn, Michigan. An attractive, dignified building, with operations well concealed from highway. (Courtesy of Michigan Department of Health.)

with three-fourths of an inch of sand or ashes and was rolled down. Full trenches were finally covered with a foot or more of soil or sand and rolled for three days. The stored material was later sold for agricultural purposes.

The use of manure as fuel, practiced in some regions, combines disposal with economic gain. Nikol'skii (1945) points out, however, that intelligent handling must be employed. In Ferghana, for example, it is the practice of the people to prepare sun-dried bricks of cow dung, called "kizyak," for this purpose. If the cakes are made not more than eight centimeters thick, and if they are turned repeatedly during drying, there is little danger that flies will breed in them during the process. It is best to utilize manure not more than five days old.

DISPOSAL OF HUMAN FECES

This subject divides itself into two categories: (1) the disposal of sewage by cities and towns, and (2) disposal by the family or private individual whose establishment is so located that connection with a public sewer is impossible.

Municipal disposal of human waste is a problem so many-sided in nature that anything approaching an adequate discussion would be impractical in

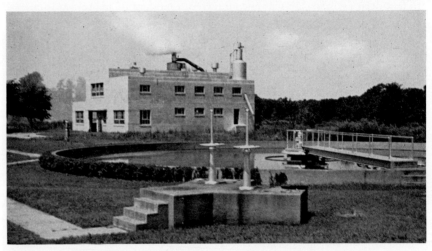

Figure 162. Sewage disposal plant in operation. This view shows primary clarifier and sewage drying house at Battle Creek, Michigan. (Courtesy of Michigan Department of Health.)

a volume of this character and size. It is sufficient to say that direct dumping of untreated sewage into rivers and lakes is being increasingly frowned upon. Sewage disposal plants, in which engineering control of bacterial action accomplishes conversion into harmless residues, are being employed by a growing number of progressive and sanitary-minded communities. Figures 160 to 163 show several such plants which have proved satisfactory in Midwestern American cities.

From a fly-hazard standpoint, the danger from dumping into natural waters is twofold. First, flies may feed upon floating bits of sewage, and later contaminate human food. Second, fluctuations in stream levels may leave sewage stranded along banks, where both fly feeding and fly breeding may ensue.

With a properly operated disposal plant, the first danger can be entirely eliminated, and the second reduced to the occasional situation in which partially digested or poor dewatering sludge may be temporarily exposed to flies. Careful study of the local situation, and intelligent handling of operations, will usually eliminate this hazard also. In a situation where fly breeding was actually in progress, in sludge of this character, Olson and Dahms (1946) succeeded in obtaining 100 per cent kill of larvae by using either borax or kerosene.

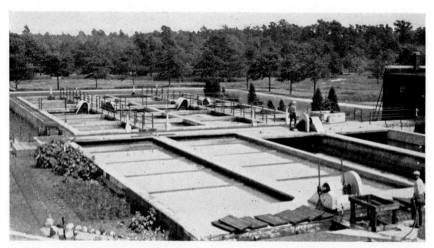

Figure 163. A practical sewage disposal plant for a small city. This view shows settling tanks and activated sludge tanks at Muskegon Heights, Michigan. (Courtesy of Michigan Department of Health.)

Private Disposal of Human Waste

Of much greater importance from the entomological standpoint is the safe disposal of human excreta under rural conditions where sewers do not exist. Farm homes, summer camps, and particularly resort areas can become not only centers of fly production but dangerous sources of epidemic disease, much of it soil- or water-borne. While planning sanitary conveniences in such a way as to eliminate fly hazards, it is therefore no more than common sense to guard against other means of contaminative dispersal.

The open latrine or unhoused privy seat is of course a violation of all good sanitary principles. It is only justified in connection with the most temporary camps and never where a considerable number of campers are likely to follow. Earth should be used to cover the feces immediately after each deposition. A generous application of powdered borax, kerosene, crude oil, or chloride of lime is recommended at least every other day during the fly season. Habitual, daily treatment is safer, as it is less likely to be neglected. The location should be carefully selected to avoid contamination of water supply.

The roofed privy is no improvement, save for added privacy and protection from the weather. The receptacle is the important feature. Lumsden, Stiles, and Freeman (1917) make this statement: "Proper disposal of human filth requires that from the time it leaves the body, to the time it is finally destroyed, none escapes to be scattered about."

Natural agencies for purification, such as microscopic organisms, sunlight,

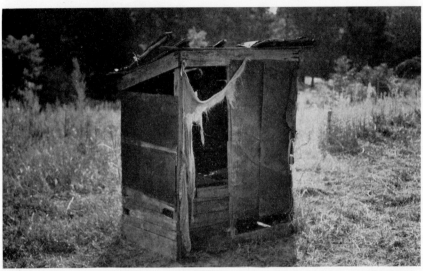

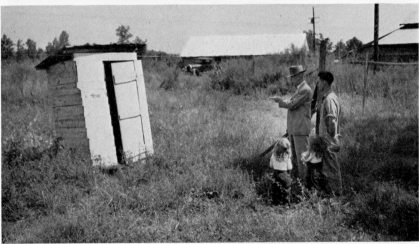

Figure 164. The insanitary privy. *Upper:* A structure that has no desirable feature, not even privacy. *Lower:* Sanitarian points out deficiencies. Privy house need not be flyproof, but seats and pit should be. (Photos supplied by the United States Public Health Service of the Federal Security Agency.)

air, soil, and water, should not be overlooked, and can be utilized to serve human need; left to themselves, however, they can no longer be relied upon to protect human health, at least where any concentration of population is likely to occur.

The proper construction of a sanitary privy is only an initial step. Proper use, proper upkeep, and proper disposal of the contents are also essential. The last requires more planning and attention than any other phase, and is most often neglected. Several types of sanitary privies will be briefly described.

The conventional pit privy, as usually constructed, is rarely sanitary. It may, however, be made so by careful planning. Two things are important. Seat holes must have tight-fitting lids, and flies must be prevented from having ingress between sills and foundation. The latter is best accomplished by pouring a reinforced floor of concrete, three inches in thickness, in which are embedded vertical bolts for anchorage of the two-by-fours that constitute the sills. A desirable type of seat consists of an iron riser sealed into the concrete and covered by a hinged lid. A horizontal vent, protected by a disc of screen, may be made to run between the riser and the outside.

A pit forty-two inches square and five feet or more in depth is adequate. In looser soils, especially, it will be found necessary to brace the sides of the pit with boards, to prevent caving. The earth obtained by excavation may be used to provide a radial slope, by which rain water is drained away from the foundation on all sides. Assuming a single-slope roof, one may guard against erosion at the rear by arranging against the wall of the privy a sloping rack of wood, covered by a panel of sheet metal. If a gable roof is used, it will be necessary to provide two of these, one on either side.

Since the bottom of the pit is of earth, there is nothing in this arrangement to prevent pollution of the soil or nearby underground waters. Such a privy, therefore, should never be located within one hundred yards of a well or upon a slope above a well or spring. Low ground will be found desirable, in most instances, but if too low a point is chosen, the pit may come to contain standing water. When this occurs, oiling may prove necessary to prevent the breeding of mosquitoes, which, because of their smaller size, sometimes gain access through apertures too small to admit flies.

When the pit is nearly filled with excrement, the house is moved and placed over another pit. The old concrete floor is usually left in place, the riser removed, and the hole permanently sealed. If the floor is removed, as will always be the case where the floor is of wood, the pit should be filled up with earth.

Surface privies with open backs (and no pits) are malodorous and certainly unsightly, but even these can be rendered flyproof by closing in the open side with screen. If this is toward the south, the sunshine will aid greatly in drying and deodorizing the material.

The simplest type which guards against soil pollution consists of a heavy, watertight can fitted with a wooden cover which also serves as a seat. The hole in the latter is covered with a hinged lid which may be provided with a

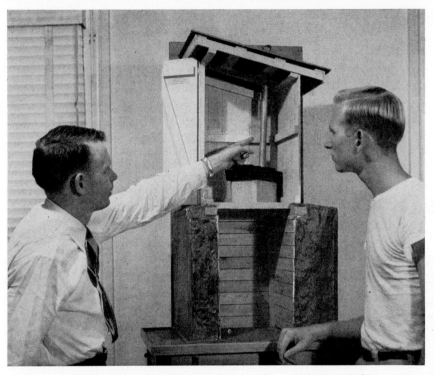

Figure 165. Scale model of sanitary pit privy, with vertical vent. Such a structure comes very close to being 100 per cent flyproof. (Photo supplied by the United States Public Health Service of the Federal Security Agency.)

screened center, to insure constant ventilation. A modification of this scheme is the boxed can, where the actual receptacle is set within a fly-tight box, the top of which serves as a seat. Two, or even three, sides of the box may be screened for ventilation, while the fourth swings on hinges for removal of the can. Both ventilation and removal will be facilitated if approximately two inches of clearance are provided between the can and the box top. The hinged lid which closes the hole should be arranged to drop into place when the privy is not in use. Either type of convenience described above may be installed in any suitable outbuilding, but a separate privy house is more satisfactory under most circumstances. The receptacle box may be a separate unit or it may be built into the wall of the privy itself, in which case removal of the receptacle may be from outside. All outside surfaces should be painted, to guard against weathering, warping, and loss of a flyproof fit. Almost any existing privy, no matter how unsanitary, can be rendered safe by the method described above. A ventilating flue, from box to outside, preferably through the roof, aids greatly in reducing offensive odors. Odors should be further reduced by the use of lime or other drying or deodorizing agencies, so that the privy will not become a center of attraction for flies seeking contact with the fecal material.

A galvanized can or bucket of one-bushel capacity makes a good receptacle. Its life will be prolonged if the interior is painted with coal tar, which also makes cleaning easier. At each emptying the can should be inspected for possible leaks. In northern latitudes the contents may freeze, particularly if much liquid is present. If this occurs, the application of a very moderate amount of heat, by pouring hot water against the sides, will cause the mass to slide out in a solid block.

Permanent Receptacles

To avoid the frequent handling of waste material, permanent receptacles of larger size are often used. The simple vault privy is widely known. The chief problem here is to design the vault so that periodic removal of excrement is not too difficult. A concrete pit with sloping walls front and rear is recommended. By having the rear slope extend well beyond the back wall of the privy, provision can be made for an inclined trap door, which may be lifted out of the way when cleaning is in progress.

Final disposal of privy contents may be by burning, by discharge into a sewer, usually through a manhole, or by burial, with or without the use of a disinfectant.

The L.R.S. Privy

This design was proposed by Lumsden, Roberts, and Stiles in 1910, to take advantage of natural fermentation as an agent in the reduction of human wastes. The pit consists of a watertight barrel, tank, or vault approximately three-fourths filled with water. At this level a T-shaped pipe, two inches or more in diameter, is installed, with the stem of the T leading horizontally from the tank. Its destination is a watertight chamber, pot, or barrel, which receives the liquid effluent. Both ends of the vertically disposed portion of

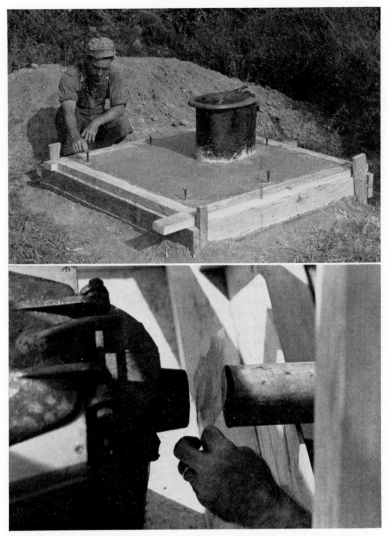

Figure 166. Construction of sanitary pit privy. *Upper:* Toilet seat, sealed in cement floor, over pit. Embedded bolts are for anchoring superstructure to foundation. *Lower:* Flyproofing the horizontal vent. Flies may be attracted into vent pipe by odors, but can get no farther than the screen. (Photo supplied by the United States Public Health Service of the Federal Security Agency.)

the T are covered with wire screen. Splashing may be avoided by a layer of floating chips or by a horizontal board, just below the surface, the position of which may be controlled by a vertical rod which passes through the seat. After use, the antisplash board should be lowered to permit paper and fecal matter to float free in the water. It was recommended that a pound or two of old manure be added to the water to initiate fermentation, and that a film of petroleum be poured over the surface of the liquid in each container, to repel insects.

The fecal material ferments in the water and gradually becomes liquid. Some is converted to gas. The liquid in the vault rises and the excess passes into the effluent tank. The residue is much less in volume than the original solid matter and needs to be cleaned out only at long intervals. The effluent is potentially dangerous and must be disposed of in some safe fashion.

In its original design the L.R.S. privy required too much intelligent attention to prove generally popular or effective. An improved model, however, in which both tanks were of concrete, gave better service. A convenient method of disposing of the effluent is to pipe it into drain tile, with open joints, and thus permit it to seep into the topsoil. Contamination of water supplies may be avoided by adding chemical disinfectants to the effluent at frequent intervals.

The modification of the L.R.S. design known as the Kentucky Sanitary Privy employs three tanks and thus makes provision for more than one stage of decomposition. Such devices were the forerunners of our modern septic tanks, which usually discharge their effluent either into "dry wells" or distributing tile.

Special Problems

In India, caste prejudices must be taken into account in providing sanitary facilities. Jolly (1923) succeeded in designing an automatic, flyproof latrine seat which met this need. Dhondy (1940) describes a greatly improved seat, which avoids mechanisms difficult for children to operate. This is controlled by a pair of foot rests, connected by levers and pulleys with sheet-metal lids, centered on pivots. When the latrine is not in use, the lids close the container. When the foot rests are depressed, the lids move into such a position that they cannot be fouled. Release of foot pressure permits the lids to return to the closed position by their own weight.

Under tropical conditions night soil is usually buried under too little earth to give adequate protection. Stiles and Gardner (1910) showed that when flyblown fecal material was buried under 48 inches of clear sand, *Musca domestica* issued from the surface. Certain undetermined muscoids issued through 72 inches. Austin and Mayne (1935) recommend dumping into pits twenty feet deep, which are covered except for a small opening which is flyproof. On the Gold Coast Otway (1926) used deep, covered pits, with a flytrap near one end, at least six feet from the filling hole. A thatched-roof structure protected the pit from torrential rains.

McMahon (1935) advocates the use of repellents in pit latrines. Naphthalene is effective, paradichlorbenzene much more so. Two pounds of the latter in powder form is recommended at the beginning of use, to be followed by the addition of four ounces every week. If maggots are already present, deterrents are of no value, however, as they tend merely to drive the larvae to the sides and edges of the pit, where many are able to transform (Corfield, 1919).

Phalen (1917) found daily burning out of military latrines a useful control measure. The box was turned back, hay or straw was thrown into the pit, and a sprinkling of crude oil was added before applying fire. An alternative method, in which the interior of the pit was sprayed with a suspension of lamp black in coal oil, was used when circumstances made it undesirable or impractical to move the box. King (1918) also records the practice of daily burning out of latrines in East Africa. He likewise reported that breeding of flies could be prevented by use of a smoking wood fire in a perforated kerosene tin, suspended halfway down by means of wires. It was necessary to renew the fire twice a day. Deep trenches were treated by spraying daily with a sodium arsenite bait.

The use of the chemical closet scarcely comes within the province of this volume, as families which employ this means of waste disposal usually move the toilet indoors, so that fly control becomes a matter of screening the premises. As with all disposal methods short of a sewer connection, the success of the chemical toilet depends upon conscientious and careful attention.

With the availability of a reliable supply of running water, the rural home is no longer dependent upon the foregoing methods of waste disposal. Indoor flush toilets should be installed and septic tanks employed. The ever-expanding program of rural electrification is rapidly reducing the magnitude of the fly problem in more heavily populated areas, at least in the United States.

MISCELLANEOUS CONSIDERATIONS RELATING TO PLANNED CONTROL

Long-range control procedures cannot always approach the ideal which ample funds, elaborate machinery, and expensive or highly trained labor make possible. Under less favorable economic conditions, one must do the best he can. The exact procedure will vary with geographical and climatic factors. Thus Pruthi (1946) developed a control method in Delhi by preparing pits of sufficient size to receive a week's supply of dung, litter, and garbage, which was gathered daily from the vicinity of human dwellings. Care was taken that no debris should be overlooked. At the end of the week, the pit was sealed by applying three layers of earth, each four inches in depth. Each layer was well pressed down, and the top two inches were converted into a plaster by watering. When sealed in by this method, no larvae lived more than six hours. The method failed only in very wet weather, when all the earth used was oozing water. A little care in providing earth not oozing wet accomplished control even in the rainy season. Pruthi found weekly sealing more effective than the older method of covering each daily accumulation with six inches of soil. It was also cheaper. The dung was later dug up and used as fertilizer.

In dry weather the spreading of fresh cow dung in the sun, in layers not to exceed two inches in depth, caused all larvae to die, and no new oviposition took place. Six species of the genus *Musca* were involved in Pruthi's experiments, with *M. nebulo* and *M. domestica vicina* the most abundant.

Deoras and Arjan Singh Jandu (1943) point out that *Musca nebulo* is the commonest housefly in India. Others of importance besides *M. domestica vicina* are *M. sorbens, M. ventrosa,* and *M. conducens.* To control all five, these authors recommend a combination of maggot trap and fermentation for large-scale disposal, but for the small farms they advocate spreading the manure in the sun, about one inch thick, with a sprinkling of dry, powdered lime to repel flies. Daily raking for four days is followed by storage in pits.

As mentioned previously, the high temperature generated in compost masses under certain environmental conditions is itself destructive to fly larvae, a fact which makes it possible to effect a certain amount of control in India merely by careful handling of refuse dumps (Joshi and Dnyansagar, 1945). In the rainy season, however, the lower temperature of such masses and the higher relative humidity permit large numbers of larvae to develop. The above-mentioned workers found that either crude oil or bleaching powder could be used during the monsoon season to offset this condition, resulting in 85 to 90 per cent control without too great expense.

One and one-half pounds of crude oil per 100 square feet proved sufficient, as did 12 pounds of bleaching powder for the same area. In either case the material was applied in two doses, one on the first day following the fill, the second a week later. Bleaching powder was less satisfactory than oil, as it deteriorates in storage under monsoon conditions and is also more expensive.

Prophylactic Use of DDT

Methods ordinarily regarded as emergency ones may be used in long-range planning when conditions warrant. In military cantonments, when it is anticipated that fly populations, originating largely in areas outside military jurisdiction, may become an annoyance, the routine use of DDT is strongly indicated. Experiments reported in the bulletin of the U.S. Army Medical Department for 1946 showed the comparative values of painting, dipping, and spraying fly screens with a 5 per cent solution of DDT. Painting the screens with wide-shouldered brushes at intervals of sixty days was found to produce an effective deposition of crystals with only reasonable expenditure of time and labor, and was adopted as standard procedure. For garbage racks, however, spraying at monthly intervals proved most satisfactory. The experiments were carried on at a military camp in Georgia during the summer of 1945. Special tools have recently been devised to replace paintbrushes in the treatment of screens. A wool-felt strip, held rigid in a slot and continually moistened by DDT solution fed through holes in a rectangular container, is very efficient. The entire device is mounted on an adjustable pole. Somewhat less popular is a metal cylinder covered with carpet. The solution in this case escapes from the cylinder through feed holes and keeps the fabric wet.

It should be remembered that DDT is not effective against ova, larvae, or pupae, but when sprayed about potential breeding areas, it does inhibit oviposition, and young adults die soon after emergence because of contact.

Scudder (1949) justifies prophylactic application of DDT by pointing out that heavy breeding of flies in certain areas results in such intense competition that long-distance migration of a portion of the fly population inevitably follows. A hitherto uninfested area may thus find itself heavily invaded, unless protective measures are instituted in advance. A reverse form of such precautionary treatment is illustrated by DDT treatment of airplanes to prevent survival of noxious insects which may be picked up at stopovers. Madden, Lindquist, and Knipling (1945) found that surfaces which had received an application of 100 mg. of DDT per square foot remained lethal after being wiped with a dry cloth.

Use of DDT as a preventive measure has thus largely superseded the employment of arsenic bait sprays, so popular between 1915 and 1945, especially in Italy. The disadvantage of arsenical preparations (usually sodium arsenite) lay, of course, in the danger to children and domestic animals through chance ingestion of the poison.

Zymothermic Cells

In 1938(c) De La Paz suggested a new method of disposing of refuse in Manila. In place of dumping he proposed systematic fermentation and reduction in zymothermic cells. Such procedure generates a temperature of 140°–

158°F (60°–70°C), which is lethal to all stages of flies as well as to most pathogenic organisms. Offensive odors are eventually abolished and the residue makes a satisfactory fertilizer.

Isaac (1944) places both fresh dung and garbage in a deep, open pit for seven days, during which time flies are free to oviposit. On the seventh day he adds a four-inch layer of heavy soil, which is rammed down and watered. Two additional four-inch layers are later added, in the same manner, producing a compaction through which the maggots are unable to emerge. The fertilizing value is retained.

USE OF NATURAL AGENTS IN PLANNED CONTROL

Some potential agencies for natural control have not as yet been thoroughly developed. The first bacterial organism to be isolated capable of causing infection in houseflies was *Bacterium delendae-muscae,* described by Roubaud and Descazeaux in 1923. The organism was obtained first from *Stomoxys calcitrans,* of which all infected specimens perished in from two to thirty days. The infection was not fatal to adults of *Musca domestica* if contracted after emergence, but when acquired by the larvae, the organisms caused death at the end of the pupal period. Blowflies were more susceptible, dying at the beginning of pupation. *Stomoxys,* when infected in the same manner, usually transformed, only to die in the adult state. These authors raised the question as to whether the newly discovered organism might be of practical use in fly control, but so far no serious effort has been made to test such methods.

The well-known appetite of barnyard fowl for living maggots can be exploited as a control factor where complete prevention of fly breeding is more or less out of the question. Thus Baranov (1939) observed that in the village of Mratzlin, Serbia, considerable numbers of *Musca domestica, Stomoxys calcitrans* and *Fannia canicularis* emerged from dung piled in sheds, but few or none from dung heaps piled in the open. The latter were accessible to barnyard fowl, which were very numerous in the village and which he believed responsible for general destruction of the maggots. Strauss (1922b) advocated spreading manure in thin layers so that poultry might pick out the larvae.

A modern report on the handling of hymenopterous parasites with a view to combatting *Musca domestica* is given by De Bach (1943), who worked with *Mormoniella vitripennis* and *Muscidifurax raptor.* Cold storage of both larvae and pupae of these species was found feasible for from one to several months, that is, until needed for release against an increasing fly population. De Bach used storage temperatures ranging from 0° to 23°C (32° to 73.5°F). The adults emerged at 27.5°C (81.5°F). In general, the fecundity was highest in those adults which resulted from larvae and pupae maintained at lowest storage temperatures.

Noel (1913) succeeded in trapping large numbers of flies by use of meat traps, from which the resulting larvae were fed to fishes in connection with a fish-culture establishment. The fly population was reduced, and Noel suggested that the practice might well be employed as a method of extermination.

It would seem that use of the natural enemies of houseflies in planned control work has but little future value, since it can only be effective where the fly population is already considerable, and proper control of potential breeding areas should eliminate this contingency.

DIVERSION TECHNIQUE

Vanskaya (1942a) impregnated various substances with ammonium carbonate, thereby rendering them much more attractive to ovipositing flies. Out of this work has come the suggestion that such material might be useful in attracting flies to cheap artificial media, which could then be destroyed. To my knowledge however, no large-scale, practical use of such a method has been tried.

AID TO INVESTIGATION

Long-range planning must be based on research, and the collection of specimens in quantity for subsequent laboratory study is a necessary part of the program. The ordinary insect net is not too practical, as it usually disturbs more flies than it captures. Furthermore, the necessary transference of the specimens to containers for transport is difficult and time-consuming. Field traps are far better, but the baits must be carefully selected so as to compete with other attractive materials in the surroundings, and when the investigator desires to study the bacterial flora of the captured flies, sterile bait must be provided. Another disadvantage of the conventional trap is that the catch is accumulated over a period of hours, and while some of the specimens are of desirable freshness, others are in a dead or dying state. The separation of the healthy flies is tedious and difficult. Again, traps must be more or less constantly supervised, lest they be stolen or knocked over.

Maier and Dow (1949) succeeded in devising a conical type of net which meets most of these objections. This consists of a cone of 18-mesh screening seventeen inches high and thirty inches in diameter at the base, with a circular opening three and a quarter inches in diameter at the top. Upon the latter is fitted a removable, cylindrical cage of the approximate dimensions of a standard No. 3 can. A flattened cone of screening with a central aperture three-quarters of an inch in diameter extends upward a short distance into the cylinder. The apparatus may be used in various ways, but is ordinarily lowered upon flies which have concentrated in some naturally attractive area. Skillfully operated, this device permits very few to escape. The collecting cylinder, if not already in position, is then fitted into place and a cloth cape of dark material is draped about the cone. The captured flies move toward the only source of available light and soon find themselves in the collecting cage. As the latter is lifted, a closing disc is slipped into place and secured by clamps. The cages with their content of living flies should be placed in a humid container for transport to the laboratory, where the flies may be anaesthetized and sorted for species and sex.

CHAPTER XIX

Newer Insecticides:
Uses and Dangers

There webs were spread of more than common size, And half-starved spiders prey'd on half-starved flies.—Charles Churchill, The Prophecy of Famine

DDT was the atomic bomb of the biologists' world. First demonstrated as an insecticide of more than common merit by Dr. Paul Müller, in Switzerland, dichloro-diphenyl-trichloroethane rose to prominence during World War II as superior to all hitherto discovered substances for the control of medically important arthropods. This was particularly true for mosquitoes and filth-feeding flies. Because DDT is rather slow in its knockdown effect, the immediate reduction in fly population was not always apparent, but a few days after application, barns, fish stalls, open privies, and other situations that had never been known to be other than fly-ridden since the dawn of history became essentially fly-free. Thus was opened a new chapter in the evolution of insect control, a chapter which seems destined to be fraught with considerable controversy and which may well record not a few gigantic errors in human judgment, should we proceed to the unrestricted use of this and similar materials without due regard for the possible secondary effects involved.

DDT owes its unusual reputation first to the fact that it is *not* a repellent. Surfaces treated with 5 per cent DDT in kerosene are, after the evaporation of the latter, quite as attractive to flies as they were before the application was made. Thus there is nothing to interfere with the utilization of such surfaces as resting places by all manner of insects, including flies. A very brief contact, in the case of *Musca domestica,* is usually sufficient for irreversible damage to the nervous system, leading to almost certain death within a few minutes, or at most a few hours, after exposure. The only insects recorded as being able to sense the presence of DDT from afar and which usually alter their path to avoid contact with it, are termites (order Isoptera). These highly specialized destroyers of buildings and furniture are thus clever enough to save themselves from the new destruction; but flies are not so clever.

The second, and distinctive, feature of DDT is found in its *residual* effect. The wall or screen which has been rendered lethal to flies by application of DDT remains so for an astonishingly long period of time. Dairy barns have been rendered fly-free for 60, 90, or even 120 days by a single spraying with a 5 per cent solution in a proper carrier.

The discussion which follows treats of DDT from five approaches: (1) historical notes on its discovery and development, (2) its usefulness as a military insecticide in World War II, (3) special data concerning its toxicity to domestic flies, (4) possible danger to the health of man, and precaution in its use, and (5) its possible disturbance of the balance of nature.

HISTORICAL DEVELOPMENT

DDT was first synthesized by Othmar Zeidler, a young German chemist, in Strasbourg in 1874. Its preparation was described in six lines of type in the *Berichte der Chemischen Gesellschaft* for that year. Neither its discoverer nor his contemporaries appear to have entertained any concept of its properties as an insecticide.

An appreciation of its economic value was the result of deliberate investigations by the research staff of the J. R. Geigy Company of Basle, Switzerland, for the purpose of discovering and developing new insecticides. The work began about 1934, but it was not until 1939 that Dr. Paul Müller, one of the investigators concerned, synthesized a product which showed remarkable insecticidal properties. Dr. Müller did not at first know that his substance was identical with Zeidler's dichloro-diphenyl-trichloroethane. Its first practical test, against the Colorado potato beetle, was carried out under the direction of Dr. R. Wiesmann, entomologist at the Swiss Federal Experimental Agricultural Station at Waederswill. Preliminary testing led to general use, and the Swiss potato crop, which had been seriously threatened that year—due partly to international conditions which limited the importation of standard insecticides—was saved.

Further experimentation demonstrated that DDT was equally effective against the body louse. The Swiss product thus appeared on the market under two names, "Gesarol" for use as a general insecticide, and "Neocid" for the control of lice on the body and in clothing.

In 1942 the Geigy Company called the attention of the American Army to the availability of Gesarol, and sent a small quantity to its American subsidiary, Geigy Company, Inc., of New York, for investigation by American authorities. Under the direction of Dr. F. C. Bishopp and Dr. F. C. Roark, of the U.S. Department of Agriculture, Bureau of Entomology and Plant Quarantine, small-scale experiments were performed which abundantly confirmed the claims of the manufacturers. This led to the organization of a full-scale research program under military direction, which was to result in general and successful use of DDT by the armed forces during the later years of the war.

A special laboratory was established at Orlando, Florida, with a staff of twenty-nine men. Dr. E. F. Knipling, of the Bureau of Entomology and Plant Quarantine, was placed in charge. Dr. Walter E. Dove, chief of the Division of Insects Affecting Man and Animals, directed the procedure from Washington. The most urgent problem was to find an adequate substitute for pyrethrum in the preparation of louse powder for army use. There had been failure of the pyrethrum crop in Africa (Kenya Colony), and both the American and British governments were in a state of anxiety concerning an adequate supply of appropriate insecticides for military purposes. Within less than a year an excellent delousing powder had been developed, consisting of 10 per cent DDT in pyrophyllite, the availability of which enabled the Army to suppress quickly the serious epidemic of typhus fever in Naples in December, 1943.

By use of emulsions, it was found that garments could be treated with DDT so that they would remain louse-free for as many as eight washings with army soap!

The laboratory next turned its attention to mosquito control, especially the possibility of spraying mosquito-breeding areas by airplane. Both solutions and emulsions were used and devices were eventually perfected which would permit distribution by fast-flying combat planes. Both larvae and adult mosquitoes were killed by exceedingly small quantities of material, and thus a new technique became available for the protection of troops from malaria, filariasis, yellow fever, dengue, and mosquito-borne encephalitis.

The use of DDT against bedbugs, cockroaches, silver fish, and other household and agricultural pests was also investigated, and respect for the new insecticide increased rapidly. Flies proved particularly susceptible to its action, especially because of the residual effect, and both Army and Navy made extensive use of DDT not only about military establishments but also in and around war plants, wherever the fly nuisance had become severe.

A total of fifteen American chemical companies were given military contracts for synthesizing DDT, and by the end of the war there was assured a practically unlimited supply, not only for military but also for civilian use.

It is a fitting conclusion to the story of DDT that in the fall of 1948, on recommendation of the Caroline Institute of the University of Medicine in Stockholm, Dr. Paul Müller was awarded the Nobel Prize in Physiology and Medicine, for his part in saving the lives of hundreds of thousands, perhaps millions, who without DDT might have perished from insect-borne diseases during the preceding five-year period.

SPECIAL REMARKS ON THE PART PLAYED BY DDT IN WORLD WAR II

As soon as the U.S. Department of Agriculture had demonstrated the promising nature of Gesarol, the findings were reported to Major General Norman T. Kirk, Surgeon General of the Army, and to Brigadier General James S. Simmons, then Chief of Preventive Medicine. There followed the extensive research activity already alluded to. Colonel William P. Stone, as Director of Sanitation and Hygiene, became personally responsible for the work which was to be so ably carried out by the Bureau of Entomology and Plant Quarantine. Colonel Stone was later succeeeded by Lieutenant Colonel A. L. Ahnfeldt, who had the satisfaction of seeing the most optimistic conjectures of his predecessor justified.

Most dramatic was the conquest of the typhus epidemic in Naples, previously mentioned. Mass-dusting stations were set up in many parts of the city, each with a crew of from six to twenty persons. DDT powder was forced under the clothing either by hand pumps or by use of compressed air. Some stations handled as many as 5,000 persons per day. Within three months over 2,250,000 persons had been deloused, the epidemic had been stopped, and the advance into Italy had been made safe for American soldiers, not one of whom contracted the disease.

Further research continued under the Army Committee for Insect and Rodent Control, with Colonel Ahnfeldt in an executive capacity. This body co-operated with the U.S. Public Health Service, the U.S. Navy, the U.S. Department of Agriculture, the U.S. Department of the Interior, the National Research Council, and the Office of Scientific Research and Development. Laboratory and field tests were rapidly made the basis of general operations for the control of mosquitoes, bedbugs, roaches, and flies, as a part of the program for disease prevention among the troops.

DDT first appeared on Army supply lists in May, 1943, and on those of the Navy in January, 1944. Toward the close of the war the Army Supply Schedule carried nine different preparations of DDT. By this time the production of DDT in the United States had reached a monthly output of

3,000,000 pounds. Nearly all of this was purchased by the armed forces. As pointed out by Leary, Fishbein, and Salter (1946), DDT thus made possible the return of many "thousands of young men who would otherwise have died somewhere far away of infectious disease."

Yielding to popular demand, the War Production Board of the United States Government released DDT for general civilian use in September, 1945. The extensive research immediately carried on by chemical manufacturers, who during the war were permitted to divert only 5 per cent of their output into civilian channels, has added greatly to our present knowledge and understanding of this remarkable and useful compound. This is especially true in connection with agricultural needs. Research in relation to military problems is also actively maintained.

DDT IN THE CONTROL OF FLIES

Effects on the Fly

Houseflies have proved particularly susceptible to the effects of DDT. Already established as a favorite test insect for the standardization of insecticides, *Musca domestica* came in for immediate and extensive investigation in determining the properties of the new material.

Among recent studies on the toxicity of DDT to *Musca domestica* are those of Parkin and Green (1945a,b), who used a concentrate 74.6 per cent pure. Sprays containing 0.05, 0.1, and 0.5 per cent of the concentrate by weight, in kerosene, were fed by atomizer into a small chamber at the rate of 2.5 ml. per 18 cubic feet. The least kill by the weakest solution was 95.8 per cent in 24 hours. The 0.5 per cent vapor always gave 100 per cent. The knockdown was slow in all these concentrations, but became complete in ten minutes when a one per cent preparation was used.

Experiments on a larger scale, utilizing a room of 8,400 cubic feet capacity in which 12,000 flies had been released, gave similar results. Eighty per cent of the flies were knocked down in ten minutes and 99.5 per cent at the expiration of an hour. Essentially complete kill (99.5 per cent) was achieved at the end of thirty hours. These results followed release of 200 ml. of the one per cent preparation described above.

Walls thoroughly treated with DDT in kerosene and not exposed to weather proved toxic to flies one year later. Action was much slower, of course, some three hours from the moment of contact being required before the flies became incapacitated; the remarkable residual effect was nevertheless clearly demonstrated.

Since the knockdown effect of DDT is so slow, many investigators recommend combining it with a small amount of standard insecticide, such as pyrethrum. The latter paralyzes the insects almost at once, so that they remain immobile, while the slower-acting DDT accomplishes their death. DDT can be dissolved in methyl alcohol, but in this vehicle it acts even more slowly than in kerosene.

Parkin and Green also recorded some interesting observations on the behavior of the flies exposed to treatment. They state that within one minute of being sprayed in a small chamber with 2 ml. of 0.05 to 1.0 per cent DDT in "Pool burning oil," the flies moved about excitedly. Shortly afterwards those alighting on the glass front of the chamber lost their grip and began to slide slowly downward. They continued, however, to run actively on the floor of the chamber, stopping frequently to clean front and hind legs, wings, and head. These movements were very vigorous. At this stage the flies would take short flights if disturbed. All of these effects, however, may be produced by oil alone, and cannot rightly be attributed to DDT. The first true DDT symptom which these investigators observed was the failure of the legs to support the weight of the body, plus definite loss of co-ordination in their use. Sometimes all or some of the legs on one side of the body were much more severely paralyzed than those on the other side. The affected flies often rolled to their backs and kicked their legs frantically in the air, tending at the same time to extrude the proboscis. A few were able to take off from their backs for very short, uncontrolled flights, and even after they could no longer take to the air, their wings would still be vibrated forcefully, resulting in a loud buzzing, a symptom usually noted by those who use DDT in fly control work. After the general convulsive activity had subsided, the flies sometimes lay for several hours in a comatose state, with continuous, marked tremors and occasional spasms of the legs, which were strongly flexed at the femorotibial joints. A drop of clear regurgitated fluid often appeared at the tip of the proboscis, which was more or less extended in most specimens. The tremors slowly became less marked, and death finally supervened. Parkin and Green did not record autotomy of the legs, a phenomenon stated to occur by Läuger, Martin, and Müller (1944) and Wiesmann and Fenjves (1944). It should be remarked that about 30 per cent of the females usually died with the ovipositor more or less extruded.

The manner in which DDT affects the insect's nervous system is but incompletely understood. Yeager and Munson (1945), working on cockroaches, obtained evidence that the site of action for DDT lies somewhere in the nerve trunks between their origin in the ventral ganglia and their termination in the muscles of the leg. Neither the point of origin nor the myoneural junctions appear to be involved. This is quite in contrast with the action of nicotine, for example, which has been shown to affect the ganglia directly.

METHODS OF APPLYING DDT

Zimmerman and Lavine (1946), in their popular and entertaining volume *DDT—Killer of Killers,* summarize the methods of applying DDT in fly control under six heads: space sprays, aerosols, residual sprays, emulsions, wettable powders, and paints.

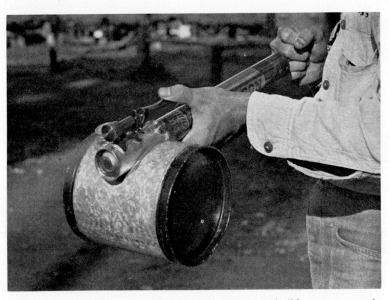

Figure 167. Hand sprayer, modern type. Pumping builds up pressure in the atomizer head. Release of liquid is controlled by a lever near the nozzle. This type of dispenser was used in field applications of DDT oil sprays for malaria control in Guadalcanal in 1944. (U.S. Army photograph.)

Space Sprays

These are for the purpose of contacting the fly directly, usually while on the wing. Since immediate knockdown is the objective desired, such sprays usually contain a rather heavy concentration of pyrethrum or of the organic thiocyanates, such as lethane or thanite. The DDT content of these sprays may be as little as 0.25 per cent, sufficient to accomplish the eventual death of flies actually contacted by it but not capable of imparting to walls and ceilings a residual lethal effect. It should be remarked that such a result may sometimes be built up by repeated spraying on successive days, due to the cumulative effect; however, this is not the purpose of such sprays, and must be considered merely an occasional, incidental result. Space sprays are applied with hand spray guns, knapsack sprayers, or power devices, depending on the volume of space to be sprayed and the facilities available.

Aerosols

These are dispensed in special bomblike containers, and may be described as space sprays in which the particles are so finely divided that these continue to float in the atmosphere for an unusually long time, being carried to all parts of the room before settling occurs. The secret of the "aerosol bomb" goes back to the work of Thomas Midgley of General Motors Corporation. In his search for a refrigerant which would be nontoxic to man, Dr. Midgley developed a substance known as Freon-12. This gas, known chemically as dichlorodifluoromethane, liquifies at $-22°F$, at ordinary atmospheric pressure. At room temperature, considerable pressure is, of course, required to keep it in a liquid state. Approximately 3 per cent DDT and 2 per cent pyrethrum extract are dissolved in Freon-12, and the solution is held captive in the metal container known as the "aerosol bomb," the walls of which are made strong enough to contain the really very great pressure within. By manipulating a valve, the operator releases the charge through a very small opening. The spray is released at such high velocity that it breaks up into an exceedingly fine mist, the particles of which are much smaller than can be delivered by the conventional nozzles of ordinary spray guns.

The freon evaporates at once, leaving the particles of pyrethrum and DDT floating in the air. During the early years of World War II, only activated pyrethrum was utilized in the bombs, and this in such small amounts that its use was practically limited to mosquito control. With pyrethrum again more abundant, and DDT generally available, the present formula has replaced the emergency solution and the modern aerosol bomb promises to be exceedingly useful in the control not only of flies but of all manner of household pests. A one-pound bomb contains sufficient spray to treat approximately 25,000 cubic feet of space. Users should calculate the size of rooms to be treated and keep the valve open only the necessary number of seconds to provide for the release of a proper amount of insecticide. Directions are usually printed on the bomb itself or on the wrapper. There is no danger to man from releasing an excessive amount of the aerosol, but the packaging is rather expensive, and there is no point in wasting good material.

The basic DDT aerosol formula for use against both mosquitoes and houseflies contained 5 per cent DDT plus 10 per cent cyclohexanone. For quick knockdown, however, pyrethrum is considered essential, and modern aerosols contain a mixture of pyrethrum and DDT. Madden *et al.* (1946) developed a formula containing 3 per cent DDT, 5 per cent cyclohexanone, 5 per cent motor oil, and 0.3 per cent pyrethrins. This is fairly stable at low temperatures and is safe to use in the presence of plastics. These authors state that the motor oil is quite as effective as the oil of sesame used in earlier pyrethrum sprays, and that, like the latter, it increases the effectiveness of the DDT.

Residual Sprays

This is the type of application in which DDT finds its best use. Five per cent DDT in deodorized kerosene has become the standard preparation. This is about the highest concentration which can be produced by direct solution in the kerosene, and even then it may require days to render the solution complete. But it is sufficient. Walls, ceilings, doors, screens, and other surfaces are sprayed with the solution, the object being to render toxic any and all surfaces on which the flies are prone to alight. One quart of spray to 250 square feet of surface is the proper amount to apply. Workmen accustomed to applying older types of garden sprays may be inclined to consider this insufficient and will tend to waste materials. The men should be cautioned and supervised until they become accustomed to the handling of DDT.

The solvent soon evaporates, leaving the DDT as an invisible deposit on all surfaces treated. Such surfaces remain toxic for an extended period of time; several months in enclosed situations, at least weeks in surfaces exposed to weather. The concentration recommended above is in reality greatly in excess of the minimum required to kill flies. In one of the original experiments performed by the Geigy Company, a box with glass walls was sprayed inside with a 0.1 per cent solution of DDT in acetone. After allowing time for evaporation, the experimenter wiped the treated surfaces 200 times with a woolen cloth. Flies introduced into the box died in a few hours. It has been calculated that only 0.0006 to 0.002 grams of DDT per kilogram of insects treated are required to bring about death. An average fly might, therefore, be killed by somewhat less than a billionth of a gram.

The spraying of 5 per cent DDT in kerosene at the rate of one quart per 250 square feet allows for penetration into the pores of wood, plaster, and similar surfaces, since only that which remains on the surface is in a position to be contacted by the flies.

For houseflies alone, only light applications of a 5 per cent solution of DDT are necessary. A *light* spray may be defined as one in which only enough spray material is used to moisten effectively the surface treated. A *heavy* application, such as might be used against ants, carpet beetles, or clothes moths, is one in which the operator uses all the spray material that will remain on the surface without running or dripping.

Oil sprays are, of course, inflammable, and should not be used near open fires. They also are less desirable for use on livestock than are the emulsions.

Emulsions

These are the ideal preparations for treating outbuildings and barns. The fire hazard is eliminated, as the amount of oil used is insignificant compared with the amount of water present.

The stock solution consists of 25 to 30 per cent DDT in xylene or some other effective solvent. Kerosene would be useless for this purpose, as only about 5 per cent of DDT can be put into solution in kerosene directly. An emulsifying agent is then added, and the concentrate is ready for use. A number of reliable emulsifiers are on the market under special trade names. Tegin, Tween, Chovis, Mulag, and Emulphor are examples. A desirable concentrate may be made up as follows:

> 4 parts emulsifying agent
> 66 parts xylene
> 30 parts DDT

To prepare the spray, one part of concentrate is mixed with five parts of water and the two are thoroughly stirred together. This gives a five per cent emulsion which may then be sprayed on ceiling, doors, and walls. It has a milky appearance. Because water is the carrier (dispersion medium or continuous phase), there is some tendency for the emulsion to run and streak the walls, and a whitish deposit usually remains. For this reason, emulsions are not used in houses, as a rule, but this feature is rarely objected to in stables and barns. Emulsion sprays may be used on livestock and even on plants (with a lesser concentration of DDT).

The solution of DDT in xylene is the dispersed phase of the mixture, its particles being uniformly distributed throughout the water. The emulsifying agent prevents this mechanical mixture from separating.

Emulsions have been used successfully for dipping cattle, as a protection against flies. The dip should contain DDT in a concentration of approximately 0.25 per cent.

Deenate 25-R is a 25 per cent emulsion of DDT.

Wettable Powders

A suspension of pulverized DDT in water has real advantages under certain circumstances, but it is not particularly easy to achieve. Pure crystals of DDT are somewhat waxy and tend to cohere, forming lumps. This makes it

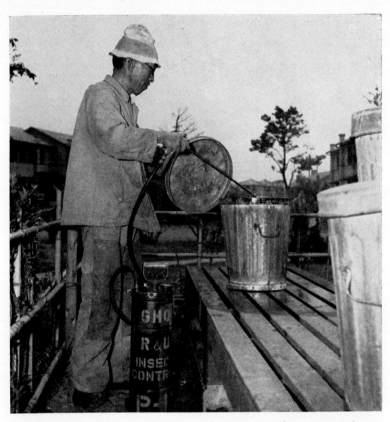

Figure 168. Sanitation in postwar Japan. Japanese worker sprays trash cans with DDT in Washington Heights area, Tokyo. (U.S. Army photograph.)

impossible to grind DDT into a sufficiently fine powder to make suspension possible. The equivalent can be accomplished, however, by grinding DDT with some inert substance, such as clay, pyrophyllite, or talc. Commercial preparations may contain up to 50 per cent DDT. To make the powder disperse readily in water, small quantities of some wetting agent are added before mixing. Also, in anticipation of the fact that it will be desirable to have the particles of DDT adhere to the sprayed surface for a considerable time, a sticking agent is added to the powder at the time of preparation.

A 50 per cent wettable powder (Deenate 50-W) may be made into a desirable spray by merely mixing one pound with about five gallons of water. Like the emulsions, it may be used directly on livestock and, of course, there is no fire hazard. As with the emulsions, there is a white, residual deposit, which limits its use to barns and similar places. The actual concentration of DDT in the above-described suspension is about 2.5 per cent. A higher concentration is not needed, as none penetrates the pores of wood or plaster and all is available to make the surface toxic to flies. Such sprays should be applied at the rate of one gallon to approximately 300 square feet. In spraying cattle, one quart per adult horse or cow should control flies for perhaps two weeks. The duration of the protection is considerably cut down by exposure to rain. Careful attention should be given to the belly, rump, and back.

Paints

The residual effects obtained with DDT, gave rise to the suggestion that this principle might be incorporated in the manufacture of paints, so that newly decorated surfaces might, for a time, at least, possess insecticidal powers.

In this connection, it has been found that conventional oil paints and varnishes can be made to carry DDT, but the dried surface is not particularly lethal to insects. It appears that the surface film traps or covers the DDT in such a way that the flies do not make contact with the poison. Certain types of paints, however, have been manufactured which render a surface lethal to flies about as long as one treated with the usual residual sprays. For interior finishes, this is probably practical. Oil-bound water paints and synthetic resin finishes lend themselves to this purpose. The DDT is believed to migrate gradually to the surface, replacing the exposed particles which become lost through abrasion and evaporation. Among the earlier studies in this connection were those of Campbell and West (1944), who incorporated from 0.5 to 5.0 per cent of DDT in oil-bound water paints and found the film lethal, by contact, for flies over a period of at least two months. These authors were not successful, however, with oil or synthetic varnish paints.

One of the most illuminating studies of the toxicity to houseflies of paints containing DDT is that carried out by Gilmour (1946). Five types of paint were used: glossy enamel, flat oil paint (containing clay and whiting), ordinary oil paint, emulsion type (to be mixed with water), and ordinary water paint. Various concentrations of DDT, containing 70 per cent p, p′ isomer, were ground up with the paint during its preparation. Flies were permitted contact with the painted surfaces for different periods of time, the mortality being recorded twenty-four hours after first exposure. A 50 per cent mortality was found to result from eight seconds' contact with 5 per cent DDT in flat oil paint. Three per cent required an exposure of twelve seconds for similar results, while with a 10 per cent mixture two seconds were sufficient. For emulsion-type paint, thirty-five seconds of contact were necessary for the same result, the DDT in this instance being in concentration of 2 per cent. Reduction to 1 per cent required contact of sixty minutes for a 50 per cent mortality at the end of twenty-four hours. The tests were made fourteen to forty days after application of the paint.

A 10 per cent DDT preparation of glossy enamel failed to give 50 per cent mortality in an hour, but 20 per cent was effective with an exposure of seven to ten minutes in the case of a freshly painted surface. Only a few seconds' exposure proved necessary after the film became aged. The insecticidal power of the surface film was thus shown to increase markedly with a lapse of time. The same was true of a 3 per cent preparation of flat oil paint. Such increased effectiveness was always accompanied by an increase in visible DDT crystals on the surface of the paint. The nature of the solvent would appear to be important in the initiation of such crystallization. In general, Gilmour's experiments tend to bear out the theory that DDT must be added to the paint in excess of the saturation level of the solvents before crystallization can take place in the film. There is evidence that crystallization may proceed somewhat more rapidly with crude DDT than with the pure p, p' isomer.

SPECIAL DEVICES AND PROCEDURES

Impregnated wallpaper has also been found effective, and may prove of very practical value in decorating the walls of nurseries, playrooms, and bedrooms used by infants and young children. Rather extensive tests have been made by the Institute of Paper Chemistry, at Appleton, Wisconsin, and the results are gratifying. A quick-acting insecticide such as "chlordane" is commonly used in combination with DDT.

Certain insecticide manufacturers have also placed on the market novelty control units in the form of crepe paper rolls, to be applied as short strips on table legs, lamp shades, chair backs, and similar situations. These are impregnated with DDT, and also contain a "fly-lure" which is intended to induce concentration of the flies on the poisoned surface. These are offered in various colors, apparently without regard to possible color preference on the part of the insects!

PRACTICAL EXPERIENCE IN FLY CONTROL

As already mentioned, some of the earliest practical tests were carried out by Wiesmann, who, in 1943, reported very satisfactory results from the use of Gesarol. One of the first tests extended over a twenty-day period and involved a problem of fly control in stables. Each evening from one hundred to two hundred flies managed to enter the stable from outside sources. None survived until morning, as the walls, floors, and ceilings, previously treated, remained toxic to all flies which came to rest upon them.

A practical test by Smit (1945a) showed the residual effect of DDT on window glass. Forty square feet of the inside surface of kitchen windows were sprayed with approximately 10 cc. of a 5 per cent solution of DDT in kerosene. Every fly that entered the kitchen was killed until the windows were washed, 68 days later, and some mortality was noticed for a considerable period after that.

Among postwar uses is the extensive employment of DDT in well-known resort areas hitherto pestered by an undesirable abundance of flies. In northern Michigan, for example, at Blaney Park, where the maintenance of riding stables has always favored the production of both house and stable flies, an almost complete control was achieved by the use of DDT in various forms. A 5 per cent solution in oil was employed on screens of windows and doors, aerosol bombs were used inside, and wettable powder was sprayed about stables, eaves, and porches. Control of spiders was usually achieved along with control of flies. Since spiders are not markedly susceptible to DDT, their disappearance was probably due in part to the removal of their principal food supply.

Equally satisfactory results were achieved on Mackinac Island, where, in accordance with tradition, only horse-drawn vehicles have been in use for many years. The relief from the fly nuisance, especially during the late summer, was little short of striking. A noticeable diminution in the number of songbirds, however, has been reported, indicating that many insects in addition to flies were doubtless eliminated, to the point where the former bird population could no longer be sustained. The possibility of the birds' being poisoned by feeding freely on the dying insects should also not be overlooked.

In New York State, the use of residual-type DDT sprays, combined with other control procedures, virtually eliminated flies from the administration area of Bear Mountain State Park. Two spraying operations, one in late spring and the other in early fall, proved sufficient.

Cities threatened with epidemics of poliomyelitis have not infrequently made use of fast-flying high-powered airplanes to control fly populations over considerable areas, in the belief that the fly factor in the spread of infantile paralysis might thus be largely eliminated. While it has been impossible to evaluate correctly the results of such a procedure, the considerable sums of money expended in these projects are indicative of the confidence which civilian populations have come to feel in the effectiveness of DDT for the control of dipterous forms.

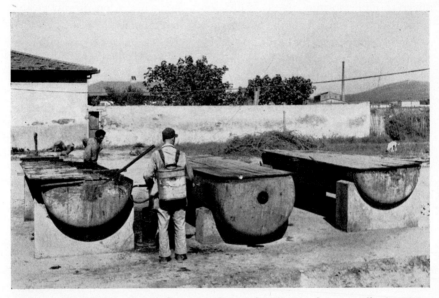

Figure 169. DDT to control flies in garbage tubs. Picture shows a collection point near refuse dump at Leghorn, Italy. Knapsack-type sprayer is being used. (U.S. Army photograph.)

The fishing port of Crisfield, Maryland, became one of the early examples of benefit to a civilian community after the termination of the war. Utilizing a crew of German prisoners of war, the Bureau of Entomology and Plant Quarantine arranged for the treatment, with pressure sprayers, of every fishery in Crisfield during the last of August, 1945. On October 8, the Washington *Evening Star* reported the fly population inside the plants reduced from 95 to 99 per cent, a continuation of the same low level obtained immediately after application. All outside toilets in Crisfield were likewise sprayed, with the result that the fly population of the entire city was reduced by at least 75 per cent.

Practical tests of DDT in the Province of Moscow are described by Derbeneva-Ukhova (1947). Dusts, suspensions, and emulsions were used. The most satisfactory results were obtained by application of a suspension to work-men's huts in a certain village during the second week of June. Application was at the rate of 0.3 g. of DDT per square meter of surface. Shops and restaurants in the same village were treated in the same manner on the ninth of July. By August first the fly population was determined as only 10.2 per cent of that in an untreated village in which natural increase had been per-mitted. The author states that the toxic effect continued for the remainder of the season.

A Russian preparation known as pentachlorin paste was tested by Okulov in Crimea (1947). The paste, which contains 40 per cent DDT, is used as the basis of a spray, the application being at the rate of 10 ml. per square meter of surface. Specimens of *Musca domestica* died if in contact with freshly treated surfaces for 5 minutes. Eighteen to twenty hours usually elapsed be-fore death. Twenty-seven days after treatment, an exposure of 380 minutes was required for complete mortality. The residual effect of this material is obviously less satisfactory than that of other DDT preparations previously discussed.

In Fiji, Lever (1946) made use of a 5 per cent solution of DDT in benzene diluted with water (1:6). Windows sprayed with this preparation remained toxic to *Musca domestica vicina* for ten weeks. The flies dropped after twenty-five minutes and were dead in two and a half hours.

In the veterinary field, E. M. Hanawalt (1945) reported investigations on control of flies at Michigan State College in barns, autopsy room, surgery rooms, and similar situations. Power sprayers, hand pumps, electric atomizers, and hand guns were used. A 0.3 per cent water suspension of DDT in pyro-phyllite remained effective for 28 days in a well-ventilated and well-lighted pig barn, while a 0.6 per cent suspension continued effective for 42 days in a poorly lighted autopsy room. A supplementary spraying around windows and doors with a 5 per cent solution in kerosene, five weeks after the applica-tion of the water suspension, proved a beneficial procedure. Fly control for at least 42 days was secured by adding 3.6 per cent DDT to a cold-water gypsum-base paint.

Practical farmers and dairymen have also been interested in the direct ap-plication of DDT to the bodies of living animals. As indicated earlier in this chapter, emulsions and wettable powders are suitable for this purpose. How-ever, the use of DDT on living cattle raises two important questions: "Is there likely to be danger to the animals?" and "How long may the residual effect be relied upon?" In this connection, Hackman (1947) gives interesting data on the factors which cause removal of DDT from sprayed cattle, thereby shortening its period of usefulness. This author reports that preparations not exceeding 2 per cent in concentration remain effective at best from one to two weeks. The greatest loss is by licking, either on the part of the sprayed animal or by another. Of much less significance are rain, sun, and mechanical rubbing. Of almost no consequence are flaking of the epithelium, absorption by skin and hair, secretions of the skin, growth and loss of hair.

For this reason, 2 per cent is but little more enduring than 1 per cent, since the animals themselves remove the spray. In spite of this habit, the animals are not affected by the amount ingested.

A question that sometimes arises in connection with chance ingestion of DDT by farm animals is whether or not the milk of a lactating animal might thereby be made to contain a significant amount of toxic substance. Although the amount involved is probably never sufficient to jeopardize the well-being of the female's own young, the presence of DDT in milk has been demonstrated beyond question. For example, an interesting experiment is described by Telford (1945) in which milk, cream, and butter, from goats which had been fed measured quantities of DDT, were tested for toxicity to laboratory animals. Houseflies were killed by feeding on milk from a goat that had received 1 gram of DDT per 8 to 9 pounds of body weight. Sprays that contained butter from such animals were likewise much more toxic than similar sprays with an equivalent content of normal goat's butter.

Schechter, Haller, and Pogorelskin (1946) have done work on the quantitative determination of the DDT content of milk by colorimetric methods. They demonstrated that DDT can occur in cow's milk up to twenty-five parts per million, or even higher, depending on the animal's intake of DDT. This is largely concentrated in the butterfat, as shown by the fact that butter manufactured from milk containing 25 p.p.m. contained as much as 532 p.p.m. of DDT. The affinity of DDT for fats was further demonstrated by the analysis of a sample of fat T-bone steak. DDT proved to be present to the extent of 178 p.p.m., but when the fatty portions were trimmed away, the remaining lean meat showed a concentration of only 4 p.p.m.

EFFECTS OF NATURAL SELECTION

The remarkable success of DDT as a destroyer of flies under almost every conceivable condition led naturally to the most optimistic predictions concerning the eventual elimination of houseflies and similar forms. Such enthusiasm, however, has been proved somewhat premature by the discovery that not all individuals are equally susceptible to the poison and that the descendants of surviving flies may be relatively resistant to exposure.

Suspicion was first aroused in Italy and Greece when flies that seemed to thrive on DDT appeared in numbers, shortly after the conclusion of World War II. Saccà (1947) suggested that the DDT-resistant strain which was becoming conspicuous in Italy be considered a new variety, for which he proposed the name *Musca domestica tiberina*. Since resistant strains have since appeared in nearly all countries where DDT is extensively used, the concept of a geographically limited insecticide-resistant race is probably untenable.

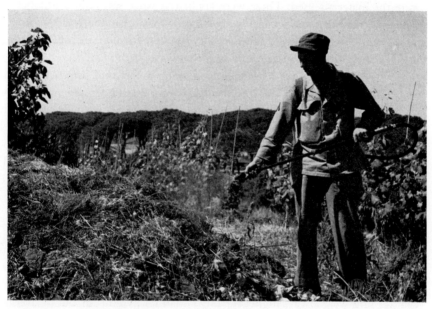

Figure 170. Knapsack-type sprayer in use. Operator is applying DDT to a manure pile on an Italian farm. (U.S. Army photograph.)

To determine whether flies that survived exposure to DDT might give rise to races more resistant than ordinary stocks, Lindquist and Wilson conducted a series of experiments at Orlando, Florida, in 1948. Approximately 300 houseflies were exposed to a fine-mist spray in a 100-cubic-foot chamber designed by Lindquist and Madden. The flies were exposed for two minutes to 1 ml. of a 1 per cent DDT-kerosene spray. Approximately 10 per cent of the flies survived, and with these a special colony was established. For fourteen generations the procedure was repeated. Four-day-old flies, from each generation beginning with the third, were tested against flies from the ordinary laboratory colony. All proved more resistant than the unselected stock. A series of paired tests was made on the fourteenth generation, involving approximately 1,600 four- and five-day-old flies. The regular stock averaged 69 per cent mortality; the special stock, 34 per cent. Selective breeding had obviously produced a strain of flies appreciably more resistant to DDT.

This resistance, however, is not specific for DDT. Wilson and Gahan (1948) studied the resistance of the above-described stock to a considerable number of proved insecticides and in every case the survival rate was greater than with ordinary flies simultaneously exposed. Thanite, rotenone, chlorinated camphene, chlordane, and pyrethrins (plus 5 per cent piperonyl cyclonene) were the materials used. These were applied as space sprays in a number of different concentrations. These workers concluded that the selection based on resistance to DDT had resulted in the development of an unusually strong stock of flies, rather than one specifically resistant to DDT.

It will probably prove impossible to develop a chemical insecticide, non-toxic to mammals, which is 100 per cent lethal for flies under any and all conditions. And where a few survive, an insecticide-resistant strain is always in the making. The implications of these findings are significant, as indicated by a popular account of certain of the above-described experiments which appeared in the St. Louis *Post Dispatch*. After stating that twice as much DDT was required to obtain a significant kill in the thirty-sixth generation as in the first, and three times as much in the forty-third, the article concludes dubiously: "The hope of a flyless millennium is dimmer than ever."

Before leaving this aspect of the subject, it should be pointed out that resistance to insecticides is not wholly dependent on constitutional vigor in the genetic sense. McGovran and Gersdorff (1945) report appreciable differences in the susceptibility of flies nourished on different types of food. Percentage kills were always higher for DDT than for pyrethrum, but by averaging the kills for the two insecticides, a single set of figures was obtained for comparing results with six different food preparations. Flies were fed the test food both before and after exposure to the insecticide, which was applied as a spray by the turntable method.

Mortality, in 24 hours, for flies fed on equal parts of fresh skimmed milk and water was 42 per cent. With one part of formalin added to 1,500 parts of diluted milk, the average was 41; with spray-dried milk powder, 43; with powdered milk, 57; with dried whey powder, 71; and with granulated sugar, 77. The last four items were fed in water, as 5 per cent solutions or suspensions.

DDT AS A LARVICIDE

It is usually stated that DDT is relatively ineffective against pupae, larvae, or eggs of common flies, and that its use should therefore be restricted to the control of adult forms. While this is generally true, the experiments of de Oliveira and Moussatche (1947) are of interest in showing to what extent immature stages may be susceptible. These authors sprayed water suspensions of DDT on horse dung in which larvae and pupae of *Musca domestica* were developing. Concentrations of 2,000:1, 1,000:1, and 500:1 were used. From 75 to 99 per cent of the immature forms were either killed or developed abnormally. Dead larvae of all stages were abundant in the treated manure, and many of the pupae from which no flies emerged presented an abnormal appearance. In these experiments a 10 per cent preparation (Neocid M) was used as a basis for the various suspensions employed.

DANGER TO MAN AND WARM-BLOODED ANIMALS

DDT is a poison that, if taken into the human body in sufficient amount, can cause toxic symptoms or even death. When used as recommended, however, insecticides containing DDT are not harmful to human health, though certain reasonable precautions should be taken to guard against possible ill effects.

Dr. F. C. Bishopp (1946a,b) has summarized the findings of a number of investigators who have studied the toxicology and pharmacology of DDT. Essential points may be tabulated as follows:

(1) Although DDT is toxic to all higher animals, its toxicity is less than that of common arsenical and nicotinic preparations long used as insecticides.

(2) The dose necessary to produce death in 50 per cent of a test group of animals varies both for species and for individuals. For example, this "median lethal dose" (MLD), which ranges from 150 to 250 milligrams per kilogram of body weight in mice or rats, runs closer to 1,000 milligrams for sheep and goats. Cats and dogs, which are about as susceptible as rats and mice, are somewhat less tolerant than horses and cows. Guinea pigs and rabbits require from 300 to 500 milligrams, while monkeys are more susceptible and succumb to an MLD of slightly over 200. Among domestic animals, chickens are most resistant, surviving, in most cases, a dosage of 1,300 milligrams of DDT per kilogram of body weight.

(3) A cumulative dose is sometimes more dangerous than a single exposure to large amounts, as shown by the fact that small quantities, given daily, may cause death before the amount of a single, acute, lethal dose has been received.

(4) When applied to the skin in powder form, DDT is not toxic, as demonstrated by the thousands who made use of DDT louse powder during World War II.

(5) DDT in oil solutions may be absorbed through the skin, with resultant toxic effects.

(6) DDT is a nerve poison, as indicated by muscular tremors and other symptoms soon after a toxic dose is swallowed or absorbed.

(7) Apparently an animal may not become sensitized to DDT. Complete recovery occurs when dosing ceases.

Experimental data on toxicity to man are not available, but selected clinical observations may be cited in lieu thereof.

Mackerras and West (1946) record mild poisoning of twenty-five men who ate tarts in which DDT powder had been used by mistake in place of baking powder. All recovered within 48 hours. Another individual was made blind for two weeks as a result of getting DDT powder in his eyes. He also recovered completely.

Chit Thoung (1946) records the case of seventy-two members of a frontier force constabulary in Burma, who experienced diarrhea, vomiting, bradycardia, dizziness, and dilated pupils after consuming contaminated rice. The latter proved to contain approximately 16 per cent DDT. All the affected individuals recovered.

Medical literature reports a number of scattered instances in which human death has followed (sometimes by many days) ingestion or absorption of DDT. Almost all of these cases, however, either involve the ingestion of other poisons along with DDT or lack complete authenticity for other reasons. The only record of human death by DDT poisoning which does not seem to have been challenged is the case of a Negro child, nineteen months of age, at a British base in West Africa. As reported by Hill and Robinson (1945), the child drank perhaps an ounce of a 5 per cent kerosene solution of DDT. Initial symptoms, involving coughing and vomiting, appeared within ten minutes. Collapse was complete at the end of two hours, and death followed two hours later. Autopsy revealed that the immediate cause of death was edema of the lungs. Other findings included congestion of the liver, enlargement of the spleen, and edema of the brain.

Allowing for differences in physiology and anatomy, the symptoms shown by warm-blooded animals do not differ essentially from those exhibited by flies. Smith and Stohlman (1944) refer to "hyperexcitability and generalized fine and coarse tremors ending in flaccid or spastic paralysis with occasional tonic and clonic convulsions preceding death by respiratory failure."

When solutions of DDT in oil are permitted to contact the skin over a period of time, symptoms of general poisoning may ensue, such as headache, vomiting, and elevation of temperature. Numbness, weakness, and swelling of the exposed region are also characteristic.

Besides poisoning through contact with the skin and by being swallowed, DDT is sometimes inhaled in dangerous amounts, either as a dust or in the form of mists or sprays. Both oil and water preparations are applied as sprays and may be taken into the lungs in such a manner. Few persons will be ex-

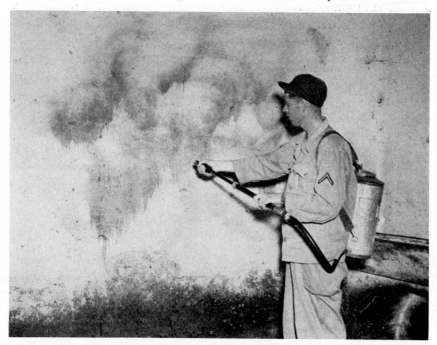

Figure 171. Treating barn with knapsack-type sprayer. Soldier is applying DDT to interior of barn on a farm near Leghorn, Italy. (U.S. Army photograph.)

posed to sprays in confined places for a sufficient period to suffer deleterious effects, but if one's work requires it, protective masks may be employed.

It should be pointed out that water emulsions are not dangerous when spilled upon the skin, as these are very difficult to absorb. It has already been indicated, however, that oil solutions are dangerous in this respect, and workmen who apply oil sprays do well to wear gloves and protect the skin in other ways.

HANDLING AND WORKING WITH DDT

In the light of the preceding paragraphs, general precautions in the use and handling of DDT are obviously necessary and desirable. The well-considered opinion of a number of agencies of the United States Government is summarized as follows: (1) Take ordinary precautions in handling and storing any DDT insecticide. (2) Avoid applying it on eating utensils and on food. (3) Store it out of reach of children, and where it will not be used by accident for flour, baking powder, or similar foods. (4) Wash your hands when you have finished applying DDT. (5) Never use oil preparations of DDT on animals. (6) Do not spray oil solutions near open fires, because they may catch fire. (7) Remove from the room (or cover) house plants, fish, and pets, when applying DDT.

The United States Food and Drug Administration has ruled (1945) that the degree of toxicity possessed by DDT does not place it in a class with the caustic poisons and that packages containing this substance need not bear the skull and crossbones label. In certain states, however, the law requires coloring of the product as a protection against accidental use.

At the time of this writing there is no known antidote for DDT poisoning. A physician should be called at once, so that appropriate symptomatic treatment may be initiated. Phenobarbitol usually reduces the severity of the reactions. Stomach lavage followed by a saline cathartic has been found helpful.

DDT AND THE "BALANCE OF NATURE"

When DDT is used on a large scale, as for the control of mosquitoes and flies over a considerable area, a certain amount of damage to beneficial forms of life is almost inevitable. Various numbers of birds, fish, frogs, and crustaceans may be destroyed. Since fly control is largely a terrestrial affair, the greatest problem is perhaps the menace to bird life. It has been shown that distribution by airplane at the rate of five pounds of DDT per acre will destroy large numbers of birds, especially if it is applied during the nesting season. Insects already paralyzed by action of the DDT are easy to catch, and the birds not only feed freely on these forms but carry prey to their young in generous quantity. Both adults and nestlings are presumably poisoned by such food. It has been demonstrated, however, that an application of two pounds per acre is not detrimental to bird life.

Beneficial insects are also destroyed, to some extent. Lacewing flies, which prey on plant lice, and many dipterous and hymenopterous parasites are rather susceptible to DDT. Fortunately, honeybees are probably more tolerant of DDT than they are of the well-known arsenates in general use.

A special report of the Fish and Wildlife Service of the U.S. Department of the Interior (1949) summarizes the work of Hoffman and Surber, who used insects that had been sprayed with DDT to feed various species of fresh-water fish. Both larvae and adults of *Musca domestica* were employed in the experiments, along with tendipedid midge larvae collected in the field. These were fed to large- and smallmouthed black bass, bluegills, and crappies. Some fish were killed; others showed no ill effects; still others developed marked tremors, but recovered. The spray was applied in a 0.1-milliacre chamber at a rate equivalent to one pound of DDT per acre, thus paralleling the results of large-scale treatment of forest areas by airplane.

Oil-sprayed insects did more harm than those sprayed with a *suspension* of DDT. In general, small fish appeared more sensitive than larger ones. The physiological condition of the fish proved relatively more important than the amount of DDT consumed, as shown by the fact that well-nourished indi-viduals invariably survived the effects of engorgement on poisoned insects much better than those which had been kept in holding ponds with neither natural nor artificial food. In a special test smallmouthed bass proved con-siderably more susceptible to DDT than goldfish.

As an example of disturbed biological balance due to area-wide employ-ment of DDT, the report of M. S. Shane (1948), of the Water Department of Wilmington, Delaware, may be significant. To control flies during an epi-demic of poliomyelitis, the entire city was sprayed at intervals over a thirty-day period during the late summer of 1947. The preparation used was a 30 per cent solution of DDT in oil. Filtered water in a certain uncovered reser-voir which lay within the area was observed to develop a marked cloudiness within five days after the application. Microscopic counts showed 1,200 organ-isms per milliliter, which soon increased to nearly 10,000. The diatomaceous genus *Synedra* was found to be practically in pure culture. Microcrustacea such as *Daphnia* and *Cyclops,* which normally feed on *Synedra,* seemed to have been eliminated. During the previous four years the microscopic count in this reservoir for the corresponding month (September) had been well under 100. After the water had been drawn off, a white deposit became visible on the dry walls. This proved to consist of DDT.

The susceptibility of Crustacea to relatively low concentrations is borne out by the observations of E. J. Wason in New South Wales (1947). DDT spray was allowed to drain into a reservoir to give a concentration of 1:25,-000,000. The next day hundreds of dead crayfish (*Parachaeraps*) were col-lected, and more showed signs of being affected. A high death rate among carp (*Carassius*) was also noted. Since crayfish are sometimes considered a nuisance, these observations suggest a possible method of control.

In the United States it has been shown that spray washed from trees into a reservoir by rain killed both fish and frogs when the concentration of DDT reached something less than 1:10,000,000.

Bishopp (1946a,b) points out that such detrimental effects may usually be minimized by confining the use of DDT to the control of forms for which it has been proved to be an effective remedy and by using the least dosage and smallest number of applications consistent with satisfactory results. This, of

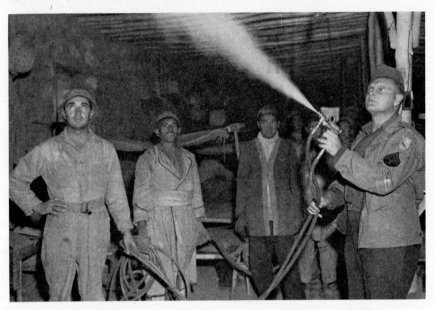

Figure 172. Treating barracks with power sprayer. Pressure line has been run into building from pump mounted on vehicle outside. These barracks at Khurramabad, Iran, were rendered free from mosquitoes, bedbugs, and flies by use of DDT residual spray. (U.S. Army photograph.)

course, requires a certain amount of guidance by qualified, professional personnel. Municipalities or engineering companies employed by them may usually secure competent advice from state or federal agencies with offices in the region concerned. Generous application over large areas without guidance should obviously be discouraged.

Regardless of these and similar problems, the fact remains that DDT has many advantages over any other insecticide thus far developed. This portion of our discussion may well conclude with a summary of its more desirable qualities: (1) DDT can be prepared synthetically; that is, its availability does not depend upon the survival of a growing crop. (2) It is extremely toxic to most races of flies. (3) It has great residual effect. (4) It is not irritating to operators during dispensation. (5) It is almost odorless. (6) It will not stain fabrics.

THE CHEMICAL NATURE OF DDT

The DDT molecule may best be understood if one considers first a molecule of ethane, an aliphatic hydrocarbon consisting of two atoms of carbon and six of hydrogen:[1]

$$
\begin{array}{c}
H \\
| \\
H-C-H \\
| \\
H-C-H \\
| \\
H
\end{array}
$$

By adding an atom of oxygen to two of the hydrogen atoms associated with one of the carbons, and substituting chlorine for all hydrogen atoms attached to the other, we can produce a molecule of chloral hydrate (trichloroacetic aldehyde):

$$
\begin{array}{c}
H \\
| \\
OH-C-OH \\
| \\
Cl-C-Cl \\
| \\
Cl
\end{array}
$$

This forms the core or central portion of the DDT molecule, which, however, to be complete must have in addition two identical "wings," each of which replaces one of the two OH groups. The wings, which have a rather elaborate structure, are based on the well-known benzene ring:

$$
\begin{array}{c}
H \quad H \\
| \quad | \\
C = C \\
\diagup \qquad \diagdown \\
H-C \qquad\qquad C-H \\
\diagdown\diagdown \qquad \diagup\diagup \\
C - C \\
| \quad | \\
H \quad H
\end{array}
$$

[1] The five structural formulas here presented are taken from Leary, Fishbein, and Salter, *DDT and the Insect Problem* (New York and London: McGraw-Hill Book Company, Inc., 1946) by permission of the publishers. Certain of the accompanying explanatory material is likewise adapted from this source.

Benzene may be converted to monochlorobenzene by replacing one of the lateral hydrogen atoms by a single atom of chlorine:

```
          H   H
          |   |
          C = C
         /     \
   Cl — C       C — H
         \\     //
          C  —  C
          |     |
          H     H
```

The corresponding hydrogen atom on the opposite side is then dropped out as the associated carbon atom links on to the chloral hydrate molecule in place of the OH group. Since this takes place on both sides of the chloral hydrate molecule, the result is a bisymmetrical molecule, as shown below:

```
      H   H                H   H
      |   |                |   |
      C = C       H        C = C
     /     \      |       /     \
Cl — C      C  — C — C        C — Cl
     \\     //    |    \\     //
      C  — C  Cl — C — Cl  C — C
      |   |        |        |   |
      H   H        Cl       H   H
```

The older method of manufacturing DDT involved the mixing of chloral hydrate and monochlorobenzene in the presence of sulphuric acid. By this procedure only about 75 per cent of the molecules turned out to be correctly formed. The remainder, with slightly different association of atoms, represent for the most part isomers of the desired compound. These isomers are of little or no value as insecticides and, if the manufacturer desires, may be eliminated by extracting the pure DDT with alcoholic crystallization. Their removal is not necessary, however, if the product bears a statement giving the percentage of pure DDT present.

In 1942, the British Government issued a patent to the J. R. Geigy, A. G. for the manufacture of dichloro-diphenyl-trichloroethane according to the following procedure:

225 parts chlorobenzene

147 parts chloral (or corresponding amount of chloral hydrate)

1,000 parts of sulphuric acid monohydrate

The chlorobenzene and chloral are first mixed together and the sulphuric acid monohydrate is added by stirring. The temperature of the mixture rises to 60°C, then falls slowly to equal that of the surrounding air. Solid parts appear. The mixture is then poured into a large quantity of water and the product separates in solid form. This is washed thoroughly, then crystallized from ethyl alcohol.[2]

Relatively pure DDT (p-Cl C_6 H_4)$_2$ CHCl$_3$ is marketed either in the form of fine, white, needlelike crystals or as a powder, with a waxy appearance and a mild, neutral, or fruity odor.

The melting point will depend upon the degree of purity. The so-called "technical" grade usually melts at 110°C (230°F). This contains approximately 70 per cent of the para-pará isomer (1-trichloro-2, 2-bis [p-chlorophenyl] ethane). The ortho-para isomer is present to the extent of about 25 per cent and the remaining 5 per cent represents impurities.

The "aerosol" grade, which is considerably more refined, has a melting point of 103°C (217.4°F). This is used chiefly in aerosol bombs.

DDT is fairly stable but is acted upon by ferric chloride and certain other metallic salts. Choice of container is therefore of some importance. Exposure to sunlight and to high temperatures weakens its value as an insecticide and therefore limits the duration of residual effects. DDT is soluble in fats and oils, but enters into solution in water only to the extent of about one part per million.

The commonly accepted name for this substance is "dichloro-diphenyl-trichloroethane," but a more specific designation is 2, 2-bis (paradichlorophenyl)-1, 1, 1-trichlorethane." Use of the somewhat nonscientific term "chlorinated diphenylethane" should be discouraged.

Considerable investigation has been carried on to determine the suitability of various emulsifiers for use with DDT. Jones and Fluno (1946) tested more than a hundred substances and finally selected an aralkyl polyether alcohol known as Triton x-100. For military use the following proportions are recommended:

DDT	25 per cent
Xylene (solvent)	65 per cent
Triton x-100 (emulsifier)	10 per cent

Emulsion results from a minimum of agitation with almost any type of water: hard, distilled, or saline. Such emulsions remain fairly stable through various dilutions ranging from 10 to 0.1 per cent DDT.

[2] Modern preparation is both simpler and more efficient. Chloral hydrate, chlorobenzene, and chlorosulfonic acid are mixed, in proper (metathetic) quantities for the desired exchange of atoms. A much purer product is obtained. Other modifications also are in use.

MODERN INSECTICIDES OTHER THAN DDT

The following quotation is from a paper by Prill, Synerholm, and Hartzell published in 1946.

Since the outstanding insecticidal activity of 2, 2-bis (p-chlorophenyl)-1, 1, 1-trichloroethane ("DDT") has become generally known, the synthesis and testing of related compounds have been actively pursued in many laboratories with the object of finding insecticidal compounds possibly better than "DDT" itself, par-

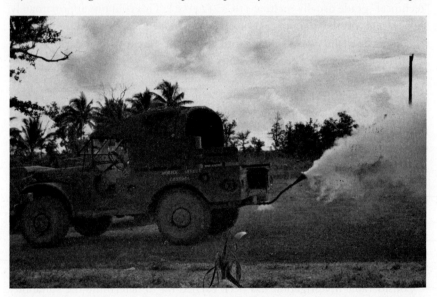

Figure 173. Truck sprayer in use. Such equipment was used to control insects, including flies, in the MARBO Base Command Area, Guam, M.I., in 1947. (U.S. Army photograph.)

ticularly compounds with faster knockdown ability, less toxicity toward warm-blooded animals, less phytotoxicity, greater specificity of action against harmful rather than beneficial insects, and with more nearly ideal physical properties; as well as the object of finding correlations between chemical structure and insecticidal activity.

Of the analogs of DDT, these authors found only a few alkoxy analogs really superior to DDT in any important respect, such as knockdown or killing power. All were tested against houseflies as well as mosquito larvae. In regard to the chemistry of these compounds, Prill and his associates find that a compound of the DDT type must have certain substituents in the 4, 4' positions in order to have a high degree of activity. The presence of additional substituents in other positions appears to cause a reduction in the desired activity.

So far, we may say that none of the compounds closely related to original DDT has been shown to exceed that substance *significantly* in insecticidal power.

Knipling (1949) has pointed out, however, that several new insecticides are superior *in some respects* to DDT. Important among these are benzene hexachloride, chlordane, toxaphene, methoxychlor, DDD(TDE), and several compounds which have a synergistic effect when combined with pyrethrum.

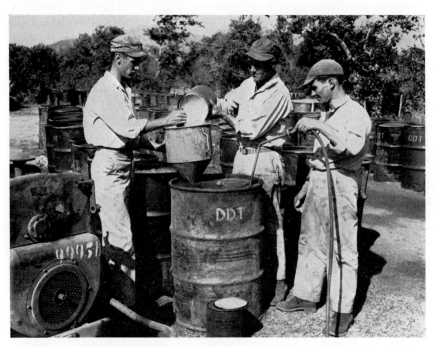

Figure 174. Preparing insecticide for dispensation by airplane. Military personnel are here shown mixing DDT powder with Diesel oil, in preparation for spraying the city of Manila, Luzon, P.I. (U.S. Army photograph.)

BENZENE HEXACHLORIDE (BHC)

This substance, also called Gammexane or 666, is produced by the reaction of chlorine with benzene in the presence of sunlight. The correct chemical designation is 1, 2, 3, 4, 5, 6-hexachlorocyclohexane. The toxic principle is the gamma isomer, which usually constitutes 10 to 12 per cent, by weight, of the crude hexachlorocyclohexane. It is soluble in most organic solvents. Preparations of the gamma isomer of benzene hexachloride, the purity of which is not less than 99 per cent, qualify under the official name, lindane.

Benzene hexachloride has been suggested as a possible competitor of DDT, principally because of its faster knockdown effect. Lepage, Giannotti, and Pereira (1945) made comparative studies of these two insecticides and showed that whereas this was true when the insects were exposed to surfaces just treated, the benzene hexachloride (666) quickly lost its superiority when treated surfaces were exposed to air or light.

In their first series of tests, solutions of DDT (or of 666) in acetone were applied to glass plates in sufficient quantity to give a residue of 0.019 mg. of insecticide per square centimeter, and were allowed to dry. The plates were then slid into frames that contained a determined number of flies. At one, two, four, and eight minutes, the plates were replaced with clean ones. The results are summarized in Table 20.

Table 20. Average time required for knockdown after various exposures.

Exposure	1 minute	2 minutes	4 minutes	8 minutes
DDT	166.5 min.	62.0 min.	25.0 min.	16.5 min.
666	40.0 min.	30.0 min.	16.0 min.	10.0 min.

The second series of experiments tested the retention of insecticidal properties after the treated surfaces had been exposed to air and sunlight. Tables 21 and 22 show these findings.

Table 21

Plates exposed to air at 25°–29°C (77°–84.2°F)	24 hours	48 hours	116 hours
For knockdown with DDT (flies exposed 4 min.)	15 min.	17 min.	16 min.
For knockdown with DDT (flies exposed 8 min.)	10 min.	8 min.	11 min.
For knockdown with 666 (flies exposed 4 min.)	40 min.	85 min.	123 min.
For knockdown with 666 (flies exposed 8 min.)	48 min.	70 min.	90 min.

Table 22

Plates exposed to sunlight at 40°–45° C (104°–113° F)	4 hours	8 hours
For knockdown with DDT (flies exposed 4 min.)	17 min.	10 min.
For knockdown with DDT (flies exposed 8 min.)	6 min.	5 min.
For knockdown with 666 (flies exposed 4 min.)	290 min.	{ not within { 5 hours
For knockdown with 666 (flies exposed 8 min.)	150 min.	{ not within { 5 hours

The symptoms displayed by the affected flies are practically the same with 666 as with DDT, except that the convulsive motions are more violent.

The physiological action of contact insecticides is not completely understood. It is probable that the ability to penetrate the cuticle is of great importance, as indicated by the work of Dresden and Krijgsman (1948). These authors compared the effects of DDT, rotenone, and the γ (gamma) isomer of benzene hexachloride. The order of toxicity was different when the substances were injected than when they were applied externally. With vertebrates, however, where no chitin is present, the order remained the same, regardless of mode of application. Thus γ benzene hexachloride, which has a greater insecticidal action than DDT, presumably owes this property to the fact that it penetrates more readily.

Once penetration has been accomplished, the chemical nature of the substance of course determines its effectiveness. This is shown by the fact that the three other isomers of benzene hexachloride, α, β, δ (alpha, beta, delta) have relatively little insecticidal action, though they seem to penetrate the chitin readily enough. Of these three the δ isomer is most toxic, with α and β following in the order named (Gomeza Ozamiz, 1945). Andrews and Simmons (1948) state that BHC may act as a contact poison, a stomach poison, a fumigant, or as a combination of any two or all three. An early suggestion that γ benzene hexachloride accomplishes its toxic effect by competing in cell metabolism with meta-inositol has not been borne out by recent investigation. All authorities report this insecticide less toxic to man and other warm-blooded animals than DDT.

Munro, Post, and Colberg (1947) found 666 equally effective with DDT and DDD in controlling flies about farm buildings and livestock. A concentration of 0.5 per cent of the actual toxic agent was used in each case.

DDT-resistant strains of houseflies usually succumb rather easily to benzene hexachloride, and early reports from the California Agricultural Experiment Station at Riverside indicated satisfactory control of houseflies over a period of several weeks in dairy barns, where DDT had failed. On the other hand, observers in Egypt report that houseflies in that country are already becoming resistant to benzene hexachloride, while March and Metcalf (1949) record a particularly resistant strain, from a poultry ranch in California, that could not be controlled with DDT, benzene hexachloride, or dieldrin (another organic insecticide of considerable promise).

CHLORDANE (CHLORDAN)

Although developed primarily for the control of ants and cockroaches, this insecticide is also useful against houseflies. When applied in the form of a space spray, it is somewhat more effective than DDT.

For at least two years chlordane was used very successfully in Sardinia to control DDT-resistant strains of *Musca domestica,* but, as with DDT, natural selection once more became operative, so that by 1950 a chlordane-resistant

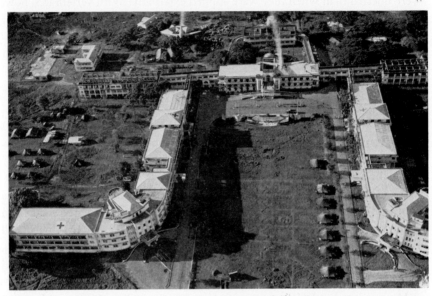

Figure 175. City sprayed from the air. Two C-47s are here shown spraying the city of Manila with DDT insecticide for control of mosquitoes and flies. (U.S. Army photograph.)

strain had appeared in considerable numbers.[3] Investigations are still in progress concerning its toxicity to various domestic animals and further trial, under a wide range of conditions, will be necessary in order to determine the true value of chlordane in fly control. Against the horn fly (*Siphona irritans*), DDT does a somewhat better job.

Chlordane shows much greater solubility in various carriers than DDT, DDD, or benzene hexachloride. Its proper chemical designation is 1, 2, 4, 5, 6, 7, 8, 8-octachloro-4, 7-methano-3a, 4, 7, 7a-tetrahydroindane. The empirical formula may be given as $C_{10}H_6Cl_8$. This insecticide is also known under the trade names Octa-Klor and Velsicol 1068.

[3] Personal communication from Dr. Paul F. Russell.

TOXAPHENE

This is a chlorinated camphene believed to have the empirical formula $C_{10}H_{10}Cl_8$. Like DDT, it has one labile chlorine atom. As available commercially, toxaphene is a waxy solid with a melting point somewhere between 65° and 90°C (149°–194°F). It stores well in solid form without deterioration. It is soluble in most organic solvents but is insoluble in water. Since toxaphene gives practically no knockdown, it has been combined, in experimental work, with thanite, for solution in deodorized kerosene. Tests in dairy barns by Parker and Beacher (1947) against *Musca domestica* and other flies demonstrated a very satisfactory residual effect. Bruce (1949) in a series of careful experiments found toxaphene superior to chlordane and benzene hexachloride in this regard, but inferior to Rothane and DDT.

One per cent toxaphene emulsions applied to manure at the rate of 100 to 200 mg. per square foot are considerably more effective against maggots than DDT but are less efficient than either chlordane or benzene hexachloride.

Toxaphene is somewhat slower in its action against horn flies than DDT. Investigators have been conservative in recommending its use because of the lack of complete information regarding its toxic effects on warm-blooded animals. Carelessly prepared dips have been known to cause the death of young calves.

When first available, toxaphene was known as Hercules Synthetic 3956.

METHOXYCHLOR

To higher animals, this is the least toxic of the newer hydrocarbon insecticides. It is somewhat more costly than DDT, but certain advantages seem to offset this. Unlike DDT, methoxychlor does not penetrate the hide of the animal, nor is it stored in adipose tissue or in the butterfat of milk. It is only slightly less effective against horn flies than DDT. Michigan State College recommends spraying cattle with a preparation made up by combining eight pounds of 50 per cent wettable powder with one hundred gallons of water. Thorough wetting of the animals does no harm, but contamination of feeds, water, or drinking cups should be avoided.

This methoxy analog of DDT is almost as effective as the latter when used against houseflies. It may be applied either as a space spray or for its residual effect. Methoxychlor is particularly recommended for trial where DDT has failed to control insecticide-resistant strains.

DICHLORO–DIPHENYL–DICHLORETHANE

This chemical ally of DDT, usually referred to as DDD or TDE,[4] has been found quite as effective against horn flies as methoxychlor. Its toxicity to warm-blooded animals is intermediate between that of the latter and DDT. Careful investigations have shown that whereas DDT may appear in the milk of dairy cattle up to 0.6 or 0.7 part per million during a season's use, the average for TDE is only 0.4 part per million, with equivalent applications. Muma and Hixson (1949) found DDD equally effective with DDT, methoxychlor, toxaphene, and chlordan in controlling both houseflies and stable flies on Nebraska farms. Sweetman (1947) recorded equivalent results for DDT and DDD in Massachusetts. Another name for this insecticide is Rothane D-3. The correct chemical designation is 2, 2′ bis (parachlorophenyl) 1, 1-dichloroethane. It is soluble in the same solvents as DDT, but differs in having a higher vapor pressure and a lower melting point.

THIOCYANOACETATES

The trade name *thanite* has become fairly well known as a result of war-time effort to find substitutes for pyrethrum, rotenone (derris), or cubé. An interesting report by Pierpont (1945b) tells of early work with fenchyl thiocyanoacetate, which, though effective, could not be produced by insecticide manufacturers in sufficient quantity because of the limited supply of natural pine oil. Attention was then directed to bornyl and isobornyl thiocyanoacetates, as there was no shortage of terpenes from which the isobornyl ester can be produced. Since the chemical, physical, and insecticidal properties of the three thiocyanoacetates are essentially the same, the term *thanite* was applied to all three or to any mixture thereof. It was soon demonstrated that tertiary as well as secondary alcohols can be used as raw material, so that thanite is now defined as "a blend of thiocyanoacetates of secondary and tertiary terpene alcohols." Large-scale production is entirely feasible.

The report indicates that thanite gives a more complete knockdown than pyrethrum, though its action is slightly slower. For livestock sprays, an oil with a viscosity rating of from 40 to 60 is recommended as a carrier. Oils with a lower viscosity may harm the animals, while too high a viscosity interferes with application by spraying apparatus ordinarily available. Thanite stores well in most types of containers and does not lose toxicity when exposed to light.

[4] Based on tetrachlorodiphenylethane.

PYRETHRUM STILL IMPORTANT

Pyrethrum has, of course, been an important insecticide for the control of flies for many years. As pointed out earlier in this chapter, it was the shortage of this useful material which stimulated extensive research on insecticides during World War II and resulted in the disclosure that DDT was an even more valuable substance. Parkin and Green (1945a) comment at some length

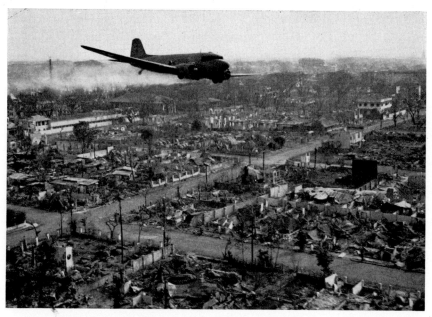

Figure 176. C-47 over Manila. This first spraying of an entire city from the air was carried out by the Fifth Air Force in 1945. This picture was made from another plane that took part in the operation. (U.S. Army photograph.)

on the relative merits of pyrethrum and DDT, and on the behavior of flies treated with a mixture of the two. Their more important observations are summarized below.

As compared with DDT, the action of pyrethrum is much more rapid. Flies knocked down with pyrethrum thus have much less opportunity to move about and continue their distribution of filth-borne organisms than flies marked for destruction by DDT. The leg movements, it has been noted, are slow and intermittent, quite unlike the continuous, vigorous kicking observed with DDT. With pyrethrum all movements slowly subside, until death finally supervenes. Treatment with restricted doses of pyrethrum and

DDT in combination results in two distinct patterns of behavior, one following the other. The first episode, which lasts from one to two hours, is marked only by pyrethrum poisoning. There may even be partial recovery from this, only to be followed by the second episode, in which the fly relapses, manifests symptoms of DDT toxemia, and dies.

A mixture containing as little as 0.03 per cent w/v total pyrethrins and 0.1 percent w/v DDT in kerosene will serve as a fly spray for practical use. Toxicity may be increased by the addition of a suitable activator, such as sesame oil or isobutylundecylenamide. The relative abundance characteristic of the postwar years has, of course, made such extreme economies unnecessary.

Synthetic equivalents of natural pyrethrins are also becoming available. One preparation of promise is allethrin, the toxicity of which approaches that of pyrethrins found in nature. This pyrethrumlike compound is the allyl homolog of cinerin I.

PIPERONYL BUTOXIDE

A very promising modern insecticide is piperonyl butoxide, an almost odorless substance which is well tolerated by warm-blooded animals. The MLD 50 for rabbits is given as 5 ml. per kg. of body weight, and for rats and dogs as from 7.5 to 10 ml. This insecticide has an advantage over piperonyl cyclohexanone (now piperonyl cyclonene), as it does not require an auxiliary solvent when used in oil sprays or liquefied gas-propelled aerosols. Both are very effective when used in combination with pyrethrins.[5] For example, a suitable mixture of pyrethrum and piperonyl butoxide has been found to be ten times as toxic to houseflies as pyrethrum used alone. The residual properties of pyrethrum are likewise greatly improved by the presence of butoxide.

Various proportions of pyrethrins and piperonyl butoxide were tested by Dove (1947) against houseflies and other pests. In standard Peet-Grady chambers 40 mg. of pyrethrins gave a mortality of 34 per cent with houseflies, while 400 mg. of piperonyl butoxide gave 65 per cent mortality. A combination of the two gave a mortality percentage of 94. The same combination gave a 98 per cent knockdown in ten minutes' time. A proportion of one part of pyrethrins to 8 parts of butoxide proved most efficient for aerosols and household sprays. Dove treated a plywood panel with a concentration of 100 mg. of butoxide and 5 mg. of pyrethrins per square foot. One hundred thirty-one days later, he obtained 100 per cent knockdown within one hour after flies were exposed. Twenty-four hours gave complete mortality.

[5] Another synergist now being used with pyrethrum is N-propylisome.

It can truly be said that applied entomology has never enjoyed so important and so respected a place in human understanding as at the present time, a position which has been made possible only by the combined scholarship and industry of medical, physical, and biological scientists, all working for the ultimate health, comfort, and security of humankind.

Such co-operative endeavor must obviously continue if we are to solve the problems of future years. The evolution of successive strains of insecticide-resistant flies is but one evidence of the futility of placing all confidence in a single new discovery, and shows clearly that it is never the part of wisdom to abandon the *proven* sanitary practices which have brought us to our present level of achievement in matters of public health. Similarly, it is important that no *new* area be left unexplored which, by its proper exploitation, might bring benefit to man. Already, the use of radioactive isotopes has given us a new understanding of the biology of many noxious forms and of the action of chemical substances employed to control them. We are a part of the atomic age, and it is vital that we harness this new knowledge to constructive ends. The hope of the world may now be said to center in the laboratories of those investigators and teachers who are fortunate enough to be permitted full academic freedom in the discovery and interpretation of scientific truth.

Bibliography

The following references have been selected from a working list approximately three times as large. All but a few are cited in the text.

ANONYMOUS 1915 Public Stable in Panama. Canal Record, Balboa, 8: 288–289.

ANONYMOUS 1918 Guarding Soldiers' Camps against Flies and Mosquitoes. Science, 48, no. 1229: 63–64.

ANONYMOUS 1938 Report of the Puerto Rico Experiment Station, 1937. Washington, D.C.

ANONYMOUS 1938–1946 Peet-Grady Method. (A succession of publications dealing with this important biological method for the determination of the effectiveness of household insecticides.) Soap and Sanit. Chem. Blue Book, 1938: 147–149, 151; 1939: 177, 179, 181–183; 1942: 1–5; 1944: 201–204; 1946: 211–214.

ANONYMOUS 1945 DDT—Safe and Efficient Use. Bull. U.S. Army Med. Dept., 4: 515–516.

ANONYMOUS 1945 DDT Used in Experimental Fly-Control. Program on Mackinac Island, Summer of 1945. Michigan Public Health, 33: 145.

ANONYMOUS 1946 Fly Control with DDT. Bull. U.S. Army Med. Dept., 5: 22–23.

ANONYMOUS 1947 DDT—For Control of Household Pests. Prepared by the Bureau of Entomology and Plant Quarantine, Agric. Res. Adm., U.S.D.A., and U.S.P.H.S., Fed. Sec. Agency, Washington, D.C. Issued March 1947.

ABBOTT, C. E. 1945 The Mechanics of Digestion in the Calliphorid Flies. Ent. News, 56: 44–47.

ACHARYA, C. N., AND KRISHNA RAO, K. S. 1945a Control of Fly-Breeding in Compost Heaps. Indian Med. Gaz., 80: 272–273.

ACHARYA, C. N., AND KRISHNA RAO, K. S. 1945b Experiments on the Control of Fly-Breeding in Compost Trenches. Indian J. Agric. Sci., 15: 318–327. Published in 1946.

ACKERT, J. E. 1918 On the Life Cycle of the Fowl Cestode, *Davainea cesticillus* (Molin). J. Parasit., 5: 41–43.

ADERS, W. M. 1916 Entomology in Relation to Public Health and Medicine. Zanzibar Protectorate Med. and Publ. Health Repts. for 1916: 47–49.

Aksinin, J. S. 1929 The Output of Free Ammonia by House-Fly Larvae (*Musca domestica* L.). Plant Protection, 6: 379–382.

Aldrich, J. M. 1905 A Catalogue of North American Diptera (or Two-winged Flies). Smithsonian Misc. Coll., 46 (no. 1444): 1–680.

Aldrich, J. M. 1916 *Sarcophaga* and Allies in North America. Lafayette, Ind.

Allen, T. C., Dicke, R. J., and Brooks, J. W. 1943 Rapid Insecticide Testing. Use of the Settling Mist Method for Testing of Vaporized Contact Insecticides against Houseflies. Soap and Sanit. Chem., 19: 94–96, 121.

Allnutt, E. B. 1926 Some Experiences in the Control of Fly-Breeding. J. R. Army Med. Corps, 47: 105–120.

Almeida, J. L. de 1933 Nouveaux agents de transmission de la berne (*Dermatobia hominis* L., Junior, 1781) au Brésil. Compt. Rend. Soc. Biol., 113: 1274–1275.

Alpatov, W. W. 1929 Growth and Variation of the Larvae of *Drosophila melanogaster*. J. Exp. Zool., 52: 407–432.

Alston, A. M. 1920 The Life History and Habits of Two Parasites of Blowflies. Proc. Zool. Soc. London, 1920: 195–243.

Andrews, H. W. 1925 Flies and Disease. Proc. S. London Ent. and Nat. Hist. Soc., 1924–1925: 45–62.

Andrews, J. M., and Simmons, S. W. 1948 Developments in the Use of the Newer Organic Insecticides of Public Health Importance. Am. J. Publ. Health, 38: 613–631.

Anduze, P. J. 1945 Breve nota sobre miasis humanas en Venezuela. Bol. Ent. Venezolana, Caracas, 4: 37–40.

Ara, F., and Marengo, U. 1932 Sull' Importanza della mosca nella diffusione della febbre tifoide. Nota I. Bull. Soc. Ital. Biol. Sper., 7: 150–154.

Arizumi, S. 1934 On the Potential Transmission of *Bacillus leprae* by Certain Insects. (In Japanese.) J. Med. Ass. Formosa, Taihoku, 33: 634–661. (English summary.)

Ark, P. A., and Thomas, H. E. 1936 Persistence of *Erwinia amylovora* in Certain Insects. Phytopath., 26: 375–381.

Armstrong, D. B. 1914a Flies and Diarrhoeal Disease. Publ. No. 79, New York Ass. for Improving the Conditions of the Poor, Bur. Public Health and Hyg., Dept. Local Welfare.

Armstrong, D. B. 1914b The House-Fly and Diarrhoeal Disease among Children. J. Am. Med. Ass., 62: 200–201.

Atkeson, F. W., Shaw, O. A., Smith, R. C., and Borgmann, A. R. 1943 Some Investigations of Fly Control in Dairy Barns. J. Dairy Sci., 26: 219–232.

Atkinson, E. L. 1916 The Fly Pest in Gallipoli. J. R. Naval Med. Service, London, 2: 147–152.

Attimonelli, R. 1940 Reperti parasitologici nell'acqua di lavaggio delle mosche. Pathologica, 32: 111–112.

AUSTEN, E. E. 1910a Some Dipterous Insects Which Cause Myiasis in Man. Trans. Soc. Trop. Med. and Hyg., 3: 215-242.

AUSTEN, E. E. 1910b A New Indian Species of *Musca*. Ann. Mag. Nat. Hist., 5: 114–117.

AUSTEN, E. E. 1913 The House-Fly as a Danger to Health. Its Life-History and How to Deal with It. Brit. Mus. (Nat. Hist.) Econ. Ser., no. 1.

AUSTEN, E. E. 1926 The House-Fly, Its Life History, Importance as a Disease Carrier and Practical Measures for Its Suppression. Brit. Mus. (Nat. Hist.) Econ. Ser., no. 1a, ed. 2.

AUSTIN, T. A., AND MAYNE, L. C. 1935 A Review of the Incidence of Amoebiasis in Zomba, with Special Reference to European Cases. Ann. Med. Rept. Nyasaland, 1934: 73–82.

AWATI, P. R. 1916a Studies in Flies. II. Contributions to the Study of Specific Differences in the Genus *Musca*. Indian J. Med. Res., 3: 510–529.

AWATI, P. R. 1916b Studies in Flies. II. Contribution to the Study of Specific Differences in the Genus *Musca*. 2. Structures Other than Genitalia. Indian J. Med. Res., 4: 123–139.

AWATI, P. R. 1920a Bionomics of House-Flies. IV. Some Notes on the Life History of *Musca*. Indian J. Med. Res., 8: 80–88.

AWATI, P. R. 1920b A Note on the Genitalia of Portchinsky's Species *M. corvina* (vivipara) and *M. corvina* (ovipara). Indian J. Med. Res., 8: 89–92.

AWATI, P. R. 1920c Bionomics of Houseflies. I. Outdoor Feeding Habits of Houseflies with Special Reference to *Musca promiscua* (*angustifrons*). Indian J. Med. Res., 7: 548–552.

AWATI, P. R. 1920d Bionomics of Houseflies. II. Attraction of Houseflies to Different Colours. Indian J. Med. Res., 7: 553–559.

AWATI, P. R., AND SWAMINATH, C. S. 1920 Bionomics of Houseflies. III. A Preliminary Note on Attraction of Houseflies to Certain Fermenting and Putrefying Substances. Indian J. Med. Res., 7: 560–567.

BABER, E. 1918 A Method of Trapping Fly Larvae in Manure Heaps. Lancet, 1 (4935): 471.

BABER, E. 1925 Fly Control by Means of the Fly-Larval-Trap Manure Enclosure. J. R. Army Med. Corps, 45: 443–452.

BACOT, A. W. 1911a On the Persistence of Bacilli in the Gut of an Insect during Metamorphosis. Trans. Ent. Soc. London, 1911: 497–500.

BACOT, A. W. 1911b The Persistence of *Bacillus pyocyaneus* in Pupae and Imagines of *Musca domestica* Raised from Larvae Experimentally Infected with the Bacillus. Parasitology, 4: 68–73.

BAER, W. S. 1929 The Use of a Viable Antiseptic in the Treatment of Osteomyelitis. Southern Med. J., 22: 582–583.

BAER, W. S. 1931 The Treatment of Chronic Osteomyelitis with the Maggot (Larva of the Blow Fly). J. Bone Joint Surg., 13: 438.

BAHR, P. H. 1914 A Study of Epidemic Dysentery in the Fiji Islands. Brit. Med. J., London, 1914: 294–296.

BALL, S. C. 1918 Migrations of Insects to Rebecca Shoal Light-Station and the Tortugas Islands, with Special Reference to Mosquitoes and Flies. Pap. Dept. Marine Biol. Carnegie Inst. Washington, 12: 193–212.

BANCROFT, E. 1769 An Essay on the Natural History of Guiana in South America. London.

BANG, F. B., AND GLASER, R. W. 1943 The Persistence of Poliomyelitis Virus in Flies. Am. J. Hyg., 37: 320–324.

BANKS, N. 1905 A Treatise on the Acarina or Mites. Proc. U.S. Nat. Mus., 28: 1–114.

BARANOV, N. 1939 Dung Heaps as Breeding Places of Flies in the Village of Mratzlin. (In Serbian.) Vet. Arhiv., Zagreb, 9: 280–287. (German summary.)

BARBER, G. W. 1919 A Note on Migration of Larvae of the House Fly. J. Econ. Ent., 12: 466.

BARBER, G. W. 1948 The Lethal Lines of the House Fly. J. Econ. Ent., 41: 292–295.

BARTSCH, A. F., AND SCOTT, R. H. 1949 The Mississippi River Sanitation Survey (Excerpts from the Progress Report for 1948). Health (bimonthly bull. of the Wisconsin State Board of Health), 8: 389–392.

BASDEN, E. B. 1947 Breeding the House-Fly *Musca domestica* L. in the Laboratory. Bull. Ent. Res., 37: 381–387.

BAXTER, G. R. 1940a The House-Fly, Public Enemy No. 1. Agric. J. Fiji, 11 (3): 66–70.

BAXTER, G. R. 1940b The Control of the Fly Nuisance. Agric. J. Fiji, 11 (4): 96–98.

BAYON, H. 1915 Leprosy: A Perspective of the Results of Experimental Study of the Disease. Ann. Trop. Med. Parasit., 9: 1–90.

BEACHLEY, R. G., AND BISHOPP, F. C. 1942 Report of a Case of Nasal Myiasis Due to a Bot Fly Larva (*Cuterebra* sp.). Virginia Med. Monthly, 69: 41–42.

BEAL, W. P. 1915 Verminous Enteritis among Sheep from Senegal. Annual Report for 1914. London. (Abstract, Rev. Appl. Ent., ser B., 4: 12, 1916.)

BEATTIE, M. V. F. 1928 Observations on the Thermal Death Points of the Blow-Fly at Different Relative Humidities. Bull. Ent. Res., 18: 397–403.

BECKER, E. R. 1923a Observations on the Morphology and Life-History of *Herpetomonas muscae-domesticae* in North American Muscoid Flies. J. Parasit., 9: 199–213.

BECKER, E. R. 1923b Transmission Experiments on the Specificity of *Herpetomonas muscae-domesticae* in Muscoid Flies. J. Parasit., 10: 25–34.

BECKER, E. R. 1923c Studies on the Relationship between Insect Flagellates and *Leishmania*. Am. J. Hyg., 3: 462–468.

BÉCLARD, J. 1858 Note relative à l'influence de la lumière sur les animaux. Compt. Rend. Acad. Sci., 46: 441–443.

BEDFORD, G. A. H. 1926 Check-List of the Muscidae and Oestridae Which Cause Myiasis in Man and Animals in South Africa. Union So. Africa Dept. Agric. Dir. Vet. Ed. and Res. Repts. 11 and 12, pt. 1: 483–491.

BEDFORD, G. A. H. 1929 Anoplura (*Siphunculata* and *Mallophaga*) from South African Hosts. 15th Rept. Vet. Serv. So. Africa, 1: 501–549.

BELLOSILLO, G. C. 1937 *Herpetomonas muscarum* (Leidy) in *Lucilia sericata* Meigen. Philipp. J. Sci., 63: 285–305.

BEQUAERT, J. 1945 Cutaneous Myiasis Due to *Cuterebra* in Massachusetts. Psyche, 52: 175–176.

BERESOFF, W. F. 1914 Die Schlafenden Fliegen als Infektionsträger. Centralbl. Bakt. Parasit. Infekt., I Abt. Orig., 74: 244–250.

BERLESE, A. 1902 L'accoppiamento della mosca domestica. Rev. Patolog. veget., 9: 345–357.

BERLESE, A. 1912 Gli insetti. Milan. 2: 18.

BERNSTEIN, J. M. 1914 Repts. Local Govnt. Bd. Publ. Health and Med. Subjects, n.s. 102, ii. The Destruction of Flies by Means of Bacterial Cultures, pp. 27–31.

BERTARELLE, E. 1910 Verbreitung des Typhus durch die Fliegen. Centralbl. Bakt. Parasit. Infekt., 53: 486–495.

BEVAN, E. W. 1926 Southern Rhodesia: Report of the Director of Veterinary Research for the Year 1925. Salisbury, Rhodesia. Fol. 9 pp.

BICKOFF, E. 1943 House Fly. *In* Laboratory Procedures in Studies of the Chemical Control of Insects, p. 74. Publ. Am. Ass. Adv. Sci., no. 20.

BIGOT, J. M. F. 1887a Diptères nouveaux ou peu connus. Muscidi. Bull. Soc. Zool. Fr., 12: 581–617.

BIGOT, J. M. F. 1887b Diptères nouveaus provenant de l'Amerique du Nord. Bull. Soc. Ent. Fr. (ser. 6), 7: clxxx–clxxxii.

BISHOPP, F. C. 1946a Present Position of DDT in the Control of Insects of Medical Importance. Pests, 14: 14–28.

BISHOPP, F. C. 1946b Present Position of DDT in the Control of Insects of Medical Importance. Am. J. Publ. Health, 36: 593–606.

BISHOPP, F. C. 1946c New Insecticides. A Progress Report on Results Being Obtained in Preliminary Test Studies. Agric. Chem., 1: 19–22, 39–40.

BISHOPP, F. C., DOVE, W. E., AND PARMAN, D. C. 1915 Notes on Certain Points of Economic Importance in the Biology of the House Fly. J. Econ. Ent., 8: 54–71.

BISHOPP, F. C., AND LAAKE, E. W. 1919 The Dispersion of Flies by Flight. J. Econ. Ent., 12: 210–211.

BISHOPP, F. C., AND LAAKE, E. W. 1921 Dispersion of Flies by Flight. J. Agric. Res., 21: 729–766.

BISHOPP, F. C., LAAKE, E. W., BRUNDRETT, H. M., AND WELLS, R. W. 1926 The Cattle Grubs or Ox Warbles, Their Biologies and Suggestions for Control. U.S. Dept. Agric. Bull. 1369.

BLAIR, D. M. 1945 Baited Fly Traps. Rhod. Agric. J., 42: 488–492.

BLAIR, K. G. 1942 How Does a Housefly Alight on the Ceiling? Entomol. Mon. Mag., London, 78: 40–41.

BLIESNER, E. R., AND BROWN, S. T. 1945 Eye Appeal Is Not Sanitation. Wisc. State Board of Health. Quar. Bull., 7: 16–18.

BODENHEIMER, F. S. 1924 Über die Voraussage der Generationenzahl von Insekten. II. Die Temperaturentwicklungskurve bei medizinisch wichtigen Insekten. Centralbl. Bakt. Parasit. Infekt., I Abt. Orig., 93: 474–480.

BODENHEIMER, F. S. 1925 On Predicting the Development Cycles of Insects. I. Ceratitis capitata Wied. Bull. Soc. R. Ent. Egypte, 1924: 149–157.

BODENHEIMER, F. S. 1931 Erfahrung über die Biologie der Hausfliege (Musca domestica L.) in Palästina. Zeit. Angew. Ent., 18: 492–504.

BODKIN, G. E. 1917 Report of the Economic Biologist. Brit. Guiana Dept. Sci. and Agric. Rept. for 1916.

BODKIN, G. E. 1923 Report of the Government Economic Biologist. Brit. Guiana Dept. Sci. and Agric. Rept., App. 3: 36–40.

BOGDANOW, E. A. 1906 Über das Züchten der Larven der gewöhnlichen Fleischfliege (Calliphora vomitoria) in sterilisierten Nahrmitteln. Pflügers Arch. Ges. Physiol., 113: 97–105.

BOGDANOW, E. A. 1908 Über die Abhängigkeit des Wachstums der Fliegenlarven von Bacterien und Fermenten und über Variabilität und Vererbung bei den Fleischfliegen. Arch. Anat. Physiol. Jahr., 1908 (Suppl.): 173–200.

BOLLINGER, O. 1874 Experimentelle Untersuchungen über die Entstehung der Milzbrandes. 46 Versamml. d. D. Naturf. u. Aerzte zu Wiesbaden. September, 1873. And "Milzbrand," in von Ziemssen's Handb. d. spec. Pathol. u. Therapie, 3: 282, 457.

BORRE, P. DE 1873a Note on Parasites of Musca domestica. Nature, 8: 263.

BORRE, P. DE 1873b Musca domestica with Chelifer panzeri Koch Attached Parasitically. Sitzungsber. Z.-G. Wien., 23: 36.

BOYD, J. E. M. 1922a The Botany and Natural History of Dyke-Land near Sandwich, Kent, as Far as They Concern Medical Entomology. J. R. Army Med. Corps, 38: 41–47, 117–130.

BOYD, J. E. M. 1922b Entomological Notes: On a Muscid Fly Breeding on a Ship at Sea. J. R. Army Med. Corps, 38: 378–379.

BRAIN, C. K. 1918 Storage of Manure and Fly Suppression at Durban Remount Depot. J. Econ. Ent., 11: 339–341.

BRAZIL, V. 1926 A defeza contra a mosca. Mem. Inst. Butantan, São Paulo, 3: 189–203. (French summary.)

BRESCIA, F., LA MER, V. K., WILSON, I. B., ROWELL, J. C., AND HODGES, K. C. 1946 Relative Toxicity of DDT Aerosols to Mosquitoes and Musca domestica. Insect Balance. Ent. News, 57:180–183.

BRÈTHES, J. 1915 Sur la Prospalangia platensis (n. gen. n. sp.) (Hymen.) et sa biologie. Anales Soc. Cien. Argentina, 79: 314, 320.

BRIDWELL, J. C. 1918 Certain Aspects of Medical and Sanitary Entomology in Hawaii. Trans. Med. Soc. Hawaii for 1916–1917, Honolulu, Mar. 1918: 27–32.

BROWN, A. W. A. 1936 Excretion of Ammonia and Uric Acid in Muscid Larvae. J. Exp. Biol., 13: 131–139.

BROWN, F. M. 1927 Descriptions of New Bacteria Found in Insects. Am. Mus. Novit., no. 251.

BRUCE, W. G. 1939 Some Observations on Insect Edaphology. J. Kans. Ent. Soc., 12: 91–93.

BRUCE, W. N. 1949 Characteristics of Residual Insecticides Toxic to the House Fly. Bull. Ill. Nat. Hist. Surv., 25: 1–32.

BRUES, C. T. 1942 Insects as Carriers of Poliomyelitis Virus. Science, 95: 169–170.

BUDDENBROCK, W. VON 1919 Function of Halteres. Arch. Ges. Physiol., 175: 125–164.

BUDDENBROCK, W. VON 1937 Grundriss der vergleichenden Physiologie. Berlin.

BUICHKOV, V. A. 1932 Über die Aufbewahrungs-dauer von *Bacterium prodigiosum* durch die Fliegen. (In Russian.) Mag. Paras. Inst. Zool. Acad. Sci. URSS, 3: 149–159.

BULL, L. 1910 Sur les inclinaisons du voile de l'aile de l'insecte pendant le vol. Compt. Rend. Acad. Sci., 150: 129–131.

BULL, L. B. 1919 A Contribution to the Study of Habronemiasis: A Clinical, Pathological and Experimental Investigation of a Granulomatous Condition of the Horse—Habronemic Granuloma. Trans. R. Soc. S. Australia, 43: 85–141.

BULL, L. B. 1922 Habronemic Conjunctivitis in Man Producing a "Bung Eye." Med. J. Australia, 9th year, ii, no. 18: 499–500.

BURNETT, W. I. 1851–1852 The Organic Relations of Some of the Infusoria, Including Investigations Concerning the Structure and Nature of the Genus *Bodo* (Ehr.). Boston Soc. Nat. Hist., 4 (1851–1854), 1851: 124 (extract); Boston J. Nat. Hist., 6 (1850–1857), 1852: 319.

BUSHNELL, L. D., AND HINSHAW, W. R. 1924 Prevention and Control of Poultry Diseases. Kansas Agric. Expt. Sta. Circ. 106.

BUSVINE, J. R., AND BARNES, S. 1947 Observations on Mortality among Insects Exposed to Dry Insecticidal Films. Bull. Ent. Res., 38: 81–90.

BUXTON, P. A. 1920 The Importance of the House-Fly as a Carrier of *E. histolytica*. Brit. Med. J., London, no. 3083: 142–144.

BUXTON, P. A., AND MELLANBY, K. 1934 The Measurement and Control of Humidity. Bull. Ent. Res., 25: 171–175.

CAMERON, J. W. M. 1938 The Reactions of the Housefly, *Musca domestica* L. to Light of Different Wave-Lengths. Canad. J. Res. (D), 16: 307–342.

CAMERON, J. W. M. 1939 Reactions of House-Flies to Light of Different Wave-Lengths. Nature, London, 143: 208.

CAMPBELL, F. L., AND SULLIVAN, W. N. 1938 Testing Fly Sprays: A Metal Turntable Method for Comparative Tests of Liquid Contact Insecticides. Soap and Sanit. Chem., 14: 119–125, 149.

CAMPBELL, G. A., AND WEST, T. F. 1944 Persistence of DDT in Oil-bound Water-Paint. Nature, London, 154: 512.

CAO, G. 1898 Sul passaggio dei micro-organismi attraverso l'intestino di alcuni insetti. Ufficiale Sanitario, Rivista d'Igiene e di Medicina Pratica, Anno 11: 337–348, 385–397.

CAO, G. 1906a Nuove osservazioni sul passagio dei microorganismi a traverso l'intestino di alcuni insetti. Ann. Igiene Sper., 16: 339–368.

CAO, G. 1906b Sul passaggio dei germi attraverso le larve di alcuni insetti. Ann. Igiene Sper., 16: 654.

CARMENT, A. G. 1922 Report on Experiment of Fly Breeding from Stable Manure with a Short Account of the Finding of a Parasite. Agric. Circ. Dept. Agric. Fiji, 3: 1–5.

CARR, E. C. 1927 Flies and Their Eradication. U.S. Nav. Med. Bull., 25: 528–542.

CASE, A. A., AND ACKERT, J. E. 1939 Intermediate Hosts of Chicken Tape-Worms Found in Kansas. Trans. Kans. Acad. Sci., 42: 437–442.

CASTELLANI, ALDO 1907 Experimental Investigation on *Framboesia tropica* (Yaws). J. Hyg., 7: 558–569.

CATTANI, G. 1886 Study sul colera. Gazz. Ospedali Milano, 7: 611.

CAUSEY, O. R. 1938 Experimental Intestinal Myiasis. Am. J. Hyg., 28: 481–486.

CELLÍ, A. 1888 Trasmissibilità dei germi patogeni mediante le dejecione delle mosche. Bull. Soc. Lancisiana d. Ospedali Roma, Fasc. 1, pl. 1.

CHANG, K. 1943 Domestic Flies as Mechanical Carriers of Certain Human Intestinal Parasites in Chengtu. J. W. China Border Res. Soc. (B), 14: 92–98.

CHAPMAN, R. K. 1944 An Interesting Occurrence of *Musca domestica* L. Larvae in Infant Bedding. Canad. Ent., 76: 230–232.

CHARLES, V. K. 1941 A Preliminary Check List of the Entomophagous Fungi of North America. Bur. Entomol., Insect Pest Survey Bull. (Suppl. to no. 9), 21: 707–785.

CHIT THOUNG, U. 1946 Poisonous Effects of DDT on Humans. Indian Med. Gaz., 81: 432.

CLAPHAM, P. A. 1939 On Flies as Intermediate Hosts of *Syngamous trachea*. J. Helminth., 17: 61–64.

CLELAND, J. B., CAMPBELL, A. W., AND BRADLEY, B. 1919 The Australian Epidemics of an Acute Polio-encephalo-myelitis (X Disease). Rept. Director-Gen. Public Health New S. Wales for Year Ended December 31, 1917: 173–174.

COBB, N. A. 1910a Notes on the Distances Flies Can Travel. Nat. Geog. Mag., 21: 380–383.

COBB, N. A. 1910b The House Fly. Nat. Geog. Mag., 21: 371–380.

COCHRANE, E. W. W.   1912   A Small Epidemic of Typhoid Fever in Connection with Specifically Infected Flies.   J. R. Army Med. Corps, 18: 271–276.

COMPERE, G.   1912   A Few Facts concerning the Fruit-Flies of the World. iii. Monthly Bull. State Bd. Hort., Calif., U.S.A., 1: 907–911.

COMSTOCK, J. H.   1940   An Introduction to Entomology. 9th ed., rev. Ithaca, N.Y.

COMSTOCK, J. H., AND NEEDHAM, J. G.   1898   The Wings of Insects.   Am. Nat., 32: 43–48, and continued through the volume into Vol. 33.

CONNAL, A.   1922   Medical Entomology. (Nigeria.)   Ann. Rept. Med. Res. Inst. 1920: 17–22.

CONVERSE, G. M.   1910   Amoebiasis. Bull. Cal. State Bd. of Health, October 1910.

COOK, F. C., HUTCHISON, R. H., AND SCALES, F. M.   1914   Experiments in the Destruction of Fly Larvae in Horse Manure.   U.S. Dept. Agric. Bull. 118.

COOK-YOUNG, A. W.   1914   The Prevalence of Flies in Delhi and Their Reduction.   Proc. Third All-India Sanitary Conf., Lucknow, Jan. 19–27, 1914, II: 141–147. (Suppl. to Indian J. Med. Res.)

COPEMAN, S. M.   1913   Hibernation of House-Flies (Preliminary Note).   Repts. Local Govnt. Bd. Publ. Health and Med. Subjects, n.s. 85; Further Repts. (no. 6) on Flies as Carriers of Infection: 14–19.

COPEMAN, S. M.   1916   Prevention of Fly-Breeding in Horse-Manure.   Lancet, no. 4841 (1916, Vol. 1): 1182–1184.

COPEMAN, S. M., AND AUSTEN, E. E.   1914   Repts. Local Govnt. Bd. Publ. Health and Med. Subjects, n.s. 102.   (I. Do House-Flies Hibernate? pp. 6–26.)

COPEMAN, S. M., HOWLETT, F. M., AND MERRIMAN, G.   1911   An Experimental Investigation on the Range of Flight of Flies.   Repts. Local Govnt. Bd. Publ. Health and Med. Subjects, n.s. 53; Further Repts. (no. 4) on Flies as Carriers of Infection, pp. 1–10.

CORFIELD, W. F.   1919   Some Experiments upon the Control of Fly-Breeding Areas in Camps.   J. R. Army Med. Corps, London, 33: 415–418.

CORNWALL, J. W., AND PATTON, W. S.   1914   Some Observations on the Salivary Secretion of the Commoner Blood-sucking Insects and Ticks.   Indian J. Med. Res., 2: 569–593.

CORY, E. N.   1918   The Control of House Flies by the Maggot Trap.   Maryland State Coll. Agric. Expt. Sta. Bull. 213: 103–126.

CORY, E. N., AND LANGFORD, G. S.   1947   Fly Control in Dairy Barns and on Livestock by Cooperative Spray Services.   J. Econ. Ent., 40: 425–426.

COTTERELL, G. S.   1940   Preliminary Investigations on the Fly Population of Stable Manure Heaps and Measures for the Prevention of Breeding.   Pap. 3d W. Afr. Agric. Conf. Nigeria June 1938, Sect. Gold Coast, Lagos, 1: 118–125.

COUSIN, G.   1932   Etude expérimentale de la diapause des insectes.   Bull. Biol. France Belg., Suppl. 15.

COX, A. J.   1944   Insecticide Testing. A Review of Testing Procedure for Evaluating Household Insecticides for Use in the Control of Flies, Clothes Moths, Roaches and Rodents. Soap and Sanit. Chem., 20 (no. 6): 114–117, 149; (no. 7): 123, 125, 129.

COX, G. L., LEWIS, F. C., AND GLYNN, E. F. 1912 The Number and Varieties of Bacteria Carried by the Common House Fly in Sanitary and Insanitary City Areas. J. Hyg., 12: 290–319.

CRAGG, F. W. 1920 The Maggot Trap: A Means for the Safe Disposal of Horse Manure and Similar Refuse. Indian J. Med. Res., Calcutta, spec. Ind. Sci. Congress no. (1920): 18–21.

CRAIG, C. F. 1917 The Occurrence of Endamebic Dysentery in the Troops Serving in the El Paso District from July 1916 to December 1916. Military Surgeon, 40: 286–302; 423–434.

CRAMPTON, G. C. 1941 The Terminal Abdominal Structures of Male Diptera. Psyche, 48: 79–94.

CRAMPTON, G. C. 1942 The External Morphology of the Diptera. In Guide to the Insects of Connecticut. Part IV. The Diptera or True Flies of Connecticut. Conn. State Geol. and Nat. Hist. Surv. Bull., 64: 10–165.

CRUMB, S. E., AND LYON, S. C. 1917 The Effect of Certain Chemicals upon Oviposition in the House-Fly (*Musca domestica* L.). J. Econ. Ent., 10: 532–536.

CRUMB, S. E., AND LYON, S. C. 1921 Further Observations on the Effect of Chemicals upon Oviposition in the House Fly. J. Econ. Ent., 14: 461–465.

CURRAN, C. H. 1934 The Families and Genera of North American Diptera. New York.

CURRIE, D. H. 1910 Mosquitoes in Relation to the Transmission of Leprosy. Flies in Relation to the Transmission of Leprosy. U.S. Publ. Health Bull. 39.

CURRY, D. P. 1935 Report of Assistant Chief Health Officer. Rept. Health Dept. Panama Canal, 1934: 12–16.

CUTHBERTSON, A. 1934a Biological Notes on Some Diptera in Southern Rhodesia. Proc. Rhod. Sci. Ass., 33: 32–50.

CUTHBERTSON, A. 1934b The Life History of the Screw-Worm Fly. (*Chrysomyia bezziana* Villen. in Southern Rhodesia.) Rhod. Agric. J., 31: 256–258.

CUTHBERTSON, A. 1942 The Skin Maggot Fly. Life History and Preventive Measures. Rhod. Agric. J., 39: 149–151.

DAKSHINAMURTY, S. 1948 The Common House-Fly, *Musca domestica* L. and its Behaviour to Temperature and Humidity. Bull. Ent. Res., 39: 339–357.

DARLING, S. T. 1912a Murrina, a Trypanosomal Disease of Horses, in Panama, and the Means Used in Controlling an Outbreak. Trans. 15th Intern. Congr. Hyg. and Demog., Washington, 5: 619–631.

DARLING, S. T. 1912b Experimental Infection of the Mule with *Trypanosoma hippicum* by Means of *Musca domestica*. J. Exp. Med., 15: 365–366.

DARLING, S. T. 1913 The Part Played by Flies and Other Insects in the Spread of Infectious Diseases in the Tropics, with Special Reference to Ants and to the

Transmission of *Tr. hippicum* by *Musca domestica*. Trans. 15th Intern. Congr. Hyg. and Demog., Washington, 5: 182–185.

DAVAINE, C. 1868 Expérience relatives à la durée de l'incubation des maladies charbonneuses. Bull. Acad. Méd., 33: 816.

DAVAINE, C. 1870a Etudes sur la contagion du carbon chez les animaux domestiques. Bull. Acad. Méd., 35: 215–235.

DAVAINE, C. 1870b Etudes sur la genèse et la propagation du charbon. Bull. Acad. Méd., 35: 471–498.

DAVID, W. A. L. 1946 The Quantity and Distribution of Sprays Collected by Insects Flying through Insecticidal Mists. Ann. Appl. Biol., 33: 133–141.

DAVIDSON, J. 1918 Some Practical Methods Adopted for the Control of Flies in the Egyptian Campaign. Bull. Ent. Res., 8: 297–309.

DAVIDSON, J. 1944 On the Relationship between Temperature and Rate of Development of Insects at Constant Temperatures. J. Anim. Ecol., 13: 26–38.

DE BACH, P. 1939 A Hormone Which Induces Pupation in the Common House Fly, *Musca domestica*. Ann. Ent. Soc. Am., 32: 743–746.

DE BACH, P. 1943 The Effect of Low Storage Temperatures on Reproduction in Certain Parasitic Hymenoptera. Pan Pacific Ent., 19: 112–119.

DE BACH, P. 1944 Environmental Contamination by an Insect Parasite and the Effect on Host Selection. Ann. Ent. Soc. Am., 37: 70–74.

DEENY, J., AND MacCORMACK, J. D. 1946 The Control of Poliomyelitis. Lancet, 251: 8–9.

DEONIER, C. C. 1938 Effects of Some Common Poisons in Sucrose Solutions on the Chemoreceptors of the Housefly, *Musca domestica*. J. Econ. Ent., 31: 742–745.

DEONIER, C. C. 1939 Responses of the Blowflies, *Cochliomyia americana* and *Phormia regina* to Stimulations of the Tarsal Chemoreceptors. Ann. Ent. Soc. Am., 32: 526–532.

DEONIER, C. C. 1940 Carcass Temperatures and Their Relation to Winter Blowfly Populations and Activity in the Southwest. J. Econ. Ent., 33: 166–170.

DEONIER, C. C., AND RICHARDSON, C. H. 1935 The Tarsal Chemoreceptor Response of the Housefly, *Musca domestica* L. to Sucrose and Levulose. Ann. Ent. Soc. Am., 28: 467–474.

DEORAS, P. J., AND ARJAN SINGH JANDU 1943 The House-Fly and Its Control. Indian Fmg., 4: 565–568.

DERBENEVA-UKHOVA, V. P. 1935a Die Einwirkung der Imaginalen Ernährungsbedingungen auf die Entwicklung der Ovarien von *Musca domestica* L. (In Russian.) Med. Parasit., 4: 394–403.

DERBENEVA-UKHOVA, V. P. 1935b Über die Zahl der Generationen bei *Musca domestica* L. (In Russian.) Med. Parasit., 4: 404–407.

DERBENEVA-UKHOVA, V. P. 1937 Die Oekologie der Larven von *Musca domestica* unter natürlichen Bedingungen. (In Russian.) Med. Parasit., 6: 408–417.

DERBENEVA-UKHOVA, V. P. 1940a Sur l'écologie des mouches de fumier à Kabarda. (In Russian.) Med. Parasit., 9: 323–339.

DERBENEVA-UKHOVA, V. P. 1940b Influence de la température sur les larves de *Musca domestica* L. (In Russian.) Med Parasit., 9: 521–524.

DERBENEVA-UKHOVA, V. P. 1940c Adaptation des larves de *Musca domestica* L. à des hautes températures. (In Russian.) Med. Parasit., 9: 525–527.

DERBENEVA-UKHOVA, V. P. 1942a The Fly-Maggots as Components of the Dung Biocenoses. (In Russian.) Med. Parasit., 11: 79–86.

DERBENEVA-UKHOVA, V. P. 1942b On the Ecology of *Musca domestica* L. and *Muscina stabulans* Flln. (In Russian.) Med. Parasit., 10: 534–543.

DERBENEVA-UKHOVA, V. P. 1943 The Influence of Soil Humidity and Compactness on the Emergence of the Imago of *M. domestica*. Med. Parasit., 12 (3): 72–76.

DERBENEVA-UKHOVA, V. P. 1947 The Application of DDT Preparations against Flies. (In Russian.) Med. Parasit., 16 (1): 16–28.

DERBENEVA-UKHOVA, V. P., AND KUZINA, O. S. 1938 Quelques Observations au cours de l'essai de lutte contre les mouches aux constructions nouvelles. (In Russian.) Med. Parasit., 7: 399–405. (French summary.)

DESOIL, P. 1924 Valeur de l'hypothèse de l'infestation par oeufs de mouches myasiques dans le cas de myase intestinale chez l'homme. Compt. Rend. Soc. Biol., 91, no. 32: 1079–1081.

DEVOE, ALAN 1945 House Flies. The American Mercury, Oct. 1945: 473–477. (One of a series of popular articles dealing with natural history subjects, published monthly in American Mercury under the section title "Down to Earth.")

DEWS, S. C., AND MORRILL, A. W. 1946 DDT for Insect Control at Army Installations in the Fourth Service Command. J. Econ. Ent., 39: 347–355.

DEXLER, G. 1918 Observations on Certain Flies Infecting Meat and Causing Human Myiasis. Agric. Gaz. Canada, Ottawa, 5: 99.

DHONDY, B. S. 1940 Automatic Flyproof Latrine Seat. Indian Med. Gaz., 75: 466–468.

DIGUET, L. 1915a The "Mosquero" or Spiders' Nest Used in Mexico as a Fly Trap. Bull. Soc. Nat. Acclimat., Paris, 62: 170–171.

DIGUET, L. 1915b Nouvelles Observations sur le mosquero ou nid d'araignées sociales employé come piège à mouches dans certaines localités du Mexique. Bull. Soc. Nat. Acclimat., Paris, 62: 240–249.

DOANE, R. W. 1910 Insects and Disease. A Popular Account of the Way in Which Insects May Spread or Cause Some of Our Common Diseases. American Nature Series. New York. (Houseflies, pp. 57–75.)

DOANE, R. W. 1914 Disease-bearing Insects in Samoa. Bull. Ent. Res., 4: 265–269.

DOLINSKAYA, T. Y., KLECHETOVA, A. M., AND TREGUBOV, A. N. 1946 The Use of Chloride of Lime for the Control of Flies. (In Russian.) Med. Parasit., Moscow, 15 (6): 81–82.

Dönhoff. 1872 Beiträge zur Physiologie. I. Ueber das Verhalten Kaltblütiger Thiere gegen Frosttemperatur. Arch. Anat. Phys. und Wiss. Med. von Reichert und Du Bois-Reymond, 1872: 724–727.

Donovan, E. 1797 Natural History of British Insects. 6: 84.

Dorman, S. C., Hale, W. C., and Hoskins, W. M. 1938 The Laboratory Rearing of Flesh Flies and the Relations beween Temperature, Diet and Egg Production. J. Econ. Ent., 31: 44–51.

Dove, W. E. 1916 Some Notes Concerning Overwintering of the House Fly, *Musca domestica* at Dallas, Texas. J. Econ. Ent., 9: 528–538.

Dove, W. E. 1937 Myiasis of Man. J. Econ. Ent., 30: 29–39.

Dove, W. E. 1947 Piperonyl Butoxide, a New and Safe Insecticide for Household and Field. Am. J. Trop. Med., 27: 339–345.

Drbohlav, J. J. 1925 Studies on the Relation of Insect Herpetomonad and Crithidial Flagellates to Leishmaniasis. Parts I, II, III. Am. J. Hyg., 5: 580–621.

Drbohlav, J. J. 1926 The Cultivation of *Herpetomonas muscarum* (Leidy 1866) Kent 1881 from *Lucilia sericata*. J. Parasit., 12: 183–190.

Dresden, D., and Krijgsman, B. J. 1948 Experiments on the Physiological Action of Contact Insecticides. Bull. Ent. Res., 38: 575–578.

Dudgeon, L. S. 1919 The Dysenteries: Bacillary and Amoebic. Brit. Med. J., London, no. 3041: 448–451.

Duncan, J. T. 1926 On a Bactericidal Principle Present in the Alimentary Canal of Insects and Arachnids. Parasitology, 18: 238–252.

Dunn, L. H. 1930 Rearing the Larvae of *Dermatobia hominis* Linn., in Man. Psyche, 37: 327–342.

DuToit, R. and Nieschulz, O. 1933 *Musca crassirostris,* a Bloodsucking Fly, New to South Africa. J. So. Africa Vet. Med. Ass., 4: 97–98.

Eagleson, C. 1939 Insect Olfactory Responses. Construction and Use of an Olfactometer for Muscoid Flies, and a Discussion of Interpreting Results. Soap and Sanit. Chem., 15: 123, 125, 127.

Eagleson, C. 1940 Livestock Sprays. A Rapid Method for Determining Their Toxicity. Soap and Sanit. Chem., 16: 96–99, 117.

Eagleson, C. 1943 Housefly. *In* Campbell, F. L., and Moulton, F. R., ed., Laboratory Procedures in Studies of the Chemical Control of Insects. Washington, D.C. Publ. Am. Ass. Adv. Sci., 20: 74–77.

Eagleson, C., and Benke, R. 1938 A Note on Rearing Houseflies. Soap and Sanit. Chem., 14: 109, 119.

Elton, C. 1927 Animal Ecology. London.

Eltringham, H. 1916 Some Experiments on the House-fly in Relation to the Farm Manure Heap. J. Agric. Sci., Cambridge, 7: 443–457.

Emden, F. I. van 1939 Muscidae: Muscinae and Stomoxydinae. Brit. Mus. Nat. Hist. Ruwenzori Exped. 1934–1935, 2: 49–89.

Essig, E. O. 1942 College Entomology. New York.

ESTEN, W. M., AND MASON, C. J. 1908 Sources of Bacteria in Milk. Storrs Agric. Expt. Sta. Bull., 51: 65–109.

EWING, H. E. 1913 A New Parasite of the House-Fly (*Acarina, Gamasoidea*). Ent. News, 24: 452–456.

EWING, H. E. 1942 The Relation of Flies (*Musca domestica* Linnaeus) to the Transmission of Bovine Mastitis. Am. J. Vet. Res., 3: 295–299.

EWING, H. E., AND HARTZELL, A. 1918 The Chigger-Mites Affecting Man and Domestic Animals. J. Econ. Ent., 11: 256–264.

EYLES, E. D. 1945 Landing on a Ceiling. New York Times, Aug. 12, 1945.

FAICHNIE, N. 1909a Fly-borne Enteric Fever; the Source of Infection. J. R. Army Med. Corps, 13: 580–584.

FAICHNIE, N. 1909b *Bacillus typhosus* in Flies. J. R. Army Med. Corps, 13: 672–675.

FAIRCHILD, DAVID, AND FAIRCHILD, MARIAN 1914 A Book of Monsters. Nat. Geog. Mag., 26: 89–98.

FANTHAM, H. B. 1922 Some Parasitic Protozoa Found in South Africa. V. S. Afr. J. Sci., 19: 332–339.

FANTHAM, H. B., AND ROBERTSON, K. G. 1927 Some Parasitic Protozoa Found in South Africa. X. S. Afr. J. Sci., 24: 441–449.

FAY, R. W. 1939 A Control for the Larvae of Houseflies in Manure Piles. J. Econ. Ent., 32: 851–854.

FAY, R. W., BUCKNER, A. J., AND SIMMONS, S. W. 1948 Laboratory Evaluation of DDT Residual Effectiveness against Houseflies, *Musca domestica*. Am. J. Trop. Med., 28: 877–888.

FELDMAN-MUHSAM, B. 1944a A Note on the Conditions of Pupation of *Musca domestica vicina* (Diptera) in Palestine, and Its Application. Proc. R. Ent. Soc. London, Ser. A, Gen. Entomology, 19: 139–140.

FELDMAN-MUHSAM, B. 1944b Studies on the Ecology of the Levant House Fly (*Musca domestica vicina* Macq.). Bull. Ent. Res., 35: 53–67.

FELT, E. P. 1910a Control of Flies and Other Household Insects. Bull. 465, New York State Educ. Dept. (*M. domestica*, pp. 6–16.)

FELT, E. P. 1910b Methods of Controlling the House-Fly and Thus Preventing the Dissemination of Disease. New York Med. J., April 2, 1910 (no. 91): 685–687.

FELT, E. P. 1910c Typhoid or House-Fly. Twenty-fifth Report State Entomologist, Bull. 475, New York State Educ. Dept., pp. 12–17. Same observations also in J. Econ. Ent., 3: 24–26.

FENG, (LAN-CHOU) 1933 Some Parasites of Mosquitoes and Flies Found in China. Lingnan Sci. J., 12 (Suppl.): 23–31.

FERRIÈRE, C. 1920 Insectes et epidémies. Rev. Internat. de la Croix-Rouge, Geneva, 2:149–173.

FERRIÈRE. C. 1933 Note sur les parasites de *Lyperosia exigua* de Meij. Rev. Suisse Zool., 40: 637–643.

FEUERBORN, H. J. 1922 Das Hypopygium inversum und circumversum. Zool. Anz., 55: 189.

FICKER, M. 1903 Typhus und Fliegen. Arch. f. Hygiene, 46: 274–283.

FISH, W. A. 1947–1948 Embryology of *Lucilia sericata* Meigen (Diptera: Calliphoridae). Parts I and II. Ann. Ent. Soc. Am., 40: 15–28, 677–687.

FISH, W. A. 1949 Embryology of *Phaenicia sericata* Meigen (*Diptera:* Calliphoridae). Part III. The Gastrular Tube. Ann. Ent. Soc. Am., 42: 121–133.

FITCH, C. P. 1918 Animal Parasites Affecting Equines. J. Am. Vet. Med. Ass., 53 (n.s. 6): 312–330.

FLETCHER, J. 1901 Practical Entomology. (Rev. of Howard, 1900, Ins. Fauna of Human Excr.) Canad. Ent., 33: 84–88.

FLEXNER, S., AND CLARK, P. F. 1911 Contamination of the House-Fly with Poliomyelitis Virus. J. Am. Med. Ass., 56: 1717–1718.

FLU, P. C. 1911 Studien über die im Darm der Stubenfliege, *Musca domestica,* vorkommenden protozoären Gebilde. Centralbl. Bakt., 57: 522–534.

FORD, NORMA. 1932 Observations on the Behaviour of the Sarcophagid Fly, *Wohlfahrtia vigil* (Walk.) J. Parasit., 19: 106–111.

FORD, N. 1936 Further Observations on the Behaviour of *Wohlfahrtia vigil* (Walk.) with Notes on the Collecting and Rearing of the Flies. J. Parasit., 22: 309–328.

FRAENKEL, G. 1932 Untersuchungen über die Koordination von Reflexen und automatisch-nervosen Rhythmen bei Insekten. Zeit. Vergl. Physiol., 16: 371–462.

FRAENKEL, G. 1935 Hormone Controlling Pupation: *Calliphora,* Dipt. Proc. R. Soc. (B), 118: 1–12.

FRAENKEL, G. 1939 The Function of the Halteres of Flies. Proc. Zool. Soc. London (ser. A, General and Experimental) 109: 69–78.

FRAENKEL, G., AND PRINGLE, J. W. S. 1938 Halteres of Flies as Gyroscopic Organs of Equilibrium. Nature, 141: 919–920.

FRANCIS, T., JR., BROWN, G. C., AND PENNER, L. R. 1948 Search for Extrahuman Sources of Poliomyelitis Virus. J. Am. Med. Ass., 136: 1088–1092.

FREEBORN, S. B., AND BERRY, L. J. 1935 Color Preferences of the House Fly, *Musca domestica* L. J. Econ. Ent., 28: 913–916.

FRINGS, H. 1941a Rearing Blowflies in the Laboratory. J. Econ. Ent., 34: 317.

FRINGS, H. 1941b The Loci of Olfactory End-Organs in the Blowfly *Cynomyia cadaverina* Desvoidy. J. Exp. Zool., 88: 65–93.

FRINGS, H. 1948 Rearing Houseflies and Blowflies on Dog Biscuit. Science, 107: 629–630.

FRISON, T. H. 1925 Intestinal Myiasis and the Common Housefly (*Musca domestica* Linn.). J. Econ. Ent., 18: 334–336.

FROGGATT, W. W. 1917 "Policeman Flies." Fossorial Wasps That Catch Flies. Agric. Gaz. New S. Wales, Sydney, 28: 667–669.

FROGGATT, W. W. 1921 Sheep-Maggot Flies and Their Parasites. Agric. Gaz. New S. Wales, Sydney, 32: 725–731, 807–813.

FRYE, W. W., AND MELENEY, H. E. 1932 Investigations of *Endamoeba histolytica* and other Intestinal Protozoa in Tennessee. IV. A Study of Flies, Rats, Mice and some Domestic Animals as Possible Carriers of the Intestinal Protozoa of Man in a Rural Community. Am. J. Hyg., 16: 729–749.

FULLAWAY, D. T. 1917 Description of a New Species of *Spalangia*. Proc. Hawaiian Ent. Soc., 3: 292–294.

FÜSTHY, Ö. 1937 Observations Concerning the Development and Biological Characteristics of the Housefly. (In Hungarian.) Különlenyomat a "Népegeszségügy" 1937. Évi 11. Számából.

GABBI, U. 1917 Dissenteria amebica. Malaria e Malattie dei Paesi Caldi, Rome, 8: 218–240.

GAFFRON, M. 1933 Untersuchungen über das Bewegungssehen bei Libellenlarven, Fliegen und Fischen. Zeit. Vergl. Physiol., 20: 299–337.

GALAINE, C., AND HOULBERT, C. 1916 Pour chasser les mouches de nos habitations. Compt. Rend. Acad. Sci., Paris, 163 (no. 5): 132–135.

GALLIARD, H. 1934 Un nouveau Cas de myiase oculaire due à *Oestrus ovis* en France. Ann. de Parasit. Humaine et Compar., 12: 177–181.

GALTSOFF, P. S., LUTZ, F. E., WELCH, P. S., AND NEEDHAM, J. G. 1937 Culture Methods for Invertebrate Animals. Ithaca, N.Y.

GENERALI, G. 1886 Una larva di nematode della mosca commune. Atti Soc. d. Nat. di Modena, Rendic., ser. 3, 2: 88–89.

GEOFFROY, E. L. 1764 Histoire abrégée des insectes, 2: 624.

GERSTON, C. D., LANCASTER, W. E. G., LARSON, G. A., AND WHEELER, G. C. 1933 *Wohlfahrtia* Myiasis in North Dakota. J. Am. Med. Ass., 100: 487–488.

GILL, C. A., AND LAL, R. B. 1931 The Epidemiology of Cholera, with Special Reference to Transmission. Indian J. Med. Res., 18: 1255–1297.

GILMOUR, D. 1946 The Toxicity to Houseflies of Paints Containing DDT. J. Coun. Sci. Industr. Res. Aust., 19: 225–232.

GIRAULT, A. A., AND SANDERS, G. E. 1910 The Chalcidoid Parasites of the Common House or Typhoid Fly (*Musca domestica*, Linn.) and Its Allies. Psyche, 17: 9–28.

GLASER, R. W. 1922 *Herpetomonas muscae domesticae*, Its Behavior and Effect in Laboratory Animals. J. Parasit., 8: 99–108.

GLASER, R. W. 1923a The Effect of Food on Longevity and Reproduction in Flies. J. Exp. Zool., 38: 383–412.

GLASER, R. W. 1923b The Survival of Bacteria in the Pupal and Adult Stages of Flies. Am. J. Hyg., 3: 469–480.

GLASER, R. W. 1924a Rearing Flies for Experimental Purposes with Biological Notes. J. Econ. Ent., 17: 486–496.

GLASER, R. W. 1924b A Bacterial Disease of Adult House Flies. Am. J. Hyg., 4: 411–415.

GLASER, R. W. 1924c The Relation of Microorganisms to the Development and Longevity of Flies. Am. J. Trop. Med., 4: 85–107.

GLASER, R. W. 1926a Further Experiments on a Bacterial Disease of Adult Flies with a Revision of the Etiological Agent. Ann. Ent. Soc. Am., 19: 193–198.

GLASER, R. W. 1926b The Isolation and Cultivation of *Herpetomonas muscae-domesticae*. Am. J. Trop. Med., 6: 205–219.

GLASER, R. W. 1938a A Method for the Sterile Culture of Houseflies. J. Parasit., 24: 177–179.

GLASER, R. W. 1938b Test of a Theory on the Origin of Bacteriophage. Am. J. Hyg., 27: 311–315.

GODFREY, R. 1909 The False-Scorpions of Scotland. Ann. Scot. Nat. Hist., no. 69 (Jan. 1909): 22–26.

GOLDING, F. D. 1946 A New Method of Trapping Flies. Bull. Ent. Res., 37: 143–154.

GÓMEZ, L. 1946 Revisión critica de los casos de oftalmomiasis españolas. Rev. Ibér. Parasit., 6: 51–73.

GOMEZA OZAMIZ, J. M. 1945 El descubrimiento del nuero insecticida 666. Ion, 5: 745–750.

GORODETZSKII, A. S., AND SUKHOVA, M. N. 1936a Nouveaux poisons pour la destruction des stades préimaginales des mouches. (In Russian.) Med. Parasit., 5: 303–323. (French summary.)

GORODETZSKII, A. S., AND SUKHOVA, M. N. 1936b Les Dépôts de fumier et les caisses à ordures comme pièges pour les larves des mouches. (In Russian.) Med. Parasit., 5: 324–328.

GOSIO, B. 1925 Über die Verbreitung der Bubonenpesterreger durch Insekten-larven. Arch. Schiffs. u. Trop. Hyg., 29 Beiheft 1: 134–139.

GOURDON, G. 1929 La Capture et la destruction des insectes par rayons ultra-violets. Recherches Inventions, 10: 245–250.

GRADY, A. G. 1928 Studies in Breeding Insects throughout the Year for Insecti-cide Tests. I. House Flies (*Musca domestica*). J. Econ. Ent., 21: 598–604.

GRAHAM-SMITH, G. S. 1909 Preliminary Note on Examinations of Flies for the Presence of Colon Bacilli. Repts. Local Govnt. Bd. Publ. Health and Med. Subjects, n.s. 16; Further Prelim. Repts. on Flies as Carriers of Infection, pp. 9–13.

GRAHAM-SMITH, G. S. 1910 Observations on the Ways in Which Artificially Infected Flies (*Musca domestica*) Carry and Distribute Pathogenic and Other Bacteria. Repts. Local Govnt. Bd. Health and Med. Subjects, n.s. 40; Further Repts. (no. 3) on Flies as Carriers of Infection: 1–41.

GRAHAM-SMITH, G. S. 1911a Further Observations on the Ways in Which Artifi-cially Infected Flies (*Musca domestica* and *Calliphora erythrocephala*) Carry and Distribute Pathogenic and Other Bacteria. Repts. Local Govnt. Bd. Publ. Health and Med. Subjects, n.s. 53; Further Reports (no. 4): 31–48.

GRAHAM-SMITH, G. S. 1911b Some Observations on the Anatomy and Function of the Oral Sucker of the Blow-Fly (*Calliphora erythrocephala*). J. Hyg., 11: 390–408.

GRAHAM-SMITH, G. S. 1912a An Investigation of the Incidence of the Micro-Organisms Known as Non-Lactose Fermenters in Flies in Normal Surroundings and in Surroundings Associated with Epidemic Diarrhoea. *In* 41st Ann. Rept. Local Govnt. Bd., Supp. Rept. Med. Officer, 1911–1912: 304–329.

GRAHAM-SMITH, G. S. 1912b An Investigation into the Possibility of Pathogenic Micro-Organisms Being Taken Up by the Larva and Subsequently Distributed by the Fly. *In* 41st Ann. Rept. Local Govnt. Bd., Supp. Rept. Med. Officer, 1911–1912: 330–335.

GRAHAM-SMITH, G. S. 1913 Further Observation on Non-Lactose Fermenting Bacilli in Flies, and the Sources from Which They Are Derived with Special Reference to Morgan's Bacillus. Repts. Local Govnt. Bd. Publ. Health and Med. Subjects, n.s. 85; Further Rept. (no. 6) on Flies as Carriers of Infection: 43–46.

GRAHAM-SMITH, G. S. 1914 Flies in Relation to Disease: Nonbloodsucking Flies. Cambridge, Eng.

GRAHAM-SMITH, G. S. 1916 Observations on the Habits and Parasites of Common Flies. Parasitology, 8: 440–544.

GRAHAM-SMITH, G. S. 1919 Further Observations on the Habits and Parasites of Common Flies. Parasitology, 11: 347–384.

GRAHAM-SMITH, G. S. 1930a Further Observations on the Anatomy and Function of the Proboscis of the Blow-Fly, *Calliphora erythrocephala* L. Parasitology, 22: 47–115.

GRAHAM-SMITH, G. S. 1930b The Oscinidae (Diptera) as Vectors of Conjunctivitis and the Anatomy of Their Mouth Parts. Parasitology, 22: 457–467.

GRAHAM-SMITH, G. S. 1934 The Alimentary Canal of *Calliphora erythrocephala* L. with Special Reference to Its Musculature and to the Proventriculus, Rectal Valve and Rectal Papillae. Parasitology, 26: 176–248.

GRANDORI, R. 1938 L'azione disinfestante della calciocianamide contro la mosca domestica sperimentalmente dimonstrata. Boll. Zool. Agrar. Bachic., 8: 233–250.

GRANTHAM-HILL, C. 1933 Preliminary Note on the Treatment of Infected Wounds with the Larva of *Wohlfahrtia nuba*. Trans. R. Soc. Trop. Med. and Hyg., 27: 93–98.

GRASSI, B. 1879 Dei pro tozoi parassiti e specialamente di quelli che sono nell'uomo. Gaz. Med. Ital. Lombard., 39: 445–448.

GRASSI, B. 1882 Intorno ad alcuni protista endoparassitici ed appartenenti alle classi dei Flagellati, Lobosi, Sporozoi e Ciliati. Memoria de Parassitología Comparata. Atti Soc. Ital. Sci. Nat., 24: 135–224.

GRASSI, B., AND ROVELLI, G. 1892 Ricerche embriologiche sui Cestodi. Atti Accad. Gionia di Sci. Nat., Catania., 4: 1–108.

GRIFFITHS, J. T., JR. 1946 DDT Used to Control Flies in Manila. J. Econ. Ent., 39: 750–755.

GROAT, R. A.   1939   Two New Mounting Media Superior to Canada Balsam and Gum Damar.   Anat. Rec., 74: 1–6.

GUSSOW, H. T.   1917   *Empusa muscae* versus *Musca domestica,* L.   Ann. App. Biol., 3: 150–158.

HACKMAN, R. H.   1947   The Persistence of DDT on Cattle.   J. Coun. Sci. Industr. Res. Aust., 20: 56–65.

HAESER.   1899   Plague and Flies.   Geschichte der Med. u. Epidem. Krankh., 3 Aufl., Vol. 3.   (Cited by Nuttall, 1899.)

HAFEZ, H. C.   1939   Some Ecological Observations on the Insect-Fauna of Dung. Bull. Soc. Fouad ler Ent., 23: 241–287.

HAFEZ, M.   1941a   Investigations into the Problem of Fly Control in Egypt.   Bull. Soc. Fouad ler Ent., 25: 99–144.

HAFEZ, M.   1941b   A Study of the Biology of the Egyptian Common House-Fly: *Musca vicina* Macq. (Diptera: Muscidae). Bull. Soc. Fouad ler Ent., 25: 163–189.

HALL, M. C.   1929   Arthropods as Intermediate Hosts of Helminths.   Smithson. Misc. Coll., 81 (no. 15).

HAMER, W. H.   1910   Flies and Vermin. Report by the Medical Officer of Health Presenting Report by Dr. Hamer, Medical Officer (General Purposes), on Nuisance from Flies and on the Seasonal Prevalence of Vermin in Common Lodging-houses.   Report of the Public Health Committee of the London County Council for 1909, Appendix 4.

HAMILTON, A.   1903   The Fly as a Carrier of Typhoid; an Inquiry into the Part Played by the Common House Fly in the Recent Epidemic of Typhoid Fever in Chicago.   J. Am. Med. Ass., 40: 576–583.

HAMILTON, A.   1904   The Common House-Fly as a Carrier of Typhoid Fever. J. Am. Med. Ass., 42: 1034.

HAMILTON, A.   1906   The Role of the House-Fly and Other Insects in the Spread of Infectious Diseases.   Ill. Med. J., Springfield, 9: 583–587.

HAMMER, O.   1941   Biological and Ecological Investigations on Flies Associated with Pasturing Cattle and Their Excrement.   Vidensk. Medd. Dansk. Naturh. Forens.   (Summary in Danish.)   Copenhagen.

HAMMOND, A.   1881   On the Thorax of the Blow-Fly (*Musca vomitoria*).   J. Linn. Soc. (Zool.), 15: 9–31.

HANAWALT, E.   1945   The Trend in Fly Control. Mich. State Coll. Vet., 5: 163–167.

HARDY, G. H.   1924   A Blowfly and Some Parasites.   Queensland Agric. J., 22: 349–350.

HARDY, G. H.   1934   Twelfth Annual Report of the Walter and Eliza Hall Fellow in Economic Biology.   Brisbane, Australia.   (Multigraph.)

HARDY, G. H.   1935   The Positions Assumed by Copulating Diptera.   Ann. Mag. Nat. Hist., 16: 419–434.

HARDY, G. H.   1944   The Copulation and the Terminal Segments of Diptera. Proc. R. Ent. Soc. London (A), 19: 52–65.

HARGREAVES, E. 1923 Entomological Notes from Taranto (Italy), with References to Faenza, during 1917 and 1918. Bull. Ent. Res., 14: 213–219.

HARRIS, A. H., AND DOWN, H. A. 1946 Studies of the Dissemination of Cysts and Ova of Human Intestinal Parasites by Flies in Various Localities on Guam. Am. J. Trop. Med., 26: 789–900.

HARSHAM, A. 1946 Debunking a Color Theory. Food Indust., 18: 851, 984.

HARTZELL, A. 1945 Histological Effects of Certain Sprays and Activators on the Nerves and Muscles of the Housefly. Contr. Boyce Thompson Inst., 13: 443–454.

HARTZELL, A., AND SCUDDER, H. L. 1942 Histological Effects of Pyrethrum and an Activator on the Central Nervous System of the Housefly. J. Econ. Ent., 35: 428–433.

HARTZELL, A., AND STRONG, M. 1944 Histological Effects of Piperine on the Central Nervous System of the Housefly. Contr. Boyce Thompson Inst., 13: 253–257.

HARTZELL, A., AND WEXLER, E. 1946 Histological Effects of Sesamin on the Brain and Muscles of the Housefly. Contr. Boyce Thompson Inst., 14: 123–126.

HASE, A. 1935 Über Wärmeentwicklung in Massenzuchten von Insekten sowie über ein einfaches Verfahren, Stubenfliegen daurend zu züchten. Zool. Anz., 112: 291–298.

HAYDON, L. G. 1922 Memorandum on the Disposal of Animal Manure and Garbage in Relation to Fly-Breeding, and the Prevention of Enteric Fever and Other Intestinal Diseases. S. African Med. Rec., Cape Town, 20: 230–232.

HAYES, W. P., AND LIU, YU-SU 1947 Tarsal Chemoreceptors of the Housefly and Their Possible Relation to DDT Toxicity. Ann. Ent. Soc. Am., 40: 401–416.

HAYWARD, E. H. 1904 The Fly as a Carrier of Tuberculosis Infection. New York Med. J., 80: 643–644.

HENNEGUY, L. F. 1904 Les Insectes. Paris. (*M. domestica*, pp. 155, 168, 497.)

HEPWORTH, J. 1854 On the Structure of the Foot of the Fly. Quart. J. Micr. Sci., 2: 158–160.

HERMS, W. B. 1909a Essentials of House-Fly Control. Bull. Berkeley (Calif.) Bd. of Health, June 29, 1909.

HERMS, W. B. 1909b The Berkeley House-Fly Campaign. Calif. J. Technol., 14 (no. 2).

HERMS, W. B. 1909c Medical Entomology, Its Scope and Methods. J. Econ. Ent., 2: 265–268.

HERMS, W. B. 1911a The Housefly in Its Relation to the Public Health. Univ. of Calif. Agric. Exp. Sta. Bull. 215: 513–548.

HERMS, W. B. 1911b The Photic Reactions of Sarcophagid Flies etc. Contr. Zool. Lab. Mus. Comp. Zool. Harvard, no. 217.

HERMS, W. B. 1928 The Effect of Different Quantities of Food during the Larval Period on the Sex Ratio and Size of *Lucilia sericata* Meigen and *Theobaldia incidens* Thom. J. Econ. Ent., 21: 720–729.

HERMS, W. B.   1944   Medical Entomology, with Special Reference to the Health and Well-Being of Man and Animals.   3d ed.   New York.

HEROLD, W.   1922   Beobachtungen an zwei Feinden der Stubenfliege: *Mellinus arvensis,* L. und *Vespa germanica,* Fabr.   Zeit. Angew. Ent., Berlin, 8: 459.

HESSE, E.   1913   A Parasitic Mould of the House Fly.   Brit. Med. J., Jan. 4, 1913: 41.

HESSE, R., ALLEE, W. C., AND SCHMIDT, K. P.   1937   Ecological Animal Geography.   New York.

HEWITT, C. G.   1912a   House-Flies and How They Spread Disease. Cambridge, Eng.   (*In* Cambridge Manuals of Science and Literature.)

HEWITT, C. G.   1912b   *Fannia (Homalomyia) canicularis* Linn. and F. *scalaris* Fab.   Parasitology, 5: 161–174.

HEWITT, C. G.   1912d   An Account of the Bionomics and the Larvae of the Flies *Fannia (Homalomyia) canicularis* L. and F. *scalaris* Fab., and Their Relation to Myiasis of the Intestinal and Urinary Tracts.   Repts. Local Govnt. Bd. Publ. Health and Med. Subjects, n.s. 60; Further Reports (no. 5) on Flies as Carriers of Infection: 15–22.

HEWITT, C. G.   1914a   The Housefly *Musca domestica* Linn. Its Structure, Habits, Development, Relation to Disease and Control.   Cambridge, Eng.

HEWITT, C. G.   1914b   House-Flies and How They Spread Disease.   Cambridge, Eng.   (*In* Cambridge Manuals of Science and Literature.)

HEWITT, C. G.   1914c   On the Predaceous Habits of Scatophaga: A New Enemy of *Musca domestica.*   Canad., Ent., 46: 2–3.

HEWITT, C. G.   1915a   Notes on the Pupation of the House-Fly (*Musca domestica*) and Its Mode of Overwintering.   Canad. Ent., 47: 73–78.

HEWITT, C. G.   1915b   House-Fly Control.   Agric. Gaz. Canada, Ottawa, 2: 418–421.

HICKSON, S. J.   1905   A Parasite of the House-Fly.   Nature, Oct. 26, 1905.

HILL, G. F.   1918   Relationship of Insects to Parasitic Diseases in Stock.   Proc. R. Soc. Victoria, Melbourne, 31: 11–107.

HILL, G. F.   1921   *Musca domestica* L. as a "Bush Fly" in Australia.   Ann. Trop. Med. Parasit., 15: 93–94.

HILL, K. R., AND ROBINSON, G.   1945   A Fatal Case of DDT Poisoning in a Child, with an Account of Two Accidental Deaths in Dogs.   Brit. Med. J., 2: 845–847.

HINDLE, E.   1914a   Flies in Relation to Disease: Bloodsucking Flies.   Cambridge, Eng.

HINDLE, E.   1914b   The Flight of the House Fly.   Proc. Cambridge Phil. Soc., 17: 310–313.

HINDLE, E., AND MERRIMAN, G.   1914   The Range of Flight of *Musca domestica.*   J. Hyg., 14: 23–45.

HOARE, C. A.   1924   A Note on the Specific Name of the Herpetomonad of the House Fly.   Trans. R. Soc. Trop. Med. and Hyg., 17: 403–406.

HOBSON, R. P. 1932 ("Ammonia Production by Sterile *Lucilia* Larvae, Dipt.") J. Exp. Biol., 9: 128–138, 366–377.

HODGE, C. F. 1910 A Practical Point in the Study of Typhoid or Filth Fly. Nature Study Review, 6: 195–199.

HODGE, C. F. 1911a A Plan to Exterminate the Typhoid or Filth-Disease Fly. La Follette's Weekly Magazine, Madison, Wisc., 3: 7–8. (No. 15.)

HODGE, C. F. 1911b How You Can Make Your Home, Town or City, Flyless. Nature and Culture, Cincinnati, Ohio, 3: 9–23. (Nos. 2 and 3.)

HODGE, C. F. 1911c Exterminating the Fly. California Outlook, Sept. 30, 1911.

HODGE, C. F. 1913a The Distance House-Flies, Blue-Bottle and Stable Flies May Travel over Water. Science, 38: 512–513.

HODGE, C. F. 1913b A New Fly Trap. J. Econ. Ent., 6: 110–112.

HOFFMAN, C. H., AND SURBER, E. W. 1949 Effects of Feeding DDT-sprayed Insects to Fresh-Water Fish. Special Scientific Report-Fisheries, no. 3, U.S. Dept. of the Interior, Fish and Wildlife Service. Washington, D.C., Oct. 1949.

HOFFMAN, R. A., AND LINDQUIST, A. W. 1949 Fumigating Properties of Several New Insecticides. J. Econ. Ent., 42: 436–438.

HOFMANN, E. 1888 Über die Verbreitung der Tuberculose durch Stubenfliegen. Correspondenzbl. d. ärztl. Kreis-und Bezirksvereine im Königr. Sachsen, 44: 130–135.

HOLLICK, F. S. J. 1940 The Flight of the Dipterous Fly *Muscina stabulans* Fallén. Proc. R. Soc. London (B), 129: 55–56.

HOLLICK, F. S. J. 1941 The Flight of the Dipterous Fly *Muscina stabulans*. Philosoph. Trans. R. Soc. London (B), 230: 357–390.

HONEIJ, J. A., AND PARKER, R. R. 1914 Leprosy: Flies in Relation to the Transmission of the Disease. J. Med. Res., 30: 127–130.

HOPE, F. W. 1840 On the Insects and Their Larvae Occasionally Found in the Human Body. Trans. Ent. Soc. London, 2: 256–271.

HORSTMANN, D. M. 1945 The Role of Flies in the Epidemiology of Poliomyelitis. J. Bact., 50: 236.

HOSKINS, W. M., AND CALDWELL, A. H., JR. 1947 Development and Use of a Small Spray Chamber. Soap and Sanit. Chem., 23: 143–145, 161, 163, 165, 167.

HOWARD, C. W. 1917a Hibernation of the House-Fly in Minnesota. J. Econ. Ent., 10: 464–468.

HOWARD, C. W. 1917b What the House-Fly Costs? Minnesota Insect Life, St. Paul, Vol. 4.

HOWARD, C. W. 1917c A Fly Control Exhibit. J. Econ. Ent., 10: 411–412.

HOWARD, C. W., AND CLARK, P. F. 1912 Experiments on Insect Transmission of the Virus of Poliomyelitis. J. Exp. Med., 16: 850–859.

HOWARD, L. O. 1896 House-Flies, *in* The Principal Household Insects of the United States, by L. O. Howard and C. L. Marlatt, U.S. Dept. Agric., Division of Entomology. Bull. 4 (n.s.): 43–47. (Rev. ed., 1902.)

HOWARD, L. O. 1900 A Contribution to the Study of the Insect Fauna of Human Excrement (with Special Reference to the Spread of Typhoid Fever by Flies). Proc. Washington Acad. Sci., 2: 541–604.

HOWARD, L. O. 1909a Economic Loss to the People of the United States through Insects That Carry Disease. Nat. Geog. Mag., 20 (Aug. 1909): 735–749.

HOWARD, L. O. 1909b Economic Loss to the People of the United States through Insects That Carry Disease. U.S. Dept. Agric., Bur. of Ent., Bull. 78.

HOWARD, L. O. 1911a The House Fly, Disease Carrier; an Account of Its Dangerous Activities and of the Means of Destroying It. New York and London.

HOWARD, L. O. 1911b House-Flies. U.S. Dept. Agric., Farmers' Bull. 459.

HOWARD, L. O. 1911c Flies as Carriers of Infection. Science (n.s.), 34: 24–25.

HOWARD, L. O., AND HUTCHISON, R. H. 1917 The House-Fly. U.S. Dept. Agric., Farmers' Bull. 851.

HOWELL, D. E. 1942 The Use of Arsenicals for the Control of Housefly Larvae. Proc. Okla. Acad. Sci. for 1941, 22: 68–72.

HUNTER, W. 1907 Occurrence of Plague Bacilli in Alimentary Tract of Flies that had Fed on Infected Material in Hong Kong. (Quoted in article, "The Danger of the Common Fly.") Nursing Times, Sept. 28, 1907: 842. (Cited by Nuttall and Jepson, 1909.)

HUNTER, W. D. 1913 American Interest in Medical Entomology. J. Econ. Ent., 6: 27–39.

HUTCHINSON, WOODS 1911 "How Doth the Little Busy Fly?" Country Life (U.S.A.), 20 (Aug. 15, 1911): 31–33.

HUTCHISON, R. H. 1914 The Migratory Habit of House Fly Larvae as Indicating a Favorable Remedial Measure. An Account of Progress. U.S. Dept. Agric. Bull. 14.

HUTCHISON, R. H. 1915 A Maggot Trap in Practical Use; an Experiment in House-Fly Control. U.S. Dept. Agric. Bull. 200.

ILLINGWORTH, J. F. 1923a Insect Fauna of Hen Manure. Proc. Hawaiian Ent. Soc., 5 (1922): 270–273.

ILLINGWORTH, J. F. 1923b House-Flies. Proc. Hawaiian Ent. Soc., 5 (1922): 275–276.

ILLINGWORTH, J. F. 1926a The Common Muscoid Flies Occurring about Sweet-Shops in Yokohama, Japan. Proc. Hawaiian Ent. Soc., 6 (1925): 260–261.

ILLINGWORTH, J. F. 1926b Notes on *Sarcophaga fuscicauda* Böttcher (Diptera). Proc. Hawaiian Ent. Soc., 6 (1925): 262–265.

IMMS, A. D. 1938 A General Textbook of Entomology. 4th ed. London.

INGLE, L. 1943 An Apparatus for Testing Chemotropic Responses of Flying Insects. J. Econ. Ent., 36: 108–110.

ISAAC, P. V. 1944 Prevention of House-Fly Breeding. Indian Fmg., 5: 61–62.

IWANOFF, X. 1934 Über Sommerwunden beim Rinde. Arch. Tierheilk, 67: 261–270.

JACK, R. W., AND WILLIAMS, W. L. 1937 The Effect of Temperature on the Reaction of *Glossina morsitans* Westw. to Light. A Preliminary Note. Bull. Ent. Res., 28: 499–503.

JACKSON, D. D. 1907 Pollution of New York Harbour as a Menace to Health by the Dissemination of Intestinal Disease through the Agency of the Common House-Fly. A Report to the Committee on Pollution of the Merchants' Association of New York.

JACKSON, D. D. 1908 Conveyance of Disease by Flies Summarised. Boston Med. and Surg. J., 1908: 451.

JAMES, H. C. 1928 On the Life-Histories and Economic Status of Certain Cynipid Parasites of Dipterous Larvae, with Descriptions of Some New Larval Forms. Ann. Appl. Biol., 15: 287–316.

JAMES, M. T. 1944 Two Erroneous Records in American Literature of the Causative Agents of Myiasis. J. Parasit., 30: 273–274.

JAMES, M. T. 1947 The Flies That Cause Myiasis in Man. U.S. Dept. Agric. Misc. Publ. 631, Washington, D.C.

JANET, C. 1907 Sur l'origine du tissu adipeux imaginal, pendant la nymphose chez les Muscides (Dipt.) Bull. Soc. Ent. Fr., 1907: 350–351.

JANET, C. 1911 Sur l'existence d'un organe chordotonal et d'une vésicule pulsatile antennaires chez l'abeille et sur la morphologie de la tête de cette espèce. Compt. Rend. Acad. Sci., 152: 110–11.

JANISCH, E. 1928 Die Lebens-und Entwicklungsdauer der Insekten als Temperaturfunktion. Zeit. Wiss. Zool., 132.

JANISCH, E. 1933 Über die Konstanthaltung von Temperatur und Luftfeuchtigkeit im biologischen Laboratoriumversuch. Abderhaldens Handbuch d. biol. Arbeitsmethoden, Abt. V, Teil 10.

JANISCH, E., AND MAERCKS, H. 1933 Über die Berechnung der Kettenlinie als Ansdruck für die Temperatur-Abhängigkeit von Lebenserscheinungen. Arb. biol. Reichsamst. Dahlern 20.

JAUSION, H., AND DEKESTER, M. 1923 Sur la transmission comparée des kystes d'*Entamoeba dystenteriae* et de *Giardia intestinalis* par les mouches. Arch. Insts. Pasteur Afr. Nord., 3: 154–155.

JEPSON, F. P. 1915 Report of the Entomologist. Dept. Agric. Fiji, Ann. Rept. for the Year 1914, Suva, 1915: 17–27.

JOHANNSEN, O. A., AND BUTT, F. H. 1941 Embryology of Insects and Myriapods. New York and London.

JOHNSTON, T. H. 1921 The Sheep Maggot Fly Problem in Queensland. Queensland Agric. J., Brisbane, 15: 244–248.

JOHNSTON, T. H., AND BANCROFT, M. J. 1921 The Life History of *Habronema* in Relation to *Musca domestica* and Native Flies in Queensland. Proc. R. Soc. Queensland, 32 (5): 61–88.

JOHNSTON, T. H., AND TIEGS, O. W. 1922 On the Biology and Economic Significance of the Chalcid Parasites of Australian Sheep Maggot-Flies. Proc. R. Soc. Queensland, 33 (1921): 99–128.

JOLLY, G. G. 1923 An Automatic Fly-proof Latrine Seat. Indian Med. Gaz., 58 (no. 12): 575–578.

JONES, H. A., AND FLUNO, H. J. 1946 DDT-Xylene Emulsions for Use against Insects Affecting Man. J. Econ. Ent., 39: 735–740.

JOSHI, K. G., AND DNYANSAGAR, V. R. 1945 Some Observations on Fly Breeding in Compost Trenches. Indian Med. Gaz., 80: 358–361.

KALANDADZE, L. P., AND CHILINGAROVA, S. V. 1942a On the Use of Sticky Paper against Flies. (In Russian.) Med. Parasit., 10: 569–572.

KALANDADZE, L. P., AND CHILINGAROVA, S. V. 1942b The Role of Substrates in the Oviposition and Pre-imaginal Development of *Musca vicina* Macq. (In Russian.) Med. Parasit., 11: 105–112.

KAMPMEIER, O. F., AND HAVILAND, T. N. 1948 On the Mounting of Anatomical Museum Specimens in Transparent Plastics. Anat. Rec., 100: 201–231.

KATAGAI, T. 1935 Seasonal Fluctuation of the Numbers of *Musca domestica* L. in the City of Taihoku. (In Japanese.) Tokyo Iji-Shimshi, no. 2929: 1218–1223.

KEARNS, H. G. H. 1942 The Control of Flies in Country and Town. Ann. Appl. Biol., 29: 310–313.

KEILIN, D. 1916 Viviparity in Diptera. Arch. Zool., 55: 393–415.

KELEVIN, N. V., AND RUIBINA, A. D. 1940 Myase de l'oreille chez l'homme provoquée par les larves de *Musca domestica*. (In Russian.) Med. Parasit., 9: 531.

KENNEY, M. 1945 Experimental Intestinal Myiasis in Man. Proc. Soc. Exp. Biol. and Med., 60: 235–237.

KENT, W. S. 1880–1882 A Manual of the Infusoria. London.

KERR (DR.) 1906 Some Prevalent Diseases in Morocco. Paper read before the Glasgow Medico-chirurgical Society, Dec. 7, 1906.

KERR, R. W. 1948 The Effect of Starvation on the Susceptibility of Houseflies to Pyrethrum Sprays. Aust. J. Sci. Res., 1: 76–92.

KEW, H. W. 1901 Lincolnshire Pseudo-Scorpions: With an Account of the Association of Such Animals with Other Arthropods. Naturalist, no. 534 (July 1901): 193–215.

KING, H. N. 1918 Some Unusual Methods of Disposal of Excreta in Camps. Indian Med. Gaz., 53: 74–75.

KINGSBURY, B. F., AND JOHANNSEN, O. A. 1935 Histological Technique. A Guide for Use in a Laboratory Course in Histology. New York.

KINGSCOTTE, A. A. 1935 Myiasis in Man and Animals due to Infection with the Larvae of *Wohlfahrtia vigil* (Walker). Ontario Vet. Coll. Rept., 1934: 51–69.

KIRBY AND SPENCE 1826 Introduction to Entomology. 4: 228–229.

KITZMILLER, J. B. 1949 The Use of Dioxane in Insect Microtechnique. Trans. Am. Micr. Soc., 67: 227–230.

KLECHETOVA, A. M. 1946 Hexachlorethane as an Insecticide for the Destruction of the Larvae of Flies. (In Russian.) Med. Parasit., 15 (6): 77–81.

KLEIN, E. 1908 Flies as Carriers of the *Bacillus typhosus*. Brit. Med. J., 2: 1150–1151.

KLING, C., AND LEVADITI, C. 1913 Etudes sur la poliomyélite aigue épidémique. Ann. Inst. Pasteur, Paris, 27: 718–749.

KLOTS, A. B. 1932 Directions for Collecting and Preserving Insects. Ward's Natural Science Establishment. Rochester.

KNIPLING, E. F. 1949 Recent Advances in Medical and Veterinary Entomology. Bull. New York Acad. Med., 25: 388–396.

KNIPLING, E. F., AND RAINWATER, H. T. 1937 Species and Incidence of Dipterous Larvae Concerned in Wound Myiasis. J. Parasit., 23: 451–455.

KOBAYASHI, H. 1921 Overwintering of Flies. Jap. Med. World, 1 (3): 11–14.

KOBAYASHI, H. 1934a The Influence of Foods on the Fecundity of *Musca domestica*. Keijo J. Med., 5: 36–67.

KOBAYASHI, H. 1934b General Survey on the Seasonal Prevalence of the House-Fly in Chosen. Second Report: Research during 1929. Keijo J. Med., 5 (2): 69–76.

KOBAYASHI, H. 1935 The Influence of Temperature upon the Development of Larvae of *Musca domestica*. Trans. Dynam. Develop., 10: 385–395.

KOBAYASHI, H. 1940a Diapause of *Fannia canicularis*. (In Japanese.) Zool. Mag., Tokyo, 52: 118–119.

KOBAYASHI, H. 1940b Passing Winter in Flies. (In Japanese.) Rept. Jap. Ass. Adv. Sci., 15: 233–236.

KOBAYASHI, H., AND MIZUSHIMA, H. 1937 The Relationship between the Laboratory Temperature and the Development of Flies. Keijo J. Med., 8: 19–39.

KOMÁREK, J. 1936 Sur le problème de la myase intestinale. Mém. Mus. Hist. Nat. Belg. (2), Fasc. 3: 23–30.

KOZHANCHIKOV, I. V. 1947 Nutritional Value of Proteins in the Growth of Blow-Fly Larvae. (In Russian.) Rev. Ent. URSS, 28: 57–63.

KRAMER, S. 1948 A Staining Procedure for the Study of Insect Musculature. Science, 108: 141–142.

KRAMER, S. D. 1915 The Effect of Temperature on the Life Cycle of *Musca domestica* and *Culex pipiens*. Science, 41: 874–877.

KRYZHANOVSKII, O. 1944 Predatory Beetles of Tadjikistan Which Destroy the Larvae of Flies. Med. Parasit. and Parasitic Dis., 13: 73–78.

KUHN, P. 1922 Untersuchungen über die Fliegenplage in Deutschland. Centralbl. Bakt. Parasit. Infekt., Jene, I Abt. Orig. 88 (no. 3): 186–204.

KUHNS, D. M., AND ANDERSON, T. G. 1944 A Fly-borne Bacillary Dysentery Epidemic in a Large Military Organization. Am. J. Publ. Health, 34: 750–755.

KUNCKEL D'HERCULAIS, J. 1875–1881 Récherches sur l'organisation et le développement des Volucelles, insectes diptères de la famille des Syrphides. Part I. Paris.

Kuzina, O. S. 1936 Fertilität und präimaginale Mortalität bei *Musca domestica* L. (In Russian.) Med. Parasit. Moscow, 5: 329–339.

Kuzina, O. S. 1938 The Choice of Egg-Laying by the House Fly (*Musca domestica* L.). (In Russian.) Med. Parasit., 7: 244–257.

Kuzina, O. S. 1940 Rôle des organes sensitifs chez la *Musca domestica* L. dans la recherche du fumier et dans la ponte des oeufs. (In Russian.) Med. Parasit., 9: 340–349.

Kuzina, O. S. 1942 On the Gonotrophic Relationships in *Stomoxys calcitrans* L. and *Haematobia stimulans* L. (In Russian.) Med. Parasit., 11: 70–78.

Kvasnikova, P. A. 1931 Flies Observed in Human Dwellings and Outhouses in the Town of Tomsk. (In Russian.) Wiss. Ber. Biol. Fak. Tomsk. St.-Univ., 1: 9–47.

Laake, E. W., Parman, D. C., Bishopp, F. C., and Roark, R. C. 1931 The Chemotropic Responses of the House Fly, the Green-Bottle Flies and the Black Blowfly. U.S. Dept. Agric. Techn. Bull. 270.

Laing, J. 1935 On the Ptilinum of the Blow-Fly (*Calliphora erythrocephala*). Quart. J. Micr. Sci., 77: 497–521.

Lal, R. B., Ghosal, S. C., and Mukherji, B. 1939 Investigations on the Variation of Vibrios in the House Fly. Indian J. Med. Res., 26:597–609.

Lamb, C. G. 1922 The Geometry of Insect Pairing. Proc. R. Soc. (B) 94: 1–11.

Lamborn, W. A. 1935a The Annual Report of the Medical Entomologist for 1934. Ann. Med. Rept. Nyasaland, 1934: 65–69.

Lamborn, W. A. 1935b The Passage of Leprosy Bacilli through the Intestine of the Fly, *Musca sorbens* Wied. Trans. R. Soc. Trop. Med. and Hyg., 29: 3–4.

Lamborn, W. A. 1936a Annual Report of the Medical Entomologist for 1935. Ann. Med. Rept. Nyasaland, 1935: 50–52.

Lamborn, W. A. 1936b The Experimental Transmission to Man of *Treponema pertenue* by the Fly *Musca sorbens* Wd. J. Trop. Med. Hyg., 39: 235–239.

Lamborn, W. A. 1937 The Hematophagous Fly, *Musca sorbens,* Wied., in Relation to the Transmission of Leprosy. J. Trop. Med. Hyg., 40: 37–42.

Lamborn, W. A. 1939 Annual Report of the Medical Entomologist for 1938. Ann. Med. Sanit. Rept. Nyasaland, 1938: 40–48.

Lamborn, W. A. 1940 Annual Report of the Medical Entomologist for 1939. Ann. Med. Sanit. Rept. Nyasaland, 1939: 26–31.

Lamborn, W. A., and Howat, C. H. 1936 A Possible Reservoir Host of *Trypanosoma rhodesiense.* Brit. Med. J., no. 3935: 1153–1155.

Lampa, S. 1887 Om Fluglarvers Förekomst I Tarmkanalen hos Menniskau (Sur le présence de larves de mouches dans le canal intestinal de l'homme.) Ent. Tidskr., 8: 5–20. (In Swedish; French résumé, pp. 136–153.)

Larrousse, F. 1921 La Myiase oculaire à *Oestrus ovis* L. dans la région parisienne. Bull. Soc. Path. Exot., 14: 595–601.

Larsen, E. B. 1943 Problems of Heat Death and Heat Injury. Experiments on

Some Species of Diptera. K. Danske Vidensk. Selskab. Biol. Medd., 19: 1–52.

LARSEN, E. B., AND THOMSEN, M. 1940 The Influence of Temperature on the Development of Some Species of Diptera. Repr. fr. Vidensk. Medd. fra Dansk Naturh. Foren, Bd. 104.

LATREILLE, P. A. 1795 *Astoma parasiticum,* Parasitic Mite of Houseflies. Magazin Encyclopédique, 4: 15.

LATREILLE, P. A. 1810 Considérations générales sur l'ordre naturel des animaux composant les classes des crustacés, des arachnides, et des insectes. Paris.

LÄUGER, P., MARTIN, H., AND MÜLLER, P. 1944 Über Konstitution und toxische Wirkung von natürlichen und neuen synthetischen insektentötenden Stoffen. Helv. Chim. Acta, 27: 892–928.

LEACH, J. G. 1940 Insect Transmission of Plant Diseases. New York.

LEARY, J. C., FISHBEIN, W. I., AND SALTER, L. C. 1946 DDT and the Insect Problem. New York and London.

LEBAILLY, C. 1924 Le Mouches ne jouent pas de rôle dans la dissémination de la fièvre aphteuse. Compt. Rend. Hebdom. Acad. Sci., 179 (no. 21): 1225–1227.

LEBOEUF, A. 1912 Dissémination de bacille de Hansen par le mouche domestique. Bull. Soc. Path. Exot., 5: 860–868.

LEBOEUF, A. 1914 La Lèpre en Nouvelle Calédonie et dépendences. Ann. Hyg. Med. Colon., 17: 177–197.

LECLERCQ, M. 1948a La Transmission de la poliomyélite par les insectes. Rev. Méd. Liége, 3 (7): 154–156; (8): 197; (11): 279–281.

LECLERCQ, M. 1948b Les Myiasis. Rev. Méd. Liége, 3: 133–140.

LEDINGHAM. J. G. 1911 On the Survival of Specific Microorganisms in Pupae and Imagines of *Musca domestica* Raised from Experimentally Infected Larvae. Experiments with *Bacillus typhosus.* J. Hyg., Cambridge, 11: 333–340.

LEDINGHAM, J. C. G. 1920 Dysentery and Enteric Disease in Mesopotamia from the Laboratory Standpoint. J. R. Army Med. Corps, London, 34: 306–320.

LEIDY, J. 1856 A Synopsis of Entozoa and some of Their Ectocongeners Observed by the Author. Proc. Acad. Nat. Sci. Phila., 8: 42–58.

LEIDY, J. 1871 Flies as a Means of Communicating Contagious Diseases. Proc. Acad. Nat. Sci. Phila., 1871: 297.

LEIKINA, L. I. 1942 The Role of Various Substrata in the Breeding of *Musca domestica.* (In Russian.) Med. Parasit., 11: 82–86.

LELEAN, P. S. 1904 Notes on Myiasis. Brit. Med. J., 1: 245–246.

LEON, N. 1920 Quelques observations sur les Pédiculides. J. Parasit., 6: 144–147.

LEON, N. 1921 A Case of Urethral Myiasis. J. Parasit., 7: 184–185.

LEPAGE, H. S., GIANNOTTI, O., AND PEREIRA, H. F. 1945 Técnia para o ensáio de inseticidas residuais. Biológico, 11: 320–325.

LEVER, R. J. A. W. 1934 Entomology and Agriculture in the British Solomon Islands. Trop. Agric., 11: 36–37.

LEVER, R. J. A. W. 1938 Entomological Notes. 3. A Javanese Beetle to Control Houseflies. Agric. J. Fiji, 9: 15, 18.

LEVER, R. J. A. W. 1944 Entomological Notes. Agric. J. Fiji, 15: 45–50.

LEVER, R. J. A. W. 1945 Entomological Notes. Agric. J. Fiji, 16: 88–90.

LEVER, R. J. A. W. 1946 Entomological Notes. Agric. J. Fiji, 17: 9–15.

LEWIS, E. A. 1933 Observations on Some Diptera and Myiasis in Kenya Colony. Bull. Ent. Res., 24: 263–269.

LIEBERMANN, A. 1925 Correlation zwischen den antennalen Geruchs-organen und der Biologie der Musciden. Zeit. Morph. u. Oekol. Tiere, 5: 1–97.

LILLY, J. H. 1931 A Preliminary Study of the Presence of Bacteria in the Blood of the House Fly *Musca domestica*. Univ. of Wisconsin, B.S. thesis.

LINDQUIST, A. 1936 Parasites of the Horn Fly and Other Flies Breeding in Dung. J. Econ. Ent., 29: 1154–1158.

LINDQUIST, A. W. 1942 Ants as Predators of *Cochliomyia americana* C. and P. J. Econ. Ent., 35: 850–852.

LINDQUIST, A. W., AND WILSON, H. G. 1948 Development of a Strain of Houseflies Resistant to DDT. Science, 107: 276.

LINNÉ, CARL VON (LINNAEUS) 1758 Systema Naturae per Regna Tria Naturae Secundum Classes, Ordines, Genera, etc. 10th ed.

LIVINGSTON, S. K., AND PRINCE, L. H. 1932 The Treatment of Chronic Osteomyelitis, with Special Reference to the Use of Maggot Active Principle. J. Am. Med. Ass., 98: 1143.

LODGE, O. C. 1916 Fly Investigation Reports. IV. Some Enquiry in the Question of Baits and Poisons for Flies, Being a Report on the Experimental Work Carried Out during 1915 for the Zoological Society of London. Proc. Zool. Soc. London, 1916: 481–518.

LODGE, O. C. 1918 An Examination of the Sense-Reactions of Flies. Bull. Ent. Res., 9: 141–151.

LORD, F. T. 1904 Flies and Tuberculosis. Boston. Med. and Surg. J., 151: 651–654.

LÖRINCZ, F., AND MAKARA, G. 1935 Observations and Experiments on Fly Control and the Biology of the House Fly. L.o.N. Health Org., C.H./Hyg. rur./E.H.5. Geneva. (Multigraph.)

LÖRINCZ, F., AND MAKARA, G. 1936 Investigations in the Fly Density in Hungary in the Years 1934 and 1935. Quart. Bull. Health Org. L.o.N., 5: 219–227.

LÖRINCZ, F., SZAPPANOS, G., AND MAKARA, G. 1936 On Flies Visiting Human Faeces in Hungary. Quart. Bull. Health Org. L.o.N., 5: 228–236.

LOWNE, B. T. 1870 The Anatomy and Physiology of the Blowfly (*Musca vomitoria*). London.

LOWNE, B. T. 1890–1895 Anatomy, Physiology and Development of the Blowfly. London.

LUBBOCK, J. 1871 The Fly in Its Sanitary Aspect. Lancet, 2: 270.

LUMSDEN, L. L., ROBERTS, AND STILES, C. W. 1910 Preliminary Note on a Simple and Inexpensive Apparatus for Use in the Safe Disposal of Night Soil. Public Health Repts., 25: 1623–1629.

LUMSDEN, L. L., STILES, C. W., AND FREEMAN, A. W. 1917 Safe Disposal of Human Excreta at Unsewered Homes. U.S. Public Health Service, Public Health Bull. 68.

LUNDBECK, W. 1898–1900 Diptera Groenlandica. I. Videnskabelige Meddelelser Naturhistoriske Forening i Kjöbenhavn, 1898: 236–314. II. *Ibid.*, 1900: 281–316.

MACALISTER, C. J. 1912 A New Cell Proliferant. Its Clinical Application in the Treatment of Ulcers. Brit. Med. J., 1: 10–12.

McDANIEL, E. I. 1942 Houseflies. Mich. State College Extension Bulletin 239.

McDONNELL, R. P., AND EASTWOOD, T. 1917 A Note on the Mode of Existence of Flies during Winter. J. R. Army Med. Corps, 29: 98–100.

McDUFFIE, W. C., LINDQUIST, A. W., AND MADDEN, A. H. 1946 Control of Fly Larvae in Simulated Pit Latrines and in Carcasses. J. Econ. Ent., 39: 743–749.

MACFIE, J. W. S. 1917 The Identifications of Insects Collected at Accra during the Year 1916, and Other Entomological Notes. Rept. Accra Laboratory for the Year 1916, London, pp. 67–75.

McGOVRAN, E. R. 1938 Insecticides to Control Blow Fly Larvae in Wounds. J. Econ. Ent., 30: 876–879.

McGOVRAN, E. R., AND ELLISOR, L. O. 1936 Repellency of Pine Tar Oil to Wound-infesting Blow Flies. J. Econ. Ent., 29: 980–983.

McGOVRAN, E. R., AND GERSDORFF, W. A. 1945 The Effect of Fly Food on Resistance to Insecticides Containing DDT or Pyrethrum. Soap and Sanit. Chem., 21: 165, 169.

MACGREGOR, M. E. 1917 A Summary of Our Knowledge of Insect Vectors of Disease. Bull. Ent. Res., 8: 155–163.

MACKERRAS, I. M., AND FULLER, M. E. 1937 A Survey of the Australian Sheep Blowflies. J. Coun. Sci. Industr. Res. Aust., 10: 261–270.

MACKERRAS, I. M., AND WEST, R. F. K. 1946 "DDT" Poisoning in Man. Med. J. Aust., March 23, 1946: 400. (Reprint, 4 pp.)

MACLOSKIE, G. 1880 The Proboscis of the House-Fly. Am. Nat., 14: 153–161.

McMAHON, J. P. 1935 Preliminary Notes on the Control of Flies. East African Med. J., 12: 128–135.

MACRAE, R. 1894 Flies and Cholera Diffusion. Indian Med. Gaz., 29: 407–412.

MADDEN, A. H., LINDQUIST, A. W., AND JONES, H. A. 1947 Fly Larvicide Test. Soap and Sanit. Chem., 23: 141, 143.

MADDEN, A. H., LINDQUIST, A. W., AND KNIPLING, E. F. 1945 DDT Treatment of Airplanes to Prevent Introduction of Noxious Insects. J. Econ. Ent., 38: 252–254.

MAIER, P. P., AND DOW, R. P. 1949 Diarrheal Disease Control Studies. II. Conical Net for Collecting Flies. Public Health Repts., 64: 604–607.

MAKARA, G. 1935 The Breeding Places of *Musca domestica* in Hungary and the Fly Control. (In Magyar.) Rep. Hung. Agric. Exp. Sta., 38: 286–291. (German, French, and English summaries.)

MALMGREN, B. 1935 Réapparition de la tularémie en Suède au cours de l'année 1934. Bull. Off. Int. Hyg. Publ., Paris, 27: 2184–2191.

MANINE, A. 1941 Un cas de myiase oculaire à *Oestrus ovis* Linné dans le Sahara central (Fort-Flatters Sahara Constantinois). Arch. Inst. Pasteur Algérie, 19: 287–289.

MANSON-BAHR, P. H. 1919 Bacillary Dysentery. Trans. R. Soc. Trop. Med. and Hyg., 13: 64–72.

MARCH, R. B., AND METCALF, R. L. 1949 Development of Resistance to Organic Insecticides Other than DDT by Houseflies. J. Econ. Ent., 42: 990.

MARCHIONATTO, J. B. 1945 Nota sobre algunos hongos entomógenos. (Publ.) Inst. Sanid. Veg. (A), 1 (8).

MARCHOUX, E. 1916 Transmission de la Lèpre par les mouches (*Musca domestica*.) Ann. Inst. Pasteur, 30: 61–68.

MARCOVITCH, S., AND ANTHONY, M. V. 1931 A Preliminary Report on the Effectiveness of Sodium Fluosilicate as Compared with Borax in Controlling the House Fly *Musca domestica* Linné. J. Econ. Ent., 24: 490–497.

MARETT, P. J. 1915a Fly Prevention Measures. J. R. Army Med. Corps, 25: 456–460.

MARETT, P. J. 1915b Sanitation in War. J. R. Army Med. Corps, London, 24: 359–366.

MAREY, U. 1901 La Locomotion animale. Paris.

MARGARINOS TORRES, C. 1925a Déterminisme de la libération spontanée des larves d'*Habronema muscae* (Carter, 1861) par la trompe de la mouche domestique: Importance de l'hématotropisme. Compt. Rend. Soc. Biol., 93 (no. 20): 33–35.

MARGARINOS TORRES, C. 1925b L'Hématotropisme des larvae mûres d'*Habronema muscae* (Carter, 1861). Compt. Rend. Soc. Biol., 93 (no. 20): 38–39.

MARGARINOS TORRES, C. B. DE, DA FONSECA, O., AND DE ARÊA LEAO, A. E. 1923 Sur la "Esponja" (Habronémose cutaneé des equidés). Du parasitisme des mouches par l'*Habronema muscae* (Carter). Compt. Rend. Soc. Biol., 89 (no. 27): 767–768.

MARPMANN, G. 1897 Bakteriologische Mitteilungen. III. Ueber den Zusammenhang von pathogenen Bakterien mit Fliegen. Zentralbl. Bakt. Parasit. Infekt. I, 22: 122–132.

MARTIN, A. W. 1903 Flies in Relation to Typhoid Fever and Summer Diarrhoea. Public Health, London, 15: 652–653.

MARTIN, C. J. 1913 Horace Dobell Lectures on Insect Porters of Bacterial Infections, Delivered before the R. Coll. of Physicians. Brit. Med. J., Jan. 4, 1913: 1–8; Jan. 11, 1913: 59–68.

MATHESON, R. 1944 Entomology for Introductory Courses. Ithaca, N.Y.

MATHESON, R. 1950 Medical Entomology. 2d ed. Ithaca, N.Y.

MATTHYSSE, J. G. 1945 Observations on Housefly Overwintering. J. Econ. Ent., 38: 493–494.

MAYNE, B. 1929 The Nature of the "Black Spores" Associated with the Malaria Parasite in the Mosquito and Their Relationship to the Tracheal System. Indian J. Med. Res., 17: 109–134.

MAZZA, S., AND JÖRG, M. E. 1939 *Cochliomyia hominivorax = americana* C. & P. Estudio de sus larvas y consideraciones sobre miasis. Publ. Mision Estud. Pat. Reg. Argent. Jujuy, Buenos Aires, no. 41: 1–46.

MAZZA, S., JÖRG, M. E., BASSO, R., *et al.* 1939 Investigaciones sobre Dipteros argentinos. I. Miasis. Buenos Aires Univ. Nac. Misión de Estud. de Patol. Región, Pub. 41: 3–86.

MEIJERE, J. H. C. DE 1925 Studies on Dipterous Larvae and Pupae. Tijdschrift voor Entomologie, 68: 211.

MELLANBY, K. 1934 The Influence of Starvation on the Thermal Death-Point of Insects. J. Exp. Biol., 11: 48–53.

MELLO, F. DE, AND CABRAL, J. 1926 Les Insectes sont-ils susceptibles de transmettre la lèpre? Bull. Soc. Path. Exot., 19: 774–777.

MELLO, F. DE, AND JACQUES, J. E. 1919 Note sur l'existence de l'*Herpetomonas muscae-domesticae* à l'Inde Portugaise. Bol. Ger. Med. e Farmacia, Nova-Goa., 5: 194–195.

MELLO, M. J. DE, AND CUOCOLO, R. 1943a Técnia para o xenodiagnóstico da habronemose gástrica dos equídeos. Arq. Inst. Biol., São Paulo, 14: 217–226.

MELLO, M. J. DE, AND CUOCOLO, R. 1943b Alguns aspetos das relações do *Habronema muscae* (Carter 1861) com a mosca domestica. Arq. Inst. Biol., São Paulo, 14: 227–234. (English summary.)

MELLO, M. J. DE, AND PEREIRA, C. 1946 Determinismo da evasão das larvas de *Habronema* sp. da tromba da mosca domestica. Arq. Inst. Biol., São Paulo, 17: 259–266. (English summary.)

MELLOR, J. E. M. 1919 Observations on the Habits of Certain Flies, Especially of those Breeding in Manure. Ann. Appl. Biol., Cambridge, 6: 53–88.

MELNICK, J. L. 1949 Isolation of Poliomyelitis Virus from Single Species of Flies during an Urban Epidemic. Am. J. Hyg., 49: 8–16.

MELNICK, J. L., AND PENNER, L. R. 1947 Experimental Infection of Flies with Human Poliomyelitis Virus. Proc. Soc. Exp. Biol. and Med., 65: 342–346.

MELVIN, R. 1934 Incubation Period of Eggs of Certain Muscoid Flies at Different Constant Temperatures. Ann. Ent. Soc. Am., 27: 406–410.

MERCIER, L. 1925 Diptères "buveurs de sang" et Diptères "succeurs de suer." Compt. Rend. Soc. Biol., 92 (no. 3): 135–136.

MERLIN, A. A. C. E. 1897 The Foot of the House-Fly. J. Quekett Micro. Club, 6: 348.

MERLIN, A. A. C. E. 1905 Supplementary Note on the Foot of the House-Fly. J. Quekett Micro. Club (2), 9: 167–168.

METCALF, C. L., AND FLINT, W. P. 1928 Destructive and Useful Insects. Their Habits and Control. New York.

METELKIN, A. 1935 The Role of Flies in the Spread of Coccidiosis in Animals and Men. (In Russian.) Med. Parasit. and Parasitic Dis., 4: 75–82.

MILLER, D. 1932 The Biology and Economic Status of New Zealand Muscidae and Calliphoridae. I. Historical Review. Bull. Ent. Res., 23: 469–476.

MILLER, D. F. 1929 Determining the Effects of Change in Temperature upon the Locomotor Movements of Fly Larvae. J. Exp. Zool., 52: 293–313.

MILLER, LA RUE L. 1948 Sanitary Land-Fill Provides for Modern Garbage Disposal. Michigan Public Health, 36: 125, 128, 136.

MILLIKEN, F. B. 1911 Another Breeding-Place for the House-Fly. J. Econ. Ent., 4: 275.

MINNICH, D. E. 1929 The Chemical Sensitivity of the Legs of the Blow-Fly, *Calliphora vomitoria,* to Various Sugars. Zeit. Vergl. Physiol., 11: 1–55.

MINNICH, D. E. 1931 The Sensitivity of the Oral Lobes of the Proboscis of the Blow-Fly, *Calliphora vomitoria* Linn., to Various Sugars. J. Exp. Zool., 60: 121–239.

MITSCHERLICH, E. 1943 Die Uebertragung der Kerato-Conjunctivitis infectiosa des Rindes durch Fliegen und die Tenazität von *Rickettsia conjunctivae* in der Aussenwelt. Dtsch. Tropenmed. Zeit., 47 (Pt. 3): 57–64.

MITZMAIN, M. B. 1916 A Digest of the Insect Transmission of Disease in the Orient with Especial Reference to the Experimental Conveyance of *Trypanosoma evansi.* New Orleans Med. and Surg. J., 69: 416–424.

MOHLER, J. R. 1919 Report of the Chief of the Bureau of Animal Industry. U.S. Dept. Agric., Washington, D.C., Sept. 29, 1919.

MONIEZ, R. 1874 Apropos des publications récentes sur le faux parasitisme des Chernétides sur différents Arthropodes. Rev. Biol. du Nord de la France, 6: 47–54.

MONTFILS, A. J. 1776 D'une maladie fréquente connue en Bourgogne sous le nom de puce maligne. J. de Médecine, 45: 500. (Cited by Nuttall.)

MOOREHEAD, S., AND WEISER, H. H. 1946 The Survival of Staphylococci Food Poisoning Strain in the Gut and Excreta of the House Fly. J. Milk Technol., 9: 253–259.

MORGAN, B. B. 1942 The Viability of *Trichomonas foetus* (Protozoa) in the House Fly *Musca domestica.* Proc. Helminth. Soc. Washington, 9: 17–20.

MORGAN, H. DE R., AND LEDINGHAM, J. C. G. 1909 The Bacteriology of Summer Diarrhoea. Proc. R. Soc. Med., 2: 133–158. (Separate pagination in reprint.)

MORISON, J., AND KEYWORTH, W. D. 1916 Flies and Their Relation to Epidemic Diarrhoea and Dysentery in Poona. Indian J. Med. Res., Calcutta, 3: 619–627.

MORRILL, A. W. 1914a Some American Insects and Arachnids Concerned in the Transmission of Disease. Arizona Med. J., Phoenix, 1914. Reprint, 12 pp.

MORRIS, H. 1919 Anthrax. Transmission of Infection by Nonbiting Flies. Agric. Expt. Sta. La., Bull. 168.

MORRIS, H. 1920 Some Carriers of Anthrax Infection. J. Am. Vet. Med. Ass., Washington, D.C., 56 (no. 6): 606–608.

MOURSI, A. A. 1946 The Effect of Temperature on the Sex Ratio of Parasitic Hymenoptera. Bull. Soc. Fouad Ier Ent., 30: 21–37.

MUMA, M. H., AND HIXSON, E. 1949 Effects of Weather, Sanitation and Chlorinated Chemical Residues on House and Stable Fly Population on Nebraska Farms. J. Econ. Ent., 42: 231–238.

MUMFORD, E. P. 1926 Three New Cases of Myiasis in Man in the North of England, with a Survey of Earlier Observations by Other Authors. Parasitology, 18: 375–383.

MUNRO, J. A., POST, R. L., AND COLBERG, W. 1947 The New Insecticides in Fly Control. Bimonthly Bull. N. Dak. Agric. Exp. Sta., 9: 123–128.

MUNROE, E. G. 1940 The Classification of the Genus *Musca* Linnaeus. A Review of Literature. Unpublished manuscript.

MURRAY, A. 1877 Economic Entomology. Aptera. London. (*Trombidium parasiticum*, p. 129.)

NAGEOTTE, J. 1943 Le Principe d'inertie dans la physiologie sensorielle: Etude sur la balancier des Diptères. Arch. Zool. Exp. et Gén., 83: 99–111.

NÁJERA ANGULO, L. 1942 Sobre un caso de oftalmomiasis producida por larvas de *Wohlfahrtia magnifica* Schiner. Bol. R. Soc. Española Hist. Nat., 40: 493–495.

NÁJERA ANGULO, L. 1947 La lucha contra las moscas. Madrid.

NATVIG, L. R. 1932 Om Myiasis samte to nye norske kasus. Norsk. Ent. Tidsskr., 3: 117–121. (German summary.)

NEIVA, A., AND GOMES, J. F. 1917 Biologia da mosca do berne *Dermatobia hominis* observada em todas as suas phases. Annaes Paulistas de Medicina e Cirurgia, São Paulo, 8: 197–209.

NEWSTEAD, R. 1907 Preliminary Report on the Habits, Life-Cycle and Breeding Places of the Common House-Fly *Musca domestica* Linn. as Observed in Liverpool, with Suggestions as to the Best Means of Checking Its Increase. Liverpool.

NEWSTEAD, R. 1908 On the Habits, Life-Cycle and Breeding-Places of the Common House-Fly. Ann. Trop. Med. Parasit. 1: 507–520.

NEWSTEAD, R. 1909 Second Interim Report on the House-Fly as Observed in the City of Liverpool.

NICHOLAS, G. E. 1873 The Fly in Its Sanitary Aspect. Lancet, 2: 724.

NICOL, G. 1946 Parasites of the Horse. J. Dept. Agric. Vict., Melbourne, 44: 53–56.

NICOLL, W. 1911a On the Varieties of *Bacillus coli* Associated with the House-Fly *Musca domestica*. J. Hyg., 11: 381–389.

NICOLL, W. 1911b On the Part Played by Flies in the Dispersal of the Eggs of

Parasitic Worms. Repts. Local Govnt. Bd. Publ. Health and Med. Subjects, n.s. 53: 13–30.

NICOLL, W. 1917a Flies and Bacillary Enteritis. Brit. Med. J., London, no. 2948: 870–872.

NICOLL, W. 1917b Flies and Typhoid. J. Hyg., Cambridge, 15: 505–526.

NICOLLE, C. 1922 État de nos connaissances d'ordre expérimental sur le trachome. Bull. Inst. Pasteur, 19: 881–894.

NICOLLE, C., CUENOD, A., AND BLANC, G. 1919 Transmission of Trachoma by Flies. Presse Méd., Dec. 20, 1919. (Abstract in Ann. d'Igiene, Rome, 31: 66.)

NIESCHULTZ [NIESCHULZ], O. 1933a Über die Bestimmung der Vorzugstemperatur von Insekten (besonders von Fliegen und Mücken). Zool. Anż., 103: 21–29.

NIESCHULTZ [NIESCHULZ], O. 1933b Über die Temperaturbegrenzung der Aktivitätsstufen von Stomoxys calcitrans. Zeit. Parasitenk., 6: 220–242.

NIESCHULZ, O. 1928 Enkele Multvuuroverbrengingsproeven met Tabaniden, Musciden en Muskieten. Veeartsenijk. Meded., Buitenzorg, no. 67: 1–23.

NIESCHULZ, O. 1934 Über die Vorzugstemperatur von Stomoxys calcitrans. Zeit. Angew. Ent., 21: 224–238.

NIESCHULZ, O. 1935 Über die Temperaturabhängigkeit der Aktivität und die Vorzugstemperatur von Musca domestica und Fannia canicularis. Zool. Anz., 110: 225–233.

NIESCHULZ, O., AND DuToIT, R. 1933 Über die Temperaturabhängigkeit der Aktivität und die Vorzugstemperatur von Stomoxys calcitrans, Musca vicina und M. crassirostris in Südafrika. Zentralbl. Bakt., Jena, 89: 244–249.

NIKOL'SKII, A. L. 1945 Rational Preparation of Kizyak as a Means of Controlling Flies. (In Russian.) Med. Parasit., 14: 70–72.

NOEL, P. 1913 La Guerre aux mouche. Bull. du Laboratoire Régional d'Entomologie Agricole, Rouen, 1913: 4–5.

NOGUCHI, H. 1926 The Differentiation of Herpetomonads and Leishmanias by Biological Tests. Science, 63: 503–504.

NOGUCHI, H., AND TILDEN, E. B. 1926 Cultivation of Herpetomonads from Insects and Plants. J. Exp. Med., 44 (no. 3): 307–325.

NUTTALL, G. H. F. 1897 Zur Aufklärung der Rolle, welche Insekten bei der Verbreitung der Pest spielen. Über die Empfindlichkeit verschiedener Thiere für dieselbe. Centralbl. Bakt., 22: 87–97.

NUTTALL, G. H. F. 1899a On the Role of Insects, Arachnids, and Myriapods, as Carriers in the Spread of Bacterial and Parasitic Diseases in Man and Animals: A Critical and Historical Study. Johns Hopkins Hospital Reports, 8: 1–155.

NUTTALL, G. H. F. 1899b Die Rolle der Insekten, Arachniden (Ixodes) und Myriapiden als Träger bei der Verbreitung von durch Bakterien und thierische Parasiten verursachten Krankheiten des Menschen und der Thiere. Hyg. Rundschau, Vol. 9. (Reprint.)

NUTTALL, G. H. F., AND JEPSON, F. P. 1909 The Part Played by *Musca domestica* and Allied (Non-biting) Flies in the Spread of Infective Diseases. A Summary of Our Present Knowledge. Repts. Local Govnt. Bd. Publ. Health and Med. Subjects, n.s. 16: 13–41.

OKULOV, V. 1947 The Results of Tests of the New Soviet Insecticide, Pentachlorin Paste. (In Russian.) Med. Parasit., 16: 33–35.

OLIVEIRA, S. J., DE, AND MOUSSATCHE, I. 1947 Acão do DDT (dichloro-difeniltricloretana) sôbre larvas e pupas de "Musca domestica" Linneu. Rev. Brasil. Biol., 7: 67–72. (Summary in German.)

OLSON, T. A., AND DAHMS, R. G. 1945 Control of Housefly Breeding in Partly Digested Sewage Sludge. J. Econ. Ent., 38: 602–604.

OLSON, T. A., AND DAHMS, R. G. 1946 Control of Housefly Breeding in Partly Digested Sewage Sludge. Public Works, 77: 5, 24.

ONO, Z. 1939 On Insects of Hygienic Importance in Shinkyo and Its Environs, Manchuria. (In Japanese.) Ent. World, Tokyo, 7: 4–11.

ONORATO, R. 1922 Le miasi in Tripolitania. Arch. Ital. Sci. Med. Colon., iii, nos. 1–12: 14–29, 33–45, 69–88, 101–117, 155–162, 188–193, 216–227, 229–259, 261–283, 293–315.

ORTON, S. F., AND DODD, W. L. 1910 Transmission of Bacteria by Flies with Special Relation to an Epidemic of Bacillary Dysentery. Boston Med. and Surg. J., Dec. 8, 1910.

OSTROLENK, M., AND WELCH, H. 1942a The House Fly as a Vector of Food Poisoning Organisms in Food Producing Establishments. Am. J. Publ. Health, 32: 487–494.

OSTROLENK, M., AND WELCH, H. 1942b The Common Housefly *Musca domestica* as a Source of Pollution in Food Establishments. Food Res., 7: 192–200.

OTWAY, A. L. 1926 A Method of Excreta Disposal in the Tropics Which Entirely Prevents Fly Dissemination. J. R. Army Med. Corps, 46 (no. 1): 14–22.

PACKARD, A. S. 1874 On the Transformation of the Common Housefly, with Notes on Allied Forms. Proc. Boston Soc. Nat. Hist., 16: 136–140.

PACKCHANIAN, A. A. 1944 Malaria Thick Films Contaminated with Excretion of Flies Containing Flagellates (*Herpetomonas*). Am. J. Trop. Med., 24: 141–143.

PAILLOT, A. 1933 L'Infection chez les insectes. Trévoux.

PAINE, J. H. 1912 The House-Fly in Relation to City Garbage. Psyche, 19: 156–159.

PARAF, J. 1920a The Spread of Bacillary Dysentery by Flies. Rev. d'Hyg. et de Police Sanitaire, 1920: 24. (Abstr. in Ann. d'Igiene, Rome, 31 [1921]: 66.)

PARAF, J. 1920b Etude expérimentale de rôle des mouches dans la propagation de la dysenterie bacillaire. Rev. Hyg., 62: 241–244.

PARAMONOV, S. J. 1934a Dipterenlarven zur biologischen Behandlung von Osteomyelitis und Gasbrand. Zeit. Wiss. Insektbiol., 27: 82–85.

PARAMONOV, S. YA 1934b Dipterenlarven als Mittel gegen die Gangräne, Osteomyelitis u.s.w. (In Ukrainian.)   J. Cycle Bio-Zool. Acad. Sci. Ukr., no. 3: 73–83.

PARISOT, J., AND FERNIER, L.   1934   The Best Methods of Treating Manure-Heaps to Prevent the Hatching of Flies.   Quart. Bull. Health Org. L.o.N. 3, Extract no. 1.

PARKER, H. L., AND THOMPSON, W. R.   1928   Contribution à la biologie des Chalcidiens entomophages.   Ann. Soc. Ent. Fr., 97: 425–465.

PARKER, K. G.   1936   Fire Blight: Overwintering Dissemination, and Control of the Pathogen.   Cornell Agric. Exp. Sta. Mem. 193.

PARKER, R. R.   1914   Summary of "Report to the Montana State Board of Entomology concerning Fly Investigations Conducted in the Yellowstone Valley During the Summer of 1914."   1st Bienn. Rept. Montana State Bd. Ent. 1913–1914: 35–50.

PARKER, R. R.   1915   New Evidence concerning the Dispersal of the House-Fly.   Bull. Dept. Publ. Hlth. Helena, Montana, 9 (7–8): 3–7.

PARKER, R. R.   1916a   The House-Fly in Relation to Public Health in Montana. Article 1. Some Facts concerning Its Habits.   Bull. Dept. Publ. Hlth. Helena, Montana, 9 (9–10): 6–11.

PARKER, R. R.   1916b   The House-Fly in Relation to Public Health in Montana. 2. The House-Fly as a Disease Carrier.   Bull. Dept. Publ. Hlth. Helena, Montana, 9 (11): 5–11.

PARKER, R. R.   1916c   Dispersion of *Musca domestica* Linn. under City Conditions in Montana.   J. Econ. Ent., 9: 325–354.

PARKER, R. R.   1916d   The House Fly and the Control of Flies.   2d Bienn. Rept., Montana State Bd. Ent., 1915–1916: 57–66.

PARKER, R. R.   1917   Seasonable Abundance of Flies in Montana.   Ent. News, 28: 278–282.

PARKER, W. L., AND BEACHER, J. H.   1947   Toxaphene, a Chlorinated Hydrocarbon with Insecticidal Properties.   Bull. Del. Agric. Exp. Sta., 264 (Technical, no. 36).

PARKES, L. C.   1911   The Common House-Fly.   J. R. Sanit. Inst., May 1911.

PARKIN, E. A., AND GREEN, A. A.   1944   Activation of Pyrethrins by Sesame Oil.   Nature, London, 154: 16–17.

PARKIN, E. A., AND GREEN, A. A.   1945a   The Toxicity of DDT to the Housefly *Musca domestica* L.   Bull. Ent. Res., 36: 149–162.

PARKIN, E. A., AND GREEN, A. A.   1945b   Residual Films of DDT.   Nature, 155 (3944): 668.

PARMAN, D. C.   1920   Observation on the Effect of Storm Phenomena on Insect Activity.   J. Econ. Ent., 13: 339–343.

PARROTT, P. J.   1927   Progress Report on Light Traps for Insect Control. New York.

PATTON, W. S.   1920a   Some Notes on Indian Calliphorinae. I. *Chrysomyia bezziana* Villeneuve, the Common Indian Calliphorinae Whose Larvae Cause Cutaneous Myiasis in Man and Animals.   Indian J. Med. Res., 8: 17–29.

PATTON, W. S.   1920b   Some Notes on the Arthropods of Medical and Veterinary

Importance in Mesopotamia, and Their Relation to Disease. II. Mesopotamian House Flies and Their Allies. Indian J. Med. Res., 7: 751–777.

PATTON, W. S. 1920c Some Notes on the Arthropods of Medical and Veterinary Importance in Mesopotamia, and on Their Relation to Disease. III. The Bot Flies of Mesopotamia. Indian J. Med. Res., 8: 1–16.

PATTON, W. S. 1921a Studies on the Flagellates of the Genera *Herpetomonas, Crithidia* and *Rhynchoidomonas*. 7. Some Miscellaneous Notes on Insect Flagellates. Indian J. Med. Res., 9: 230–239.

PATTON, W. S. 1921b Notes on the Myiasis-producing Diptera of Man and Animals. Bull. Ent. Res., 12: 239–261.

PATTON, W. S. 1922a Notes on the Species of the Genus *Musca* Linnaeus. I. Bull. Ent. Res., 12: 411–426.

PATTON, W. S. 1922b Some Notes on Indian Calliphorinae. II. Indian J. Med. Res., 9: 548–574.

PATTON, W. S. 1922c Some Notes on Indian Calliphorinae. VI. How to Recognize the Indian Myiasis-producing Flies and Their Larvae, Together with Some Notes on How to Breed Them and Study Their Habits. Indian J. Med. Res., 9: 635–653.

PATTON, W. S. 1922d Some Notes on Indian Calliphorinae. VII. Additional Cases of Myiasis Caused by the Larvae of *Chrysomyia bezziana* Vill., Together with Some Notes on the Diptera Which Cause Myiasis in Man and Animals. Indian J. Med. Res., 9: 654–682.

PATTON, W. S. 1922e Notes on Some Indian Aphiochaetae . . . Whose Larvae Cause Cutaneous and Intestinal Myiasis in Man and Animals. Indian J. Med. Res., 9: 683–691.

PATTON, W. S. 1922f Note on the Occurrence of the Larvae of *Philaematomyia crassirostris*, Stein, in the Human Intestine. Indian J. Med. Res., 10: 57–59.

PATTON, W. S. 1923a Some Philippine Species of the Genus Musca. Philipp. J. Sci., 23: 309–322.

PATTON, W. S. 1923b A New Oriental Species of the Genus *Musca* with a Note on the Occurrence of *Musca dasyops*, Stein, in China and a Revised List of the Oriental Species of the Genus *Musca*, Linnaeus. Philipp. J. Sci., 23: 323–335.

PATTON, W. S. 1930 Insects, Ticks, Mites and Venomous Animals of Medical and Veterinary Importance. II. Public Health. Croydon, Eng.

PATTON, W. S. 1933a Studies on the Higher Diptera of Medical and Veterinary Importance. A Revision of the Genera of the Tribe Muscini, Subfamily Muscinae, Based on a Comparative Study of the Male Terminalia. I. The Genus *Musca* Linnaeus. Ann. Trop. Med. Parasit., 27: 135–156.

PATTON, W. S. 1933b Studies on the Higher Diptera of Veterinary and Medical Importance. A Revision of the Species of the Genus *Musca*, Based on a Comparative Study of the Male Terminalia. II. A Practical Guide to the Palaearctic Species. Ann. Trop. Med. Parasit., 27: 327–345, 397–430.

PATTON, W. S. 1933c Studies on the Higher Diptera of Medical and Veterinary

Importance. A Revision of the Tribe Muscini, Subfamily Muscinae, Based on a Comparative Study of the Male Terminalia. II. The Genus *Stomoxys* Geoffroy (Sens. lat.). Ann. Trop. Med. Parasit., 27: 501–537.

PATTON, W. S. 1935 Classification of the Myiasis-producing Diptera of Man and Animals. *In* Parasites, Transmetteurs, Anim. Venimeux. Rec. Trav. 25e Anniv. Sci. Pavlovsky 1909–1934, pp. 269–271.

PATTON, W.S. 1937a Studies on the Higher Diptera of Medical and Veterinary Importance. A Revision of the Species of the Genus *Musca,* Based on a Comparative Study of the Male Terminalia. IV. A Practical Guide to the Oriental Species. Ann. Trop. Med. Parasit., 31: 127–140, 195–213.

PATTON, W. S. 1937b Male Genitalia of *Musca dasyops.* Ann. Trop. Med. Parasit., 31: 209.

PATTON, W. S., AND COOKSON, H. A. 1925 Cutaneous Myiasis in Man Caused by *Musca domestica.* Lancet, 1 (June 20): 1291.

PATTON, W. S., AND CRAGG, F. W. 1913a On Certain Haematophagous Species of the Genus *Musca* with Descriptions of Two New Species. Indian J. Med. Res., 1: 11–25.

PATTON, W. S., AND CRAGG, F. W. 1913b A New Species of *Philaematomyia,* with Some Remarks on the Genus. Indian J. Med. Res., 1: 26–33.

PATTON, W. S., AND CRAGG, F. W. 1913c A Text-Book of Medical Entomology. London, Madras, and Calcutta.

PATTON, W. S., AND EVANS, A. M. 1929 Insects, Ticks, Mites and Venomous Animals of Medical and Veterinary Importance. I. Medical. Croydon, Eng.

PAUL, J. R., TRASK, J. D., BISHOP, M. B., MELNICK, J. L., AND CASEY, A. E. 1941 The Detection of Poliomyelitis Virus in Flies. Science, 94: 395–396.

PAVLOVSKI(Y), E. N., AND STEIN, A. K. 1924 Die Gastrophilus-larve als Gastparasit in der Menschenhaut. Parasitology, 16: 32–43.

PAVLOVSKII, E. N., STEIN, A. K., AND BUICHKOV, V. A. 1932 Experimentelle Untersuchungen über die Wirkung einiger Verdauungssekrete von *Musca domestica* auf die Hautdecken des Menschen. (In Russian.) Mag. Paras. Inst. Zool. Acad. Sci., URSS, 3: 131–147. (German summary.)

PAZ, G. C. DE LA 1938a The Bacterial Flora of Flies Caught in Foodstores in the City of Manila. Monthly Bull. Bur. Health. Philipp. I., 18: 393–412.

PAZ, G. C. DE LA 1938b The Breeding of Flies in Garbage and Their Control. Monthly Bull. Bur. Health. Philipp. I., 18: 515–519.

PAZ, G. C. DE LA 1938c The Fly Problem in Relation to Refuse Disposal in Manila. Monthly Bull. Bur. Health. Philipp. I., 18: 521–539.

PEAIRS, L. M. 1927 Some Phases of the Relation of Temperature to the Development of Insects. Coll. Agric. West Virginia Univ., Agric. Exp. Sta. Bull. 208.

PECKHAM, G. W., AND PECKHAM, E. G. 1905 Wasps, Social and Solitary. Boston.

PÉDOYA, C. 1941 Un Cas de myiases oculaire à *Oestrus ovis* à Beni Ounif (Sud oranais). Arch. Inst. Pasteur Algérie, 19: 362–363.

PEREIRA, C. 1947 A luta contra as moscas. Biológico, São Paulo, 13 (2): 25–43.

PEREIRA, C., AND CASTRO, M. P. DE 1945 Contribuição para o'conhecimento da espécie tipo de *Macrocheles* Latr. (Acarina): *M. muscaedomesticae* (Scopoli, 1772) emend. Arq. Inst. Biol., São Paulo, 16: 153–186.

PÉREZ, C. 1910 Metamorphosis of Blowfly. Arch. Zool. Exp., 4: 1–274.

PETRISHCHEVA, P. A. 1932 Zur Biologie der Hausfliege in den Bedingungen der Stadt Samara. (In Russian.) Mag. Paras. Inst. Zool. Acad. Sci., URSS, 3: 161–182.

PHALEN, J. M. 1917 U.S. Army Methods of Disposal of Camp Refuse. Am. J. Publ. Health, 7: 481–484.

PHÉLOUKIS, T., AND KNITHAKIS, E. 1932 L'Habronémose cutanée en Grèce. Bull. Acad. Vét. Fr., 4: 121–124, 1931. (Absts. in Vet. Bull., 2: 19; Weybridge, Surrey, Imp. Bur. Anim. Health, Jan. 1932.)

PICKARD-CAMBRIDGE, O. 1892 On the British Species of False-Scorpions. Proc. Dorset Nat. Hist. and Antiq. Field Club, 13: 199–231.

PIERCE, W. D., *et al.* 1921 Sanitary Entomology. (A series of lectures by various authorities, including W. D. Pierce, who served as editor.) Boston.

PIERPONT, R. L. 1945a Terpin Diacetate as an Activator for Pyrethrum. J. Econ. Ent., 38: 123–124.

PIERPONT, R. L. 1945b Development of a Terpene Thiocyano Ester (Thanite) as a Fly Spray Concentrate. Bull. Del. Agric. Exp. Sta., no. 253.

PINKUS, H. 1913 The Life-History and Habits of *Spalangia muscidarum* Richardson; a Parasite of the Stable-Fly. Psyche, 20: 148–158.

PIPKIN, A. C. 1942 Filth Flies as Transmitters of *Endamoeba histolytica*. Proc. Soc. Exp. Biol. and Med., 49: 46–48.

PIPKIN, A. C. 1943 Experimental Studies on the Role of Filth Flies in the Transmission of Certain Helminthic and Protozoan Infections of Man. Absts. theses Tulane Univ., 44: 9–13.

PIPKIN, A. C. 1949 Experimental Studies on the Role of Filth Flies in the Transmission of *Endamoeba histolytica*. Am. J. Hyg., 49: 255–275.

PLACE, F. C. 1915 Flies, a Factor in a Phase of Filariasis in the Horse. Adelaide, N.D. (Abstr. in Rev. App. Ent., 3: 209–210.)

PODYAPOLSKAYA, V., AND GNEDINA, M. 1934 Sur le rôle des mouches dans l'épidémiologie des helminthoses. (In Russian.) Med. Parasit. and Parasitic Dis., 3: 179–185. (French summary.)

POKROVSKII, S. N., AND ZIMA, G. G. 1938 Mouches comme transporteurs des oeufs des helminthes dans les conditions naturelles. (In Russian.) Med. Parasit., 7: 262–264.

PORTCHINSKY, I. A. 1906 Le Taon russe (*Rhinoestrus purpureus* Br.) parasite du cheval. Larves éjaculées dans les yeux des gens. (In Russian.) Trav. Bur. Ent. Comm. Sci. Min. Agric. St. Petersbourg, 6: 1–44.

PORTCHINSKY, I. A. 1910 Recherches biologiques sur le *Stomoxys calcitrans* L.

et biologie comparée des mouches coprophagues. (In Russian.) Publ. Ent. Bur. Russian Dept. Land Adm. and Agric., Vol. 8, no. 8.

PORTCHINSKY, I. A. 1913a *Hydrotaea dentipes;* Its Biology and the Destruction by Its Larvae of the Larvae of *Musca domestica.* Mem. Bur. Ent. Sci. Comm. Cent. Bd. Russian Dept. Land Adm. and Agric., Vol. 9, no. 5.

PORTCHINSKY, I. A. 1913b *Muscina stabulans* Fall., mouche nuisible à l'homme et à son ménage, en état larvaire destructeuse des larves de *Musca domestica.* Publ. Ent. Bur. Russian Dept. Land Adm. and Agric., Vol. 10, no. 1.

PORTCHINSKY, I. A. 1913c *Oestrus ovis,* sa biologie et son rapport à l'homme. Publ. Ent. Bur. Russian Dept. Land Adm. and Agric., Vol. 10, no. 3.

PORTCHINSKY, I. A. 1915 *Rhinoestrus purpureus* Br., a Parasite of the Horse, Injecting Its Larvae into the Eyes of Men. (In Russian.) Mem. Bur. Ent. Sci. Comm. Cent. Bd. Land Adm. and Agric., Vol. 6, no. 6.

PORTCHINSKY, I. A. 1916 *Wohlfahrtia magnifica* Schin. Sa Biologie et son rapport à l'homme et aux animaux domestiques. (In Russian.) Mem. Bur. Ent. Sci. Comm. Min. Agric., Vol. 11, no. 9.

PRELL, H. 1914 Die Lebensweise der Raupenfliegen. Zeit. Angew. Ent. 1: 172–195.

PRILL, E. A., SYNERHOLM, M. E., AND HARTZELL, A. 1946 Some Compounds Related to the Insecticide "DDT" and Their Effectiveness against Mosquito Larvae and Houseflies. Contr. Boyce Thompson Inst., 14: 341–353.

PRUTHI, H. S. 1946 Studies on House-Fly and Other Diptera. Abridg. Sci. Rept. Agric. Res. Inst. New Delhi 1941–1944: 69–70.

PRYOR, M. G. M. 1940 On the Hardening of the Cuticle of Insects. Proc. R. Soc. (B), 128: 393–407.

PURI, I. M. 1943 The House-frequenting Flies, Their Relation to Disease and Their Control. Health Bull. 31. 2d ed. Simla, India.

RAIMBERT, A. 1869 Recherches expérimentales sur la transmission du charbon par les mouches. Compt. Rend. Acad. Sci. Paris, 69: 805–812. See also Paris Acad. Méd. Bull., 35 (1870): 50, 215, 417; Union Méd. Paris, 9 (1870): 209, 350, 507, 709.

RAMAKRISHNA IYER, T. V. 1935 The Housefly Nuisance and Its Control with Maggot Traps. Madras Agric. J., 23: 96–98.

RAMSBOTTOM, J. 1914 Repts. Local Govt. Bd. Publ. Health and Med. Subjects, n.s. 102, iii. An Investigation of Mr. Hesse's Work on the Supposed Relationship of *Empusa muscae* and *Mucor racemosus,* pp. 31–32.

RANSOM, B. H. 1911 The Life-History of a Parasitic Nematode (*Habronema musca*). Science, n.s. 34: 690–692.

RANSOM, B. H. 1913 The Life History of *Habronema muscae* (Carter), a Parasite of the Horse Transmitted by the House Fly. U.S. Dept. Agric. Bur. Animal Ind. Bull. 163.

RAO, G. R. 1929 Myiasis in Lepers. Indian Med. Gaz., 63: 201–202; 64: 380–382.

RÉAUMUR, R. A. F. DE 1738 Mémoires pour servir à l'histoire des insectes, Paris, 4: 384.

REED, W. 1899 Flies the Cause of Typhoid Outbreak in Army in 1899. War Dept. Ann. Rept., Washington, 1899: 627–633.

REED, W., VAUGHAN, V. C., AND SHAKESPEARE, E. O. 1904 Report on the Origin and Spread of Typhoid Fever in U.S. Military Camp during the Spanish War of 1898. Vol. 1, text; Vol. 2, maps and charts.

REID, W. M., AND ACKERT, J. E. 1937 The Cysticercoid of *Choanotaenia infundibulum* (Bloch) and the Housefly as Its Host. Trans. Am. Micro. Soc., 56: 99–104.

RENDTORFF, R. C., AND FRANCIS, T. 1943 Survival of the Lansing Strain of Poliomyelitis Virus in the Common House Fly, *Musca domestica* L. J. Infect. Dis., 73: 198–205.

RENNIE, J. 1927 A Case of Intestinal Myiasis in a Breast-fed Infant. Parasitology, 19: 139–140.

RICHARDS, O. W. 1927 Sexual Selection and Allied Problems in the Insects. The Mechanical Relation of the Male and Female Genitalia. Biol. Rev., 2: 322–328.

RICHARDSON, C. H. 1913a An Undescribed Hymenopterous Parasite of the House-Fly. Psyche, 20: 38–39.

RICHARDSON, C. H. 1913b Studies on the Habits and Development of a Hymenopterous Parasite, *Spalangia muscidarum*, Richardson. J. Morph., 24: 513–549.

RICHARDSON, C. H. 1915 Fly Control on the College Farm. Rept. Ent. Dept., N.J. Agric. Coll. Exp. Sta. for 1914, Paterson, pp. 382–399.

RICHARDSON, C. H. 1916a The Response of the House-Fly (*Musca domestica* L.) to Ammonia and Other Substances. N.J. Agric. Exp. Sta. Bull. 292.

RICHARDSON, C. H. 1916b A Chemotropic Response of the House-Fly (*Musca domestica* L.). Science, 43: 613–616.

RICHARDSON, C. H. 1917a The Response of the House-Fly to Certain Foods and Their Fermentation Products. Rept. Ent. Dept., N.J. Agric. Exp. Sta. for 1916, New Brunswick, pp. 511–519. (Also publ. in J. Econ. Ent., 10: 102–109.)

RICHARDSON, C. H. 1917b The Domestic Flies of New Jersey. N.J. Agric. Exp. Sta. Bull. 307.

RICHARDSON, C. H., AND RICHARDSON, E. H. 1922 Is the Housefly in Its Natural Environment Attracted to Carbon Dioxide? J. Econ. Ent., 15: 425–430.

RICHARDSON, H. H. 1932a An Efficient Medium for Rearing House Flies throughout the Year. Science, 76: 350–351.

RICHARDSON, H. H. 1932b Insecticidal Studies of Midcontinent Distillates as Bases for Pyrethrum Extracts. Industr. Engng. Chem. Ind. Ed., 24: 1394–1397.

RILEY, W. A. 1939 The Possibility of Intestinal Myiasis in Man. J. Econ. Ent., 32: 875–876.

RILEY, W. A., AND JOHANNSEN, O. A. 1938 Medical Entomology. 2d ed. New York.

ROBERTS, E. W. 1947 The Part Played by the Faeces and Vomit-drop in the Transmission of *Entamoeba histolytica* by *Musca domestica*. Ann. Trop. Med. and Parasit., 41: 129–142.

ROBERTSON, J. 1917 Flies and Stable Litter. Public Health, London, 30: 245–246.

ROBINEAU-DESVOIDY, J. B. 1830 Essai sur les Myodaires. Mémoires des savants étrangers de l'Academie des Sciences de Paris. Vol. II. Paris.

ROBINSON, W. 1935 Stimulation of Healing in Nonhealing Wounds by Allantoin Occurring in Maggot Secretions and of Wide Biological Distribution. J. Bone Joint Surg., 17: 267–271.

ROBINSON, W. 1937 The Healing Properties of Allantoin and Urea Discovered through the Use of Maggots in Human Wounds. Smithson. Inst. Publ., Rept. 3471: 451–461.

ROBINSON, W. 1940a Ammonium Bicarbonate Secreted by Surgical Maggots Stimulates Healing in Purulent Wounds. Am. J. Surg., n.s. 47: 111–155.

ROBINSON, W. 1940b Ammonia as a Cell Proliferant and Its Spontaneous Production from Urea by the Enzyme Urease. Am. J. Surg., 49: 319–325.

ROBINSON, W., AND NORWOOD, V. H. 1933 The Role of Surgical Maggots in the Disinfection of Osteomyelitis and Other Infected Wounds. J. Bone Joint Surg., 15: 409–412.

ROBINSON, W., AND NORWOOD, V. H. 1934 Destruction of Phygenic Bacteria in the Alimentary Tract of Surgical Maggots Implanted in Infected Wounds. J. Lab. Clin. Med., 19: 581–586.

RÖDEL, H. 1886 Über das vitale Temperaturminimum wirbelloser Tiere. Zeit. Naturw., 59: 183–214.

ROMANOV, A. N. 1940 L'Écologie des mouches synanthropes du Tadjikestan méridional. (In Russian.) Med. Parasit., 9: 355–363.

ROOT, F. M. 1921 Experiments on the Carriage of Intestinal Protozoa of Man by Flies. Am. J. Hyg., 1: 131–153.

ROSENAU, M. J. 1927 Preventive Medicine and Hygiene. 5th ed. New York.

ROSS, I. C. 1929 Observations on the Hydatid Parasite (*Echinococcus granulosus*) and the Control of Hydatid Disease in Australia. Bull. Coun. Sci. Ind. Res. Aust., no. 40.

ROSS, J. N. M. 1916 Medical Impressions of the Gallipoli Campaign from a Battalion Medical Officer's Standpoint. J.R. Naval Med. Serv., London, 2: 313–324.

ROSS, W. C., AND HUSSAIN, M. 1924 On the Life History of *Herpetomonas muscae-domesticae*. A Preliminary Note. Indian Med. Gaz., 59 (no. 12): 614–615.

ROSTRUP, S. 1922 Stuefluens Bekaempelse. Almanak 1922 Kjøbenhavns Observ., Copenhagen.

ROUBAUD, E. 1911 Sur la biologie et la viviparite poecilogoniques de la mouche des bestiaux (*Musca corvina* Fab.) en Afrique tropicale. Compt. Rend. Acad. Sci., Paris, 152: 158–160.

ROUBAUD, E. 1914 Les Producteurs de myiases et agents similaires chez l'homme et les animaux. *In* Bouet, G., et Roubaud, E., Etudes sur la faune parasitaire de l'Afrique Occidentale Française. Fasc. 1. Paris.

ROUBAUD, E. 1915a Etudes biologiques sur la mouche domestique. Méthode biothermique de destruction des oeufs dans le tas de fumier. Compt. Rend. Soc. Biol., Paris, 78: 615–616.

ROUBAUD, E. 1915b Production et auto-destruction par le fumier de cheval des mouches domestiques. Compt. Rend. Acad. Sci., Paris, 161 (no. 11): 325–327.

ROUBAUD, E. 1918 Le Rôle des mouches dans la dispersion des amibes dysentériques et autres protozoaires intestinaux. Bull. Soc. Path. Exot., 11: 166–171.

ROUBAUD, E. 1922a Recherches sur la fécondité et la longévité de la mouche domestique. Ann. Inst. Pasteur, 36: 765–783.

ROUBAUD, E. 1922b Etudes sur le sommeil d'hiver pré-imaginal des Muscides. Bull. Biol. France Belg., 56 (no. 4): 455–544.

ROUBAUD, E. 1936 The Biothermic Method of Fly Destruction and the Ease with Which It Can Be Adapted to Rural Conditions. Quart. Bull. Health Org. L.o.N., 5: 214–218.

ROUBAUD, E., AND COLAS-BELCOUR, J. 1936 Observations biologiques sur les glossines. . . . Bull. Soc. Path. Exot., 29: 691–696.

ROUBAUD, E., AND DESCAZEAUX, J. 1921 Contribution à l'histoire de la mouche domestique comme agent vecteur des habronémoses d'equidés. Cycle évolutif et parasitisme de l'*Habronema megastoma* (Rudolphi 1819) chez la mouche. Bull. Soc. Path. Exot., Paris, 14: 471–506.

ROUBAUD, E., AND DESCAZEAUX, J. 1922a Evolution de l'*Habronema muscae,* Carter, chez la mouche domestique et de l'*H. microstomum,* Schneider, chez le Stomoxe. (Note préliminaire.) Bull. Soc. Path. Exot., Paris, 15: 572–574.

ROUBAUD, E., AND DESCAZEAUX, J. 1922b Deuxième contribution à l'étude des mouches dans leurs rapports avec l'évolution des habronèmes d'equidés. Bull. Soc. Path. Exot., 15: 978–1001.

ROUBAUD, E., AND DESCAZEAUX, J. 1923 Sur un agent bactérien pathogène pour les mouches communes: *Bacterium delendae-muscae* n. sp. Compt. Rend. Acad. Sci., Paris, 177 (no. 16): 716–717.

ROUBAUD, E., AND TREILLARD, M. 1935 Un Coccobacille pathogène pour les mouches tsétsés. Compt. Rend. Acad. Sci., Paris, 201: 304–306.

ROY, D. N., AND SIDDONS, L. B. 1939 A List of Hymenoptera of Superfamily Chalcidoidea Parasites of Calyptrate Muscoidea. Rec. Indian Museum, 41: 223–224.

ROY, D. N., SIDDONS, L. B., AND MUKHERJEE, S. P. 1940 The Bionomics of *Dirhinus pachycerus* Masi (Hymenoptera: Chalcidoidea), a Pupal Parasite of Muscoid Flies. Indian J. Ent., 2: 229–240.

RUHLAND, H. H., AND HUDDLESON, I. F. 1941 The Role of One Species of Cockroach and Several Species of Flies in the Dissemination of *Brucella*. Am. J. Vet. Res., 2: 371–372.

RUSSO, C. 1930 Recherches expérimentales sur l'épidémiogenèse de la peste bubonique par les insectes. Bull. Off. Int. Hyg. Publ. 22 (no. 11): 2108–2120.

SABIN, A. B., AND WARD, R. 1941 Flies as Carriers of Poliomyelitis Virus in Urban Epidemics. Science, 94: 590–591.

SABIN, A. B., AND WARD, R. 1942 Insects and Epidemiology of Poliomyelitis. Science, 95: 300–301.

SACCÀ, G. 1947 Sull'esistenza di mosche domestiche resitenti al DDT. Riv. di Parassitol., 8: 127–128.

SACEGHEM, R. VAN 1917 Contribution à l'étude de la dermite granuleuse chez des equidés. Bull. Soc. Path. Exot., Paris, 10: 726–729.

SACEGHEM, R. VAN 1918 Cause étiologique et traitement de la dermite granuleuse. Bull. Soc. Path. Exot., 11: 575–578.

SACEGHEM, R. VAN 1919 Cause étiologique et traitement de la dermite granuleuse. Ann. Méd. Vét., Brussels, 64 (nos. 5–6): 151–154.

SALLES, J. F. DE, AND HATHAWAY, C. R. 1944 Nota sobre a infestação de *Musca domestica* Linneu, 1758, per um ficomiceto do genero *Empusa*. Mem. Inst. Osw. Cruz, 41: 95–99.

SANDERS, D. A. 1940 *Musca domestica* a Vector of Bovine Mastitis (Preliminary Report). J. Am. Vet. Med. Ass., 97: 120–122.

SANDERS, G. E. 1942 House Fly Control in Relation to Poliomyelitis. Pests, 10: 22–26.

SARKARIA, D. S., AND PATTON, R. L. 1949 Histological and Morphological Factors in the Penetration of DDT through the Pulvilli of Several Insect Species. Trans. Am. Ent. Soc., 75: 71–82.

SAUNDERS, W. H. 1916a Fly Investigations Reports. I. Some Observations on the Life-History of the Blow-Fly and of the House-Fly made from August to September, 1915, for the Zoological Society of London. Proc. Zool. Soc., London, 1916 (Part 3): 461–463.

SAUNDERS, W. H. 1916b Fly Investigations Reports. II. Trials for Catching, Repelling and Exterminating Flies in Houses, Made during the Year 1915 for the Zoological Society of London. Proc. Zool. Soc., London, 1916 (Part 3): 465–468.

SCHARFF, J. W. 1940 Composting. J. Malay Branch Brit. Med. Ass., 4 (no. 1, June).

SCHECHTER, M. S., HALLER, H. L., AND POGORELSKIN, M. A. 1946 Colorimetric Determination of DDT in Milk. Agric. Chem., New York, 1: 27, 46.

SCHUCKMANN, W. VON 1923 Über Mittel zur Fliegenbekämpfung. Zeit. Angew. Ent., 9: 81–101.

SCHWARTZ, B., AND CRAM, E. B. 1925 Horse Parasites Collected in the Philippine Islands. Philipp. J. Sci., 27: 495–505.

Scott, J. R. 1917a Studies upon the Common House-Fly (*Musca domestica* Linn.). I. A General Study of the Bacteriology of the House-Fly in the District of Columbia. J. Med. Res., 37: 101–119.

Scott, J. R. 1917b Studies upon the Common House-Fly (*Musca domestica* Linn.). II. Isolation of B. *cuniculicida,* a Hitherto Unreported Isolation. J. Med. Res., 37: 121–124.

Scudder, H. I. 1947 A New Technique for Sampling the Density of Housefly Populations. Public Health Repts., 62: 681–686. (Reprint no. 2785.)

Scudder, H. I. 1949 Some Principles of Fly Control for the Sanitarian. Am. J. Trop. Med., 29: 609–623.

Séguy, W. 1929 Etude sur les diptères à larves commensales ou parasites des oiseaux de l'Europe occidentale. Encyc. Ent., sér B, II. Dipt. V, pp. 63–82.

Sen, S. K., and Minett, F. C. 1944 Experiments on the Transmission of Anthrax through Flies. Indian J. Vet. Sci. and An. Hus., 14: 149–158.

Sergent, Ed., and Sergent, Et. 1934 Fly-free Manure Heaps. Quart. Bull. Health Org. L.o.N., 3: 299–303.

Shane, M. S. 1948 Effect of DDT Spray on Reservoir Biological Balance. J. Am. Water Works Ass., 40: 333–336.

Sharpy-Schafer, E. 1938 Essentials of Histology. Ed. H. M. Carleton. 14th ed. Philadelphia.

Shelford, V. E. 1929 Laboratory and Field Ecology. Baltimore.

Shinoda, O., and Ando, T. 1935 Diurnal Rhythm of Flies. (In Japanese.) Bot. and Zool., 3: 117–121.

Shircore, T. O. 1916 A Note on Some Helminthic Diseases, with Special Reference to the House-Fly as a Natural Carrier of the Ova. Parasitology, 8: 239–243.

Shooter, R. A. and Waterworth, P. M. 1944 A Note on the Transmissibility of Haemolytic Streptococcal Infection by Flies. Brit. Med. J., no. 4337: 247–248.

Shope, R. E. 1927 Bacteriophage Isolated from the Common House Fly (*Musca domestica*). J. Exp. Med., 45: 1037–1044.

Showalter, W. J. 1914 Redeeming the Tropics. Nat. Geog. Mag., 25: 344–364.

Shuzo, Asami. 1933 Propagation de la lèpre par les insectes. La Lèpre No. 1. (Abstr. in Bull. Off. Int. Hyg. Publ., Paris, 25 [Nov. 1933]: 2006.)

Sibthorpe, E. H. 1896 Cholera and Flies. Brit. Med. J., Sept. 1896: 700.

Siddons, L. B., and Roy, D. N. 1940 The Early Stages of *Musca inferior* Stein. Indian J. Med. Res., 27: 819–822.

Sieyro, Luis. 1942 Die Hausfliege (*Musca domestica*) als Uebertrager von *Entamoeba histolytica* und anderen Darmprotozoen. Dtsch. Tropenmed. Zeit., 46: 361–372.

Sikes, E. K., and Wigglesworth, V. B. 1931 The Hatching of Insects from the Egg and the Appearance of Air in the Tracheal System. Quart. J. Micr. Sci., 74: 165–192.

SILER, J. F.   1931   Report of the Health Department of the Panama Canal for the Calendar Year 1930. Balboa Heights, C.Z.

SILVERTHORNE, N., AND BROWN, A.   1934   Cutaneous Myiasis in Infants. Arch. Dis. Childhood, 54: 339–342.

SIMITCH, T., AND KOSTITCH, D.   1937   Rôle de la mouche domestique dans la propagation du *Trichomonas intestinalis* chez l'homme. Ann. Parasit. Hum. Comp., 15: 324–325.

SIMMONDS, H. W.   1922   Entomological Notes. Agric. Circ. Dept. Agric. Fiji, 3: 24.

SIMMONDS, H. W.   1925   House Fly Pest and Its Control in Fiji. Agric. Circ. Dept. Agric. Fiji, 5: 85–86.

SIMMONDS, H. W.   1928   The House Fly Problem in Fiji. Agric. J. Fiji, 1 (no. 1): 12–23.

SIMMONDS, H. W.   1929a   Introduction of *Spalangia cameroni*, Parasite of the Housefly, into Fiji. Agric. J. Fiji., 2 (1): 35.

SIMMONDS, H. W.   1929b   Introduction of Natural Enemies against the House Fly in Fiji. Agric. J. Fiji, 2 (2): 46.

SIMMONDS, H. W.   1932   The House-Fly Problem in Fiji. Fiji Ann. Med. and Health Rept. for Year 1932: 46–53.

SIMMONDS, H. W.   1940   Investigations with a View to the Biological Control of Houseflies in Fiji. Trop. Agric., 17: 197–199.

SIMMONDS, M.   1892   Fliegen und Choleraübertragen. Dtsch. Med. Wochenschr., no. 41: 931.

SIMMONS, P.   1923   A House-Fly Plague in the American Expeditionary Force. J. Econ. Ent., 16: 357–363.

SIMMONS, S. W.   1935a   The Bactericidal Properties of Excretions of the Maggot of *Lucilia sericata*. Bull. Ent. Res., 26: 559–563.

SIMMONS, S. W.   1935b   A Bactericidal Principle in Excretions of Surgical Maggots Which Destroys Important Etiological Agents of Pyogenic Infections. J. Bact., 30: 253–267.

SIMMONS, S. W., AND DOVE, W. E.   1942   Waste Celery as a Breeding Medium for the Stable Fly or "Dog Fly," with Suggestions for Control. J. Econ. Ent., 35: 709–715.

SKINNER, H.   1913   How Does the House-Fly Pass the Winter? Ent. News, 24: 303–304.

SKINNER, H.   1915   How Does the House-Fly Pass the Winter? (Dipt.) Ent. News, 26: 263–264.

SMART, J.   1942   *Simulium* as a "Swarming Housefly." The Entomologist, 75: 262–263.

SMART, J.   1943   A Handbook for the Identification of Insects of Medical Importance. London.

SMIRNOV, E. S.   1937   Résultats sommaires du travail du laboratoire dans sa lutte contre les mouches. (In Russian.) Med. Parasit., 6: 872–879.

SMIRNOV, E. S. 1940 Le Problème des mouches à Tadjikistane. (In Russian.) Med. Parasit., 9: 515–517.

SMIRNOV, E., AND KUZINA, O. 1933 Experimentalökologische Studien an Fliegenparasiten. I. Teil. (In Russian.) Zool. J., 12: 96–108.

SMIRNOV, E., AND WLADIMIROW, M. 1934 Studien über die Vermehrungsfähigkeit der Pteromalide *Mormoniella vitripennis* Wlk. Zeit. Wiss. Zool., 145: 507–522.

SMIT, B. 1945a The New DDT Insecticide. Fmg. in S. Afr., 20: 337–340, 356.

SMITH, M. I., AND STOHLMAN, E. F. 1944 Pharmacologic Action of 2, 2-bis (p-Chlorphenyl)-1, 1, 1-Trichlorethane and Its Estimation in the Tissues and Body Fluids. Public Health Repts., Washington, 59: 984–993.

SNODGRASS, R. E. 1935 Principles of Insect Morphology. New York and London.

SOLBERG, A. N. 1939 The Preparation of Plaster of Paris Embedding Boxes. Stain Tech., 14: 27–28.

SOUZA, GABRIEL SOARES DE 1587 Tratado descriptivo do Brazil em 1587: Obra de Gabriel de Souza. Rio di Janeiro. (Cited by França C., in Trans. R. Soc. Trop. Med. and Hyg., London, 15 [1–2].)

SOUZA-ARAUJO, H. C. DE 1943 Verificação da Infecção de Moscas da familia Tachinidae pela *Empusa* Cohn 1855. Essas moscus, sugando ulceras lepróticas, se infestaram com o bacilo de Hansen. Mem. Inst. Osw. Cruz, 39 (2): 201–203.

SPEYER, E. R. 1920 Notes on Chemotropism in the House-Fly. Ann. Appl. Biol., Cambridge, 7:124–140.

SPIELMAN, M., AND HAUSHALTER, M. 1887 Dissémination du bacille de la tuberculose par la mouche. Compt. Rend. Acad. Sci., 105: 352–353.

STEIN, F. R. 1878 Der Organismus des Infusionsthiere, II, and III, Abtheilungen. Leipzig.

STEINER, G. 1945 Fallenversuche zur Kennzeichnung der Verhaltens von Schmeissfliegen gegenüber verschiedenen Merkmalen ihrer Umgebung. Darmstadt.

STEINHAUS, E. A. 1946 Insect Microbiology: An Account of the Microbes Associated with Insects and Ticks with Special Reference to the Biologic Relationships Involved. Ithaca, N.Y.

STEINHAUS, E. A. 1949 Principles of Insect Pathology. New York.

STERZINGER, O. 1929 Verhalten und Umstimmungen der Stubenfliege bei Gewitter. Zeit. Psychol., 109: 229–230.

STEWART, M. A. 1929 A Case of Dermal Myiasis Caused by *Phormia regina* Meig. J. Am. Med. Ass., 92: 798–799.

STEWART, M. A. 1934 The Role of *Lucilia sericata* Meig. Larvae in Osteomyelitis Wounds. Ann. Trop. Med. Parasit., 28: 445–454.

STEWART, W. 1944 On the Viability and Transmission of Dysentery Bacilli by Flies in North Africa. J. R. Army Med. Corps, 83: 42–46.

STILES, C. W. 1917 Notice to the Zoological Profession of a Possible Suspension of the International Rules of Zoological Nomenclature in the Cases of *Musca* Linnaeus, 1758, and *Calliphora* Desvoidy, 1830 (Dipt.). Ent. News, 28: 231.

STILES, C. W.   1923   *Musca* Linnaeus, 1758 and *Calliphora* Desvoidy, 1830.   Science, 57: 176.

STILES, C. W., AND GARDNER, C. H.   1910   Further Observations on the Disposal of Excreta.   U.S. Publ. Health Repts., 25: 1825–1830.

STILES, C. W., AND LUMSDEN, L. L.   1916   The Sanitary Privy.   U.S. Dept. Agric. Farmer's Bull. 463.

STRAUSS, P.   1922a   Sur la destruction des mouches domestiques.   Circulaire du Ministre de l'Hygiene de l'Assistance et de la Prévoyance sociales.   J. d'Agric. Prat., Paris, 37: 361–362.

STRAUSS, P.   1922b   Comment détruire les mouches.   Vie Agric. et Rur., Paris, 20: 432–433.

STRICKLAND, C., AND ROY, D. N.   1940   Experimental Intestinal Myiasis.   Indian J. Med. Res., 28: 593–594.

STRICKLAND, C., AND ROY, D. N.   1941   Myiasis-producing Diptera in Man.   Indian J. Med. Res., 29: 863–865.

STRICKLAND, E. H.   1945   A Method for Permanently Reducing the Number of Blowflies in Screened Houses.   Bull. Brooklyn Ent. Soc., 40: 59–60.

SUGAI, C., AND KAWABADA, K.   1918   Leprosy and Tubercle Bacilli, Viability of, in Alimentary Tract of the Fish and Fly.   Igaku Chuo Zasshi (Central J. of Med. Sci.), no. 271.   (Abstr. in China Med. J., 34: 170.)

SURFACE, H. A.   1915   To Keep Down House Flies.   Zool. Press. Bull., Div. of Zool. Pennsyl. Dept. Agric., Harrisburg, no. 313.

SWEET, E. A.   1916   The Transmission of Disease by Flies.   Supplement no. 29 to the Public Health Repts.   2d ed., May 1916.

SWEETMAN, H. L.   1936   The Biological Control of Insects.   Ithaca, N.Y.

SWEETMAN, H. L.   1947   Comparative Effectiveness of DDT and DDD for Control of Flies.   J. Econ. Ent., 40: 565–566.

SYDENHAM, T.   1666   Sydenham's Works.   Syd. Soc. Ed., Vol. 1, p. 271.

TAGGART, R. S.   1946   DDT.   Cornell Vet., 36: 159–169.

TAO, S. M.   1927   A Comparative Study of the Early Larval Stages of Some Common Flies.   Am. J. Hyg., 7: 735–761.

TATTERSFIELD, F., AND MORRIS, H. M.   1924   An Apparatus for Testing the Toxic Values of Contact Insecticides under Controlled Conditions.   Bull. Ent. Res., 14: 223–233.

TAYLOR, J. F.   1919   The Role of the Fly as a Carrier of Bacillary Dysentery in the Salonica Command.   Med. Research Committee Nat. Health Insurance, London.   Spec. Rept., ser. 40: 68–83.

TEBBUTT, H.   1913   On the Influence of the Metamorphosis of *Musca domestica* upon Bacteria Administered in the Larval Stage.   J. Hyg., 12: 516–526.

TEICHMANN. E.   1918   Die Bekämpfung der Fliegenplage.   Zeit. Angew. Ent., Berlin, 4: 347–365.

TEISSIER, G.   1931   Growth Measurements.   Trav. Stat. Biol. Roscoff, 9: 29–238.

TELFORD, H. S. 1945 DDT Toxicity. Soap and Sanit. Chem., 21: 161, 163, 167, 169.

THAXTER, R. 1888 The Entomophthoreae of the United States. Mem. Boston Soc. Nat. Hist., 4: 133–201.

THOMAS, H. E., AND ARK, P. A. 1934 Fire Blight of Pears and Related Plants. California Agric. Exp. Sta. Bull. 586.

THOMSEN, E. 1938 Über die Kreislauf im Flügel der Musciden, mit besonderer Berücksichtigung der akzessorischen pulsierenden Organe. Zeit. Morph. u. Ökol. Tiere, 34: 416–438.

THOMSEN, E., AND THOMSEN, M. 1937 Über das Thermopräferendum der Larven einiger Fliegenarten. Zeit. Vergl. Physiol., 24: 343–380.

THOMSEN, M. 1934 Fly Control in Denmark. Quart. Bull. Health Org. L.o.N. 3: 304–324.

THOMSEN, M. 1935a The Problem of Fly Control. L.o.N., Health Org., C.H./ Hyg. rur./E.H. 4.

THOMSEN, M. 1935b A Comparative Study of the Development of the Stomoxydinae (Especially *Haematobia stimulans* Meigen) with Remarks on other Coprophagous Muscids. Proc. Zool. Soc., 1935 (Part 3): 531–550.

THOMSEN, M. 1936 Fluerne og deres Bekaempelse. Aarhus, Dansk. Mejerinforen. Faellesorganis.

THOMSEN, M. 1938 Stuefluen (*Musca domestica*) og Stikfluen (*Stomoxys calcitrans*). Beretn. Vet. og Landbohøjsk Forsøgslab. no. 176. Copenhagen.

THOMSEN, M., AND HAMMER, O. 1936 The Breeding Media of Some Common Flies. Bull. Ent. Res., 27: 559–587.

THOMSON, F. W. 1912 The House-Fly as a Carrier of Typhoid Infection. J. Trop. Med. Hyg., 15: 273–277.

THOMSON, J. G., AND LAMBORN, W. A. 1934 Mechanical Transmission of Trypanosomiasis, Leishmaniasis and Yaws through the Agency of Non-biting Haematophagous Flies. (Preliminary Note on Experiments.) Brit. Med. J., no. 3845: 506–509.

THOMSSEN, E. G., AND DONER, M. H. 1938 Breeding Houseflies: A Simplified and More Convenient Method of Rearing and Handling Flies for Peet-Grady Tests. Soap and Sanit. Chem., 14: 89–90, 101.

TISCHLER, N. 1931a Reproductivity of Flies Exposed to Pyrethrum Sprays. J. Econ. Ent., 24: 558.

TISCHLER, N. 1931b A Satisfactory Nutriment for Adult Houseflies. J. Econ. Ent., 24: 559.

TIZZONI, G., AND CATTANI, J. 1886 Untersuchungen über Cholera. Centralbl. f. d. Med. Wissensch., Berlin, 24: 769–771.

TOOMEY, J. A., TAKACS, W. S., AND TISCHER, L. A. 1941 Poliomyelitis Virus from Flies. Proc. Soc. Exp. Biol. and Med., 48: 637–639.

TORREY, J. C. 1912 Numbers and Types of Bacteria Carried by City Flies. J. Infect. Dis., 10: 166–177.

TOWNSEND, C. H. T.   1915   Correction of the Misuse of the Generic Name *Musca* with Descriptions of Two New Genera.   J. Washington Acad. Sci., 5:433–436.

TOWNSEND, C. H. T.   1942   Manual of Myiology. Part XII. General Consideration of the Oestromuscaria.   Itaquaquecetuba, São Paulo.

TRASK, J. D., AND PAUL, J. R.   1943   The Detection of Poliomyelitis Virus in Flies Collected during Epidemics of Poliomyelitis. II. Clinical Circumstances under Which Flies Were Collected.   J. Exp. Med., 77: 545–556.

TRASK, J. D., PAUL, J. R., AND MELNICK, J. L.   1943   The Detection of Poliomyelitis Virus in Flies Collected during Epidemics of Poliomyelitis. I. Methods, Results and Types of Flies Involved.   J. Exp. Med., 77: 531–544.

TRAVIS, B. V., AND BOHART, R. M.   1946   DDT to Control Maggots in Latrines. J. Econ. Ent., 39: 740–742.

TULLY, E. J.   1945   Sanitary Garbage Disposal.   Wisconsin State Board of Health Quart. Bull., 7: 3–7.

UNDERHILL, G. W.   1940   Some Factors Influencing the Feeding Activity of Simuliids in the Field.   J. Econ. Ent., 33: 915–917.

UNDERHILL, G. W.   1944   Blackflies Found Feeding on Turkeys in Virginia. Virginia Exp. Sta. Tech. Bull. 94.

URIBE, C.   1926   A New Invertebrate Host of *Trypanosma cruzi* Chagas.   J. Parasit., 12: 213–215.

UVAROV, B. P.   1931   Insects and Climate.   Trans. Ent. Soc., London, 79: 1–247.

VAILLARD, (DR.)   1913   Au sujet des measures à prendre contre les mouches. Bull. Mens. Office Internat. d'Hyg. Publique, Paris, Aug. 1913: 1313–1336.

VAILLARD, (DR.)   1914   Pour lutter contre les mouches.   Vie Agric. et Rur., Paris, 3: 373–378.

VANDENBERG, S. R.   1930   Report of the Entomologist.   Rept. Guam Agric. Exp. Sta., 1928: 23–31.

VANDENBERG, S. R.   1931a   Report of the Entomologist.   Rept. Guam Agric. Exp. Sta., 1929: 16–17.

VANDENBERG, S. R.   1931b   Report of the Entomologist.   Rep. Guam Agric. Exp. Sta., 1930: 23–25.

VANSKAYA, R. A.   1942a   The Use of Ammonium Carbonate for the Control of *Musca domestica* L. (In Russian.)   Med. Parasit., 10: 562–567.

VANSKAYA, R. A.   1942b   Hibernation of *Musca domestica* L. (In Russian.) Med. Parasit., 11: 87–90.

VARTIAINEN, O.   1946   Über Myiasis intestinalis.   Ann. Med. Intern. Fenniae, 35: 68–73.

VAUGHAN, V. C.   1899   Some Remarks on Typhoid Fever among Our Soldiers during the Late War with Spain.   Am. J. Med. Sci., 118: 10–24.

VEEDER, M. A.   1898a   Flies as Spreaders of Sickness in Camps.   Medical Record, 54: 429–430.

VEEDER, M. A.   1898b   The Spread of Typhoid and Dysenteric Diseases by Flies. Public Health (U.S.A.), 24: 260–262.

VEITCH, R., AND GREENWOOD, W. 1924 The Food Plants or Hosts of Some Fijian Insects. II. Proc. Linn. Soc. New S. Wales, 49, Part 2, no. 196: 153–161.

VENABLES, E. P. 1914 A Note upon the Food Habits of Adult Tenthredinidae. Canad. Ent., 46: 121.

VLADIMIROVA, M. S., AND SMIRNOV, E. S. 1938 Concurrence vitale dans une population homogène de *Musca domestica* L. de *Phormia groenlandica* et entre ces deux espèces. (In Russian.) Med. Parasit., 7: 755–777. (French summary.)

VOSS, F. 1913 Vergleichende Untersuchungen über die Flugwerkzeuge der Insekten. Verhandl. Dtsch. Zool. Ges., 23: 118–142.

WALKER, E. M. 1920 *Wohlfahrtia vigil* (Walker) as a Human Parasite. (Diptera-Sarcophagidae). J. Parasit., 7: 1–7.

WALKER, E. M. 1922 Some Cases of Cutaneous Myiasis, with Notes on the Larvae of *Wohlfahrtia vigil* (Walker). J. Parasit., 9: 1–5.

WALKER, E. M. 1922 The Larval Stages of *Wohlfahrtia vigil* (Walker). J. Parasit., 23: 163–174.

WALSH, B. D. 1870 Larvae in the Human Bowels. Am. Ent., 2: 137–141.

WARD, R., MELNICK, J. L., AND HORSTMAN, D. M. 1945 Poliomyelitis Virus in Fly-contaminated Food Collected at an Epidemic. Science 101: 491–493.

WARE, F. 1924 A Case of Habronemiasis in England. J. Comp. Path. and Therap., 37: 160–162.

WASHBURN, F. L. 1910 The Typhoid Fly on the Minnesota Iron Range. 13th Report of the State Entomologist of Minnesota, 1909–1910: 135–141.

WASON, E. J. 1947 Fish and Yabbies Killed with DDT. Agric. Gaz. New S. Wales, 58: 637–638.

WATERHOUSE, D. F. 1947 An Examination of the Peet-Grady Method for the Evaluation of Household Fly Sprays. Aust. Coun. Sci. Indust. Res. Bull. 216: 1–24.

WATERHOUSE, D. F. 1948 The Effect of Colour on the Numbers of Houseflies Resting on Painted Surfaces. Aust. J. Sci. Res. (B), 1: 65–75.

WATERSTON, J. 1916 On the Occurrence of *Stenomalus muscarum* Linn. in Company with Hibernating Flies. Scottish Naturalist, Edinburg, no. 54 (June 1916): 140–142.

WATT, J., AND LINDSAY, D. R. 1948 Diarrheal Disease Control Studies. I. Effect of Fly Control in a High Morbidity Area. Reprint no. 2890, Public Health Repts., 63: 1319–1334.

WAYSON, N. E. 1914 Plague and Plague-like Disease: A Report on Their Transmission by *Stomoxys calcitrans* and *Musca domestica*. Public Health Repts., Washington, D.C., 29: 3390–3393.

WEBSTER, J. D. 1945 Intestinal Myiasis with *Lucilia*. J. Parasit., 31: 151.

WEINLAND, E. 1906 Ammonia Production in *Calliphora* Larvae. Zeit. Biol., 47: 232–250.

WEINLAND, E. 1907 Weitere Beobachtungen an *Calliphora*. IV. Über chemische Momente bei der Metamorphose (und Entwicklung). Zeit. Biol., 49: 486–493.

WEINLAND, E. 1909 Ammonia Production in *Calliphora* Larvae, Dipt. Biol. Centralbl., 29: 564–577.

WEISMANN, A. 1863 Die Entwicklung der Dipteren im Ei, nach Beobachtungen an *Chironomus* spec., *Musca vomitoria* und *Pulex canis*. Zeit. Wiss. Zool., 13: 107–220.

WEISMANN, A. 1864a Die nachembryonalen Entwicklung der Musciden nach Beobachtungen an *Musca vomitoria* und *Sarcophaga carnaria*. Zeit. Wiss. Zool., 14: 185–336.

WEISMANN, A. 1864b Die Entwicklung der Dipteren. I. Die Entwicklung der Dipteren im Ei. II. Die nachembryonalen Entwicklung der Musciden. Leipzig.

WELANDER. 1896 Gonorrhoeal Ophthalmia Conveyed by Flies. Wien. Klin. Wochenschr., no. 52. (Cited by Abel, 1899.)

WELCH, E. V. 1939 Insects Found on Aircraft at Miami, Fla., in 1938. Public Health Repts., 54: 561–566.

WELDON, L. 1946 Shoo Fly. The American Girl, June 1946, p. 30.

WELLINGTON, W. G. 1944 Barotaxis in Diptera and Its Possible Significance to Economic Entomology. Nature, 154: 671–672.

WELLINGTON, W. G. 1945 Conditions Governing the Distribution of Insects in the Free Atmosphere. Canad. Ent., 77: 7–15, 21–28, 44–49.

WELLINGTON, W. G. 1946a The Effects of Variations in Atmospheric Pressure upon Insects. Canad. J. Res., sect. D, Zool. Sci., 24: 51–70.

WELLINGTON, W. G. 1946b Some Reactions of Muscoid Diptera to Changes in Atmospheric Pressure. Canad. J. Res., sect. D, Zool. Sci., 24: 105–117.

WENYON, C. M., AND O'CONNOR, F. W. 1917a The Carriage of Cysts of *Entamoeba histolytica* and Other Intestinal Protozoa and Eggs of Parasitic Worms by House-Flies with Some Notes on the Resistance of Cysts to Disinfectants and Other Agents. J. R. Army Med. Corps, 28: 522–527.

WENYON, C. M., AND O'CONNOR, F. W. 1917b An Inquiry into Some Problems Affecting the Spread and Incidence of Intestinal Protozoal Infections of British Troops and Natives in Egypt. . . . IV. Experimental Work with the Human Intestinal Protozoa, Their Carriage by House-Flies and the Resistance of Their Cysts to Disinfectants and Other Agents. J. R. Army Med. Corps, 28: 686–698.

WENYON, C. M., AND O'CONNOR, F. W. 1917c Human Intestinal Protozoa in the Near East. Wellcome Bureau of Scientific Research. London.

WEST, L. S. 1923 Immunity to Parasitism in *Samia ceropia* Linn. (Lep.: Saturniidae; Dipt.: Tachinidae). Ent. News, 34: 23–25.

WEST, L. S. 1924 New Northeastern Dexiinae (Diptera: Tachinidae). Psyche, 31: 184–192.

WEST, L. S. 1925a The Phasiidae and Tachinidae of New York and Adjacent States. Doctoral dissertation, deposited in Library of Cornell University, Ithaca, N.Y. (Contains review of literature, host-parasite catalog, and taxonomic keys.)

WEST, L. S. 1925b New Phasiidae and Tachinidae from New York State. J. New York Ent. Soc., 33: 121–135.

WEST, L. S. 1945 The Order Diptera; Myiasis. *In* Manual of Tropical Medicine, by T. T. Mackie, G. W. Hunter, and C. B. Worth. Philadelphia and London. Pp. 569–646.

WEST, L. S. 1946 Distribution. *In* Practical Malariology, by P. F. Russell, L. S. West, and R. D. Manwell. Philadelphia and London.

WEST, L. S. 1948 The Status of *Rhynchiodexia* (*Dinera*) *robusta* Curran Together with a Consideration of Certain Cephalic and Other Characters Useful in Muscoid Taxonomy. Papers Mich. Acad., 34: 109–117.

WIESMANN, R. 1943 Fly Control in Stables. Use of "Gesarol" or the New "DDT" in the Control of Stable Flies. Soap and Sanit. Chem., 19 (12): 117, 119, 141, 143. (Translation of "Eine Neue Methode der Bekämpfung der Fliegenplagen in Stallen," Anz. Schädlingsk., Berlin, 19: 5–8.

WIESMANN, R. 1947 Untersuchungen über das physiologische Verhalten von *Musca domestica* L. verschiedener Provenienzen. Mitt. Schweiz. Ent. Ges., 20: 484–504.

WIESMANN, R., AND FENJVES, P. 1944 Autotomie bei Lepidopteren und Dipteren nach Berührung mit Gesarol. Mitt. Schweiz. Ent. Ges., 19: 179–184.

WIETING, J. O. G., AND HOSKINS, W. M. 1939 The Olfactory Responses of Flies in a New Type of Insect Olfactometer. II. Responses of the Housefly to Ammonia, Carbon Dioxide and Ethyl Alcohol. J. Econ. Ent., 32: 24–29.

WIGGLESWORTH, V. B. 1934 Insect Physiology. London.

WIGGLESWORTH, V. B. 1939 The Principles of Insect Physiology. 2d ed., 1944; 3d ed., 1947. London.

WILLISTON, S. W. 1908 Manual of North American Diptera. 3d ed. New Haven, Conn.

WILSON, H. G., AND GAHAN, J. B. 1948 Susceptibility of DDT-resistant Houseflies to Other Insecticidal Sprays. Science, 107: 276–277.

WLADIMIROW, M., AND SMIRNOV, E. 1934 Über das Verhalten der Schlupfwespe *Mormoniella vitripennis* Wlk. zu verschiedenen Fliegenarten. Zool. Anz., 107: 85–89.

WOLLMAN, E. 1911 Sur l'élevage des mouches steriles: Contribution à la connaissance du rôle des microbes dans les voies digestive. Ann. Inst. Pasteur, 25: 79–88.

WOLLMAN, E. 1921a Le Rôle des mouches dans le transport de germes pathogènes étudié par la technique des élevages aseptiques. Compt. Rend. Hebdom. Acad. Sci. Paris, 72 (no. 5): 298–301.

WOLLMAN, E. 1921b La Méthode des élevages aseptiques en physiologie. Arch. Intern. Physiol., 18: 194–199.

WOLLMAN, E. 1922 Biologie de la mouche domestique et des larves de mouches à viande, en élevages aseptiques. Ann. Inst. Pasteur, 36: 784–788.

Woodcock, H. M. 1918 Note on the Epidemiology of Dysentery. J. R. Army Med. Corps, 30: 110–111.

Woodcock, H. M. 1919 Note on the Epidemiology of Amoebic Dysentery. J. R. Army Med. Corps, 32: 231–235.

Yao, H. Y., Huan, I. C., and Huie, D. 1929 The Relation of Flies, Beverages and Well Water to Gastro-intestinal Diseases in Peiping. Nat. Med. J. China, 15: 410–418.

Yatsenko, F., Paretskaya, M., and Kipritch, S. 1934 A Case of Myiasis of the Urethra. Med. Parasit. and Parsitic Dis., Moscow, 3: 348.

Yeager, J. F., and Hendrickson, G. O. 1933 A Simple Method of Demonstrating Blood Circulation in the Wings and Wing-pads of the Cockroach, *Periplaneta americana* Linn. Proc. Soc. Exp. Biol. and Med., 30: 858–860.

Yeager, J. F., and Hendrickson, G. O. 1934 Circulation of Blood in Wings and Wing Pads of the Cockroach, *Periplaneta americana* Linn. Ann. Ent. Soc. Am., 27: 257–272.

Yeager, J. F., and Munson, S. C. 1945 Physiological Evidence of a Site of Action of DDT in an Insect. Science, 102: 305–307.

Zanini, E. 1930 E l'*Holostaspis badius* (Koch) parassita della mosca domestica? Contributo alla lotta contro la mosca domestica. Boll. Lab. Zool. Agrar. Bachic. Milano, i (1928–1929): 59–73.

Zimin, L. S. 1939–1941a A Survey of the Synanthropic Diptera of Tadzhikistan. Conf. on Parasit. Probl. Summaries of Reports. (In Russian.) Moscow, Izd. Akad. Nauk SSSR, 1939–1941: 35–38.

Zimin, L. S. 1939–1941b An Experiment in the Control of Flies under the Conditions of Southern Tadzhikistan. Conf. on Parasit. Probl. Summaries of Reports. (In Russian.) Moscow, Izd. Akad. Nauk SSSR, 1939–1941: 38–39.

Zimmerman, O. T., and Lavine, Irvin 1946 DDT—Killer of Killers. Dover, N.H.

Zmeev, G. Ya 1939–1941 The Importance of the Large Hornet (*Vespa orientalis*) in the Epidemiology of Dysentery. Conf. on Parasit. Probl., Dec. 1939 (Moscow-Leningrad), Nov. 1940 (Leningrad), March 1941 (Moscow). Summaries of Reports. (In Russian.) Izd. Akad. Nauk SSSR, pp. 34–35.

Zwölfer, W. 1934 Die praktische Bedeutung der verbesserten Temperatursummenregel in der Forstentomologie. Verhandl. Dtsch. Ges. Angew. Ent., 9: 20–27. Berlin.

Index